McCracken's
Removable Partial Prosthodontics

McCracken's
Removable Partial Prosthodontics

DAVIS HENDERSON, B.S., D.D.S., F.A.C.D.

Professor Emeritus, University of Florida College of Dentistry, Gainesville, Florida;
Formerly Chairman, Department of Prosthodontics, University of Kentucky
College of Dentistry, Lexington, Kentucky; Fellow and Past President,
Academy of Denture Prosthetics; Life Member, American Prosthodontic Society;
Life Member and Past President, Southeastern Academy of Prosthodontics;
Life and Charter Member, American College of Prosthodontists; Life and Charter
Member and Past President, Carl O. Boucher Prosthodontic Conference;
Diplomate and Past President, American Board of Prosthodontics; Captain, DC,
United States Navy (Ret.)

GLEN P. McGIVNEY, D.D.S., F.A.C.D.

Professor and Chairman, Department of Removable Prosthodontics, Marquette University
School of Dentistry, Milwaukee, Wisconsin; Fellow, Academy of Denture Prosthetics;
Charter Member, American College of Prosthodontists; President, Federation of
Prosthodontic Organizations; Member and Past President, Midwest Academy of
Prosthodontics; Member, American Prosthodontic Society; Member, Advisory Committee on
Advanced Education in Prosthodontics, American Dental Association; Diplomate,
American Board of Prosthodontics

DWIGHT J. CASTLEBERRY, B.S.Ed., D.M.D., M.S., F.A.C.D.

Professor and Chairman, Department of Removable Prosthodontics, University of Alabama
School of Dentistry, Birmingham, Alabama; Fellow, American College of Prosthodontics;
Fellow, American Academy of Maxillofacial Prosthetics; Member, American
Prosthodontic Society; Member, Southeastern Academy of Prosthodontics;
Diplomate, American Board of Prosthodontics

SEVENTH EDITION

with **951** illustrations

The C. V. Mosby Company

ST. LOUIS • TORONTO • PRINCETON   1985

MOSBY

A TRADITION OF PUBLISHING EXCELLENCE

Editor: Darlene Warfel
Assistant editor: Melba Steube
Editing supervisor: Elaine Steinborn
Manuscript editor: Barry Thornell
Book design: Staff
Cover design: Mick Monahan
Production: Judith Bamert, Barbara Merritt, Russ Till

SEVENTH EDITION

The C.V. Mosby Company
11830 Westline Industrial Drive, St. Louis, Missouri 63146

Library of Congress Cataloging in Publication Data

McCracken, William L.
  McCracken's Removable partial prosthodontics.

  Bibliography: p.
  Includes index.
  1. Partial dentures, Removable.   I. Henderson,
Davis. II. McGivney, Glen P. III. Castleberry,
Dwight J. IV. Title. V. Title: Removable partial
prosthodontics. [DNLM: 1. Denture, Partial,
Removable. WU 515 M132p]
RK665.M38 1985   617.6′92   84-20572
ISBN 0-8016-2171-2

GW/VH/VH 9 8 7 6 5 4 3 2 1   03/B/367

To
STUDENTS OF DENTISTRY

PREFACE to seventh edition

The emphasis on preventive dentistry by the profession is responsible for saving many teeth that otherwise would have been lost. Thus a need for removable partial dentures as a physiologically sound treatment for many partially edentulous patients is seemingly increasing.

Fundamentals of dental restorative disciplines rarely change; only materials, methods, and technical procedures change. The science of removable partial prosthodontics cannot be considered static. Constant revising and updating are necessary to keep the study dynamic—a justification for this seventh edition.

The greatest possible number of clinical skills and related factors are involved in treating patients with removable partial dentures. The practice of removable partial prosthodontics involves all the basic and dental clinical sciences, laws and effects of leverages, consideration of supports, occlusal contacts, direction of forces, relative health of all oral structures, and dental materials, to name only a few.

The contents of this textbook extend from initial contact with the patient to postplacement care of oral structures. Steps of treatment are covered in normal sequence. Chapters are arranged in an orderly sequence of learning; that is, components and their biomechanical characteristics, denture bases, surveying, and principles of design of restorations precede diagnosis, treatment planning, and treatment.

An endeavor has been made in this edition, as well as in former editions, to carry out the original objectives of the late Dr. William L. McCracken. He intended that the book, although encompassing both clinical and laboratory aspects, should provide predoctoral and postdoctoral students, as well as practicing dentists, with basic principles and time-tested, practical procedures in the treatment of partially edentulous patients with removable restorations.

Several changes have been made in this revision of the sixth edition. The physical layout of the text is more amenable to a reader's retention of information. Key words and phrases (sometimes sentences) have been set in boldface type to enhance recognition and retention. Appropriate chapters have been structured to reinforce the logical sequence of clinical concepts and philosophies for the practice of removable partial prosthodontics. The number of explicit examples and illustrations has been noticeably increased to make the written material more readily understood by the student. The Selected Reading Resources section of the text has been updated to reflect a current review of textbooks and dental periodical literature. We have tried to enhance the reading level of this edition, and we believe it contains the element of scholarship that is so necessary to excellence in education and in the practice of dentistry.

The guidance and counsel of the late Dr. Victor L. Steffel, coauthor of editions 3 to 6, are missed, as well as the contributions of the late Dr. John J. Sharry. On a happier note, important pluses for this seventh edition are the new coauthors, Drs. Glen McGivney and Dwight Castleberry. The continued involvement of Dr. Samuel Low is most appreciated. Dr. William R. Laney is a welcome contributor to this seventh edition.

Grateful acknowledgment is extended to those who offered constructive criticism of the sixth edition. Many of the changes in this edition resulted from their suggestions.

Davis Henderson

PREFACE to first edition

Although I welcomed the invitation to author a textbook on the subject of partial denture construction, I realized from the outset that such a book would follow closely in the wake of several excellent textbooks on this subject. I therefore approached the task with a sense of great responsibility. However, I would not have accepted the challenge had I not felt sincerely that I could add something to what had already been written and thus produce a text in this field which is sorely needed and which provides the dental student, the dental practitioner, and the dental laboratory technician with the information necessary to produce a partial denture that is in itself a definitive restorative entity. It is my sincere hope that this textbook will be used not only by teachers of prosthetic dentistry but also by practicing dentists and dental technicians, and that in this book the dentist and dental technician may find a common meeting ground for better solution of the problems associated with the partially edentulous patient.

I am deeply grateful for the opportunities that I have had to combine private practice with teaching and for the knowledge that has evolved from this experience. Although I have attempted to present various philosophies and techniques in order that the reader may select that which to him seems most applicable, it is inevitable that certain preferences will be obvious. These are based upon convictions evolved through experience both in private practice and in the teaching of clinical prosthodontics. It is only logical, then, that I should therefore state my own personal beliefs, which are as follows:

1. I believe that the practice of prosthetic dentistry must forever remain in the hands of the dentist and that he must therefore be totally competent to render this service. In the fabrication of a partial denture restoration, the dentist must be competent to render a comprehensive diagnosis of the partially edentulous mouth and, utilizing all of the mechanical aids necessary, plan every detail of treatment. He must either personally accomplish whatever mouth preparations are necessary or delegate to his colleagues such specialized services as surgical, periodontal, and endodontic treatment. In any case, primary responsibility for adequate mouth preparations remains his alone. He must undertake whatever impression procedures are necessary and must be primarily responsible for the accuracy of any casts of the mouth upon which work is to be fabricated. He must provide the laboratory technician with an adequate prescription in the form of diagrams and written instructions and with a master cast which has been completely surveyed with a specific design outlined upon it. He must be solely responsible for the accuracy and adequacy of any jaw relation records and must specify all materials and, in many instances, the exact method by which occlusion is to be established on the finished restoration. Finally, he must be competent to judge the excellence of the finished restoration or recognize its inadequacies and must assume the responsibility for demanding a degree of excellence from the technician that will continually raise rather than lower the standards of dental laboratory service.

2. I believe that the dental laboratory technician has a responsibility to his profession to demand a quality of leadership from the dentist which he can respect and follow without question. The responsibility for providing adequate prosthetic dentistry service to the patient must be shared by both dentist and technician, and each has not only a right to expect that the other do his part competently but also an obligation to demand a quality of service from the other

that will not jeopardize the finished product. The technician therefore would do dentistry a great service if he would reject inadequate material from the dentist and respectfully suggest whatever improvements are necessary for him to produce an acceptable piece of work. As long as the technician accepts inadequate material from the dentist and the dentist is willing to place an inadequate product in the patient's mouth, the quality of removable prosthetic appliances will continue to be, as it all too frequently is, a far poorer service than the dentist and technician together are capable of rendering.

I believe also that dental laboratories should always be willing to adopt newer techniques and philosophies developed by the dental profession and being taught to dental graduates. Too often the commercial dental laboratory insists upon using stereotyped techniques that suit its production methods and actively attempts to discourage the recent graduate from putting into practice modern methods and techniques that were painstakingly taught to him in dental school by instructors whose knowledge of the subject far exceeds that of the laboratory technician who depreciates it.

3. I believe that any free-end partial denture must have the best possible support from the underlying edentulous ridge and that the design of the abutment retainers must apply a minimum of torque to the adjacent abutment teeth. I believe that some kind of secondary impression is necessary to obtain adequate support for the denture base, both through tissue placement and from the broadest possible coverage compatible with biologic requirements and limitations.

4. I believe in the functional, or dynamic, registration of occlusal relationships rather than in relying upon intraoral adjustment of an established centric occlusion or upon the ability of an instrument to simulate articulatory movements. I believe that the occlusion on a partial denture, be it fixed or removable, should be made to harmonize with the existing adjusted natural occlusion, and that this can best be accomplished by the registration of functional occlusal paths. For this to be done adequately, occlusion on the partial denture must be established upon either the final denture base(s) or upon an accurate substitute for the final base(s). The practice of attempting to submit jaw relation records to the technician prior to the fabrication of the denture framework is therefore, with few exceptions, strongly condemned.

5. I believe that a partial denture, when properly designed, carefully made, and serviced when needed, can be an entirely satisfactory restoration and can serve as a means of preserving remaining oral structures as well as restoring missing dentition. Unless a partial denture is made with adequate abutment support, with optimal base support, and with harmonious and functional occlusion, it should be clear to all concerned that such a denture should be considered only a temporary treatment, or interim denture rather than a restoration representative of the best that modern prosthetic dentistry has to offer.

W. L. McCracken

CONTENTS

1 INTRODUCTION AND TERMINOLOGY

Introduction
Terminology

INTRODUCTION

A **prosthesis** is the replacement of an absent part of the human body by some artificial part such as an eye, a leg, or a denture. **Prosthetics,** then, is the art and science of supplying missing parts of the human body.

When applied to dentistry, the term **prosthetics** becomes **prosthodontics** and denotes the branch of dental art and science that deals specifically with the replacement of missing dental and oral structures. **Prosthodontics** may be defined as "that branch of dentistry pertaining to the restoration and maintenance of oral func-

tions, comfort, appearance, and health of the patient by replacement of missing teeth and contiguous tissues with artificial substitutes."

The replacement of missing teeth in a partially edentulous arch may be accomplished by a fixed, or cemented, prosthesis or by a removable prosthesis. A fixed prosthesis is not designed to be removed by the patient (Fig. 1-1). This type of restoration is a **fixed partial denture.** On the other hand, a **removable partial denture** is designed so that it can be removed conveniently from the mouth and replaced by the patient (Fig. 1-2).

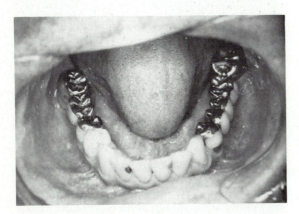

Fig. 1-1. Fixed partial dentures restore patient's missing posterior teeth. Teeth bounding edentulous spaces are used as abutments.

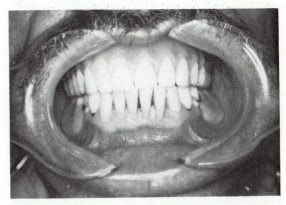

Fig. 1-2. Patient's missing mandibular first and second molars are restored with clasp-type removable partial denture. It is opposed by maxillary complete denture.

1

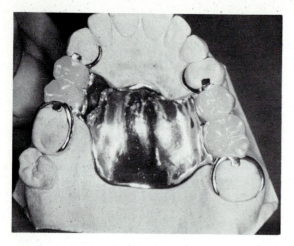

Fig. 1-3. Tooth-borne removable partial denture restoring missing posterior teeth. Teeth bounding edentulous spaces provide support, retention, and stability for restoration.

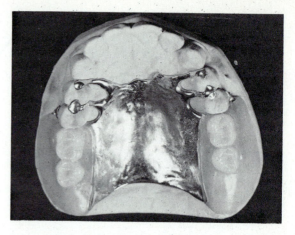

Fig. 1-4. Maxillary bilateral distal extension removable partial denture restoring missing first and second molars. Support, retention, and stability are shared by abutment teeth and residual ridges.

A removable partial denture may be entirely tooth supported or may derive its support from both the teeth and the tissues of the residual ridge. The denture base of a tooth-borne removable partial denture derives its support from teeth at each end of the edentulous area(s) (Fig. 1-3). A tooth-tissue-supported removable partial denture has at least one denture base that extends anteriorly or posteriorly, terminating in a denture base portion that is not tooth supported (Fig. 1-4). Such a base extending posteriorly on a removable partial denture qualifies the restoration as a **distal extension denture.**

It is perhaps only natural, when beginning the study of removable partial prosthodontics, to think primarily in terms of **construction** of restorations. However, if students would direct their thinking primarily to the **promotion** of oral health and **preservation** of remaining oral structures for patients in their care, a better perspective of the study would be developed.

The objectives of prosthodontic treatment of partially edentulous individuals with removable restorations are (1) the elimination of oral disease to the greatest extent possible, (2) the preservation of the health and relationships of the teeth and the health of oral and paraoral structures, and (3) the restoration of oral functions with an esthetically pleasing end result.

Subsequent to the conscientious study of removable partial prosthodontics in the treatment of partially edentulous patients, success and professional happiness may be more readily obtained by following these guidelines:

1. Establish a genuine rapport to promote trust and confidence.
2. Demonstrate thoroughness in diagnosis and treatment planning.
3. Make an empathic identification of problems and their causes.
4. Make the patients fully aware of the correlation between dental and general health as adjuncts to total well-being.
5. Explain the suggested treatment plan and alternate plans including time commitments for treatment.
6. Make the patients fully aware of their responsibilities in the success of the treatment by conscientious home care and periodic recall visits.
7. Avoid an overly optimistic prognosis.
8. Plainly state anticipated compromises from the ideal based on inherent factors that cannot be altered by treatment.

9. Arrive at a just and considerate fee for the proposed treatment by taking into account the values, desires, financial position, and other constraints of the patients, and adjust each plan, as may be required, in the best interest of each patient under the given circumstances.
10. Have the highest respect for the dignity, comfort, and well-being of each patient at all times.

TERMINOLOGY

Familiarity with accepted prosthodontic terminology should be acquired by the predoctoral student-dentist because once a vocabulary is established, it is difficult to change. However, it is unrealistic to expect a student-dentist to memorize terms as an introduction to the study of removable partial prosthodontics. Therefore this section should be looked on as an overview of prosthodontic terminology and as an explanation (justification) for the choice of such terminology.

Significant strides have been made in prosthodontic terminology in recent years, eliminating much confusion created by conflicting terms. A *Glossary of Prosthodontic Terms* is available to the profession through the continuing efforts of the Academy of Denture Prosthetics.* The third edition of a glossary of accepted terms in all disciplines of dentistry, *Boucher's Clinical Dental Terminology*, is also available.† Both glossaries provide excellent bases for dignified spoken and written communication in prosthetic dentistry.

The conflicting or indefinite terms in common usage in prosthodontics require definition and clarification. Many of these are used synony-

---

* This glossary first appeared in the March, 1956, issue of *The Journal of Prosthetic Dentistry* (published by The C. V. Mosby Co., St. Louis, Mo.) The lastest reprint (fourth edition), published in 1977, may be obtained from the Education and Research Foundation of Prosthodontics, Dr. Thomas A. Curtis, Graduate Prosthodontics, C-634, University of California, School of Dentistry, San Francisco, CA 94143.
† Zwemer, T.J., editor: Boucher's clinical dental terminology, a glossary of accepted terms in all disciplines of dentistry, ed. 3, St. Louis, 1982, The C. V. Mosby Co.

mously; even today others are used incorrectly. Whereas the following is not meant to be a complete glossary of removable partial prosthodontic terminology, some definitions will be given, based on available reference material. The discussion type format does not lend itself to alphabetical arrangement of defined words or terms, hopefully creating only a minor inconvenience to students.

The term **appliance** is correctly applied only to a device worn by the patient in the course of treatment, such as splints, orthodontic appliances, and space maintainers. A denture, an obturator, a fixed partial denture, or a crown is properly called a **prosthesis**. The terms **prosthesis, restoration,** and **denture** are equally acceptable terms and will be used synonymously in this book.

Stability is defined as the quality of a denture to be firm, that is, not subject to change of position, when forces are applied. Stability becomes more meaningful when thought of as a denture base to supporting bone relationship.

Retention is spoken of as that quality inherent in the denture that resists the force of gravity, the adhesiveness of foods, and the forces associated with opening of the jaws.

A temporary **denture** is a dental prosthesis to be used for a short time for reasons of esthetics, mastication, occlusal support, and convenience until more definite prosthetic dental treatment can be provided or for conditioning the patient to accept an artificial substitute for missing natural teeth.

A **complete denture** is a dental prosthesis that replaces all of the natural dentition and associated structures of the maxillae or mandible. It is entirely supported by the tissues (mucous membrane, connective tissues, and underlying bone) to which it is attached.

An **abutment** is a tooth used for the support of a fixed or removable prosthesis.

The term **height of contour** is defined as a line encircling a tooth, designating its greatest circumference at a selected position.

The term **undercut,** when used in reference to an abutment, is that portion of a tooth that lies between the height of contour and the gingivae; when it is used in reference to other oral structures, undercut means the contour or cross section of a residual ridge or dental arch that would prevent the placement of a denture.

The **angle** of **cervical convergence** is an angle viewed between a vertical rod contacting an abutment tooth and the axial surface of the abutment. It is an apical angle having its apex at the height of the contour of the abutment. Discerning this angle is important in developing uniform retention through clasps.

Two or more parallel axial surfaces of abutment teeth so shaped as to direct a prosthesis during placement and removal are called **guiding planes.** Guiding plane surfaces are parallel to the path of the placement; however, they may or may not face each other. Preferably these surfaces are made parallel to the long axes of abutment teeth.

In a description of the various components of the partial denture, conflicting terminology must be recognized and the preferred terms defined. A **retainer** is defined as "any type of clasp, attachment, or device used for the fixation or stabilization of a prosthesis." Thus the attachment may be either intracoronal or extracoronal and may be used as a means of retaining either a removable or a fixed restoration. The term **internal attachment** will be used in preference to precision attachment, frictional attachment, and other terms to describe any mechanical retaining device that depends on frictional resistance between parallel walls of male and female (key and keyway) parts. Precision attachment is discarded because its usage implies that all other types of retainers are less precise in their design and fabrication.

Clasp (direct retainer) will be used in conjunction with the words **retainer, arm,** or **assembly** whenever possible. The clasp assembly will consist of a **retentive clasp arm** and a **reciprocal** or **stabilizing clasp arm** plus any minor connectors and rests from which they originate or with which they are associated. **Bar clasp arm** will be used in preference to Roach's name to designate this type of extracoronal retainer and is defined as a clasp arm that originates from the base or framework, traverses soft tissue, and approaches the tooth undercut area from a gingival direction. In contrast, the term **circumferential**

clasp arm will be used to designate a clasp arm that originates above the height of contour, traverses part of the suprabulge portion of the tooth, and approaches the tooth undercut from an occlusal direction. Both types of clasp arms terminate in a retentive undercut lying gingival to the height of contour, and both provide retention by the resistance of metal to deformation rather than frictional resistance of parallel walls.

A **major connector** is the part of a removable partial denture that connects the components on one side of the arch to the components on the opposite side of the arch.

A **continuous bar retainer** is a component of the partial denture framework that augments the major connector and lies on the lingual or facial surface of several teeth. It is most frequently used on the middle third of the lingual slope of lower anterior teeth. If attached to the lingual bar major connector by a thin, contoured apron, the major connector is then designated as a **linguoplate.**

Any thin, broad palatal coverage used as a major connector is called a **palatal major connector** or if of lesser width, a **palatal bar.** A palatal major connector may be further described according to its anteroposterior location on the palatal surface, for example, an anterior palatal major connector or a posterior palatal bar. The differentiation between a palatal bar and a palatal strap is somewhat subjective. As we interpret it, a palatal strap is proportionally thinner and broader than a palatal bar. In this textbook a palatal major connector component less than 8 mm in width will be referred to as a **bar.** The term **anatomic replica** will be used to designate cast metal palatal major connectors that duplicate the topography of that portion of the patient's mouth. This is in keeping with a desire to use descriptive terminology whenever possible.

The term **indirect retainer** denotes a part of a removable partial denture that assists the direct retainers in preventing displacement of distal extension denture bases by functioning as part of the resistance arm of a lever on the opposite side of the fulcrum line.

The term **rest** will be used to designate any component of the partial denture that is placed on an abutment tooth, ideally in a rest seat prepared to receive it, so that it limits movement of the denture in a gingival direction. When a rest is placed on the occlusal surface of a posterior tooth, it is designated as an **occlusal rest.** If the rest occupies a position on the lingual surface of an anterior tooth, it is referred to as a **lingual rest.** A rest placed on the incisal edge of an anterior abutment tooth is called an **incisal rest.** All these rests function to prevent movement of the denture toward the soft tissues and to assist in providing occlusal support for the prosthesis.

Denture base will be used to designate the part of a denture, whether of metal or of a resinous material, that holds the artificial teeth and that receives support from the abutment teeth, the residual ridge, or both. The word **saddle** is considered objectionable terminology when used to designate the base of a removable partial denture.

The structures underlying the denture base will be mentioned as the **residual ridge** or **edentulous ridge,** referring to the residual bone with its soft tissue covering. The exact character of this soft tissue covering may vary, and it includes the mucous membrane and the underlying fibrous connective tissue.

Resurfacing of a denture base with new material to make it fit the underlying tissues more accurately will be spoken of as **relining. Rebasing** refers to a process that goes beyond relining and involves the refitting of a denture by the replacement of the denture base with new material without changing the occlusal relations of the teeth. The oral tissues and structures of the residual ridge supporting a denture base will be referred to as the **basal seat.**

To describe an impression and the resulting cast of the supporting form of the edentulous ridge, **functional impression** and **functional ridge form** will be used in the absence of a more descriptive terminology. These terms have become accepted as meaning the form of the edentulous ridge when it is supporting a denture base. It is artifically created by means of a specially molded (individualized) tray or an impression material, or both, that displaces those tissues that can be readily displaced and that would be incapable of rendering support to the denture base. Firm areas are not displaced because of the flow characteristics of the impression material. Thus the tissues are recorded more nearly in the form they will assume when supporting a functional load. In contrast, the static form of the edentulous ridge, as often recorded in a soft impression material such as hydrocolloid, rubber-base material, or metallic oxide impression paste, is referred to as the **anatomic ridge form** and results when an impression tray is uniformly relieved. This is the surface form of the edentulous ridge when at rest or when not supporting a functional load.

Perhaps no other terms in prosthodontics have been associated with more controversy than have **centric jaw relation** and **centric occlusion.** All confusion could be terminated by acceptance of one definition of centric relation and one definition of centric occlusion and then using these respective positions as references for other horizontal locations of the mandible or other relationships of opposing teeth. The following definitions, which are given in the *Glossary of Prosthodontic Terms*, are selected as meaningful:

centric jaw relation the most posterior relation of the mandible to the maxillae at the established vertical dimension.

centric occlusion the centered contact position of the occlusal surfaces of the mandibular teeth against the occlusal surfaces of the maxillary teeth.

For complete dentures, centric occlusion should be made to coincide with centric relation for that patient. In an adjustment of natural occlusion the objective may be to establish harmony between centric relation and centric occlusion. With removable partial dentures the objective is to make the artificial occlusion coincide and be in harmony with the remaining natural occlusion. Ideally the natural occlusion has been adjusted to harmonious contact in centric relation and is free of eccentric interference before a similar occlusion is established on the partial denture.

Balanced occlusion is a term that describes the contact of opposing teeth. It is defined as the simultaneous contacting of maxillary and mandibular teeth on the right and left in the anterior and posterior occlusal areas in centric or any eccentric position.

Functional occlusal registration is sufficiently descriptive and is used to designate a dynamic registration of opposing dentition rather than the recording of a static relationship of one jaw to another. While centric position is found somewhere in a functional occlusal registration, eccentric positions are also recorded, and the created occlusion is made to harmonize with all gliding and chewing movements the patient is capable of making.

The word **cast** may be used as a verb (to cast) or as an adjective (cast framework or cast metal base). It is used most frequently in this text as a noun to designate a positive reproduction of a maxillary or mandibular dental arch made from an impression of that arch. Such an objective is further designated according to the purpose for which it is made, such as **diagnostic cast, master cast,** or **investment cast.** An investment cast also may be referred to as a **refractory cast,** since it is compounded to withstand high temperatures without disintegrating and, incidentally, to perform certain functions relative to the burnout and expansion of the mold. A **refractory investment** is an investment material that can withstand the high temperatures of casting or soldering. Plaster of paris and artificial stone also may be considered **investment** if either is used to invest any part of a dental restoration for processing it.

Cast in dentistry should always imply that it is an accurate reproduction of the tissues being studied or on which a restoration may be fabricated. Any cast that is admittedly inaccurate is unpardonable and unacceptable in modern dentistry because of the excellence of impression and cast materials available today.

The word **cast** is preferable to the term **model,** which should be used only to designate a reproduction for display or demonstration purposes. A model of a dental arch or any portion thereof may be made of durable and attractive material. It need not be an accurate reproduction but should be a reasonable facsimile of the original. It is frequently made of tooth- and tissue-colored acrylic resin.

Mold is also incorrect when applied to a reproduction of a dental arch or a portion thereof. It is used to indicate either the cavity into which a casting is made or the shape of an artificial tooth.

A **wax pattern** is converted to a **casting** by the elimination of the pattern by heat, leaving a mold into which the molten metal is forced by centrifugal force or other means. **Casting** is therefore used most frequently as a noun, meaning "a metal object shaped by being poured into a mold to harden." It is used primarily to designate the cast metal framework of a partial denture but also may be used to describe a molded denture base, which is also actually cast into a mold.

Dental stones are used to make an artificial stone reproduction from an impression, and they are used as an investment or for mounting purposes. All dental stones are gypsum products. Use of the word **stone** in dentistry should be applied only to those gypsum materials that are employed for their hardness, accuracy, or abrasion resistance.

A **dental cast surveyor** is an instrument used to determine the relative parallelism of two or more axial surfaces of teeth or other parts of a cast of a dental arch.

The word **wrought,** when used to describe an alloy, means worked into shape by artistry or effort. Mechanical treatment of an alloy has two primary objectives. One objective is to obtain a desired form for use, for example, wires, bands, bars, and sheets. Another objective is to enhance certain mechanical properties that are unsatisfactory in a cast alloy.

The term **canine** (tooth) and **premolar** (tooth) will be used to designate those teeth commonly called cuspid and bicuspid teeth. Denton gives the chief arguments for the use of the word **canine** as "(1) it is the term used in other sciences, and (2) other terms in standard usage can be understood only in relation to **canine** tooth: canine eminence, canine muscle, canine fossa." For the use of **premolar** he gives the following arguments: "(1) the term bicuspid is not descriptive of all teeth of that class, and (2) the acceptance of premolar makes uniform the terminology of dentistry and comparative dental anatomy."*

* From Denton, G.B.: The vocabulary of dentistry and oral science, Chicago, 1958, American Dental Association.

Some controversy exists over the use of the terms **x-ray, radiograph,** and **roentgenogram** in dentistry. The American Academy of Oral Roentgenology has indicated its preference for the use of roentgenogram, at the same time admitting that it may leave much to be desired as descriptive terminology. Examination of several recent textbooks on dental subjects finds usage divided between all three terms. However, in deference to the terminology preferred by the American Academy of Oral Roentgenology, the terms **roentgenogram, roentgenographic survey,** and **roentgenographic interpretation** are used herein.

Use of the term **acrylic** as a noun will be avoided. Instead it will be used only as an adjective, such as **acrylic** resin. The word **plastic** may be used either as an adjective or a noun; in the latter sense it refers to any of various substances that harden and retain their shape after being molded. The term **resin** will be used broadly for substances named according to their chemical composition, physical structure, and means for activation or curing, such as acrylic **resin**.

Retention, in terms of complete dentures, should be considered a denture base to soft tissue relationship. In removable partial prosthodontics we speak in terms of direct retention. **Direct retention** is the retention obtained in a removable partial denture by the use of attachments or direct retainers (clasps) that resist their removal from the abutment teeth.

Many other terms used in prosthodontics might be defined in this chapter, but such an undertaking is worthy of the efforts of those who again have recently directed their thoughts to that end. The Nomenclature Committee of the Academy of Denture Prosthetics and the Federation of Prosthodontic Organizations are to be commended for their efforts in compiling a current glossary that may be used for guidance in prosthodontic terminology.

2 CLASP-RETAINED PARTIAL DENTURE

POINTS OF VIEW

The clasp-retained partial denture utilizing the extracoronal direct retainer is probably used a hundred times more frequently than is the intracoronal, or internal attachment, partial denture (Fig. 2-1). Although the clasp-retained partial denture has disadvantages, for reasons of economy and time involved, it will probably continue to be employed because it is capable of providing physiologically sound treatment for the greatest number of patients needing partial denture restorations in keeping with their ability to pay for such treatment. Some of the **possible disadvantages** of a clasp-retained partial denture are as follows:

1. **Caries** may develop beneath clasp components, especially if the abutments are not protected with cast restorations and if the patient fails to keep the prosthesis and the abutments clean.
2. **Strain** too often is placed on the abutment teeth by improper clasp designs.
3. Clasps are often unesthetic, particularly when placed on visible tooth surfaces.

Despite these disadvantages, the use of removable prostheses may be preferred whenever there are tooth-bounded edentulous spaces of greater magnitude than can be restored safely with fixed prostheses or when cross-arch stabilization and wider distribution of forces is desirable. The removable partial denture retained by internal attachments eliminates some of the disadvantages of clasps, but it has other disadvantages, one of which is too great a cost for a large percentage of patients needing partial dentures. **Fixed partial dentures should always be used whenever indicated.**

When the alignment of the abutment teeth is favorable, the clinical crown is of sufficient length, the pulp size is diminished by tooth maturity, and the economic status of the patient permits, an internal attachment prosthesis is unquestionably preferable for esthetic reasons. In most instances, if the internal attachment denture is designed properly, this is its only advantage, since abutment protection and stabilizing components should be used with both internal and external retainers. However, economics permitting, esthetics alone may justify the use of an internal attachment denture.

We do not believe in the routine use of hinges or other types of stressbreakers for distal exten-

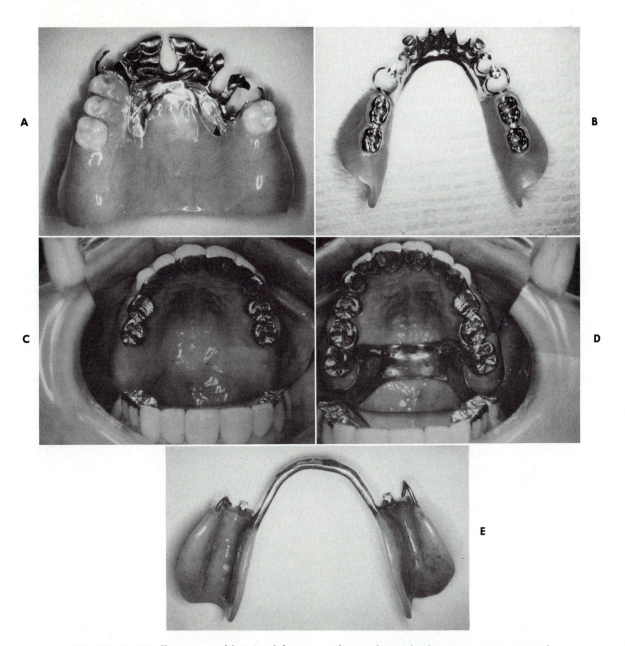

Fig. 2-1. A, Maxillary removable partial denture with complete palatal coverage. It is retained by extracoronal retainers (clasps) on terminal abutments. **B,** Mandibular removable restoration retained by clasps on terminal abutments. **C,** Maxillary arch prepared for an internal attachment restoration. Note "dovetail" preparations in distal portions of second premolars. Male portions of attachments will be attached to denture and will occupy dovetail preparations. **D,** Internal attachment restoration in patient's mouth. Note precise fit of male and female portions of attachments. **E,** Mandibular internal attachment partial denture viewed from residual ridge side. Male portions of attachments can be seen at anterior of each denture base. Buccal extracoronal retentive arms assist in retaining the denture. (**C** and **D** courtesy Dr. P. K. Thomas.)

sion partial dentures. It is not that they are ineffective, but they are more frequently misused and substituted for adequate support for the partial denture base. Particularly in the mandibular arch, in the absence of the cross-arch stabilization inherent in a rigid denture design, a stress-broken distal extension denture frequently subjects the edentulous ridge to excessive trauma from horizontal forces.

Because it must be used in conjunction with some form of stressbreaker, the locking or dove-tail-type internal attachment is not indicated when one or more distal extension edentulous spaces exist. A rigid design is preferred, and therefore some type of extra-coronal retainer must be used. Of these retainers, the clasp retainer is still the most frequently used, and it seems likely that its use will continue until a more widely acceptable retainer is devised.

Dental treatment for patients must be highly individualized. The dentist must be prepared to interpret the true meaning of optimal services and apply the concept to patients whose individual circumstances, in spite of needs, may dictate no treatment, limited treatment, or extensive treatment.

SIX PHASES OF PARTIAL DENTURE SERVICE

Partial denture service logically may be divided into six phases. The first phase is related to **patient education.** Included in the second phase are **treatment planning, design of the partial denture framework,** and **execution of mouth preparations.** The third phase is **provision of adequate support for the distal extension denture base.** The fourth phase is **establishment of harmonious occlusal relationships with opposing and remaining natural teeth.** The fifth phase involves **initial placement procedures** including adjustments to the bearing surfaces of denture bases, adjustments to assure occlusal harmony, and a review of instructions given the patient to optimally maintain oral structures and the provided restorations. The sixth and final phase of partial denture service is **follow-up services by the dentist** through recall appointments for periodic evaluation of the responses of oral tissues to restorations and of the acceptance of the restorations by the patient.

Education of patient

The term patient education is described in *Boucher's Clinical Dental Terminology*, ed. 3, 1982, as "Effective communication between the dentist (and/or auxiliaries) and the patient concerning dentistry and the principles of treatment and prevention. The procedure of increasing the patient's knowledge of the oral cavity and its care to the point where the reasons for proposed dental services are understood."

Responsibility for the ultimate success of a removable partial denture is shared by the dentist and the patient. It is folly to assume that a patient will have an understanding of the benefits of a removable partial denture unless so informed. It is also unlikely that the patient will have the knowledge to avoid misuse of the restoration or be able to provide the required oral care and maintenance procedures to ensure the success of the partial denture unless he is adequately advised.

The finest biologically oriented removable partial denture is often doomed to extremely limited success if the patient relaxes proper oral hygiene habits or fails to respond to recall appointments. One of the primary objectives for a partial denture, **preservation,** will most likely not be achieved with only token cooperation on the part of the patient.

Patient education should begin at the initial contact with the patient and continue throughout treatment. This educational procedure is especially important when the treatment plan and prognosis are discussed with the patient. The limitations imposed on the success of treatment through failure of the patient to accept responsibility must be explained before definitive treatment is undertaken. A patient will not usually retain all the information presented in the oral educational instructions. For this reason, patients should be presented with written suggestions to reinforce the oral presentations.

Treatment planning and design

After a health history and a history of past dental experiences have been obtained, and after a complete oral examination has been made, a treatment plan is evolved that is based on the support available for the partial denture. The examination must include a clinical and radio-

Clasp-retained partial denture **11**

graphic interpretation of (1) periodontal conditions, (2) responses of teeth (especially abutment teeth) to previous stress, and (3) vitality of remaining teeth. Additionally, evaluation of occlusal relations of remaining teeth (visually and by properly articulated diagnostic casts) and a survey of diagnostic casts must be meticulously accomplished.

Distal extension situations in which no posterior abutments remain and in which extension bases must derive their principal support from the underlying residual ridge require an entirely different partial denture design than does one in which total abutment support is available. This is apparent from visual examination, but roentgenographic interpretation and the surveying of abutments and soft tissue contours must take into consideration the greater torque and tipping leverages of the distal extension partial denture.

Sufficient differences exist between the tooth-supported and the tooth- and tissue-supported removable restorations to justify a distinction between them. Principles of design and techniques employed in construction may be completely dissimilar. The points of difference are as follows:

1. Manner in which the prosthesis is supported.
2. Impression methods required for each
3. Types of direct retainers best suited for each
4. Denture base material best suited for each
5. Need for indirect retention

A distinction between these two types of removable restorations is adequately made by an acceptable classification of removable partial dentures.

Basically the same principles apply to the unilateral distal extension denture as to the bilateral distal extension denture. On the other hand, entirely different principles of design, as stated above, apply to a prosthesis that is totally tooth supported. Each type must be designed according to the manner of support.

It is necessary that a specific design be planned carefully in advance of mouth preparations and that these mouth preparations be carried out with care, **as outlined on the diagnostic cast.** Then specific and exact mouth prep-

arations, including abutment restorations, will dictate the final form of the denture framework to be outlined on the master cast. This should be drawn accurately onto the master cast after surveying so that there will be no doubt in the mind of the technician as to the exact design of the partial denture framework to be constructed under guidance and supervision of a dentist.

The dental cast **surveyor** (Fig. 2-2) is necessary in any dental office in which patients are being treated with removable partial dentures. There is no more reason to justify its omission from a dentist's armamentarium than to ignore the need for roentgenographic equipment or the mouth mirror and explorer or the periodontal probe used for diagnostic purposes.

Several moderately priced surveyors that will adequately accomplish the diagnostic procedures necessary for designing the partial denture are on the market. And yet in many dental offices

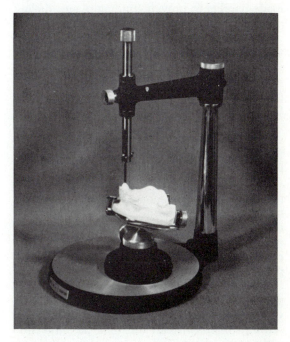

Fig. 2-2. Dental cast surveyor facilitates design of a removable restoration. It is an instrument by which parallelism or lack of parallelism of abutment teeth and other oral structures, on a stone cast, can be determined. Use of surveyor is covered in succeeding chapters.

today this most important phase of dental diagnosis is delegated to the commercial dental laboratory because of the absence of a single necessary piece of equipment or apathy on the part of the dentist who does include removable partial prosthodontics in the practice. This is a deplorable and degrading situation, which makes no more sense than relying on the technician to interpret roentgenograms and to render a diagnosis therefrom.

After treatment planning, mouth preparations may be performed with a definite goal in mind. Through the aid of diagnostic casts on which the tentative design of the partial denture has been outlined and the mouth changes have been indicated in colored pencil, occlusal adjustments, abutment restorations, and abutment modifications can be accomplished, providing for adequate support and retention and a harmonious occlusion for the partial denture.

Selected **proximal tooth surfaces** should be made parallel to provide guiding planes during placement and removal of the prosthesis. **Occlusal rest seats** that will direct occlusal forces along the long axis of the supporting teeth as nearly as possible should be established so that neither the tooth nor the denture will be displaced under occlusal loading. This dictates that the floor of the rest preparation be made to incline apically from the marginal ridge and be spoon shaped, with the marginal ridge lowered to permit sufficient bulk without occlusal interference from the rest.

Retentive areas must be identified or created that will provide, as far as is feasible, for relatively equal and uniform retention on all abutment teeth, sufficient only to resist reasonable dislodging forces. **Tooth surfaces on which reciprocal and stabilizing clasp arms may be placed also must be identified or created.**

After mouth preparations are believed completed, an impression should be made in irreversible hydrocolloid and a cast poured in quick-setting stone. This cast can then be surveyed, with the patient still present, to ascertain whether the planned abutment contours have been accomplished or if additional recontouring is necessary. When mouth preparations have been completed, the impression for the master cast should be made and the cast poured immediately. The master cast must then be surveyed so that the design of the denture framework can be drawn on it.

The final design of the denture framework should be outlined with colored pencils on the master cast, including the location of the clasp arms. It must be remembered that the location of the clasp arms will be determined by the height of contour of the abutment teeth and that this exists for a given path of placement only; hence proximal guiding planes and accurate blockout of proximal tooth surfaces are desirable. The position of the cast in relation to the surveyor must be recorded so that the technician may similarly place the cast on his surveyor to parallel the blockout material. This is easily done by scoring the base of the cast on three sides parallel to the path of placement or by tripoding the cast, but this must be done before the cast is removed from the surveyor.

Surveying the master cast, recording the relationship of the cast to the surveyor, and drawing a definite outline on the master cast are still not enough. It is difficult to draw all the details of the denture design on the master cast. This should be done by labeling a colored pencil drawing on a chart, which provides the technician with an outline of the partial denture framework and allows for instructions for the technician to follow in fabricating the denture. From this information it is possible for the technician to return a casting **that the dentist can superimpose** on the outline as drawn on the master cast. From any lesser instructions the technician cannot be criticized for returning a more stereotyped partial denture design.

The dentist should be responsible for the design of the partial denture framework from the beginning to the finish; therefore he is accountable for providing the technician with all the information needed. It is the responsibility of the technician to follow the written instructions given by the dentist, but at the same time it is his prerogative to demand that these instructions be so informative that he can follow them without question.

Up to this point the treatment planning and preliminary design of the partial denture, the mouth preparation procedures, and the design of the denture framework have been accomplished by the dentist. Given thorough written instructions and the master cast on which the dentist has drawn precisely the denture design, the technician then may fabricate the metal framework. The finished framework should be returned to the dentist so that he can evaluate its fit in the mouth and make any necessary adjustments on the framework.

When laboratory procedures are correctly executed, the framework should fit the master cast as planned. If the framework does not fit the mouth as planned, the dentist then can determine whether the error is the result of a faulty impression on his part, or an inaccurate master cast, or a laboratory procedure. In any event, adequate support for distal extension denture bases and the need for exacting occlusal records make it necessary for the denture framework to be returned to the dentist for further records before completion of the restoration.

Support for distal extension denture bases

The third of the six phases in the treatment of a patient with a partial denture is obtaining adequate support for distal extension bases; therefore it does not apply to tooth-borne removable partial dentures. In the latter, support comes entirely from the abutment teeth through the use of rests.

For the distal extension partial denture, however, a base made to fit the anatomic ridge form does not provide adequate support under occlusal loading (Fig. 2-3). Neither does it provide for maximum border extension nor accurate border detail. Therefore some type of correction impression is necessary. This may be accomplished by several means, all of which satisfy the requirements for support of any distal extension partial denture base.

Foremost is the requirement that certain soft tissues should be recorded or related under some loading so that the base may be made to fit the form of the ridge when under function, thereby providing support and assuring a maintenance of that support for the longest possible time. This requirement makes the distal extension partial denture unique in that the support from the tissues underlying the distal extension base must be made as equal to and compatible with the tooth support as is possible.

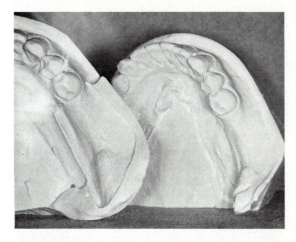

Fig. 2-3. Cast on right was made from impression that recorded anatomic form of residual ridge. On the left is same cast, with residual ridge recorded in a functional, or supporting, form by a secondary impression. Note that supporting form of ridge clearly delineates the extent of coverage available for a denture base.

A complete denture is entirely tissue supported, and the entire denture can move tissueward under function. In contrast, any movement of a partial denture base is inevitably a rotational movement, which may result in a loss of planned occlusal contacts and the application of undesirable forces to the abutment teeth. Therefore every effort must be made to provide the best possible support for the distal extension base to minimize these forces.

Usually no single impression technique will adequately record the anatomic form of the teeth and adjacent structures and at the same time record the supporting form of the lower edentulous ridge. However, the same relative results can be accomplished, provided an individualized acrylic resin tray is used and is so prepared that placement of the soft tissue on the buccal shelf (the primary stress-bearing area) is accomplished. Some method should be used that will record these tissues either in their supporting **form** or in a supporting **relationship** to the rest of the denture (Fig. 2-3). This may be accomplished by one of several methods, which will be discussed in Chapter 15.

Establishment of occlusal relations

Whether the partial denture is tooth borne or has one or more distal extension bases, the recording of occlusal relationships comprises a most important step in the construction of a partial denture. For the tooth-borne partial denture, ridge form is of less significance than the tooth- and tissue-supported prosthesis, since it is not called on to support the prosthesis. For the distal extension base, however, jaw relation records should be made only after obtaining the best possible support for the denture base. This necessitates the making of a base or bases that will provide the same support as the finished denture. Therefore jaw relations cannot be recorded until after the denture framework has been returned to the dentist and a secondary impression has been made. Then either a new resin base or a corrected base must be used to record jaw relations.

Occlusal records for a removable partial denture may be made by the various methods described in Chapter 16.

Initial placement procedures

The fifth phase of treatment occurs when the patient is given possession of the removable restoration(s). Inevitably it seems that minute changes in the planned occlusal relationships occur during processing of the dentures. Not only must occlusal harmony be assured before the patient is given possession of the dentures, but the processed bases must be reasonably perfected to basal seats. It must also be assured that the patient understands the suggestions and recommendations given by the dentist for care of the dentures and oral structures, as well as expectations in the adjustment phases and use of the restorations. These facets of treatment are discussed in detail in Chapter 19.

Periodic recall

Initial placement and adjustment of the restoration(s) are certainly not the end of treatment for the partially edentulous patient. Periodic recall of the patient to evaluate the oral tissues, their response to the restorations, and the restorations themselves is a part of total treatment responsibility. Changes in the oral structures or the dentures must be ascertained rather soon to avoid compromised oral health. This can be accomplished by periodic recall. Although a 6 months' recall period is adequate for most patients, a more frequent evaluation may be required for some patients. Chapter 19 contains some suggestions concerning this sixth phase of treatment.

REASONS FOR FAILURE OF CLASP-RETAINED PARTIAL DENTURES

Experience with the clasp-retained partial denture made by the methods outlined has proved its merit and justifies its continued use. The occasional objection to the visibility of retentive clasps can be minimized through the use of wrought-wire clasp arms. There are few contraindications for use of a properly designed clasp-retained partial denture. Practically all objections to this type of denture can be disposed of by pointing to (some, but not all inclusive) deficiencies in its design and fabrication and to deficiencies related to patient education. These are as follows:

Diagnosis and treatment planning
1. Inadequate diagnosis
2. Failure to either use the surveyor or to use it properly during treatment planning

Mouth preparation procedures
1. Inadequate mouth preparations, usually resulting from insufficient planning of the design of the partial denture

Design of the framework
1. Incorrect use of clasp designs
2. Use of cast clasps that have too little flexibility, too broad tooth coverage, and too little consideration for esthetics
3. Flexible or incorrectly located major and minor connectors
4. Failure to use properly located multiple rests

Laboratory procedures
1. Problems in master cast preparation
   a. Inaccurate impression
   b. Poor cast-forming procedures
   c. Incompatible impression materials and gypsum products
2. Failure to provide the technician with a specific design and the necessary information for executing it
3. Failure of the technician to follow the design and written instructions

Support for denture bases

1. Failure to return supporting tissues to optimum health before impression procedures
2. Inadequate coverage of basal seat tissues
3. Failure to record basal seat tissues in a supporting form

Occlusion

1. Failure to develop a harmonious occlusion
2. Failure to use compatible materials for opposing occlusal surfaces

Patient-dentist

1. Failure of dentist to provide adequate dental health care information, including care and use of restorations
2. Failure of dentist to provide recall opportunities on a periodic basis
3. Failure of patient to exercise a dental health care regimen and respond to recall

A removable partial denture designed and fabricated so that it avoids the errors and deficiencies listed previously is one that proves the clasp-type partial denture can be made functional, esthetically pleasing, and long lasting without damage to the supporting structures. The proof of the merit of this type of restoration lies in the knowledge that (1) it permits treatment for the largest number of patients, as the need for this service increases with advances in other phases of dentistry, and is made economically possible by the avoidance of elaborate mechanical devices and high laboratory costs; (2) it provides restorations that are comfortable and efficient over a long period of time, with adequate support and maintenance of occlusal contact relations; (3) it provides for healthy abutments, free of caries and periodontal disease; (4) it provides for the continued health of restored, healthy tissues of the basal seats; and (5) it makes possible a partial denture service that is definitive and not merely an interim treatment.

Removable partial dentures thus made contribute to a concept of prosthetic dentistry that has as its goal the promotion of oral health, the restoration of partially edentulous mouths, and **an elimination of the ultimate need for complete dentures.**

SELF-ASSESSMENT AIDS

1. In chronologic order of accomplishment give the six sequential, correlated phases in treating a partially edentulous patient with removable restorations.
2. If responsibility for the success of treatment is shared by the dentist and the patient, what must be undertaken to prepare patients to accept their responsibility?
3. Since treatment planning is the sole responsibility of the dentist, which of the following may be omitted as noncontributory to total treatment: (1) a complete health history, (2) a history of past dental experiences, (3) an oral examination, (4) a roentgenographic examination, (5) an evaluation of occlusal relations of remaining teeth, or (6) a survey of diagnostic casts?
4. A specific design of the removable restoration must be planned before mouth preparation procedures. The dentist (can) (should not) delegate the responsibility for the design to a dental laboratory technician.
5. Stability in a removable restoration is desirable to help maintain the health of oral structures. A tooth-borne restoration usually (can) (cannot) be made more stable than a restoration supported by teeth and residual ridges.
6. When a removable partial denture is supported both by teeth and residual ridges, support by the residual ridge should be made as equal as possible to the support given by the teeth. This may be accomplished by recording which form of the residual ridge in making impressions—anatomic or functional?
7. Recording of jaw relations to properly orient master or opposing casts to an articulator should be delayed until the framework has been fitted and a secondary impression has been made. True or false?
8. In the fifth phase of treatment (initial placement of the restoration(s)) three things are done before the patient is given possession of the denture(s). Two of these are correction of occlusal discrepancies as a result of processing, and review of patient education including adjustment expectations. What other step must be accomplished during the appointment?
9. What is the purpose of periodic recall of patients treated with removable partial dentures?
10. What is the one predominant reason why the clasp-type partial denture is used much more frequently in most practices than is the internal attachment–type restoration?
11. Deficiencies in design and fabrication and those related to patient education are the culprits of limited success in treatment with removable restorations. Avoiding these deficiencies will make the goal of prosthetic dentistry obtainable. This goal is _____, _____, and _____.

3 CLASSIFICATION OF PARTIALLY EDENTULOUS ARCHES

Requirements of an acceptable method of
  classification
Kennedy's classification
  Applegate's rules for applying the Kennedy
    classification

Several methods of classification of partially edentulous arches have been proposed and are in use today. This has led to much confusion and disagreement concerning which method should be adopted and which best classifies all possible combinations.

It has been estimated that there are over 65,000 possible combinations of teeth and edentulous spaces in opposing arches. It is obvious that no single method of classification can be descriptive of any except the most basic types. Therefore a basic classification should be sufficient. It is unfortunate that no single method has been universally adopted by the profession. This fact probably has done more to prevent a comprehensive approach to the principles of partial denture design than has any other single factor.

Although classifications are actually descriptive of the partially edentulous arches, the removable partial denture restoring a particular class arch is described as a denture of that class. For example, we speak of a Class III or Class I removable partial denture. Certainly this is acceptable and promotes an economy of words. It is simpler to say "a Class II partial denture" than to say "a partial denture restoring a Class II partially edentulous arch."

The most familiar classifications are those originally proposed by Kennedy, Cummer, and Bailyn. Classifications have also been proposed by Beckett, Godfrey, Swenson, Friedman, Wilson, Skinner, Applegate, Avant, Miller, and others. It is evident that an attempt should be made to combine the best features of all classifications so that a universal classification can be adopted in the future.

Kennedy's method of classification is probably the most widely accepted classification of partially edentulous arches today. Any method that will satisfy the requirements of a classification is acceptable. In an attempt to simplify the problem and encourage more universal usage of a classification and in the interest of adequate communication, the Kennedy classification will be used in this textbook. The student is referred to the Selected Reading Resources section for information relative to other classifications.

REQUIREMENTS OF AN ACCEPTABLE METHOD OF CLASSIFICATION

The classification of a partially edentulous arch should satisfy the following requirements:
1. It should permit immediate visualization of the type of partially edentulous arch being considered.
2. It should permit immediate differentiation between the tooth-borne and the tooth- and tissue-supported removable partial denture.
3. It should be universally acceptable.

KENNEDY'S CLASSIFICATION

The Kennedy method of classification was originally proposed by Dr. Edward Kennedy in 1925. Like the Bailyn classification and also the Skinner classification, it attempts to classify the partially edentulous arch in a manner that will suggest certain principles of design for a given situation (Fig. 3-1).

Kennedy divided all partially edentulous arches into four main types. Edentulous areas other than those determining the main types were designated as **modification spaces** (Fig. 3-2).

The Kennedy classification is as follows:

CLASS I. Bilateral edentulous areas located posterior to the remaining natural teeth

CLASS II. A unilateral edentulous area located posterior to the remaining natural teeth

CLASS III. A unilateral edentulous area with natural teeth remaining both anterior and posterior to it

CLASS IV. A single, but bilateral (crossing the

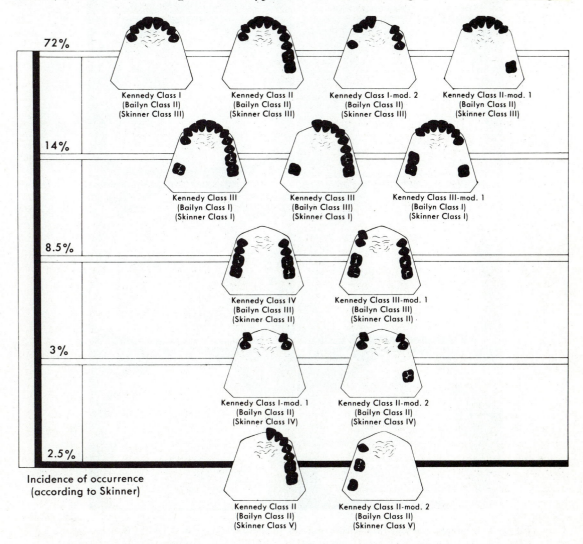

Fig. 3-1. Representative examples of partially edentulous arches classified by the Kennedy, Bailyn, and Skinner methods of classification.

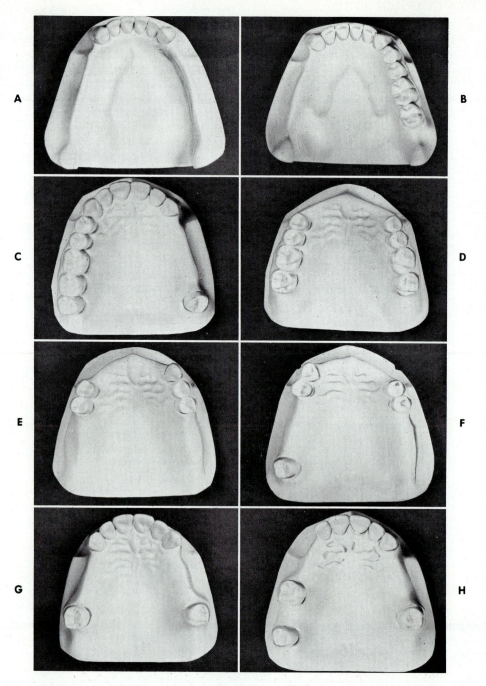

Fig. 3-2. Kennedy classification with examples of modifications. **A,** Class I; **B,** Class II; **C,** Class III; **D,** Class IV; **E,** Class I, modification 1; **F,** Class II, modification 2; **G,** Class III, modification 1; **H,** Class III, modification 2.

midline), edentulous area located anterior the remaining natural teeth

One of the principal advantages of the Kennedy method is that it permits immediate visualization of the partially edentulous arch. Those schooled in its use and in the principles of partial denture design may immediately compartmentalize their thinking concerning the basic partial denture design that will be employed. It permits a logical approach to the problems of design. It makes possible the application of sound principles of partial denture design and is therefore a logical method of classification. However, a classification system should not be used to stereotype design.

Applegate's rules for applying the Kennedy classification

The Kennedy classification would be difficult to apply to every situation without certain rules for application. Applegate has provided the following eight rules governing the application of the Kennedy method:

RULE 1. Classification should follow rather than precede any extractions of teeth that might alter the original classification.

RULE 2. If a third molar is missing and not to be replaced, *it is not considered in the classification.*

RULE 3. If a third molar is present and is to be used as an abutment, *it is not considered in the classification.*

RULE 4. If a second molar is missing and is not to be replaced, *it is not considered in the classification* (for example, if the opposing second molar is likewise missing and is not to be replaced).

RULE 5. The *most posterior edentulous area* (or areas) always determines the classification.

RULE 6. Edentulous areas other than those determining the classification are referred to as *modifications* and are designated by their number.

RULE 7. The *extent* of the modification is not considered, only the *number* of additional edentulous areas.

RULE 8. There can be no modification areas in Class IV arches. (Another edentulous area lying posterior to the "single bilateral area crossing the midline" would instead determine the classification.)

One suggested change in the order of the Kennedy classification is an attempt to correlate the Class I and Class II partially edentulous arches with the number of edentulous areas involved. Thus Class I would be a unilateral edentulous area posterior to the remaining teeth, and Class II would be a bilateral edentulous area posterior to the remaining teeth.

Whereas it is true that there is some confusion in the mind of the student initially as to why Class I should refer to two edentulous areas and Class II should refer to one, the principles of design make this position logical. Either by design or by accident, presumably the former, Kennedy placed the Class II unilateral distal extension type between the Class I bilateral distal extension type and the Class III toothbounded classification. Any change in this order would be illogical for the following reasons. The Class I partial denture is designed as a tooth- **and** tissue-supported denture. Three of the features necessary for the success of such a denture are adequate support for the distal extension bases, flexible direct retention, and some provision for indirect retention. The Class III partial denture is designed as a tooth-borne denture, without need generally (but not always) for indirect retention, without base support from the ridge tissues, and with direct retention, the only function of which is to retain the prosthesis. An entirely different design is therefore common to each class because of the difference in support.

However, the Class II partial denture must embody features of both, especially when tooth-borne modifications are present. Having a tissue-supported extension base, it must be designed similarly to a Class I denture, but frequently there is a tooth-supported, or Class III, component elsewhere in the arch. Thus the Class II partial denture rightly falls between the Class I and the Class III because it embodies design features common to both. In keeping with the principle that design is based on the classification, the application of such principles of design is simplified by retaining the original classification of Kennedy.

SELF-ASSESSMENT AIDS

1. Would you agree that the primary purpose of a classification is to enhance communication among dentists?

2. Many classification systems have been proposed; however, the most widely accepted system in the United States is the one proposed by _____ in 1925.
3. A classification of partially edentulous arches should satisfy at least three requirements. Can you recall these three requirements?
4. Kennedy divided all partially edentulous arches into _____ main types.

5. What is meant by a modification space?
6. Which two classes of partially edentulous arches have the greatest incidence?
7. Dr. O.C. Applegate contributed greatly to the application of the original Kennedy classification system. What was this contribution?
8. Classify the partially edentulous arches illustrated in Fig. 3-3.

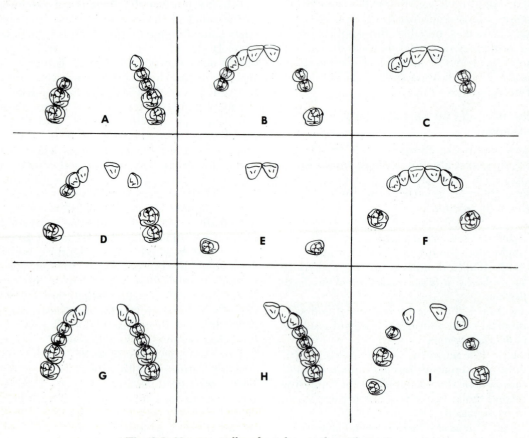

Fig. 3-3. Nine partially edentulous arch configurations.

4 MAJOR AND MINOR CONNECTORS

Components of a typical removable partial denture are illustrated in Fig. 4-1, *A*.

1. Major connector
2. Minor connector
3. Rests
4. Direct retainers
5. Reciprocal or stabilizing components (as parts of a direct retainer assembly)
6. Indirect retainers (if the prosthesis has one or more distal extension bases)
7. One or more bases, each supporting one to several replacement teeth (Fig. 4-1, *B* and *C*)

In this chapter major and minor connectors will be considered separately as to their function, location, and design criteria, keeping in mind both biologic and mechanical considerations. Other components are presented in designated chapters.

MAJOR CONNECTORS

A major connector is the unit of the partial denture that connects the parts of the prosthesis located on one side of the arch with those on the opposite side. It is that unit of the partial denture to which all other parts are directly or indirectly attached (Fig. 4-2).

The major connector may be compared with the frame of an automobile or with the foun-

dation of a building. In the construction of a removable partial denture, it is just as essential. Major connectors must be rigid so that forces applied to any portion of the denture may be effectively distributed over the entire supporting subjacent structures. Rigidity of the major connector resists flexing and torque that would otherwise be transmitted to abutment teeth in the form of leverage.

It is through the major connector that other components of the partial denture may be effective. If they are attached to, or originate from, a flexible connector, the effectiveness of components may be jeopardized to the detriment of oral structures and comfort of the patient. Failure of the major connector to provide rigidity may be manifest by traumatic damage to periodontal support of abutment teeth, injury to residual ridges, or impingement of underlying tissues.

Location. Major connectors should be designed and located with the following guidelines in mind:

1. They should be free of movable tissues.
2. Impingement of gingival tissues should be avoided.
3. Bony and soft tissue prominences should be avoided during placement and removal.
4. Relief should be provided beneath a major

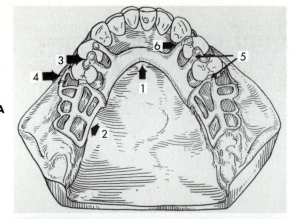

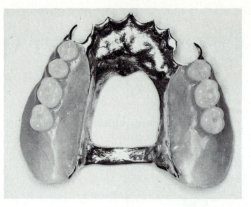

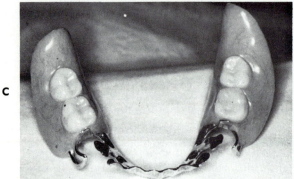

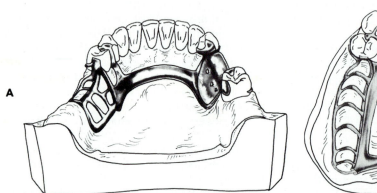

Fig. 4-1. A, Framework for mandibular removable partial denture with following components: *1,* lingual bar major connector; *2,* minor connector by which the acrylic resin denture bases will be attached; *3,* occlusal rests; *4,* direct retainer arm, which is part of the total clasp assembly; *5,* reciprocal and stabilizing components of clasp assembly (two minor connectors and two rests); and *6,* an indirect retainer consisting of a minor connector and an occlusal rest. **B,** Maxillary removable partial denture with acrylic resin denture bases supporting artificial posterior teeth. Bases are attached to metal framework by ladderlike minor connectors. **C,** Mandibular bilateral distal extension removable partial denture with acrylic resin denture bases supporting artificial posterior teeth.

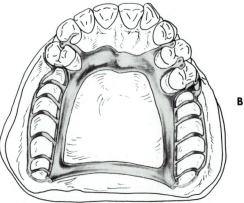

Fig. 4-2. A, Lingual bar major connector for mandibular removable partial denture framework. It rigidly joins cast base on right side to other elements of the framework on left side. **B,** Anterior-posterior strap–type maxillary major connector for a Class I partially edentulous arch. This is a rigid type of major connector and covers only a small portion of palatal tissue.

connector to prevent its settling into areas of possible interference such as inoperable tori or elevated palatal median sutures.

5. They should be located or relieved to prevent impingement of tissues as the distal extension denture rotates in function.

Planned relief beneath the major connector, when indicated, avoids the need for later adjustment to provide relief of the prosthesis after tissue damage has occurred. In addition to being time consuming, grinding to provide relief from impingement may seriously weaken the major connector, result in flexibility, or possibly lead to fracture. Major connectors should be carefully designed for proper shape, thickness, and location. Interruption of these dimensions by grinding can only be detrimental. **Relief** is covered at the end of this chapter and expanded in Chapter 10.

Margins of major connectors adjacent to gingival tissues should be located far enough from those tissues to avoid any possible impingement. The superior border of a lingual bar connector should be located at least 4 mm below the gingival margin(s) and more if possible (Fig. 4-3). The limiting factor, inferiorly, is the height of the moving tissues in the floor of the mouth. Since the connector must have sufficient width and bulk to provide rigidity, a linguoplate must be used in lieu of a lingual bar in instances of space limitation.

In the maxillary arch, since there are no moving tissues in the palate as in the floor of the mouth, the borders of the major connector may be placed well away from gingival tissues. Impingement of gingival tissues is not justifiable because adequate support for the connector is almost always available elsewhere. Structurally the tissues covering the palate are well suited for placement of the connector and have adequate deep blood supply. However, when soft tissue covering the median portion of the palate is less displaceable than the tissue covering the residual ridge, varying amounts of relief under the connectors must be provided to avoid impingement of tissue with its resulting sequelae.

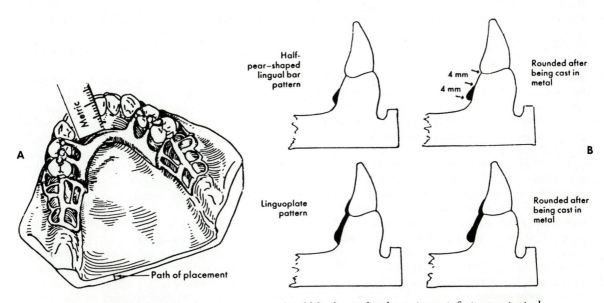

Fig. 4-3. A, Lingual bar major connector should be located at least 4 mm inferior to gingival margins and more if possible. The width of a finished lingual bar should be at least 4 mm for strength and rigidity. **B,** If less than 8 mm exists between gingival margins and movable floor of mouth, a linguoplate is preferred as a major connector. The inferior border of mandibular major connectors should be gently rounded after being cast to eliminate a sharp edge.

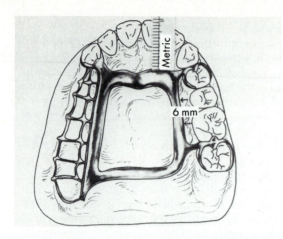

Fig. 4-4. Palatal major connector should be located at least 6 mm away from gingival margins and parallel to their mean curvature. All adjoining minor connectors should cross gingival tissues abruptly and should join major connectors at nearly a right angle.

The amount of relief required is directly proportional to the difference in displaceability of tissues covering the medial palatal raphe and tissues covering the residual ridges. The gingival tissues, on the other hand, must have an unrestricted superficial blood supply to remain healthy. The borders of the palatal connector should be placed a minimum of 6 mm away from gingival margins and should be located parallel to their mean curve. Minor connectors that must cross gingival tissues should do so abruptly, joining the major connector at nearly a right angle (Fig. 4-4). In this way the maximum freedom of gingival tissues is assured.

Except for a palatal torus or elevated median suture line, palatal connectors ordinarily require no relief, nor is relief desirable. Intimate contact between the connector and the supporting tissues adds much to the retention, stability, and support of the denture. Except for gingival areas, intimacy of contact elsewhere in the palate is not of itself detrimental to the health of the tissues, if supported against settling by rests on abutment teeth.

An anterior palatal strap or the anterior border of a palatal plate also should be located as far posteriorly as possible to avoid interference with the tongue in the rugae area. It should be **flat** or **straplike,** rather than half-oval, and should

be located so that its anterior border follows existing valleys between crests of the rugae. The anterior border of such palatal major connectors will therefore be irregular in outline as it follows the valleys between the rugae. The tongue may then pass from one rugae prominence to another without encountering the border of the denture lying between. When a rugae crest must be crossed by the connector border, it should be done abruptly, avoiding the crest as much as possible. The posterior limitation of a maxillary major connector should be just anterior to the vibrating line.

A rule to be used throughout partial denture design is as follows: **Try to avoid adding any part of the denture framework to an already convex surface. Rather, try to use existing valleys and embrasures for the location of component parts of the framework. All components should be tapered where they join convex surfaces.**

The characteristics of major connectors contributing to the maintenance of health of the oral environment and the well-being of the patient may be listed as follows:

1. Is made from an alloy compatible with oral tissues
2. Is rigid—employs the broad distribution of stress principle
3. Does not interfere with and is not irritating to the tongue
4. Does not substantially alter the natural contour of the lingual surface of the mandibular alveolar ridge or of the palatal vault
5. Does not impinge on oral tissues when the restoration is placed, is removed, or rotates in function
6. Covers no more tissue than is absolutely necessary
7. Does not contribute to retention or trapping of food particles
8. Has support from other elements of the framework to minimize rotation tendencies in function
9. Contributes to the support of the prosthesis

Mandibular major connectors

The following are four types of mandibular major connectors:

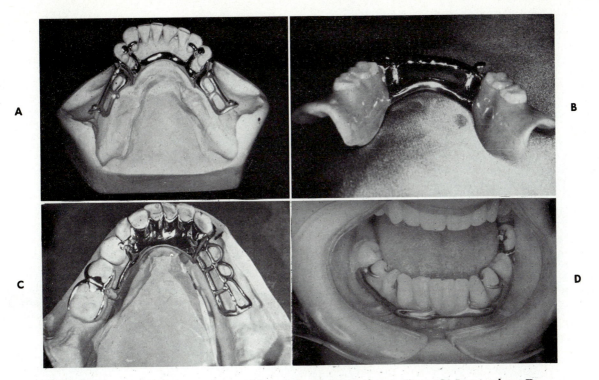

Fig. 4-5. A, Lingual bar. **B,** Lingual bar with continuous bar retainer. **C,** Linguoplate. **D,** Labial bar.

1. Lingual bar (Fig. 4-5, *A*)
2. Lingual bar with continuous bar retainer (Fig. 4-5, *B*)
3. Linguoplate (Fig. 4-5, *C*)
4. Labial bar (Fig. 4-5, *D*)

Lingual bar. The basic form of a mandibular major connector is the **half-pear–shaped lingual bar,** located above moving tissues but as far below the gingival tissues as possible. It is usually made of reinforced, **6-gauge,** half-pear–shaped wax or a similar plastic pattern (Fig. 4-6).

The major connector must be contoured so that it does not present sharp margins to the tongue and cause irritation or annoyance by its angular form. The superior border of a lingual bar connector should be tapered to the tissues above, with its greatest bulk at the lower border. This results in a contour that is known as a half-pear shape, being flat on the tissue side, tapered superiorly, and having the greatest bulk in the inferior third. Lingual bar patterns, both wax and plastic, are made in this conventional shape.

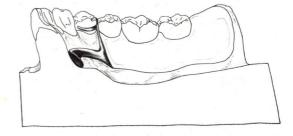

Fig. 4-6. Sagittal section showing half-pear shape of lingual bar. A taper of superior border of the bar to the soft tissues above will minimize interference with tongue and will be more acceptable to patient than would a dissimilar contour.

However, the inferior border of the lingual bar should be slightly rounded when the framework is polished. **A rounded border will not impinge on the lingual tissue when the denture bases rotate inferiorly under occlusal loads.** Frequently additional bulk is necessary to provide rigidity, particularly when the bar is long or an

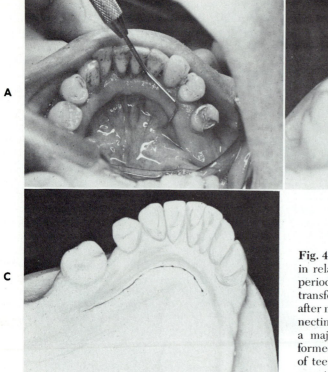

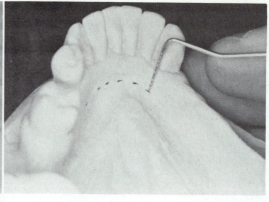

Fig. 4-7. **A,** Height of floor of mouth (tongue elevated) in relation to lingual gingival sulci measured with a periodontal probe. **B,** Recorded measurements are transferred to diagnostic cast and then to master cast after mouth preparations are completed. **C,** Line connecting marks indicates location of inferior border of a major connector. If periodontal surgery is performed, line on the cast can be related to incisal edges of teeth and the measurements recorded for subsequent use.

alloy of lesser rigidity is used. This is accomplished by underlying the ready-made form with a sheet of 24-gauge casting wax rather than altering the original half-pear shape.

The inferior border of a lingual mandibular major connector must be so located that it does not impinge on the tissues in the floor of the mouth as they change elevations during normal activity, that is, swallowing, speaking, licking the lips, and so forth. Yet at the same time it seems logical to locate the inferior border of these connectors as far inferiorly as possible to avoid interference to the resting tongue and trapping of food substances when they are introduced into the mouth. Additionally, the more inferiorly a lingual bar can be located, the farther the superior border of the bar can be placed from the lingual gingival crevices of adjacent teeth, which in itself will avoid impingement on the gingival tissue.

There are at least two clinically acceptable methods to determine the relative height of the

floor of the mouth to locate the inferior border of a lingual mandibular major connector. The first method is to measure the height of the floor of the mouth with a periodontal probe in relation to the lingual gingival margins of adjacent teeth (Fig. 4-7). During these measurements the tip of the patient's tongue should be just lightly touching the vermilion border of the upper lip. Recording of these measurements permits their transfer to both diagnostic and master casts, thus assuring a rather advantageous location of the inferior border of the major connector. The second method is to use an individualized impression tray having its lingual borders about 3 mm short of the elevated floor of the mouth and then to use an impression material that will permit the impression to be accurately molded as the patient licks his lips (Fig. 4-8). The inferior border of the planned major connector can then be located at the height of the lingual sulcus of the cast resulting from such an impression. Of the two methods, we have found the measuring of

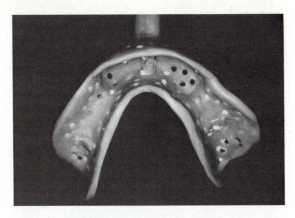

Fig. 4-8. Individualized mandibular acrylic resin impression tray. Lingual flanges should be so trimmed that elevated position of alveolar lingual sulcus can be accurately recorded in impression material when patient touches vermilion border of upper lip with tip of tongue. Tray was constructed as illustrated in Fig. 14-7.

the height of the floor of the mouth to be less variable and more clinically acceptable.

Continuous bar retainer. A continuous bar retainer located on or slightly above the cingula of the anterior teeth may be added to the lingual bar for one reason or another, but this should never be done without good reason (Fig. 4-9). **When a linguoplate is otherwise indicated, but the axial alignment of the anterior teeth is such that excessive blockout of interproximal undercuts must be made, a continuous bar retainer may be indicated.** Additionally, when wide diastemas exist between the lower anterior teeth, a continuous bar retainer may be more esthetically acceptable than a linguoplate.

Linguoplate. If the rectangular space bounded by the lingual bar, the continuous bar retainer, and the bounding minor connectors is filled in, a linguoplate results (Figs. 4-10 and 4-11). Again, this should only be done for good reason. The following rule applies: **No component of a partial denture should be added arbitrarily or conventionally. Each component should be added for a good reason and to serve a definite purpose.** The reason for adding a component may be for stabilization against horizontal rotation, retention, support, patient comfort, preservation of the health of the tissues, es-

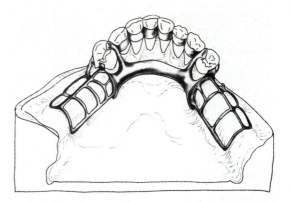

Fig. 4-9. Lingual bar and continuous bar retainer major connector. Upper portion of this major connector is located on cingula of anterior teeth. Requirement of positive support by rest seats, at least as far anteriorly as the canines, is critical. Note that superior border of bar portion must be placed objectionably close to gingival margins if sufficient rigidity is to be obtained. This type of major connector is definitely a food trap and is often much more objectionable to patient than a linguoplate from the standpoint of annoyance.

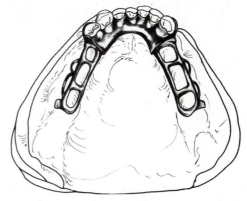

Fig. 4-10. Linguoplate is used when space between bounding connectors is better filled than left open. Such an apron does not serve to replace those connectors but, instead, is added to fundamental denture design to make major connector rigid.

thetics, or any one of several other reasons, **but the dentist alone should be responsible for the choice of design used and should have good reasons, both biologic and mechanical, for making these choices.**

A linguoplate should be made as thin as is technically feasible and should be contoured to

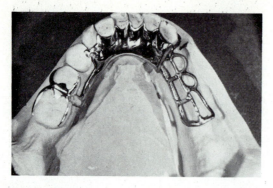

Fig. 4-11. View of mandibular Class II design with contoured linguoplate. Linguoplate is made as thin as possible and follows contours of teeth contacted, resulting in scalloped shape.

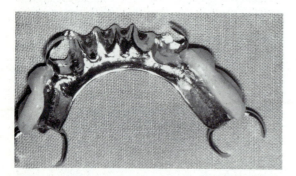

Fig. 4-12. Apron of linguoplate (tissue side) is closely adapted to teeth extending into nonundercut interproximal embrasures, resulting in scalloped form. This form will use some anterior teeth in group function to help resist horizontal rotation tendencies of the restoration.

follow the contours of the teeth and the embrasures (Fig. 4-12). The patient should be made as little aware of added bulk and altered contours in this area as is possible. The upper border should follow the natural curvature of the supracingular surfaces of the teeth and should not be located above the middle third of the lingual surface except to cover interproximal spaces to the contact points. All gingival crevices and deep embrasures must be blocked out parallel to the path of placement to avoid gingival irritation and any wedging effect between the teeth. In many instances the judicious recontouring of lingual proximal surfaces of overlapped anterior teeth

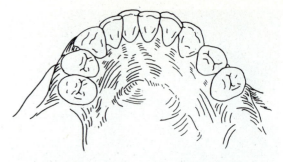

Fig. 4-13. If linguoplate major connector was indicated for this patient with overlapped anterior teeth, judicious recontouring of lingual proximal surfaces of right lateral, right central, and left lateral incisors would eliminate some gross undercuts, thereby permitting closer adaptation of lingual apron of major connector.

permits a closer adaptation of the linguoplate major connector, eliminating otherwise deep interproximal embrasures to be covered (Fig. 4-13).

The linguoplate should be something that is added to, not something replacing, the conventional lingual bar. The half-pear shape of a lingual bar should still be present, with the greatest bulk and rigidity at the inferior border. The linguoplate does not in itself serve as an indirect retainer. When indirect retention is required, **definite rests** must be provided for this purpose. Both the linguoplate and the continuous bar retainer should ideally have a terminal rest at each end regardless of the need for indirect retention. But when indirect retainers are necessary, it is incidental that these rests may serve also as terminal rests for the linguoplate or continuous bar retainer. **In such instances it is the rests—not the linguoplate or continuous bar retainer—** that function as indirect retainers.

Indications for the use of a linguoplate. The indications for the use of a linguoplate may be listed as follows:

1. **When the lingual frenum is high or the space available for a lingual bar is limited.** In either instance the superior border of a lingual bar would have to be placed objectionably close to gingival tissues. Irritation could be avoided only by generous relief, which would not only be annoying to the tongue but would also create

an undesirable food trap. Use of a linguoplate permits the gingivae to be bridged and the superior border to be tapered to tooth contact. This then permits the inferior border to be placed more superiorly without tongue and gingival irritation and without compromise of rigidity. Where a clinical measurement from the free gingival margins to the slightly elevated floor of the mouth is less than **8 mm**, a linguoplate is indicated in lieu of a lingual bar.

2. **In Class I situations in which the residual ridges have undergone excessive vertical resorption.** Flat residual ridges offer little resistance to horizontal rotational tendencies of a denture. The remaining teeth must be depended on to resist such rotation. A correctly designed linguoplate will use remaining teeth to resist horizontal rotations (Fig. 4-10).

3. **For stabilizing periodontally weakened teeth.** Although not as effective as fixed splinting and not as effective as the addition of a labial bar, lingual splinting with a linguoplate can be of considerable value when used with definite rests on sound adjacent teeth. A continuous bar retainer may be used to accomplish the same purpose, since it is actually the superior border of a linguoplate without the gingival apron. The continuous bar retainer accomplishes stabilization along with the other advantages of a linguoplate. However, it is frequently more objectionable to the patient's tongue and is certainly more of a food trap than is the contoured apron.

4. **When the future replacement of one or more incisor teeth will be facilitated by the addition of retention loops to an existing linguoplate.** Mandibular incisors that are periodontally weak may thus be retained, with provisions for future additions.

The same reasons for use of a linguoplate anteriorly apply also to its use elsewhere in the mandibular arch. If a lingual bar alone is to be used anteriorly, there is no reason for adding an apron elsewhere. However, when auxiliary splinting is used for stabilization of the remaining teeth, for horizontal stabilizing of the prosthesis, or for both, small rectangular spaces sometimes remain. **Tissue response to such small spaces** is better when bridged with an apron than when left open. Generally this is done to avoid gingival irritation or the entrap-

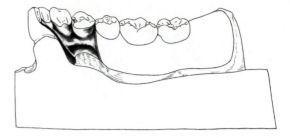

Fig. 4-14. Sagittal section through linguoplate demonstrating basic half-pear–shaped inferior border with metallic apron extending superiorly. Note that gingival crevice is "bridged" by linguoplate to avoid impingement of gingival tissue. The linguoplate receives positive support from a lingual rest (in properly prepared rest seat) on the canine and a mesiocclusal rest on the first premolar. Extension of linguoplate to height of contour on premolar was accomplished to enclose a rather large triangular interproximal space inferior to contact point between canine and premolar. Such spaces may often be bridged to eliminate obvious food traps and to provide more hygienic oral environment.

ment of food debris or to cover generously relieved areas that would be irritating to the tongue (Fig. 4-14). Sometimes a dentist is faced with a clinical situation wherein a linguoplate is indicated as the major connector of choice even though the anterior teeth are quite spaced and the patient strenuously objects to metal showing through the spaces. The linguoplate can then be so constructed that the metal will not appreciably show through the spaced anterior teeth (Fig. 4-15). Rigidity of the major connector is not greatly altered; however, such a design may be as much of a food trap as the continuous bar retainer type of major connector.

Labial bar. Fortunately there are few situations in which extreme lingual inclination of the remaining lower premolar and incisor teeth prevents the use of a lingual bar connector. By conservative mouth preparations in the form of recontouring and by blockout, a lingual connector can almost always be used. Lingually inclined teeth may sometimes have to be reshaped by means of crowns. Although the use of a labial major connector may be necessary in rare instances, this should be avoided by resorting to necessary mouth preparations, rather than ac-

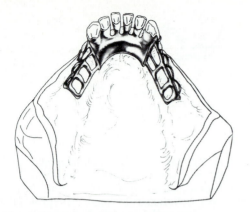

Fig. 4-15. Diastemas are not bridged by major connector. Framework must be supported by rests on canines placed in properly prepared rest seats. Rigidity of major connector is not necessarily compromised, but such a contour definitely lends itself to food being retained around teeth and under apron extensions.

cepting a condition that is otherwise correctable (Fig. 4-16). The same applies to the use of a labial bar when a mandibular torus interferes with the placement of a lingual bar. **Unless surgery is definitely contraindicated, interfering mandibular tori should be removed so the use of a labial bar connector may be avoided.**

Hinged continuous labial bar. The Swing-Lock* design consists of a labial or buccal bar that is connected to the major connector by a hinge on one end and a latch at the other end (Fig. 4-17). **Support** is provided by multiple rests on the remaining natural teeth. **Stabilization and reciprocation** are provided by a linguoplate contacting the remaining teeth and are supplemented by the labial bar with its retentive struts. **Retention** is provided by bar-type retentive clasp arms projecting from the labial or buc-

*Swing-Lock, Idea Development Company, Dallas, Texas

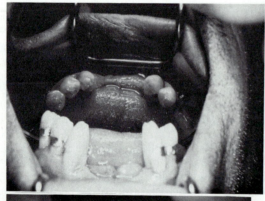

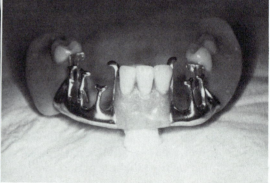

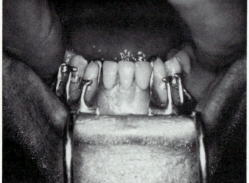

Fig. 4-16. A, Severe lingual inclinations of patient's canines and premolars preclude use of lingual bar. Advanced age of patient and economic status ruled out either orthodontic treatment or fixed restorations. **B,** Labial bar major connector was used in treatment. **C,** Retention was obtained on terminal abutments. Support and stabilization were gained by using rests, struts arising from labial bar, and well-fitting denture bases.

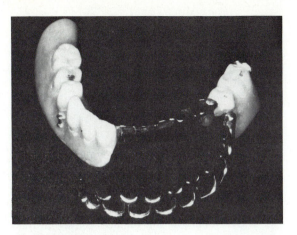

Fig. 4-17. The hinge for this continuous labial bar connector is located at buccal aspect of left second premolar. Latching mechanism can be seen on buccal flange of the denture, between the right canine and first premolar.

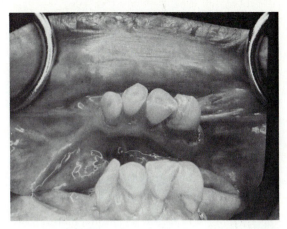

Fig. 4-18. Absence of right canine and lateral incisor requires that all remaining anterior teeth be used for retention and stabilization of replacement restoration. Swing-Lock concept can be used to ensure group function of these remaining mandibular teeth.

cal bar contacting the infrabulge areas on the labial surfaces of the teeth.

Use of the Swing-Lock concept would seem primarily indicated when there are:

1. **Missing key abutments.** By using all remaining teeth for retention and stability, the absence of a key abutment (such as a canine) may not present as serious a treatment problem with this concept as with more conventional designs (Fig. 4-18).

2. **Unfavorable tooth contours.** When existing tooth contours (uncorrectable with fixed restorations) or excessive labial inclinations of anterior teeth prevent conventional clasp designs, the basic principles of removable partial design may be better implemented with the Swing-Lock concept (Fig. 4-19).

3. **Unfavorable soft tissue contours.** Extensive soft tissue undercuts often prevent proper location of component parts of a conventional removable partial denture or an overdenture (Fig. 4-20). The hinged continuous labial bar concept may provide an adjunctive modality to accommodate such unfavorable soft tissue contours.

4. **Teeth with questionable prognoses.** The subsequent loss of a tooth (a key abutment) with a guarded prognosis seriously affects the reten-

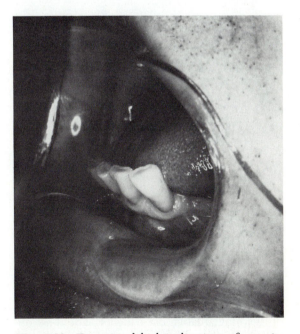

Fig. 4-19. Excessive labial inclinations of anterior teeth cannot be satisfactorily corrected with fixed restorations so that the patient can be provided a conventional restoration.

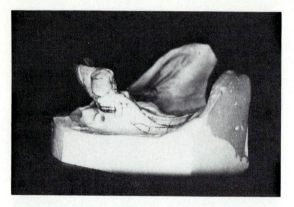

Fig. 4-20. Gross labial soft tissue undercuts obviate use of conventional clasping of terminal abutments. Therefore it seems prudent to use a group function concept of all remaining anterior teeth for this patient.

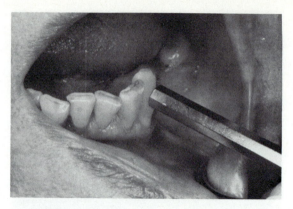

Fig. 4-21. Mobility of left canine suggests guarded prognosis for its use as a terminal abutment. If splinting cannot be accomplished, the patient might be better served with a hinged continuous labial bar in conjunction with a linguoplate major connector.

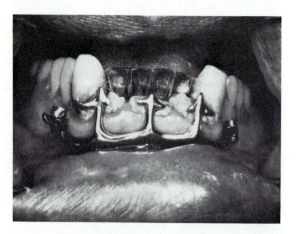

Fig. 4-22. Poor oral hygiene and lack of motivation for oral health certainly contribute to limited success of any dental treatment.

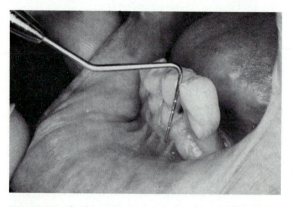

Fig. 4-23. If otherwise indicated, a hinged labial bar could not be optimally located because of shallow labial vestibule. Vestibular depth could be increased by surgical intervention.

tion and stability of a conventional prosthesis (Fig. 4-21). Since all remaining teeth function as abutments in the Swing-Lock denture, the loss of a tooth would seemingly not compromise retention and stability to such a degree.

There are obvious **contraindications** to the use of this hinged labial bar concept. The most obvious is **poor oral hygiene** or **lack of motivation for plaque control** by the patient (Fig. 4-22). Another contraindication is the presence of a **shallow buccal or labial vestibule** or a **high frenal** attachment (Fig. 4-23). Any of these factors would prevent the proper placement of components of the Swing-Lock partial denture.

The hinged labial bar type of restoration can be used satisfactorily for certain clinically compromised situations. Good oral hygiene, maintenance, and regular recall, as well as close attention to details of design, are paramount to successful implementation of this treatment con-

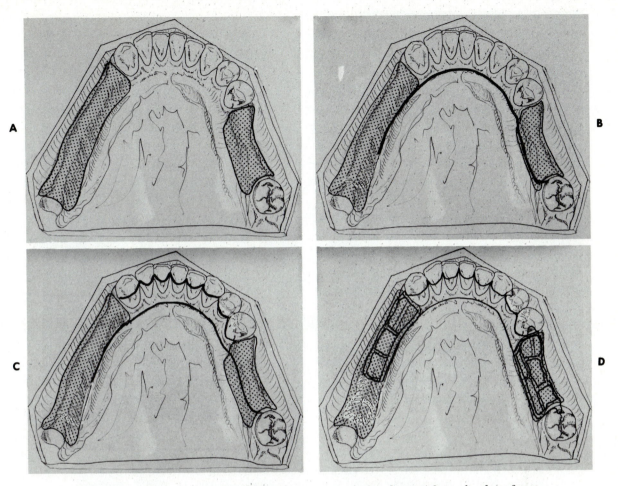

Fig. 4-24. **A,** Diagnostic cast with basal seat areas outlined. **B,** Inferior border of major connector is outlined. Location of inferior border was determined as suggested in Fig. 4-7. **C,** Superior border of major connector is outlined. Limited space for lingual bar requires use of linguoplate major connector. Linguoplate requires that rest seats be used on canines and first premolar for positive support. Lingual space between premolars is bridged by major connector to enhance its rigidity. **D,** Rest seat areas on posterior teeth are outlined, and minor connectors for retention of acrylic resin denture bases are sketched.

cept. The same statement is equally applicable to any type of removable restoration.

Design. A systematic approach to designing mandibular lingual bar and linguoplate major connectors can be readily employed with the diagnostic casts after considering the diagnostic data and relating them to the basic principles of major connector design:

STEP 1. Outline of the basal seat areas on the diagnostic cast (Fig. 4-24, *A*)

STEP 2. Outline of the inferior border of the major connector (Fig. 4-24, *B*)

STEP 3. Outline of the superior border of the major connector (Fig. 4-24, *C*)

STEP 4. Unification (Fig. 4-24, *D*)

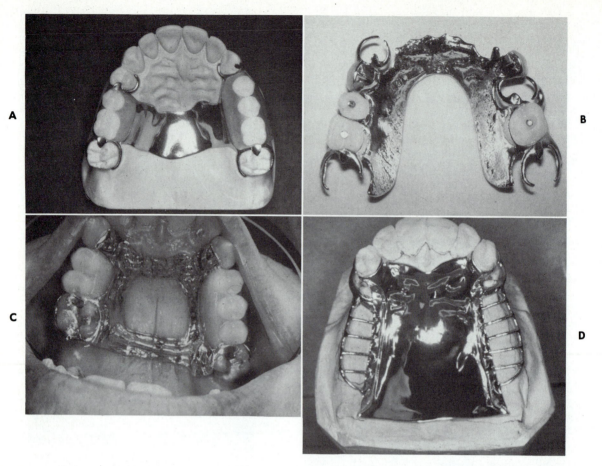

Fig. 4-25. A, Single palatal strap–type maxillary major connector. **B,** U-shaped maxillary major connector. **C,** Anterior-posterior palatal strap–type major connector. **D,** Palatal plate–type major connector.

Maxillary major connectors

Four basic types of maxillary major connectors will be considered:

1. Single palatal strap (Fig. 4-25, *A*)
2. U-shaped palatal connector (Fig. 4-25, *B*)
3. Combination anterior and posterior palatal strap–type connector (Fig. 4-25, *C*)
4. Palatal plate–type connector (Fig. 4-25, *D*)

It is again emphasized that to differentiate between a palatal bar and a palatal strap, a palatal connector component of less than 8 mm in width is referred to as a bar in this textbook.

Single palatal strap. The single palatal bar is perhaps the most widely used and yet the least

logical of all palatal major connectors (Fig. 4-26). It is difficult to say whether this or the U-shaped palatal connector is the more objectionable of palatal connectors.

For a single palatal bar to have the necessary rigidity, it must have concentrated bulk. The latter may be avoided only by ignoring the need for rigidity, which, unfortunately, is too frequently done. For a single palatal bar to be rigid enough to be effective, it must be centrally located between the two halves of the denture. This means that a single palatal bar always must be centrally located with concentrated bulk. Mechanically this practice may be sound enough,

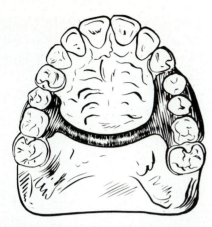

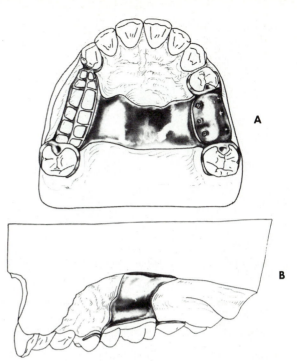

Fig. 4-26. Half-round palatal bar must be bulky to obtain rigidity required for cross-arch distribution of stress. Its bulk may make it objectionable to patient's tongue.

but from the standpoint of patient comfort and alteration of palatal contours, it is highly objectionable.

A partial denture made with a single palatal bar is frequently either too flexible or too objectionable to the patient's tongue, or both. The decision to use a single palatal strap should be based on the size of the denture areas being connected and on whether a single connector located between them would be rigid without objectionable bulk. Bilateral tooth-borne restorations of short spans may be effectively connected with a single, broad palatal strap connector, particularly when the edentulous areas are located posteriorly (Fig. 4-27). Such a connector can be made rigid, without objectionable bulk and interference to the tongue, provided its surface lies in three planes.

For reasons of torque and leverage, a single palatal connector should not be used to connect anterior replacements with distal extension bases. To be rigid enough to resist torque and to provide adequate horizontal and vertical support as well, a single strap would have to be objectionably bulky. When placed anteriorly, this bulk becomes even more objectionable to the patient, since it interferes with speech formation.

A suitable rigidity, without excessive bulk, may be obtained for a single palatal strap by

Fig. 4-27. This single palatal strap–type major connector may be used for tooth-borne restorations of bilateral edentulous areas of short span. It may also be used in tooth-borne unilateral edentulous situation with provision for cross-arch attachment by either extracoronal retainers or internal attachments. Width of palatal strap should be confined within the boundaries of supporting rests. **B,** Sagittal section through **A.** Midportion of major connector is slightly elevated to provide rigidity. Such thickness of major connector does not appreciably alter palatal contours.

using a 22-gauge matte plastic pattern. In lieu of a matte pattern, 32-gauge casting wax superimposed on a strip of 28-gauge wax as illustrated in Fig. 4-27 may be used.

U-shaped palatal connector. From both the patient's standpoint and a mechanical standpoint the U-shaped palatal connector is the least desirable of maxillary major connectors. It should never be used arbitrarily. When a large inoperable palatal torus exists and occasionally when several anterior teeth are to be replaced, the U-shaped palatal connector may have to be used (Fig. 4-28). In most instances, however, other designs will serve more effectively.

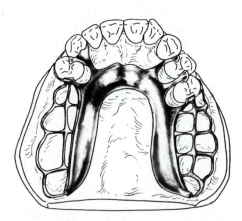

Fig. 4-28. U-Shaped palatal connector is probably the least rigid type of maxillary major connector and should be used only when large inoperable palatal torus prevents use of palatal coverage or combination anterior-posterior palatal strap–type designed framework.

The **principal objections** to use of the U-shaped connector are as follows:

1. Its lack of rigidity (compared to other designs) may induce torque or direct lateral force to abutment teeth.
2. The design fails to provide good support characteristics and may permit impingement of tissues underlying its palatal borders when subjected to occlusal loading.
3. Bulk to enhance rigidity results in increased thickness in areas most frequented by the tongue.

To be rigid the U-shaped palatal connector must have bulk where the tongue needs the most freedom, which is the rugae area. Without sufficient bulk the U-shaped design leads to increased flexibility and movement at the open ends. In distal extension dentures when posterior tooth support is nonexistent, movement is particularly noticeable and is traumatic to the residual ridge. Many maxillary partial dentures have failed for no other reason except the flexibility of a U-shaped major connector (Fig. 4-29). No matter how well the extension base is supported or how harmonious the occlusion, without a rigid major connector, the residual ridge suffers.

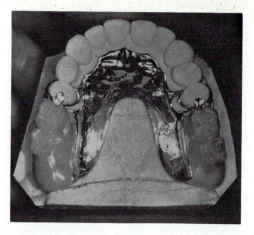

Fig. 4-29. Common partial denture design using an objectionable U-shaped palatal major connector. Such a connector lacks necessary rigidity, places bulk where it is most objectionable to patient, and impinges on gingival tissues lingual to remaining teeth, resulting in chronic inflammation. This denture failed primarily because it lacked rigidity in the major connector, provision for indirect retention, occlusal support, and consideration of gingival health in location of anterior border of major connector.

The wider the coverage of a U-shaped major connector, the more it resembles a palatal plate–type connector with its several advantages. But when used as a narrow U design, the necessary rigidity is usually lacking. A U-shaped connector may be made more rigid by providing multiple tooth support through definite rests. A common error in the design of a U-shaped connector, however, is its proximity to, or actual contact with, gingival tissues. The principle that the borders of major connectors should either be supported by rests in prepared rest seats or be located well away from gingival tissues has been given previously. The majority of U-shaped connectors fail to do either, with resulting gingival irritation and periodontal damage to the tissues adjacent to the remaining teeth.

Combination anterior and posterior palatal strap–type connector. Structurally the most rigid of palatal major connectors, the anterior and posterior palatal strap combination may be used in almost any maxillary partial denture design (Figs. 4-30 to 4-32).

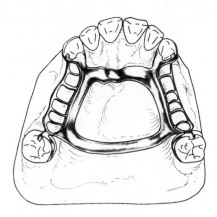

Fig. 4-30. Combination anterior-posterior palatal strap is most rigid of palatal major connectors and, when properly designed, is neither objectionable to patient nor harmful to adjacent tissues.

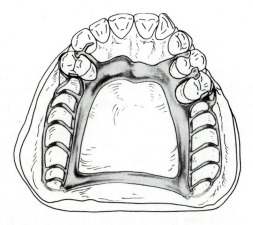

Fig. 4-31. Anterior-posterior palatal strap–type major connector. Anterior component is a flat strap located as far posteriorly as possible to avoid rugae coverage and tongue interference. Anterior border of this strap should be located just posterior to a rugae crest or in the valley between two crests. Posterior bar is half-oval (approximately 6 gauge) and is located as far posteriorly as possible, yet entirely on hard palate. It should be located at right angles to midline rather than diagonally.

Whenever it is necessary for the palatal connector to make contact with the teeth for reasons of support, definite tooth support must be provided. Anterior tooth support is sometimes necessary, particularly when the denture includes anterior replacements. This is best accomplished by establishing definite rest seats on gold restorations, using veneer crowns, three-quarter crowns, or pin-ledge restorations. These should be located far enough above the gingival attachment to provide for bridging the gingival crevice with blockout. At the same time, they should be low enough on the tooth to avoid unfavorable leverage and low enough on maxillary incisors and canine teeth to avoid incisal interference at the cingulum of the tooth.

Connector borders resting on unprepared tooth surfaces can lead only to slippage of the denture along inclines, to orthodontic movement of the tooth, or to both. In any case, settling into gingival tissues is inevitable. When the needed vertical support ceases to exist, the health of the surrounding tissues is usually impaired. Similarly, interproximal projections resting on the gingival third of the tooth and on gingival tissues that are structurally unable to render support can only cause impingement to the detriment of the health of those tissues.

A cardinal rule, then, for the location of the major connector in relation to the remaining teeth and their surrounding gingivae is this: **Either support the connector by definite rests on the teeth contacted, bridging the gingivae with adequate relief, or locate the connector far enough away from the gingivae to avoid any possible restriction of blood supply and entrapment of food debris.** All gingival crossings should be abrupt and at right angles to the major connector, and these should bridge the gingivae with adequate relief.

Creating a sharp, angular form on any portion of a palatal connector should be avoided, and all borders should be tapered slightly toward the tissues. A posterior palatal bar should be half-oval in shape. Posterior palatal connectors should be located as far posteriorly as possible to avoid interference with the tongue, but should never be placed on moving tissues. They should be located on the hard palate anterior to the line of flexure formed by the junction of the

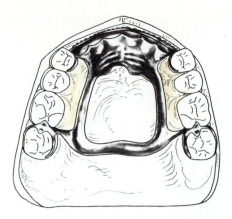

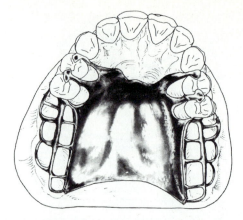

Fig. 4-32. Anterior-posterior component major connector for a Class IV partially edentulous arch. Positive support for anterior portion of major connector is furnished by "splint bar" joining the four crowned premolars. Notice that lateral portions of major connector are placed at least 6 mm from lingual gingival crevices.

Fig. 4-33. Palatal major connector covering two thirds of palate. Anterior border follows valleys between rugae and does not extend anterior to indirect retainers on first premolars. Posterior border is located at junction of hard and soft palates but does not extend onto soft palate. In bilateral distal extension situation illustrated, indirect retainers are a must to aid in resisting horizontal rotation of the restoration. Note that provisions have been made for a butt-type joint joining the denture bases and framework as denture base on each side passes through pterygomaxillary notch.

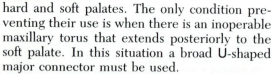

hard and soft palates. The only condition preventing their use is when there is an inoperable maxillary torus that extends posteriorly to the soft palate. In this situation a broad U-shaped major connector must be used.

The strength of this major connector design lies in the fact that the anterior and posterior components are joined together by longitudinal connectors on either side, forming a square or rectangular frame. Each component braces the other against possible torque and flexure. Flexure is practically nonexistent in such a design.

The anterior connector may be extended anteriorly to support anterior tooth replacements (Fig. 4-32). In this form a U-shaped connector is made rigid because of the added horizontal strap posteriorly. Frequently a maxillary torus may thus be encircled by the major connector without sacrificing rigidity.

The combination anterior-posterior connector design may be used with any Kennedy class of partially edentulous arch. It is used most frequently in Classes II and IV, whereas the single wide palatal strap is more frequently used in Class III situations, and the palatal plate–type or complete coverage connector is used most

frequently in Class I situations for reasons to be explained subsequently.

Both anterior and posterior connectors, and also the anterior and posterior borders of a palatal plate, should cross the midline at a right angle rather than on a diagonal. This is for reasons of symmetry. The tongue, being a bilateral organ, will accept symmetrically placed components far more readily than those placed without regard for bilateral symmetry. Therefore any curves in the connector should be placed to one side of the midline so that the connector may pass from one side to the other at right angles to the sagittal plane.

Palatal plate–type connector. For the lack of better terminology, the words **palatal plate** are used to designate any thin, broad, contoured palatal coverage used as a maxillary major connector covering one half or more of the hard palate (Fig. 4-33). The older types of thin castings, usually made of 26-gauge wax, were of indefinite thickness. This was the result of both the wax's being thinned during adaptation to the cast and to polishing with abrasive wheels. Newer techniques have resulted in the production of anatomic replica palatal castings that have uniform thickness and strength by reason of their corrugated contours. Thinner castings possessing greater rigidity are possible by this method. Through the use of electrolytic polishing, uniformity of thickness can be maintained and the anatomic contours of the palate faithfully reproduced in the finished denture.

The anatomic replica palatal major connector has several advantages over other types of palatal major connectors. Some of these follow:

1. It permits the making of a uniformly thin metal plate that reproduces faithfully the anatomic contours of the patient's own palate. Because of its uniform thinness, its familiar feel to the patient's tongue, and the thermal conductivity of the metal, the palatal plate is probably accepted more readily by the tongue and underlying tissues than any other type of connector.

2. The corrugation in the anatomic replica adds strength to the casting; a thinner casting with adequate rigidity can thus be made than could formerly be constructed with adapted sheet wax.

3. Surface irregularities are intentional rather than accidental; therefore electrolytic polishing is all that is needed. The original uniform thickness of the plastic pattern is thus maintained.

4. Interfacial surface tension between metal and tissues provides the prosthesis with greater retention. Retention must be adequate to resist the pull of sticky foods, the action of moving border tissues against the denture, the forces of gravity, and the more violent forces of coughing and sneezing. These are all resisted to some extent by the retention of the base itself in proportion to the total area of denture contact. The amount of both direct and indirect retention required will depend on the amount of retention provided by the denture base.

The palatal plate may be used in one of three ways. It may be used as a plate of varying width covering the area between two or more edentulous areas (Fig. 4-34), or it may be used as a complete or partial cast plate extending posteriorly to the junction of the hard and soft palates (Fig. 4-35 and 4-36), or it also may be used in

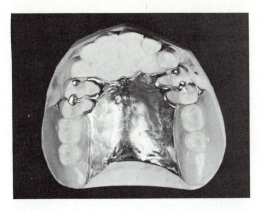

Fig. 4-34. Maxillary Class I partial denture framework with anatomic replica palatal major connector. Although retention is increased by using broad major connector, need for indirect retainers still exists, and they are placed on mesio-occlusal surfaces of first premolars. Direct retention is furnished by bar-type clasps engaging distobuccal undercuts on second premolars. Metal extension from framework contacts prepared guiding planes on distal surfaces of second premolars to complete clasp assembly.

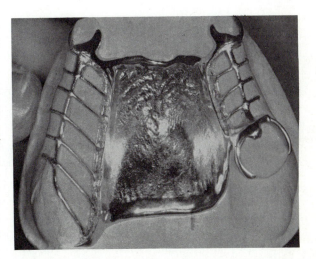

Fig. 4-35. Anatomic replica palatal major connector for a Class II, modification 1, partial denture. Anterior border avoids coverage of anterior rugae; posterior border lies well back on immovable hard palate, crossing midline at a right angle. Total contact provides excellent auxiliary retention without objectionable bulk.

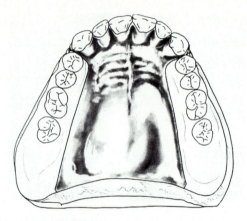

Fig. 4-36. Complete coverage palatal major connector. Posterior border terminates at junction of hard and soft palates. Anterior portion, in the form of palatal linguoplate, is supported by positive lingual rest seats on canines. Location of finishing lines is most important in this type of major connector. Unless they relatively follow line of the arch and are located just lingual to an imaginary line contacting lingual surfaces of missing natural teeth, alteration of natural palatal contour should be anticipated with its attendant detrimental effect on speech.

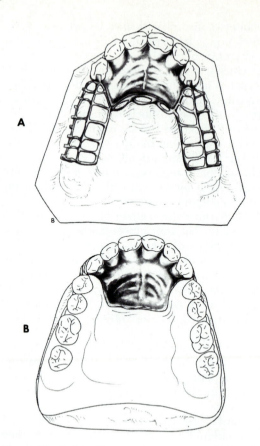

Fig. 4-37. A, Maxillary major connector in the form of palatal linguoplate with provision for attaching full-coverage acrylic resin denture base. **B,** Completed removable partial denture with acrylic resin base. Palatal linguoplate is supported by rests occupying lingual rest seats prepared in gold restorations on canines. This type of removable partial denture is particularly applicable where (1) residual ridges have undergone extreme vertical resorption and (2) terminal abutments have suffered some bone loss and splinting cannot be accomplished.

the form of an anterior palatal connector with a provision for extending an acrylic resin denture base posteriorly (Fig. 4-37).

In most situations the palatal plate will be located anterior to the posterior palatal seal area. Little posterior seal is every necessary with a metal palate because of the accuracy and stability of the cast metal. This is in contrast to the posterior palatal seal needed with resin complete denture bases. Inevitably the release of inherent strains in a processed acrylic resin base covering the palate and tuberosities requires that some provision be made for intimate contact of the posterior portion of the denture base and the tissue on which it is resting. This is accomplished by scoring the master cast to form a groove not exceeding 1×1 mm through the pterygomaxillary notches and across the junction of the hard and soft palates.

When the last remaining abutment tooth on either side of a Class I arch is the canine or first premolar tooth, complete palatal coverage is not only advisable, but is also practically mandatory when the residual ridges have undergone ex-

cessive vertical resorption. This may be accomplished in one of two ways. One method is to use a complete cast palate extending to the junction of the hard and soft palates (Fig. 4-36). The other method is to use a cast major connector anteriorly with retention posteriorly for the attachment of a resin denture base, which then extends posteriorly to the anatomic landmarks previously described (Fig. 4-37).

The several advantages of a cast palate over a complete resin palate make the complete cast

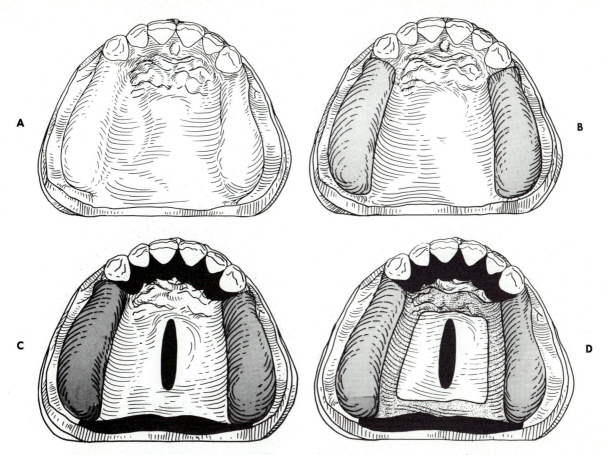

Fig. 4-38. A, Diagnostic cast of partially edentulous maxillary arch. **B,** Denture base areas are outlined. **C,** Nonbearing areas outlined in black, which include lingual soft tissue within 5 to 6 mm of teeth, an unyielding median palatal raphe area, and soft palate. The space bounded by bearing and nonbearing area outlines is available for placement of major connector. **D,** Major connector selected will be rigid and noninterfering with tongue and will cover a minimum of the palate.

palate sufficiently preferable to offset the slight additional cost. However, when the cost and fee must be held to a minimum, the former method may be used satisfactorily. The partial metal palate may also be used when later relining is anticipated. In such case the posterior beading can be redone as part of the relining procedure.

Whereas the complete palatal plate is not a connector that may be used universally, it has become accepted as the most satisfactory palatal connector for many maxillary partial dentures. In all circumstances the portion contacting the teeth must have positive support from adequate

rest seats. The dentist should be familiar with its use and, at the same time, with its limitations, so that it may be used intelligently and to fullest advantage.

Design. In 1953 Blatterfein described a systematic approach to designing maxillary major connectors. His method involves five basic steps and is certainly applicable to most maxillary removable partial denture situations. With a diagnostic cast in hand and a knowledge of the relative displaceability of the tissues covering the median palatal raphe, he recommends the following basic steps:

STEP 1. **Outline of primary bearing areas.** The primary bearing areas are those that will be covered by the denture base(s) (Fig. 4-38, *A* and *B*).

STEP 2. **Outline of nonbearing areas.** The nonbearing areas are the lingual gingival tissues within 5 to 6 mm of the remaining teeth, hard areas of the medial palatal raphe (including tori), and palatal tissues posterior to the vibrating line (Fig. 4-38, *C*).

STEP 3. **Outline of strap areas.** Steps 1 and 2, when completed, provide an outline or designate areas that are available to place components of major connectors (Fig. 4-38, *C*).

STEP 4. **Selection of strap type.** Selection of the type of connecting strap(s) is based on four factors: mouth comfort, rigidity, location of denture bases, and indirect retention. Connecting straps should be of minimum bulk and so positioned that interference with the tongue during speech and mastication is not encountered. Connecting straps must have a maximum of rigidity to distribute stress bilaterally. The double-strap type major connector provides the maximum rigidity without bulk and total tissue coverage. In many instances the choice of a strap type is limited by the location of the edentulous ridge areas. When edentulous areas are located anteriorly, the use of only a posterior strap is not possible. By the same token, when only posterior edentulous areas are present, the use of only an anterior strap is not plausible. The need for indirect retention influences the outline of the major connector: provision must be made in its location so indirect retainers may be attached.

STEP 5. **Unification.** After selection of the type straps based on the considerations in Step 4, the denture base areas and connecting straps are joined (Fig. 4-38, *D*).

The indications for the use of complete palatal coverage have been previously discussed in this chapter. Although there are many variations in palatal major connectors, a thorough comprehension of all factors influencing their design will lead to the best design for each patient.

Beading of the maxillary cast. Beading is a term used to denote the scribing of a shallow groove on the maxillary master cast outlining the palatal major connector exclusive of rugae areas (Fig. 4-39, *A* and *B*). The purposes of beading are as follows:

1. To transfer the major connector design to the investment cast (Fig. 4-40)
2. To provide a visible finishing line for the casting (Fig. 4-41, *A* and *B*)
3. To ensure intimate tissue contact of the major connector with selected palatal tissues

A 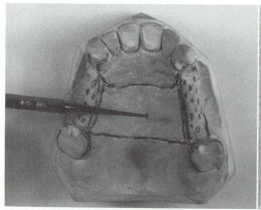 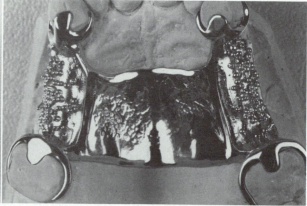 B

Fig. 4-39. **A,** Framework design on master cast before preparation for duplication in refractory investment. Shallow groove (0.5 mm) has been scribed on outline of anterior and posterior borders of major connector. Anterior outline follows valleys of rugae. Design calls for cast bases. **B,** Finished casting returned to master cast. Major connector is confined to previously scribed beading.

Beading is readily accomplished by using an appropriate instrument such as a cleoid carver. Care must be exercised to create a groove not in excess of 0.5 mm in width or depth (Fig. 4-42, *A* and *B*).

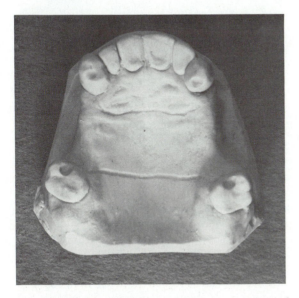

Fig. 4-40. Refractory cast. Note definitive outline of major connector transferred in duplicating master cast. Wax pattern for major connector can be accurately executed by beading.

MINOR CONNECTORS

Arising from the major connector, the minor connector joins the major connector with other parts of the denture. For example, each direct retainer and each occlusal rest are joined to the major connector by a minor connector. In many instances a minor connector may be identified even though continuous with some other part of the denture. For example, an occlusal rest at one end of a linguoplate is actually the terminus of a minor connector, even though that minor connector is continuous with the linguoplate. Similarly, the portion of a denture base frame that supports the clasp and the occlusal rest is a minor connector, joining the major connector with the clasp proper. Those portions of a denture framework by which the denture bases are attached are minor connectors.

Functions

In addition to joining denture parts, the minor connector serves two other purposes. These are diametric in function.

1. **To transfer functional stress to the abutment teeth.** Occlusal forces applied to the artificial teeth are transmitted through the base to the underlying ridge tissues if that base is primarily tissue supported. Occlusal forces applied to the artificial teeth nearer to an abutment are transferred to that tooth through the occlusal rest. Similarly, occlusal forces are transferred to

A

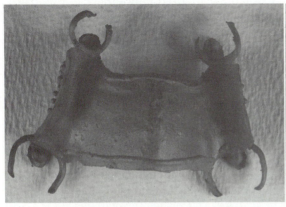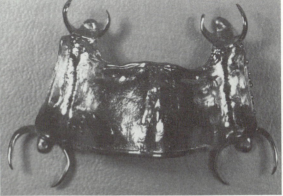

B

Fig. 4-41. A, Tissue side of casting as removed from refractory investment. Note slightly elevated ridges outlining major connector. **B,** Casting is finished to demarcated outline.

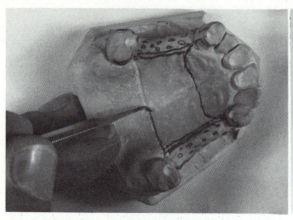

A

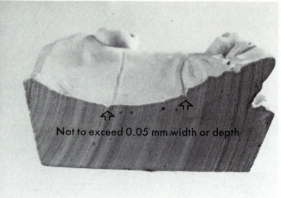

Not to exceed 0.05 mm width or depth

B

Fig. 4-42. **A,** Beading is readily accomplished with cleoid carver. Slightly rounded groove is preferred to V-shaped groove. **B,** Sagittal view of sectioned cast with width and depth of beading indicated.

other abutment teeth supporting auxiliary rests and to the abutment teeth supporting a partial denture that is entirely tooth borne. The minor connectors arising from a rigid major connector make possible this transfer of functional stress throughout the dental arch. This, then, is a **prosthesis-to-abutment** function of the minor connector.

2. **To transfer the effect of the retainers, rests, and stabilizing components to the rest of the denture.** This is an **abutment-to-prosthesis** function of the minor connector. The effect of occlusal rests on supporting tooth surfaces, the action of retainers, and the effect of reciprocal clasp arms, contacted guiding planes, and other stabilizing components are transferred to the remainder of the denture by the minor connectors and then throughout the dental arch. Thus forces applied on one portion of the denture may be resisted by other components placed elsewhere in the arch for that purpose. A stabilizing component on one side of the arch may be placed to resist horizontal forces originating on the opposite side. This is possible only because of the transferring effect of the minor connector, which supports that stabilizing component, and the rigidity of the major connector.

Form and location

Like the major connector, the minor connector must have sufficient bulk to be rigid; other-

wise the transfer of the stresses and of the effects of other components cannot be effective. At the same time, the bulk of the minor connector must be as unobjectionable as possible.

A minor connector contacting the axial surface of an abutment should not be located on a convex surface but instead should be located in an embrasure in which it will be least noticeable to the tongue. It should conform to the interdental embrasure, passing vertically from the major connector to the other components. It should be thickest toward the lingual surface, tapering toward the contact area. The deepest part of the interdental embrasure should have been blocked out to avoid interference during placement and removal and to avoid any wedging effect on the teeth contacted.

Generally the minor connector should form a right angle with the major connector so that the gingival crossing may be abrupt and cover as little of the gingival tissues as possible. All gingival crossings should be relieved by blockout of the gingival crevice on the master cast before a refractory cast is made.

When a minor connector contacts tooth surfaces on either side of the embrasure in which it lies, it should be tapered to the teeth so that the tongue may encounter a smooth surface (Fig. 4-43). Sharp angles should be avoided, and spaces should not exist for the trapping of food debris.

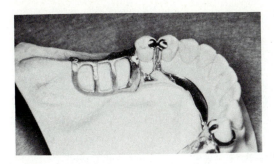

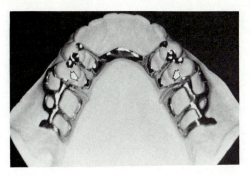

Fig. 4-43. Undercuts in lingual embrasure between premolars have been blocked out parallel to path of placement. Minor connector is V shaped to avoid bulk, with greatest depth of the V being at junction with occlusal rests.

Fig. 4-44. Minor connector (arrows) contacting guiding plane surface is as broad as about two thirds the distance between tips of adjacent buccal and lingual cusps of the abutment tooth. It extends gingivally contacting an area of the abutment from the marginal ridge to two thirds the length of the enamel crown. Viewed from above, it is triangular in shape, the apex of the triangle being bucally located and the base of the triangle located lingually. Less interference with arrangement of adjacent artificial tooth is encountered with minor connector so shaped.

It is a minor connector that contacts the guiding plane surfaces of the abutment teeth whether as a connected part of a direct retainer assembly or as a separate entity (Fig. 4-44). Here the minor connector must be wide enough to use the guiding plane to fullest advantage. When it gives rise to a clasp arm, the connector should be tapered to the tooth below the origin of the clasp. If no clasp arm is formed, as when a bar clasp arm originates elsewhere, the connector should be tapered to a knife-edge the full length of its buccal aspect.

When an artificial tooth will be placed against a proximal minor connector, the minor connector's greatest bulk should be toward the lingual aspect of the abutment tooth. This way sufficient bulk is assured with the least interference to placement of the artificial tooth. Ideally the artificial tooth should contact the abutment tooth with only a thin layer of metal intervening buccally. Lingually the bulk of the minor connector should lie in the interdental embrasure the same as between two natural teeth.

The minor connector, then, should be positioned to pass vertically in an interdental embrasure whenever possible. Its shape should conform to the interdental embrasure, with sufficient bulk to be rigid but tapered to the tooth surface when exposed to the tongue, and it should be designed so that it will not interfere with the placement of an artificial tooth.

As stated previously, those portions of a den-

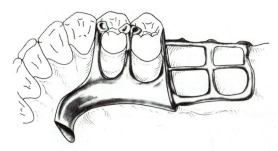

Fig. 4-45. Finishing line at junction of ladder-like minor connector and major connector blends smoothly into minor connector, contacting distal guiding plane on second premolar. Framework is "feathered" toward tissue anterior to finishing line to avoid as much bulk in this area as possible—without compromising the strength of the butt-type joint.

ture framework by which acrylic resin denture bases are attached are minor connectors. This type of minor connector should be so constructed that it will be completely embedded within the denture base.

The junctions of these mandibular minor connectors with the major connectors should be strong butt-type joints but without appreciable bulk (Fig. 4-45). Angles formed at the junctions of the connectors should not be greater than 90

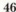

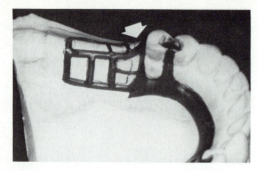

Fig. 4-46. Wax pattern for minor connector by which acrylic resin denture base will be attached. It is extended on both lingual and buccal surfaces of residual ridge and is made using 12-gauge half-round forms and 18-gauge round forms. Note that this minor connector is extended at least two thirds the length of the edentulous span.

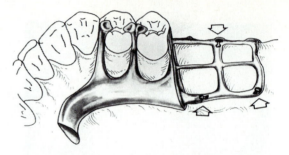

Fig. 4-47. Three small "nailhead" minor connectors (arrows) by which individualized impression trays may be attached when secondary impression is used. These nailheads are initially made of 18-gauge round wax strips on framework pattern and can be removed from framework, if desired, after impression for mast cast has been made.

degrees, thus assuring the most advantageous and strongest connection between the acrylic resin denture base and the major connector.

An open latticework or ladder type of construction is preferable and is conveniently made by using preformed 12-gauge half-round and 18-gauge round wax strips. The minor connector for the **mandibular** distal extension base should extend posteriorly about two thirds the length of the edentulous ridge and **have elements on both the lingual and buccal surfaces.** Not only will such an arrangement add strength to the denture base, but in all probability it will also minimize distortion of the cured base from its inherent strains caused by processing. The minor connector must be planned with care so that it will not interfere with the arrangement of artificial teeth (Fig. 4-46). A means to attach acrylic resin individualized trays to the mandibular framework when a secondary impression is planned must be arranged when the framework pattern is being developed. Three "nailhead" minor connectors fabricated as part of the denture base minor connector serve this purpose well (Fig. 4-47). Unless some similar arrangement is made, the resin trays may become detached or loosened during impression-making procedures. Minor connectors for maxillary distal extension denture bases should extend the entire length of the residual ridge and should also be of a ladderlike and loop construction (Fig. 4-48).

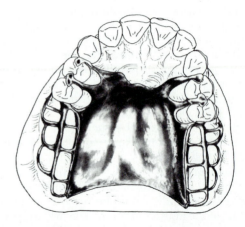

Fig. 4-48. Extension of finishing line to area of pterygomaxillary notch provides butt-type joint for attachment of border portion of acrylic resin base through pterygomaxillary notch.

Tissue stops

Tissue stops are integral parts of minor connectors designed for retention of acrylic resin bases. They provide stability to the framework during the stages of transfer and processing. They are particularly useful in preventing distortion of the framework during acrylic resin processing procedures. Tissue stops should engage buccal and lingual slopes of the residual ridge for stability (Fig. 4-49).

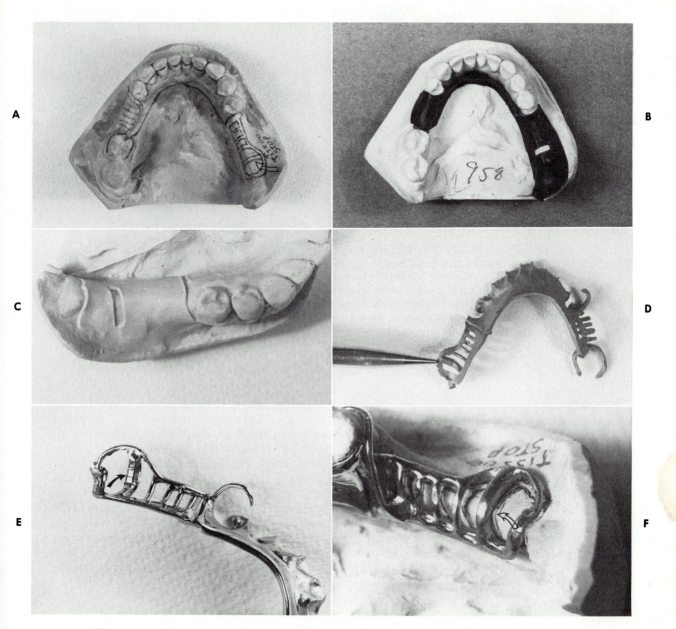

Fig. 4-49. A, Arrow points to location of tissue stop for minor connector by which acrylic resin denture base will be attached. **B,** Master cast partially prepared for duplication in refractory investment. Note posteriorly located window cut in relief wax over residual ridge for tissue stop. **C,** Window in refractory cast on which framework pattern will be developed. **D,** Pencil points to tissue stop as seen from tissue side of recovered cast framework. **E,** Finished framework. Arrow points to created tissue stop. Note that a tapered wrought wire retainer has been soldered to framework. **F,** Tissue stop on master cast contacts residual ridge. Remainder of minor connector to attach denture base is elevated from residual ridge the thickness of a sheet of baseplate wax.

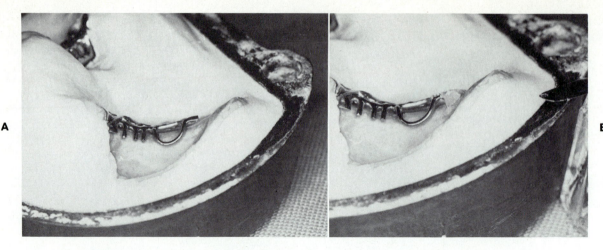

Fig. 4-50. A, Lower half of flask in which distal extension denture was invested. Note that terminal portion of minor connector (original tissue stop) is elevated from residual ridge. Framework was developed on cast with residual ridge recorded in its anatomic form. Residual ridge was later recorded in its functional form by a secondary impression, thus the elevated tissue stop. **B,** Autopolymerizing acrylic resin is painted on between tissue stop and ridge to maintain position of minor connector during packing and processing procedures for an acrylic resin denture base.

Altered cast impression procedures often require that tissue stops be placed subsequent to the development of the altered cast. This can be readily accomplished with the addition of autopolymerizing acrylic resin (Fig. 4-50).

Another integral part of the minor connector designed to retain the acrylic resin denture base is similar to a tissue stop but serves a different purpose. It is located distal to the terminal abutment and is a continuation of the minor connector contacting the guiding plane. Its purpose is to establish a definitive finishing index for the acrylic resin base after processing (Fig. 4-51).

Finishing lines

The finishing line junction with the major connector should take the form of an angle of less than 90 degrees, therefore being somewhat undercut (Fig. 4-52). Of course the medial extent of the minor connector depends on the lateral extent of the major palatal connector. Too little attention is given this finishing line location in many instances. If the finishing line is located too far medially, the natural contour of the palate will be altered by the thickness of resin supporting the artificial teeth (Fig. 4-53). If, on the other hand, the finishing line is located too far buccally, it will be most difficult to create a natural contour of the acrylic resin on the lingual surface of the artificial teeth. **The location of the finishing line at the junction of the major and minor connector should be based on restoring the natural palatal shape,** taking into consideration the presumed anterior-posterior and lateral alignment of the missing natural posterior teeth.

Just as consideration is given the junction of major and minor connectors attaching the denture base, so must equal consideration be given the junction of minor connectors and bar-type direct retainer arms (Fig. 4-54). These junctions are also butt-type joints and when so made possess the same advantages of the butt-type joint previously discussed.

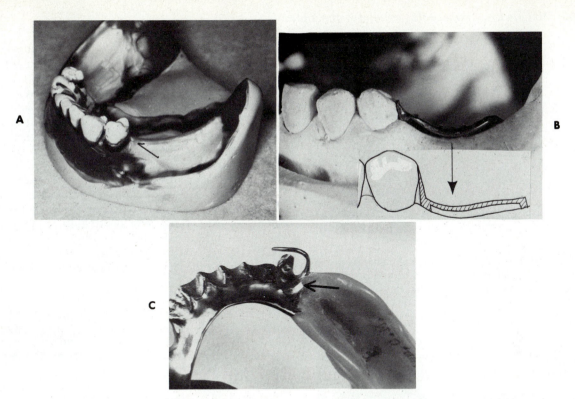

Fig. 4-51. Finishing index tissue stop. **A,** Blocked out and relieved master cast. Note small window in relief wax over residual ridge just distal to first premolar. Undercut on distal has been blocked out parallel to path of placement including gingival crevice. Anterior portion of window does not violate parallel blockout. Final casting will fill window space. **B,** Photograph of cut-away framework casing and schematic of minor connectors for attaching denture base. Note anterior portion of minor connector contacts guiding plane of abutment and residual ridge parallel to path of placement. Processing of acrylic resin bases will fill gingival undercut area on distal of premolar. **C,** View of index finishing stop from tissue side of base. Base was finished to the finishing stop, thereby maintaining planned relationship of anterior portion of denture base to abutment tooth.

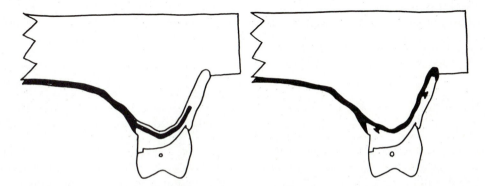

Fig. 4-52. Frontal sections through lingual finishing lines of palatal major connectors. Figure on right is through cast base; figure on left is through acrylic resin denture base. In both situations, location of finishing lines minimizes bulk of acrylic resin attaching the artificial teeth. Palatal contours are restored, enhancing speech and contributing to a natural feeling for the patient.

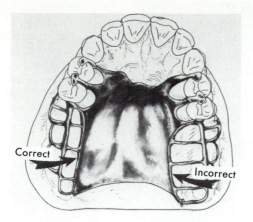

Fig. 4-53. Junction of major connector and minor connectors at palatal finishing lines should be located 2 mm medial to an imaginary line that would contact lingual surfaces of missing posterior teeth.

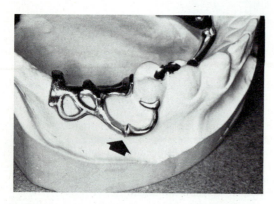

Fig. 4-54. Note direct retainer arm tapers from its tip to finishing line. Without a finishing line (arrow) at junction of direct retainer arm and minor connector for denture base, flexing of direct retainer arm would create minute cracks in anterior border of denture base—often contributing to chipping of borders as well as unhygienic condition from food particle impaction.

REACTION OF TISSUES TO METALLIC COVERAGE

The reaction of tissue to metallic coverage has been the subject of some controversy, particularly in areas at gingival crossings and broad areas of metal contact with tissues.

From the prosthodontic viewpoint, if oral tissues may not be safely covered with the framework of removable partial dentures, then all parts of the partial denture resting on or crossing soft tissues jeopardize the health of those tissues. If this is true, it is not the fact of coverage alone but several factors that jeopardize the tissues.

First of these is **pressure resulting from lack of support.** If relief over gingival crossings and other areas of contact with tissues that are incapable of supporting the prosthesis is inadequate, then impingement on those tissues is inevitable. Impingement will likewise occur if the denture settles because of loss of tooth support. This may be caused by failure of the rest areas as a result of improper design, caries involvement, or by the flow of amalgam alloy restorations, or by intrusion of abutment teeth under occlusal loading. It is the responsibility of the dentist to provide and maintain adequate relief and adequate occlusal support.

Settling of the denture also may produce pressure elsewhere in the arch, such as beneath major connectors. Again, the cause of settling must be prevented or corrected if it becomes manifest. Fisher has shown that pressure alone may have a nonspecific effect on tissues, which has been mistaken for allergic response or the effect of coverage. Pressure, then, must be avoided whenever oral tissues must be covered or crossed by elements of the partial denture.

The second reason is **uncleanliness.** It is known that tissues respond unfavorably to an accumulation of food debris and bacterial enzymes. Coverage of oral tissues with dentures that are not kept clean irritates those tissues, not because they are covered but because of the accumulation of irritating factors. This has led to a misinterpretation of the effect of tissue coverage by prosthetic restorations.

A third explanation of unfavorable tissue response to coverage is the **amount of time the denture is worn.** It is apparent that mucous membrane reverts to connective tissue if isolated from the oral environment for a long enough period of time. Evidence of this is the appearance of tissue, once mucous membrane, beneath the pontics of fixed partial dentures. A raw, denuded surface is visible on removal of the fixed restoration. The same thing can occur beneath removable prosthetic restorations if they are allowed to remain against the tissue long enough.

Some patients become so accustomed to wearing a removable restoration that they neglect to remove it often enough to give the tissues any respite from constant contact. This is frequently true when anterior teeth are replaced by the partial denture and the individual will not allow the restoration to be out of the mouth at any time except in the privacy of the bathroom during toothbrushing.

The fact remains that living tissue should not be covered all the time or changes in those tissues will occur. **Partial dentures should be removed for several hours each day, usually on retiring at night, so that the tissues may rest and be returned to a normal environment.**

Clinical experience with the use of linguoplates and complete metallic palatal coverage has shown conclusively that when factors of pressure, cleanliness, and time are controlled, tissue coverage is not in itself detrimental to the health of oral tissues.

MAJOR CONNECTORS IN REVIEW*

It is only through the **rigidity** of the major connector that all other components of the partial denture may be effective.

Design of major connectors must be determined during diagnostic and treatment planning phases because mouth preparation procedures depend in part on the contemplated design of major connectors.

Major connectors must be located in favorable relation to moving tissues and, at the same time, must avoid impingement of gingival tissues.

No component of a removable partial denture framework may engage undercuts other than the terminal portions of retentive direct retainer arms.

---

*A review of factors influencing the choice of design, definitive location, and average pattern specifications of various major connectors is now presented in a rather condensed version. It is hoped that such a presentation coming after a general discussion will be a meaningful guide to student-dentists in their decision-making processes.

Adequate but not excessive tissue relief beneath major connectors, when indicated, avoids the need for later adjustments to provide relief after tissue damage has occurred. Sufficient relief must be provided beneath major connectors to avoid any settling into hard areas such as inoperable tori, other exostoses, or prominent median palatal suture areas. The amount of such relief is determined by ascertaining the difference in displaceability of the tissues to be covered by the maxillary major connector and those of the primary stress-bearing areas of residual ridges. Additionally, the quality of support anticipated by using other elements of the framework to resist horizontal rotations and displacement toward the tissues is another factor to be considered in the amount of relief to be provided for any type of major connector.

Relief of free gingival margins must be provided for any component of the framework, in addition to denture bases. This support is derived primarily from components terminating in rest seats specifically prepared to receive them.

Anatomic replica patterns for palatal major connectors permit the rather faithful reproduction of palatal contours and are probably more readily accepted by the patient than are other types of construction and may be made thinner without sacrificing rigidity.

Operable tori or other bony exostoses should be removed to avoid compromises in the design and for optimum location of major connectors.

MANDIBULAR LINGUAL BAR

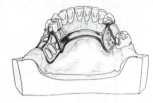

INDICATIONS FOR USE: The lingual bar should be used for mandibular removable partial dentures wherein sufficient space exists between the slightly elevated alveolar lingual sulcus and the lingual gingival tissues to place a rigid bar.

CHARACTERISTICS AND LOCATION: (1) Half-pear shaped with bulkiest portion inferiorly located. (2) Superior border tapered to soft tissue. (3) Superior border located at least 4 mm inferior to gingival margins and more if possible. (4) Inferior border located at the ascertained height of the alveolar lingual sulcus when the patient's tongue is slightly elevated.

BLOCKOUT AND RELIEF OF MASTER CAST: (1) All tissue undercuts parallel to path of placement. (2) All tissue undercuts parallel to path of placement, plus an additional thickness of 32-gauge sheet wax when the lingual surface of the alveolar ridge is either undercut or parallel to the path of placement (Figs. 10-23 and 10-24). (3) No relief necessary when the lingual surface of the alveolar ridge slopes inferiorly and posteriorly. (4) One thickness of baseplate wax over basal seat areas (to elevate minor connectors for attaching acrylic resin denture bases).

WAXING SPECIFICATIONS: (1) Six-gauge, half-pear–shaped wax form reinforced by 22- to 24-gauge sheet wax or similar plastic pattern adapted to design width. (2) Long bar bulkier than short bar; however, cross-sectional shape is unchanged.

FINISHING LINES: Butt-type joint(s) with minor connector(s) for retention of denture base(s).

MANDIBULAR LINGUOPLATE

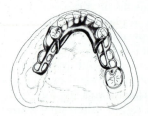

INDICATIONS FOR USE: (1) Where the alveolar lingual sulcus so closely approximates lingual gingival crevices that adequate width for a rigid lingual bar does not exist. (2) In those instances in which the residual ridges in Class I arch have undergone such vertical resorption that they will offer only minimal resistance to horizontal rotations of the denture through its bases. (3) For using periodontally weakened teeth in "group" function to furnish support to the prosthesis and to help resist horizontal (off-vertical) rotation of the distal extension-type denture. (4) When the future replacement of one or more incisor teeth will be facilitated by the addition of retention loops to an existing linguoplate.

CHARACTERISTICS AND LOCATION: (1) Half-pear shaped with bulkiest portion inferiorly located. (2) Thin metal apron extending superiorly to contact cingula of anterior teeth and lingual surfaces of involved posterior teeth at their height of contour. (3) Apron extended interproximally to height of contact

points, that is, closing interproximal spaces. (4) Scalloped contour of apron as dictated by interproximal blockout. (5) Superior border finished to continuous plane with contacted teeth. (6) Inferior border at the ascertained height of the alveolar lingual sulcus when the patient's tongue is slightly elevated.

BLOCKOUT AND RELIEF OF MASTER CAST: (1) All involved undercuts of contacted teeth parallel to the path of placement. (2) All involved gingival crevices. (3) Lingual surface of alveolar ridge and basal seat areas the same as for a lingual bar.

WAXING SPECIFICATIONS: (1) Inferior border—6-gauge, half-pear–shaped wax form reinforced with 24-gauge sheet wax or similar plastic pattern. (2) Apron—24-gauge sheet wax.

FINISHING LINES: Butt-type joint(s) with minor connector(s) for retention of denture base(s).

MANDIBULAR LINGUAL BAR WITH CONTINUOUS BAR RETAINER

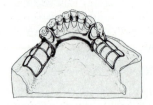

INDICATIONS FOR USE: (1) When a linguoplate is otherwise indicated but the axial alignment of anterior teeth is such that excessive blockout of interproximal undercuts would be required. (2) When wide diastemas exist between mandibular anterior teeth and a linguoplate would objectionably display metal in a frontal view.

CHARACTERISTICS AND LOCATION: (1) Conventionally shaped and located same as lingual bar major connector component when possible. (2) Thin, narrow (3 mm) metal strap located on cingula of anterior teeth, scalloped to follow interproximal embrasures with inferior and superior borders tapered to tooth surfaces. (3) Originates bilaterally from incisal, lingual, or occlusal rests of adjacent principal abutments.

BLOCKOUT AND RELIEF OF MASTER CAST: (1) Lingual surface of alveolar ridge and basal seat areas same as for lingual bar. (2) No relief for continuous bar retainer except blockout of interproximal spaces parallel to path of placement.

WAXING SPECIFICATIONS: (1) Lingual bar major connector component waxed and shaped same as lingual bar. (2) Continuous bar retainer pattern formed by adapting two strips (3 mm wide) of 28-gauge sheet wax, one at a time, over the cingula and into interproximal embrasures.

FINISHING LINES: Butt-type joint(s) with minor connector(s) for retention of denture base(s).

MANDIBULAR LABIAL BAR

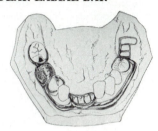

INDICATIONS FOR USE: (1) When lingual inclinations of remaining mandibular premolar and incisor teeth cannot be corrected, preventing the placement of a conventional lingual bar connector. (2) When severe lingual tori cannot be removed and prevent the use of a lingual bar. (3) When severe and abrupt lingual tissue undercuts make it impractical to use a lingual bar connector.

CHARACTERISTICS AND LOCATION: (1) Half-pear shaped with bulkiest portion inferiorly located on the labial and buccal aspects of the mandible. (2) Superior border tapered to soft tissue. (3) Superior border located at least 4 mm inferior to labial and buccal gingival margins and more if possible. (4) Inferior border located in the labial-buccal vestibule at the juncture of attached (immobile) and unattached (mobile) mucosa.

BLOCKOUT AND RELIEF OF MASTER CAST: (1) All tissue undercuts parallel to path of placement, plus an additional thickness of 32-gauge sheet wax when the labial surface is either undercut or parallel to the path of placement. (2) No relief necessary when the labial surface of the alveolar ridge slopes inferiorly to the labial or buccal. (3) Basal seat areas same as for lingual bar major connector.

WAXING SPECIFICATIONS: (1) Six-gauge, half-pear–shaped wax form reinforced with 22- to 24-gauge sheet wax or similar plastic pattern. (2) Long bar bulkier than short bar; however, cross-sectional shape unchanged. (3) Minor connectors joined with occlusal or other superior components by a labial or buccal approach. (4) Minor connectors for base attachment joined by a labial or buccal approach.

FINISHING LINES: Butt-type joint(s) with minor connector(s) for retention of denture base(s).

SINGLE PALATAL STRAP–TYPE MAJOR CONNECTOR

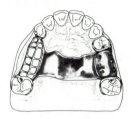

INDICATIONS FOR USE: Bilateral edentulous spaces of short span in a tooth-borne restoration.

CHARACTERISTICS AND LOCATION: (1) Anatomic replica form. (2) Anterior border follows the valleys between rugae as nearly as possible at right angles to median suture line. (3) Posterior border at right angle to median suture line. (4) Approximately as wide as the combined width of a maxillary premolar and first molar. (5) Confined within an area bounded by the four principal rests.

BLOCKOUT AND RELIEF OF MASTER CAST: (1) Usually none required except slight relief of elevated medial palatal raphe or any exostosis crossed by the connector. (2) One thickness of baseplate wax over basal seat areas (to elevate minor connectors for attaching acrylic resin denture bases).

BEADING: See Figs. 4-39 to 4-42.

WAXING SPECIFICATIONS: (1) Anatomic replica pattern equivalent to 22- to 24-gauge wax depending on arch width. (2) 22- to 24-gauge sheet wax reinforced with "faired" 14-gauge half-round wax form in the center portion when an anatomic replica pattern or matte pattern is not used.

FINISHING LINES: (1) Undercut and slightly elevated. (2) No farther than 2 mm medial to an imaginary line contacting lingual surfaces of principal abutments and teeth to be replaced. (3) Follow curvature of arch.

SINGLE BROAD PALATAL MAJOR CONNECTOR

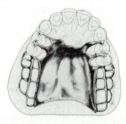

INDICATIONS FOR USE: (1) Class I partially edentulous arches having residual ridges that have undergone little vertical resorption and will lend excellent support. (2) V- or U-shaped palates. (3) Strong abutments (single or made so by splinting). (4) More teeth in arch than six remaining anterior teeth. (5) Direct retention not a problem. (6) No interfering tori.

CHARACTERISTICS AND LOCATION: (1) Anatomic replica form. (2) Anterior border following valleys of rugae as near right angle to median suture line as possible and not extending anterior to occlusal rests or indirect retainers. (3) Posterior border located at junction of hard and soft palate but not extended onto soft palate; at right angle to the median suture line; extended to pterygomaxillary notches.

BLOCKOUT AND RELIEF OF MASTER CAST: (1) Usually none required except relief of elevated median palatal raphe or any small exostosis covered by the connector. (2) One thickness of baseplate wax over basal seat areas (to elevate minor connectors for attaching acrylic resin denture bases).

BEADING: See Figs. 4-39 to 4-42.

WAXING SPECIFICATIONS: Anatomic replica pattern equivalent to 24-gauge sheet wax thickness.

FINISHING LINES: (1) Provision for butt-type joint at pterygomaxillary notches. (2) Undercut and slightly elevated. (3) No farther than 2 mm medial to an imaginary line contacting the lingual surfaces of the missing natural teeth. (4) Follow curvature of arch.

ANTERIOR-POSTERIOR STRAP–TYPE MAJOR CONNECTOR

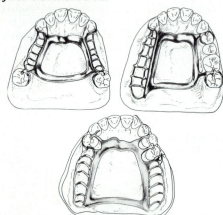

INDICATIONS FOR USE: (1) Class I and II arches in which excellent abutment support and residual ridge support exists, and direct retention can be made adequate without the need for direct-indirect retention. (2) Long edentulous spans in Class II, modification 1 arches. (3) Class IV arches in which

anterior teeth must be replaced with a removable partial denture. (4) Inoperable palatal tori that do not extend posteriorly to the junction of the hard and soft palates.

CHARACTERISTICS AND LOCATION: (1) Parallelogram shaped and open in center portion. (2) Relatively narrow (8 to 10 mm) anterior and posterior palatal straps. (3) Lateral palatal straps 7 to 9 mm broad and parallel to curve of arch; minimum of 6 mm from gingival crevices of remaining teeth. (4) Anterior palatal strap: anterior border not placed farther anteriorly than anterior rests and never closer than 6 mm to lingual gingival crevices; follows the valleys of the rugae at right angles to the median palatal suture. Posterior border, if in rugae area, follows valleys of rugae at right angles to median palatal suture. (5) Posterior palatal connector: posterior border located at junction of hard and soft palates and at right angles to median palatal suture and extended to hamular notch area(s) on distal extension side(s). (6) Anatomic replica or matte surface.

BLOCKOUT AND RELIEF OF MASTER CAST: (1) Usually none required except slight relief of elevated median palatal raphe where anterior or posterior straps cross the palate. (2) One thickness of baseplate wax over basal seat areas (to elevate minor connectors for attaching acrylic resin denture bases).

BEADING: See Figs. 4-39 to 4-42.

WAXING SPECIFICATIONS: (1) Anatomic replica patterns or matte surface forms of 22-gauge thickness. (2) Posterior palatal component—half-oval form of approximately 6-gauge thickness and width. (A strap of 22-gauge thickness, 8 to 10 mm wide may also be used.)

FINISHING LINES: Same as for single broad palatal major connector.

COMPLETE PALATAL COVERAGE MAJOR CONNECTOR

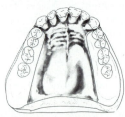

INDICATIONS FOR USE: (1) In most situations where only some or all anterior teeth remain. (2) Class II arch with a posterior modification space and some missing anterior teeth in distal extension edentulous area. (3) Class I arch with one to four premolars and some or all anterior teeth remaining, and abutment support is poor and cannot otherwise be enhanced; residual ridges have undergone extreme vertical resorption; direct retention is difficult to obtain. (4) In the absence of a pedunculated torus.

CHARACTERISTICS AND LOCATION: (1) Anatomic replica form for full palatal metal casting supported anteriorly by positive rest seats. (2) Palatal linguoplate supported anteriorly and designed for the attachment of acrylic resin extension posteriorly. (3) Contacts all or almost all the teeth remaining in the arch. (4) Posterior border: terminates at the junction of the hard and soft palates; extended to hamular notch area(s) on distal extension side(s); at a right angle to median suture line.

BLOCKOUT AND RELIEF OF MASTER CAST: (1) Usually none required except relief of elevated median palatal raphe or any small palatal exostosis. (2) One thickness of baseplate wax over basal seat areas (to elevate minor connectors for attaching acrylic resin denture bases).

BEADING: See Figs. 4-39 to 4-42.

WAXING SPECIFICATIONS: (1) Anatomic replica pattern equivalent to 22- to 24-gauge sheet wax thickness. (2) Acrylic resin extension from linguoplate the same as for a complete denture.

FINISHING LINES: As illustrated here and previously discussed.

U-SHAPED PALATAL MAJOR CONNECTOR

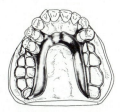

This connector should be used only in those situations where inoperable tori extend to the posterior limit of the hard palate.

The U-shaped palatal major connector is the least favorable design of all palatal major connectors because it lacks the rigidity of other types of connectors. Where it must be used, any portion of the connector extending anteriorly from the principal occlusal rests must be supported by indirect retainers. Anterior border areas of this type of connector must be kept at least 6 mm away from adjacent teeth. If for any reason the anterior border must contact remaining teeth, the connector must again be supported by rests placed in properly prepared rest seats. It should never

be supported even temporarily by inclined lingual surfaces of anterior teeth.

Waxing specifications, finishing lines, and so forth are the same as for full palatal castings or other similar major connectors previously discussed.

SELF-ASSESSMENT AIDS

1. A Class I removable partial denture will or should have six components. Can you name the components?
2. Define the term **major connector** in your own words.
3. Several desirable characteristics of major connectors are listed in the first few pages of Chapter 4. Can you recall five of these characteristics?
4. What purposes are served by rigid major connectors as contrasted to flexible connectors?
5. Major connectors should be located in a favorable relation to moving tissues, gingival tissues, and areas of bony and tissue prominences. What difficulties would the patient encounter if the preceding is not carried out?
6. Can you name and draw the cross-sectional form of the basic mandibular connector?
7. Margins of major connectors adjacent to gingival tissues should be located far enough from those tissues to avoid possible impingement when the denture rotates from functional and parafunctional forces. The superior border of a lingual bar should be located at least _____ mm from gingival crevices.
8. The inferior border of a lingual bar is located as far inferiorly as possible without encroaching on the constantly moving tissues in the alveolar lingual sulcus. Can you describe two methods by which the location of the inferior border can be accurately determined?
9. Sufficient **relief** must be provided beneath a major connector to avoid impingement and gross displacement of soft tissues resulting in an inflammatory response. What is meant by the word **relief?** Can you rationalize planned relief for a lingual bar and give quantitative rules of thumb depending on the contour of the anterior, lingual alveolar ridge?
10. Discuss those clinical observations which indicate the choice of a lingual bar as a major connector.
11. What is the form of a mandibular linguoplate major connector?
12. Give four clinical observations that indicate using a linguoplate rather than a lingual bar as a major connector.
13. Can you draw a sagittal section through a cast showing the basic form of a linguoplate?

14. Is there a difference in determining the location of the inferior borders for lingual bars and linguoplates?

15. Describe the superior extent of the apron portion of a linguoplate in relation to the lingual surfaces of teeth contacted by the major connector.

16. What are the indications for use of a lingual bar–continuous bar retainer type of major connector?

17. Interpret in your own words the rationale of the following statement made by McCracken: "No component of a partial denture should be added arbitrarily or conventionally. Each component should be added for a good reason and to serve a definite purpose."

18. How may a linguoplate be modified to avoid an overdisplay of metal when used on an arch in which wide diastemas exist between anterior teeth?

19. The dentist alone is responsible for the design of the restoration, which is based on both biologic and mechanical principles. Can you give the dimensional specifications for developing the wax patterns of mandibular major connectors?

20. At what point in treating the partially edentulous patient must the choice of maxillary and mandibular major connectors be made? Rationalize your answer.

21. There are basically four types of maxillary major connectors. Can you recall these four types of basic connectors?

22. What objections are usually manifested in use of the single palatal bar–type major connector?

23. Which type of palatal major connector is probably the most rigid and at the same time covers the smallest amount of soft tissues?

24. In what situations would you be most likely to use a single palatal strap–type major connector?

25. There are definite rules of thumb for the location of the anterior and posterior borders of all palatal major connectors. Can you relate borders to rugae, junction of hard and soft palates, gingival crevices, pterygomaxillary notches, and palatal tori?

26. Whenever it is necessary for the palatal major connector to make contact with the teeth for reasons of support, can adequate support be obtained by resting the connector on tooth inclines?

27. Rationalize this statement: "Either support the connector by definite rests on the teeth contacted, bridging the gingivae with adequate relief, or locate the connector far enough away from the gingivae to avoid any possible restriction of blood supply and entrapment of food debris."

28. Why should all gingival crossings by components of a framework be abrupt and at right angles to the major connector and bridge the gingivae with adequate relief?

29. What clinical and diagnostic observations would lead you to select an anterior-posterior palatal strap–type major connector?

30. Under what circumstances is full palatal coverage by the major connector indicated?

31. Describe a palatal linguoplate major connector and tell why you would select such a design.

32. Can you look at a diagnostic cast of a Class I maxillary arch and apply the five steps outlined by Blatterfein for the design of palatal major connectors?

33. What is a **minor** connector?

34. What are the functions of minor connectors?

35. Should minor connectors be structurally rigid or flexible? Why?

36. Can you describe the shape of a minor connector contacting axial surfaces of adjacent abutments at interproximal areas?

37. Can you identify eight minor connectors in this drawing?

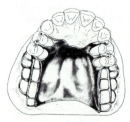

38. Minor connectors used to attach acrylic resin denture bases to major connectors should be located on both buccal and lingual sides of the residual ridge. Why?

39. State rules of thumb for the form and length of minor connectors connecting acrylic resin denture bases to major connectors.

40. What advantages accrue to the restoration by having minor connectors for acrylic resin denture bases attached to the major connector in a butt-type joint?

41. Describe the best location for palatal finishing lines at the junction of major and minor connectors. How do you determine this optimum location on a cast? Why is it important that the natural contour of the palatal vault be restored with a removable restoration?

42. In addition to a more natural feeling contour, what other factors may be achieved by using anatomic replica patterns for palatal major connectors?

43. Can you think of three probable consequences of indiscriminate use of U-shaped palatal major connectors?
44. Presence of severe and abrupt lingual tissue undercuts is one indication for considering the use of a labial bar major connector. Can you state two other indications?

The last few pages in Chapter 4 review major connectors in cookbook style. Indications for use, characteristics and location, blockout and relief of master casts, waxing specifications, and finishing lines for major connectors are condensed. Your practice of dentistry will be more rewarding if you assimilate the information presented or at least have it available as reference material.

CHAPTER

5 RESTS AND REST SEATS

Form of the occlusal rest and rest seat
Interproximal occlusal rest seats
Internal occlusal rests
Possible movements of partial denture
Support for rests
Lingual rests on canines and incisor teeth
Incisal rests and rest seats

Vertical support for a removable partial denture must be provided. Any unit of a partial denture that rests on a tooth surface to provide vertical support is called a **rest** (Fig. 5-1). Vertical support is sometimes attempted on a tooth surface inclined occlusally or incisally from its greatest convexity, but any rest so placed is subject to slipping along tooth inclines. **Rests should always be located on tooth surfaces properly prepared to receive them.** The **prepared surface** of an abutment to receive the rest is called the **rest seat**. Rests are designated by the surface of the tooth prepared to receive them, that is, **occlusal rest, lingual rest,** and **incisal rest.**

The **primary purpose** of the rest is to provide vertical support for the partial denture. In doing so it also does the following:

1. Maintains components in their planned positions
2. Maintains established occlusal relationships by preventing settling of the denture.
3. Prevents impingement of soft tissues
4. Directs and distributes occlusal loads to abutment teeth

Thus rests serve to support the position of a partial denture and to resist movement in a cervical direction. They serve to transmit vertical forces to the abutment teeth and to direct those forces along the long axes of the teeth. In this respect, tooth-borne removable partial denture rests function in a manner similar to fixed abutment retainers. It is obvious that for this degree of stability to exist, the rests must be rigid and must receive positive support from the abutment teeth.

In a removable partial denture having one or more distal extension bases, the denture becomes increasingly tissue supported as the distance from the abutment increases. Closer to the abutment, however, the occlusal load is transmitted to the abutment tooth by means of the rest. The load is thereby distributed between the abutment and the supporting residual ridge tissues.

By the rest's preventing movement of the denture in a cervical direction, the position of the retentive portion of the clasp arm is maintained in its intended relation to the tooth undercut. Although passive when in its terminal position, the retentive portion of the clasp arm should remain in contact with the tooth, ready to resist a vertical dislodging force. Then when a dislodging force is applied, the clasp arm should immediately become active to resist vertical displacement. If because of settling of the denture the clasp arm is standing away from the tooth, some vertical displacement is possible before the retainer can become functional. The rest

58

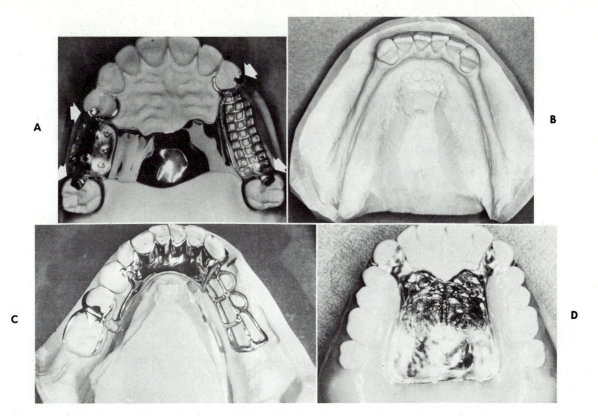

Fig. 5-1. A, Framework for tooth-supported removable partial denture. Arrows point to components (rests) located on specifically prepared areas of abutment teeth. Denture will be supported through three occlusal rests and one incisal rest on canine. **B,** Canines have been restored with ceramic-metal crowns on which lingual rest seats have been developed to support a linguoplate major connector. **C,** Tooth support for this framework is provided by rests occupying definite, prepared, lingual rest seats on canines and occlusal surfaces of posterior teeth. **D,** Maxillary bilateral distal extension removable partial denture supported by rests occupying lingual rest seats on canines. Rest seats were placed on three-quarter crowns.

serves to prevent such settling and thereby helps to maintain the vertical stability of the partial denture.

FORM OF THE OCCLUSAL REST AND REST SEAT

1. The outline form of an occlusal rest seat should be a **"rounded" triangular shape** with the apex toward the center of the occlusal surface (Fig. 5-2).
2. It should be as long as it is wide, and the base of the triangular shape (at the marginal ridge) should be at least **2.5 mm** for both molars and premolars. Rest seats of smaller dimensions do not provide for an adequate bulk of metal for rests, especially if the rest is contoured to restore the occlusal morphology of the abutment tooth.
3. The marginal ridge of the abutment tooth at the site of the rest seat must be lowered to permit a sufficient bulk of metal for strength and rigidity of the rest and minor connector. This then means that a **reduction of the marginal ridge of approximately 1.5 mm is usually necessary.**
4. The floor of the occlusal rest seat should be

apical to the marginal ridge and occlusal surface and should be concave or **spoon shaped** (Fig. 5-3). Caution should be exercised in preparing a rest seat to avoid creating **sharp edges or line-angles in the preparation.**

5. The angle formed by the occlusal rest and the vertical minor connector from which it originates should be less than 90 degrees (Figs. 5-4 and 5-5). Only in this way can the occlusal forces be directed along the long axis of the

abutment tooth. An angle greater than 90 degrees fails to transmit occlusal forces along the supporting axis of the abutment tooth. It also permits slippage of the prosthesis away from the abutment and causes orthodontic forces to be applied, which are the result of forces applied to an inclined plane (Fig. 5-6).

When an existing occlusal rest preparation on enamel or on an existing cast restoration cannot

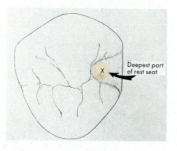

Fig. 5-2. Deepest part of an occlusal rest preparaton should be inside lowered marginal ridge at *X*. Marginal ridge is lowered to accommodate origin of occlusal rest with least occlusal interference without sacrificing bulk.

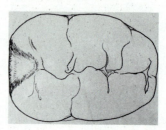

Fig. 5-3. Occlusal rest seat preparation on molar. Preparation is rounded and triangular concavity has smooth margins on occlusal surface and lowered, rounded marginal ridge.

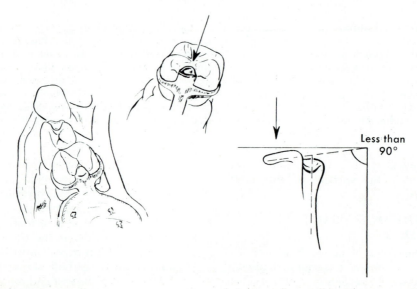

Fig. 5-4. Occlusal rest should be spoon shaped and slightly inclined apically from marginal ridge on occlusal surface properly prepared to receive it. The rest should restore occlusal morphology of tooth that existed before preparation of rest seat.

be modified or deepened because of fear of perforation of the enamel or gold, yet the existing floor is inclined apically toward the reduced marginal ridge, a secondary occlusal rest must be employed to prevent slippage of the primary rest and orthodontic movement of the abutment tooth (Fig. 5-7). Such a rest should pass over the lowered marginal ridge on the side of the tooth opposite the primary rest and should, if possible, be inclined slightly apically from the marginal ridge. However, two opposing occlusal rests on diverging tooth inclines will function to prevent unfavorable forces if all related connectors are sufficiently rigid.

In any partly tissue-supported partial denture

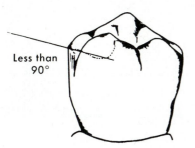

Fig. 5-5. Floor of occlusal rest seat should be inclined apically from lowered marginal ridge. Any angle less than 90 degrees is acceptable as long as preparation of proximal surface and lowering and rounding of marginal ridge precede completion of rest seat itself.

the relation of the occlusal rest to the abutment should be that of a shallow ball-and-socket joint so shaped to prevent a possible transfer of horizontal stresses to the abutment tooth. The occlusal rest should provide only occlusal support. Stabilization against horizontal movement of the prosthesis must be provided by other components of the partial denture rather than by any locking effect of the occlusal rest, which might cause the application of leverages to the abutment tooth.

INTERPROXIMAL OCCLUSAL REST SEATS

The design of a direct retainer assembly may require that interproximal occlusal rests be used (Fig. 5-8). The rest seats are prepared as adjoining occlusal rest seats with the exception that the preparations must be extended farther lingually than is ordinarily accomplished (Fig. 5-9). Adjacent rests rather than a single rest are used to avoid interproximal wedging by the framework. Additionally, the joined rests will shunt food away from contact points.

In preparing such rest seats, care must be exercised to avoid eliminating contact points of abutment teeth. Yet sufficient tooth structure must be removed to allow for adequate bulk of the component for strength and to permit the component to be so shaped that occlusion will not be altered.

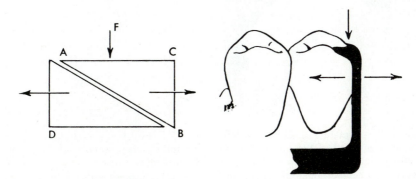

Fig. 5-6. Result of force applied to an inclined plane when floor of occlusal rest preparation inclines apically toward marginal ridge of abutment tooth. *F*, Occlusal force applied to abutment tooth. *AB*, Relationship of occlusal rest to abutment tooth when angle is greater than 90 degrees. *ABC*, Partial denture framework. *ABD*, Abutment tooth.

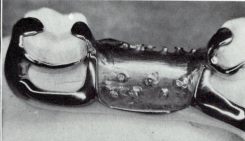

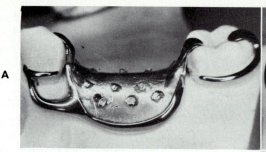

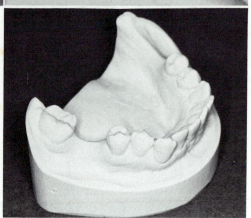

Fig. 5-7. A, Existing gold crown on molar, having previous, minimally prepared mesio-occlusal rest seat, could be recontoured only on mesial proximal surface, with slight reduction of distal marginal ridge, without fear of penetrating the crown. Mesial and distal occlusal rests (each on an unfavorable inclined plane) were used to direct forces as near axially as possible. **B,** Lingual view of **A.** Bar extension from cast base was used to attach direct retainer assembly to molar. Opposing arch was restored with complete denture. **C,** Anterior tilt of molar precludes preparation of acceptable rest seat on mesio-occlusal surface. Patient could not afford either crown to improve axial alignment or orthodontic treatment to upright the molar. Occlusal rests were used on mesio-occlusal and disto-occlusal surfaces to support restoration and direct forces over greatest root mass of abutment.

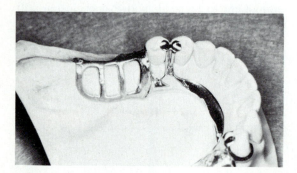

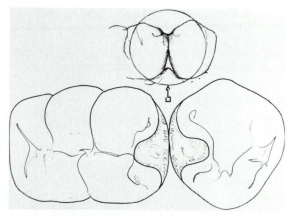

Fig. 5-8. Design of direct retainer assembly on left premolar abutments consisted of bar-type retainer arm engaging a distobuccal undercut on second premolar, a minor connector contacting guiding plane on distal of second premolar, and a reciprocal, stabilizing, supporting interproximal element. Joined occlusal rests occupy specifically prepared adjoining rest seats.

Fig. 5-9. Rest seat preparations on premolar and molar fulfill requirements of properly prepared rest seats. Preparations are extended lingually to provide strength (through bulk) without overly filling interproximal space with minor connector. This type of preparation is rather difficult, and care must be exercised to avoid violation of contact points—yet marginal ridge of each abutment should be sufficiently lowered (1.5 mm).

The lingual interproximal area requires only a modicum of preparation, and, certainly, creation of a vertical groove must be avoided to prevent a torquing effect on the abutments by the minor connector.

Analysis of mounted diagnostic casts is mandatory to assess interocclusal contact areas where rests are to be placed. Sufficient space must be present or created to avoid interference with placement of rests (Fig. 5-10).

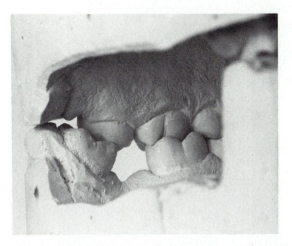

Fig. 5-10. Lingual views of mounted diagnostic casts aid in assessing interocclusal space available for properly prepared rest seats.

INTERNAL OCCLUSAL RESTS

A partial denture that is totally tooth supported by means of cast retainers on all abutment teeth may use internal occlusal rests for both occlusal support and horizontal stabilization (Figs. 5-11 to 5-13).

An internal occlusal rest is not in any way a retainer and therefore should not be confused with an internal attachment. The term **precision** is applied to both, **but any element of a partial denture should possess the accuracy and exactness synonymous with precision.**

Occlusal support is derived from the floor of the rest seat and from an additional occlusal bevel if such is provided. Horizontal stabilization is derived from the near-vertical walls. The form of the rest should be parallel to the path of placement, slightly tapered occlusally, and slightly dovetailed to prevent dislodgement proximally.

The principal advantages of the internal rest are that it facilitates the elimination of a visible clasp arm buccally and permits the location of the rest seat in a more favorable position in relation to the "tipping" axis (horizontal) of the abutment. Retention is provided by a lingual clasp arm, either cast or of wrought wire, lying in a natural or prepared infrabulge area on the abutment tooth.

Technical obstacles to the use of internal rests are gradually being overcome. Such a rest seat usually cannot satisfactorily be carved in wax or

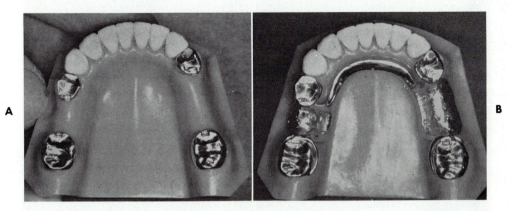

Fig. 5-11. Mandibular internal rest partial dentures. **A,** Abutment crowns with internal rests. Both dovetail design and gingival well prevent horizontal movement. **B,** Completed partial denture framework with cast lingual retention on all four abutments. Short buccal stabilizing and removal arm is used on molar abutments.

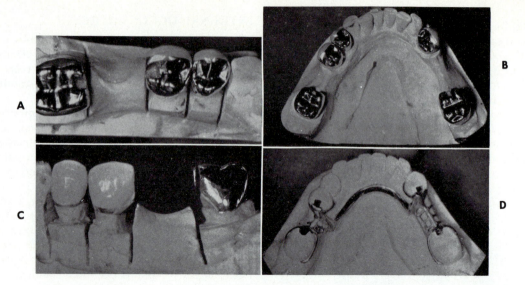

Fig. 5-12. Mandibular internal rest partial dentures. **A,** Internal rests in four abutment crowns. **B,** Occlusal view showing proximal guiding planes. **C,** Buccal view showing machined parallelism of proximal surface. **D,** Completed gold alloy casting with wrought-wire lingual retention on all four abutments. Use of buccal stablizing arm is optional.

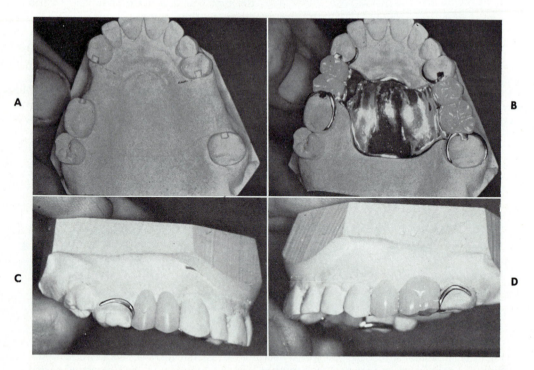

Fig. 5-13. Maxillary internal rest partial denture. **A,** Internal rest seats in four abutment crowns. **B,** Completed partial denture with lingual retentive clasp arms on canine and premolar abutments. **C and D,** Buccal views of completed restoration showing abutted resin teeth (on which gold occlusal surfaces will be fabricated) and absence of visible clasp arms on premolar abutments.

machined in gold. Ready-made plastic rest patterns are generally too bulky. Assembly of a ready-made rest similar to an internal attachment necessitates soldering operations and added cost. The best solution seems to be the use of a machined mandrel made of a chromium-cobalt alloy,* which can be waxed into the crown or inlay pattern, invested, and cast-to, having been positioned parallel to the path of placement with a dental cast surveyor. The mandrel is easily tapped out, leaving the internal rest formed in the abutment casting. Further developments of this technique promise more widespread use of the internal occlusal rest but only for tooth-supported partial dentures.

POSSIBLE MOVEMENTS OF PARTIAL DENTURE

At least three possible movements of a distal extension partial denture exist. **One is rotation**

---

* Ticon PRP mandrel and surveyor fixture, Ticonium Division, CMP Industries, Inc., Albany, N.Y.

about an axis through the most posterior abutments. This axis may be through occlusal rests or any other rigid portion of a direct retainer assembly located occlusally or incisally to the height of contour of the abutments (Fig. 5-14, A). This axis, known as the **fulcrum line,** is the center of rotation as the distal extension base moves **toward** the supporting tissues when an occlusal load is applied. The axis of rotation shifts to anteriorly placed elements, occlusal or incisal to the height of contour of the abutment, as the base moves **away** from the supporting tissues when vertical dislodging forces become effective. These dislodging forces are the vertical pull of food between opposing tooth surfaces, the effect of moving border tissues, and the forces of gravity against a maxillary denture. Presuming that the direct retainers are functional and that the supportive anterior elements remain seated, rotation rather than total displacement occurs. Vertical tissueward movement of the denture base is resisted by the tissues of the residual ridge in proportion to the supporting

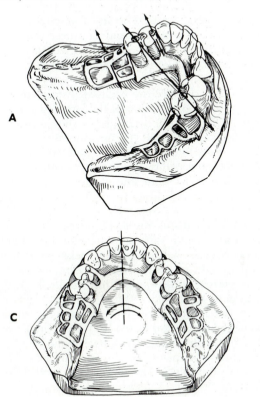

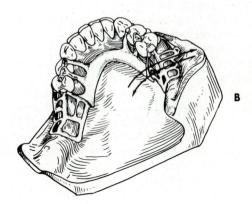

Fig. 5-14. Three possible movements of distal extension partial denture. **A,** Rotation around fulcrum line passing through two principal occlusal rests when denture base moves toward supporting residual ridges. **B,** Rotation around longitudinal axis formed by crest of residual ridge. **C,** Rotation around vertical axis located near center of arch.

quality of those tissues, the accuracy of the fit of the denture base, and the total amount of occlusal load applied. Movement of the base in the opposite direction is resisted by the action of the retentive clasp arms on terminal abutments in conjunction with seated, vertical support elements of the framework anterior to the terminal abutments acting as indirect retainers. Of course, unless supporting elements anterior to the terminal abutments are seated when a dislodging force is initiated, the axis of rotation will run through the retentive tips of direct retainers (clasps) on the terminal abutments.

A second movement is rotation about a longitudinal axis as the distal extension base moves in a rotary direction about the residual ridge (Fig. 5-14, *B*). This movement is resisted primarily by the rigidity of the major connector and its ability to resist torque. If the major connector is not rigid or if a stressbreaker exists between the distal extension base and the major connector, this rotation about a longitudinal axis either applies undue stress to the sides of the supporting ridge or causes horizontal shifting of the denture base.

A third movement is rotation about an imaginary vertical axis located near the center of the dental arch (Fig. 5-14, *C*). This movement occurs under function as diagonal and horizontal occlusal forces are brought to bear on the partial denture. It is resisted by stabilizing components, such as reciprocal clasp arms and minor connectors that are in contact with vertical tooth surfaces. Such stabilizing components are essential to any partial denture design regardless of the manner of support and the type of direct retention employed. Stabilizing components on one side of the arch act to stabilize the partial denture against horizontal forces applied from the opposite side. It is obvious that rigid connectors must be employed to make this effect possible.

Horizontal forces always will exist to some degree because of lateral stresses occurring during mastication and bruxism. These forces are accentuated by failure to consider the orientation of the occlusal plane, the influence of malpositioned teeth, and the effect of abnormal jaw relationships. The magnitude of lateral stress may be minimized by fabricating an occlusion that is in harmony with the opposing dentition and free of lateral interference during excursive jaw movements. The amount of horizontal shift occurring in the partial denture will therefore depend on the magnitude of lateral forces applied and the effectiveness of the stabilizing components.

In a tooth-borne partial denture, movement of the base **toward** the edentulous ridge is prevented primarily by the rests on the abutment teeth and to some degree by any rigid portion of the framework located occlusal to the height of contour. Movement **away** from the edentulous ridge is prevented by the action of direct retainers on the abutments, situated at each end of each edentulous space. Therefore the **first** of the three possible movements is nonexistent in the tooth-borne denture. The **second** possible movement, which is about a longitudinal axis, is prevented by the rigid components of the direct retainers on the abutment teeth as well as by the ability of the major connector to resist torque. This movement is much less in the tooth-borne denture because of the presence of posterior abutments. The **third** possible movement occurs in any partial denture; therefore stabilizing components against horizontal movement must be incorporated into any partial denture design.

The functions of the occlusal rest are not directly involved in either of the latter two movements. Instead the occlusal rest should provide occlusal support only. All movements of the partial denture other than in a gingival direction should be resisted by other components. For the occlusal rest to enter into a stabilizing function would result in a direct transfer of torque to the abutment tooth. Since three movements are possible in a distal extension partial denture, an occlusal rest for such a partial denture should not have steep vertical walls or locking dovetails, which could possibly cause horizontal and torquing forces to be applied intracoronally to the abutment tooth.

In the tooth-borne denture the only movements of any significance are horizontal, and these may be resisted by the stabilizing effect of components placed on the axial surfaces of the several abutments. Therefore in the tooth-borne denture the use of intracoronal rests is permissible. In such usage the rests provide not only occlusal support but also horizontal stabilization to some degree.

Force distribution in a tooth-supported partial denture is, or should be, such that each abutment tooth is assisted by others in the dental arch, and possible movements of the partial denture under function are held within acceptable physiologic limitations. It is therefore possible and acceptable to use an intracoronal type of occlusal rest if desired in any tooth-supported situation. In such a case vertical walls of an internal occlusal rest may be used to transfer horizontal forces to the abutment teeth and, by so doing, stabilize the partial denture against horizontal movement. An internal occlusal rest can thus be substituted for an external stabilizing clasp arm and, by using a retentive clasp arm on the lingual surface of an abutment tooth, can eliminate altogether the necessity for a visible clasp arm buccally or labially.

The use of intracoronal rests and intracoronal direct retainers is optional with the tooth-borne denture. However, with the distal extension denture the ball-and-socket type of rest or the nonlocking internal rest is preferable and should be used whenever possible.

SUPPORT FOR RESTS

Rests may be placed on sound enamel, cast restorations, or silver amalgam alloy restorations. The use of a silver amalgam alloy restoration as support for an occlusal rest is the least desirable because of its tendency to flow under pressure and also because of the comparative weakness of a marginal ridge made of this alloy.

Rests placed on sound enamel are not conducive to caries in a mouth with a low caries index, provided good oral hygiene is maintained. Proximal tooth surfaces are much more vulnerable to caries attack than are the occlusal surfaces supporting an occlusal rest. The decision to use abutment coverage is usually based on proximal and cervical vulnerability of the tooth rather than on the vulnerability of an occlusal rest area. When precarious fissures are found in the occlusal rest areas in teeth that are otherwise sound, they may be removed and restored, preferably with gold foil, without resorting to more extensive abutment protection.

Whereas it cannot be denied that the best protection from caries for an abutment tooth is full coverage, it must be presumed that such crowns will be contoured properly to provide support and retention for the partial denture and that full coverage restorations will provide subgingival protection for the tooth. Little is accomplished by the placement of full crowns if the more vulnerable cervical areas of an abutment tooth are not fully protected.

In making the decision whether to use unprotected enamel surfaces for rests, future vulnerability must be considered, for it is not easy to fabricate full crowns later to accommodate rests and clasp arms. In many instances sound enamel may be used safely for the support of occlusal rests. In such situations the patient should be advised that future caries susceptibility is not predictable and that much will depend on oral hygiene and possible future changes in caries susceptibility. Although the decision to use unprotected abutments logically should be left up to the dentist, economic factors may influence the final decision. The patient should be made aware of the risks involved and of his responsibility for maintaining good oral hygiene and for returning periodically for observation.

Rest seat preparations in sound enamel. In most instances, preparation of proximal tooth surfaces is necessary to provide proximal guiding planes and to eliminate undesirable undercuts that rigid parts of the framework must pass during its placement and removal. The preparation of occlusal rest seats **always must follow proximal preparation,** never precede it. Only after the alteration is completed may the location of the occlusal rest seat in relation to the marginal ridge be determined. When proximal preparation follows occlusal rest seat preparation, the inevitable consequence is that the marginal ridge is too low and too sharp, with the center of the floor of the rest seat too close to the marginal ridge. Therefore it is often impossible to correct the rest preparation without making it too deep, and then irreparable damage has been done to the tooth.

Occlusal rest seats in sound enamel may be prepared with diamond points of approximately the size of Nos. 6 and 8 round burs or with

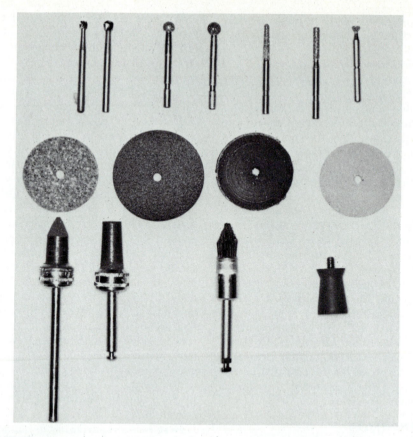

Fig. 5-15. Recontouring of axial surfaces and rest seat preparations in enamel may be readily accomplished by selected use of accessories shown (from top, left to right): round carbide burs, round diamond stones, tapered diamond stone with round end, cylindric diamond stone, inverted cone diamond stone, wet or dry sanding disks, abrasive rubber polishing disks and points, and pointed brush and polishing cup to be used with flour of pumice.

carbide burs (Fig. 5-15). The larger of the two diamonds is used first to lower the marginal ridge and to establish the outline form of the rest seat. The resulting occlusal rest seat is then complete except that the floor is not sufficiently concave. The smaller diamond point is then used to deepen the floor of the occlusal rest seat, at the same time forming the desired spoon shape inside the lowered marginal ridge. Smoothing the enamel rods by the planing action of a round bur of suitable size revolving at moderate speed, followed by the use of an abrasive rubber point, is usually the only polishing needed.

When a small enamel defect is encountered in the preparation of an occlusal rest seat, it is usually best to ignore it until the rest preparation has been completed and then, with small burs, prepare the remaining defect to receive a small gold foil restoration. This then may be finished flush with the floor of the rest preparation previously established.

A fluoride gel should be applied to abutment teeth following enamel recontouring. Application of the gel should be delayed until after impressions are made for the cast on which the framework will be fabricated. Fluoride gels and irreversible hydrocolloids are seemingly incompatible.

Occlusal rest seat preparations in existing restorations are treated the same as those in sound enamel. Any proximal preparations must be done first, for if the occlusal rest seat is placed first and then the proximal surface is disked, the outline form of the occlusal rest seat is sometimes irreparably altered.

There is always a possibility that an existing restoration may be perforated in the process of preparing an ideal occlusal rest seat. Although some compromise is permissible, the effectiveness of the occlusal rest seat should not be jeopardized for fear of perforating an existing inlay or crown. The rest seat may be widened to compensate for its shallowness, but the floor of the rest seat should still be slightly inclined apically from the marginal ridge. When this is not possible, a secondary occlusal rest should be used on the opposite side of the tooth to prevent slipping of the primary rest.

When perforation does occur, it may be filled with gold foil, but occasionally the making of a new restoration is unavoidable. In such a situation the original crown or inlay preparation should be modified to accommodate the occlusal rest, which is then placed in the wax pattern to avoid risking again the perforation of the completed restoration.

Occlusal rest seats in new restorations always should be placed in the wax pattern. The location of the occlusal rest should be known when the tooth is prepared for a crown or an inlay so that sufficient clearance may be provided in the preparation for the rest. The final step in the preparation of the tooth should be to make sure that such clearance exists and, if not, to make a depression to accommodate the depth of the rest (Fig. 5-16).

Occlusal rest seats in crowns and inlays are generally made somewhat larger and deeper than those in enamel. Those made in abutment crowns supporting tooth-borne dentures may be made slightly deeper than those in abutments supporting a distal extension base, thus approaching the effectiveness of boxlike internal rests.

Internal rest seats also should be created first in wax, either with suitable burs in a handpiece holder or by waxing around a lubricated mandrel held in the surveyor. In either situation the rest preparation must be finished on the casting with burs in a handpiece holder or with a precision

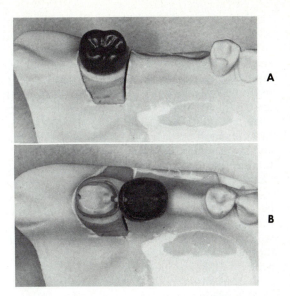

Fig. 5-16. A, Pattern for full crown on molar has been carved to meet requirements of occlusion and optimal location of direct retainer components. Occlusal rest seat has been prepared on mesio-occlusal surface. **B,** Pattern is removed from die. Note concavity in prepared abutment to accommodate adequate depth for occlusal rest seat on finished crown. Need for such procedure is determined by observation of accurately mounted diagnostic casts before abutment preparation is initiated.

drill press. Plastic and metal shoes that fit over a mandrel are also available for this purpose, thus assuring a smooth casting and eliminating the need for finishing the inside of the internal rest with burs. Sufficient clearance must have been provided in the preparation of the abutment to accommodate the depth of the internal rest.

LINGUAL RESTS ON CANINES AND INCISOR TEETH

Analysis of mounted diagnostic casts is mandatory to assess incisal and lingual contact areas where rests are to be placed. Sufficient space must be present or created to avoid interference with placement of rests.

Whereas the preferred site for an external rest is the occlusal surface of a molar or premolar, an anterior tooth may be the only abutment available for occlusal support of the denture. Also, an anterior tooth occasionally must be used to support an indirect retainer or an auxiliary rest. A canine is much preferred over an incisor for this purpose. When a canine is not present, multiple rests spread over several incisor teeth are preferable to the use of a single incisor. Root form, root length, inclination of the tooth, and ratio of the length of the clinical crown to the alveolar support must be considered in determining the site and form of rests placed on incisors.

A lingual rest is preferable to an incisal rest because it is placed nearer the horizontal axis of rotation (tipping) of the abutment and therefore will have less tendency to tip the tooth. In addition, lingual rests are more esthetically acceptable than are incisal rests.

If an anterior tooth is sound and the lingual slope is gradual rather than perpendicular, a lingual rest may sometimes be placed in an enamel seat at or just incisally to the cingulum (Fig. 5-17). **This type of lingual rest is usually confined to maxillary canines having a gradual lingual incline and a prominent cingulum.** In a few instances such a rest also may be placed on maxillary central incisors. The lingual slope of the mandibular canine is usually too steep for an adequate lingual rest seat to be placed in the enamel, and some other provision for rest support must be made. **Lingual rest seat preparations in enamel are rarely satisfactory be-** cause of a lack of thickness of enamel in which to prepare a seat of adequate form to be truly supportive.

The preparation of an anterior tooth to receive a lingual rest may be accomplished in one of two ways. These are as follows:

1. A slightly "rounded" V is prepared on the lingual surface at the junction of the gingival and middle one third of the tooth. The apex of the V is directed incisally. A preparation may be started by using an inverted cone-shaped diamond stone and progressing to smaller, tapered stones with round ends to complete the preparation. All line angles must be eliminated, and the enamel seat must be highly polished. Shaped, abrasive rubber polishing points, followed by flour of pumice, produce an adequately smooth and polished rest seat. A predetermined path of placement for the denture must be kept in mind in preparing the rest seat. The lingual rest seat must not be prepared as though it were going to be approached from a direction perpendicular to the lingual slope. The floor of the rest seat should be toward the cingulum rather than the axial wall (Fig. 5-18). Care must be taken not to create an enamel undercut, which would interfere with placement of the denture.

2. The most satisfactory lingual rest, from the standpoint of support, is one placed on a prepared rest seat in a cast restoration (Fig. 5-19). This is done most effectively by planning and executing a rest seat in the wax pattern rather than by attempting to cut a rest in a cast restoration in the mouth. The contour of the framework may then restore the lingual form of the tooth.

By accentuating the cingulum in the wax pattern, the floor of the rest seat is readily carved to be the most apical portion of the preparation. A saddlelike shape, which provides a positive rest seat located favorably in relation to the long axis of the tooth, is thus formed. The framework of the denture is made to fill out the continuity of the lingual surface so that the tongue contacts a smooth surface without the patient's being conscious of bulk or irregularities.

The lingual rest may be placed on the lingual surface of a cast veneer crown, a three-quarter crown, or some type of inlay (Fig. 5-20). The latter displays less metal than the three-quarter

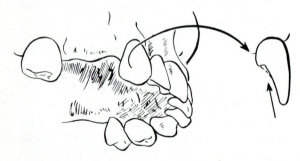

Fig. 5-17. Lingual rest seat placed in enamel just incisally to cingulum. Its preparation requires slight reduction of portion of cingulum. **Rest seat preparation should be confined to maxillary canines and central incisors that have exaggerated cingulum.**

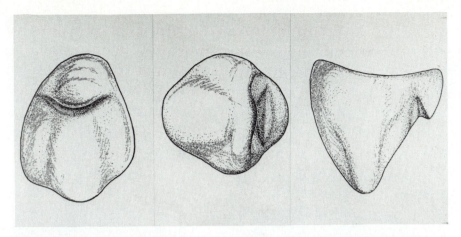

Fig. 5-18. Three views of lingual rest seat prepared in enamel of maxillary canine. The rest seat, from lingual aspect, assumes form of a broad inverted V, maintaining natural contour sometimes seen in a maxillary canine cingulum. Inverted V notch form is self-centering for the rest and at the same time directs forces rather favorably in an apical direction. Looking at preparation from incisal view, it will be noted that rest seat preparation is broadest at most lingual aspect of canine. As preparation approaches proximal surfaces of tooth, it is less broad than at any other areas. Proximal view demonstrates correct taper of floor of rest seat. It also should be noted that borders of rest seat are slightly rounded to avoid line angles in its preparation. Mesiodistal length of preparation should be a minimum of 2.5 to 3 mm, labiolingual width about 2 mm, and incisal-apical depth a minimum of 1.5 mm. **It is a risky preparation** and should not be attempted on lower anterior teeth.

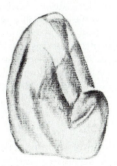

Fig. 5-19. Rest seat preparation can be exaggerated for better support when it is prepared in metallic restoration.

crown, especially on the mandibular canine where the lingual rest placed on a cast restoration is frequently used, and it is a more conservative restoration. The three-quarter crown may be used if the labial surface of the tooth is sound and retentive contours are satisfactory. However, if the labial surface presents inadequate or excessive contours for placement of a retentive clasp arm, or if gingival decalcificiation or caries is present, a veneered complete coverage crown should be used.

In some instances, ball-type rests may be used in prepared seats. Such rest seats may be cautiously prepared in tooth surfaces with overly sufficient enamel thickness or may be prepared in restorations placed in teeth where enamel thickness is inadequate (Fig. 5-20, *C*). Conservative restorations (silver amalgam, compacted gold, pin inlays, etc.) in anterior teeth may be better suited for ball-type rest seats than are the less conservative inverted V-type rest seats.

There is evidence that individually cast chromium-cobalt alloy rest seat forms may be attached to lingual surfaces of anterior teeth by using composite resin cements with acid-etched tooth preparation. If this procedure proves to be acceptable through long-term clinical observations, it may serve as a conservative approach to forming rest seats on teeth with unacceptable lingual contours.

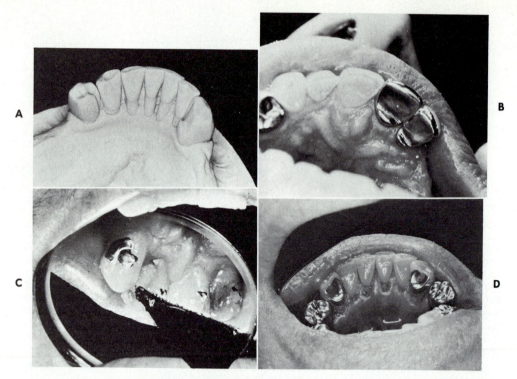

Fig. 5-20. A, Master cast from which removable partial denture framework will be constructed. Properly contoured lingual rest seat was placed in veneer crown for canine abutment. **B,** Positive vertical support for prosthesis is furnished by rest seats prepared in splinted three-quarter crowns on lateral and central incisors. These rest seats are optimally placed on incisors as near horizontal axis of rotation as possible. **C,** Lingual rest seat placed in this pin-retained inlay is cup shaped and is confined within inlay itself. **D,** Lingual rest seats on mandibular canines contained within pin onlays. Suitable rest seats could not be prepared in enamel. Pin-onlay restoration is more conservative and esthetically desirable than three-quarter crown to accomplish the same end results. (Courtesy Dr. Robert Matteson, Gainesville, Fla.)

INCISAL RESTS AND REST SEATS

Incisal rests are placed at the incisal angles of anterior teeth and on prepared rest seats. Although this is the least desirable placement of a rest seat for reasons previously mentioned, it may be used successfully for selected patients when the abutment is sound and when a cast restoration is not otherwise indicated. Therefore incisal rests generally are placed on enamel (Fig. 5-21). **Incisal rests are used predominantly as auxiliary rests or as indirect retainers.**

Although the incisal rest may be used on a canine abutment in either arch, it is more applicable to the mandibular canine. This type of

rest provides definite support with relatively little loss of tooth structure and little display of metal. Esthetically it is preferable to the three-quarter crown (Fig. 5-22). The same criteria apply in deciding whether to use unprotected enamel for an occlusal rest on a molar or premolar. An incisal rest is more likely to lead to some orthodontic movement of the tooth because of unfavorable leverage factors than is a lingual rest.

An incisal rest seat is prepared in the form of a rounded notch at an incisal angle or on an incisal edge, with the deepest portion of the preparation apical to the incisal edge (Fig.

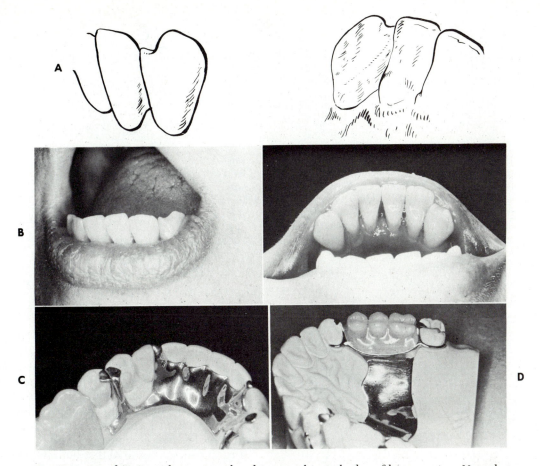

Fig. 5-21. A and **B,** Incisal rest seat placed in mesial incisal edge of lower canine. Note that contact point is not involved in preparation of rest seat to support linguoplate (as seen in **C**). **D,** Distal incisal rest on canine furnishes excellent vertical support for tooth-borne removable partial denture and is not esthetically objectionable.

Fig. 5-22. Incisal rests are used on this removable partial denture and are more esthetically acceptable than three-quarter crowns in which lingual rest seats may be placed.

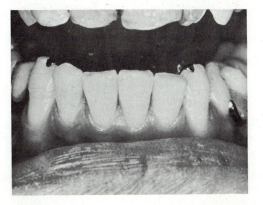

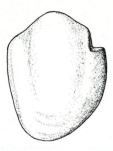
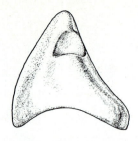
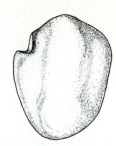

Fig. 5-23. Three views of incisal rest seat preparation on mandibular canine adjacent to a modification space. Labial view demonstrates inclination of floor of rest seat, which allows forces to be directed along the long axis of tooth as nearly as possible. Note that floor of rest seat has been extended slightly onto labial aspect of tooth. As seen from a proximal view, proximal edge of rest seat is rounded rather than straight. Lingual view shows that all borders of rest seat are rounded to avoid sharp line angles. It is especially important to avoid a line angle at junction of axial wall of preparation and floor of rest seat. The rest that occupies such a preparation should be able to move slightly in a lateral direction to avoid torquing the abutment tooth.

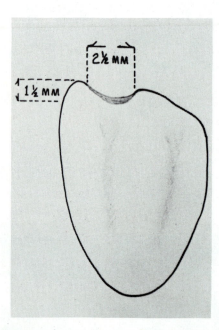

Fig. 5-24. Dimension given in illustration for incisal rest seat preparation will provide adequate strength of framework at junction of rest and minor connector. Rest seats of smaller dimension have proved unsatisfactory regardless of metal alloy from which framework is made.

5-23). The notch should be beveled both labially and lingually, and the lingual enamel should be partly shaped to accommodate the rigid minor connector connecting the rest to the framework. An incisal rest seat should be approximately 2.5 mm wide and 1.5 mm deep so that the rest will be strong without having to exceed the natural contour of the incisal edge (Fig. 5-24).

It is, of course, essential that both the master cast and the casting be accurate if the rest is to seat properly. The incisal rest should be overcontoured slightly to allow for labial and incisal finishing to the adjoining enamel in much the same manner as a three-quarter crown or inlay margin is finished to enamel. In this way minimal display of metal is possible without jeopardizing the effectiveness of the rest.

Care in selecting the type of rest seat to be used, in preparing it, and in fabricating the framework casting does much to assure the success of any type of rest. **The topography of any rest should be such that it restores the topography of the tooth existing before the rest seat was prepared.**

SELF-ASSESSMENT AIDS

1. Define the word **rest** as a component of a removable partial denture.

2. What are the functions of a rest?
3. Rests are designated by the surface of the tooth prepared to receive the rest. Therefore rests are _____rests, or _____rests, or _____ rests.
4. Can you describe the form of an adequately prepared occlusal rest seat?
5. Where is the "deepest" portion of an occlusal rest seat located?
6. Can you diagram the approximate dimensions of an occlusal rest seat on a molar? A premolar?
7. Why should the angle formed by the rest and the vertical minor connector from which it originates be less than 90 degrees?
8. Under what circumstances would you elect to prepare a secondary occlusal rest seat on the same tooth?
9. Describe the form of adjacent, interproximal occlusal rest seats.
10. What advantages are gained by using adjacent, interproximal occlusal rest seats rather than a single interproximal rest seat?
11. Can you describe an internal occlusal rest seat and relate the circumstances under which it may be used?
12. How do you go about fabricating an internal occlusal rest seat?
13. Rests may be placed on sound enamel, cast restorations, or silver amalgam alloy restorations. Which of the three structures is least desirable for support of the rests? Why?
14. When preparing occlusal rest seats immediately adjacent to a proximal surface that has to be recontoured for optimum location of other components, which is accomplished first—rest seat preparation or recontouring of axial surface of abutment? Defend your answer.
15. What is the sequence of operations in preparing an occlusal rest seat in enamel? Name the cutting and polishing instruments used.
16. How is a small enamel defect encountered in preparing a rest seat handled?
17. Suppose you expose dentin in preparing an occlusal rest seat in enamel—what then?
18. Describe the form of a lingual rest seat preparation.
19. Which unrestored teeth may sometimes have such a lingual contour that an acceptable lingual rest seat may be prepared in enamel?
20. Five morphologic or anatomic factors must be evaluated in determining whether an abutment can support a lingual rest. Can you enumerate these five factors?
21. Most often, unrestored canines and incisors should not be used for supports for lingual rests. Why?
22. For what reasons should a rounded, inverted V notch form be used for a lingual rest seat?
23. Can you state the minimum dimensions for a lingual rest seat mesiodistally, labiolingually, and incisal-apically?
24. Please give the sequence of use of rotary instruments in preparing a lingual rest seat in enamel.
25. The design of a framework is such that lingual rest seats must be placed on incisor teeth, yet dentin will knowingly be exposed in preparing acceptable rest seats. What are your options for providing adequate rest seats on the incisors?
26. The adequacy of a lingual rest seat is better accomplished with a cast restoration than a preparation confined to enamel. True or false?
27. Describe the contour of an incisal rest seat preparation.
28. What are the minimum acceptable dimensions of an incisal rest seat?
29. Can you think of several indications for the use of incisal rests?
30. Which rest is the most unfavorable in relation to a possible tipping of the tooth? Which is the most favorable to avoid unfavorable leverage factors?
31. For what reasons must a rest restore the occlusal, lingual, or incisal morphology of the abutment tooth that existed before the rest seat preparation?

6 DIRECT RETAINERS

A removable partial denture must have **support,** derived from the abutment teeth through the use of rests and from the residual ridge through well-fitting bases. It must be **stabilized against horizontal movement** through the use of rigid components such as reciprocal clasp arms and the contact of minor connectors with vertical tooth surfaces. It must be **stabilized against rotational movement and resulting torque** through the use of rigid connectors, indirect retainers, and other stabilizing components. In addition, the removable partial denture must have sufficient **retention** to resist reasonable dislodging forces.

Retention for the removable partial denture is accomplished mechanically by placing retaining elements on the abutment teeth and by the intimate relationship of denture bases and major connectors (maxillary) with the underlying tissues. The latter is similar to the retention of complete dentures and is proportionate to the accuracy of the impression registration, the accuracy of the fit of the denture bases, and the total area of contact involved.

Retention of denture bases has been described as the result of the following forces: (1) adhesion, which is the attraction of the saliva to the denture and to the tissues; (2) cohesion, which is the attraction of the molecules of the saliva for each other; (3) atmospheric pressure, which is dependent on a border seal and results in a partial vacuum beneath the denture base when a dislodging force is applied; (4) the plastic molding of the tissues around the polished surfaces of the denture; and (5) the effect of gravity on the manidbular denture. Boucher, writing on the subject of complete denture impressions, describes these forces as follows:

Adhesion and cohesion are effective when there is perfect apposition of the impression surface of the denture to the mucous membrane surfaces. These forces lose their effectiveness if there is any horizontal displacement of the dentures that breaks the continuity of this contact. Atmospheric pressure is effective primarily as a rescue force when extreme dislodging forces are applied to the denture. It depends on a perfect border seal to keep the pressure applied on only one side of the denture. The presence of air on the impression surface would neutralize the pressure of the air against the polished surface. Since each of these forces is directly proportional to the area covered by the dentures, the dentures should be extended to the limits of the oral cavity.

The plastic molding of the soft tissues around the polished surfaces of dentures helps to perfect the border seal. Also, it forms a mechanical lock at certain locations on the dentures, provided these surfaces are prepared for it. This lock is developed automatically and without effort by the patient if the impression is made with an understanding of the anatomic possibilities.*

Although few partial dentures are made without some mechanical retention, retention from the denture bases may contribute significantly to the overall retention of the partial denture and therefore must not be discounted as a retentive force. **Denture bases should be designed and fabricated so that they will contribute as much retention to the partial denture as possible.** However, it is questionable whether atmospheric pressure plays an important role in retention of removable partial dentures, since a "border seal" cannot be obtained as can be accomplished with complete dentures. Therefore adhesion and cohesion gained by excellent apposition of the denture base and soft tissues of the basal seat do play an important retentive role.

Mechanical retention of removable partial dentures is accomplished by means of direct retainers of one type or another. A direct retainer is any unit of a removable dental prosthesis that engages an abutment tooth in such a manner as to resist displacement of the prosthesis away from basal seat tissues. This may be accomplished by frictional means, by engaging a depression in the abutment tooth, or by engaging a tooth undercut lying cervically to the height of contour.

There are two basic types of direct retainers. One is the **intracoronal** retainer, which engages vertical walls built into the crown of the abutment tooth to create frictional resistance to removal (Fig. 6-1). The other type is the **extracoronal** retainer, of which there are two configurations: the manufactured retainer such as the

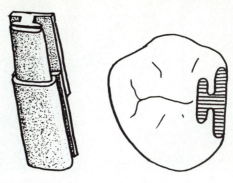

Fig. 6-1. This intracoronal retainer consists of a key and keyway system with extremely small tolerance. Keyway is placed totally within metallic crown on abutment tooth, and key is attached to removable partial denture framework. There is frictional resistance to removal and placement as well as limitation of movement of prosthesis other than placement and removal.

Dalbo (Fig. 6-2) and the clasp-type retainer (Figs. 6-3 and 6-4). The clasp type engages an external surface of the abutment tooth in an area cervical to the greatest convexity or in a depression created for that purpose. Rather than creating frictional resistance to removal, **a flexible arm is forced to deform, or a spring device is compressed, thereby generating resistance to removal.** The most common extracoronal attachment is the **retentive clasp arm.**

The intracoronal retainer is usually spoken of as an **internal attachment,** or a **precision attachment.** The principle of the internal attachment was first formulated by Dr. Herman E. S. Chayes in 1906, and the attachment manufactured commercially carries his name. Although it may be fabricated by the dental technician as a cast dovetail fitting into a counterpart receptacle in the abutment crown, the alloys used in manufactured attachments and the precision with which they are constructed make the ready-made attachment much preferable to any of this type that can be fabricated in the dental laboratory. Much credit is due the manufacturers of metals used in dentistry for their continued improvements in the design of internal attachments.

Some of the better-known internal attachments are the Ney-Chayes attachment, the

---

*Paraphrased from Boucher, C.O.: Complete denture impressions based upon the anatomy of the mouth, J. Am. Dent. Assoc. **31:**1174-1181, 1944.

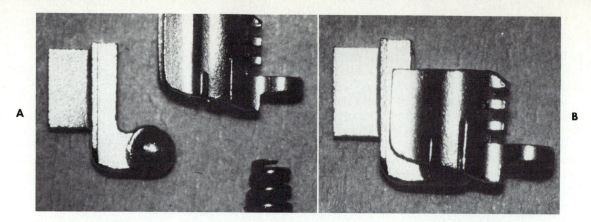

Fig. 6-2. Dalbo extracoronal attachment. **A,** Components consist of L-shaped male portion that is attached to an abutment crown, female sleeve that is placed in artificial tooth adjacent to abutment, and coiled spring that fits into female portion. **B,** Attachment is assembled. Design permits some vertical movement of denture under force through compression of coiled spring.

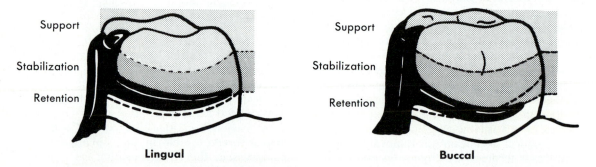

Fig. 6-3. Extracoronal circumferential direct retainer (mirror view). Assembly consists of buccal flexible retentive arm, lingual limited flexing reciprocal-stabilizing arm, and supporting occlusal rest. Terminal portion of retentive arm engages measured undercut. Assembly remains passive until activated by placement or removal of restoration or when subjected to masticatory generated forces.

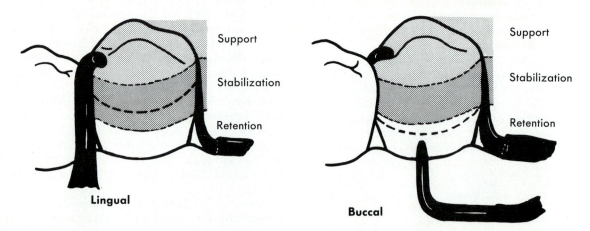

Fig. 6-4. Extracoronal bar-type direct retainer (mirror view). Assembly consists of buccal retentive arm engaging measured undercut, reciprocal-stabilizing elements (proximal plate minor connector on distal and lingually placed mesial minor connector for occlusal rest), and mesially placed supporting occlusal rest. Assembly remains passive until activated.

Stern-Goldsmith attachment, and the Baker attachment. Descriptive literature and technique manuals are available from the manufacturers.

INTERNAL ATTACHMENTS

The internal attachment has two major advantages over the extracoronal attachment: elimination of a visible retentive component and of a visible vertical support through a rest seat located more favorably in relation to the horizontal axis of the abutment tooth. For this reason the internal attachment may be preferable in selected situations. It provides some horizontal stabilization similar to that of an internal rest, but some additional extracoronal stabilization is usually desirable. It has been claimed that stimulation to the underlying tissues is greater when internal attachments are used because of intermittent vertical massage. This is probably no more than is possible with extracoronal retainers of similar construction.

Some of the disadvantages of internal attachments are that (1) they require prepared abutments and castings; (2) they require somewhat complicated clinical and laboratory procedures; (3) they eventually wear, with resulting loss of frictional resistance to denture removal; (4) they are difficult to repair and replace; (5) they are effective in proportion to their length and are therefore least effective on short teeth; and (6) they are difficult to place completely with the circumference of an abutment tooth.

Since the internal attachment must be built within the coronal limits of the tooth, a large pulp may be jeopardized by the depth of the receptacle. Because it depends on frictional resistance for retention, crown length must be sufficient to provide adequate frictional surfaces. The cost of an internal attachment prosthesis is necessarily higher than is a restoration of similar construction using extracoronal retainers, even when the latter utilizes abutment castings. Limitations to the use of internal attachments are (1) size of pulp, which is usually related to the age of the patient; (2) length of the clinical crown, which may prevent use on short or abraded teeth; and (3) greater cost to the patient.

Since the principle of the internal attachment does not permit horizontal movement, all horizontal, tipping, and rotational movements of the prosthesis are transmitted directly to the abutment tooth. **The internal attachment therefore should not be used in conjunction with tissue supported distal extension denture bases unless some form of stressbreaker is used between the movable base and the rigid attachment.** Whereas stressbreakers may be used, they do have some disadvantages, which will be discussed later, and their use adds further to the cost of the partial denture. It is doubtful that the possible advantages of the stress-broken, internal-attachment denture are available to but a small percentage of the population needing a removable partial denture service.

EXTRACORONAL DIRECT RETAINERS

Although the extracoronal or clasp direct retainer is used many times more frequently than the internal attachment, it is also all too frequently misused. It is hoped that a better understanding of the principles of clasp design will lead to more intelligent use of this retainer in the future.

Critical areas of an abutment that provide for retention, stabilization, reciprocation, and guiding planes can only be identified with the use of a dental cast surveyor (Table 6-1). To enhance

Table 6-1. *Function and position of clasp assembly parts*

Component part	Function	Location
Rest	Support	Occlusal, lingual, incisal
Minor connector	Stabilization	Proximal surfaces extending from the prepared marginal ridge to the junction of the middle and gingival third of abutment crown
Clasp arms	Stabilization	Apical portion of middle third of crown
	Reciprocation	Apical portion of middle third of crown
	Retention	Gingival third of crown in measured undercut

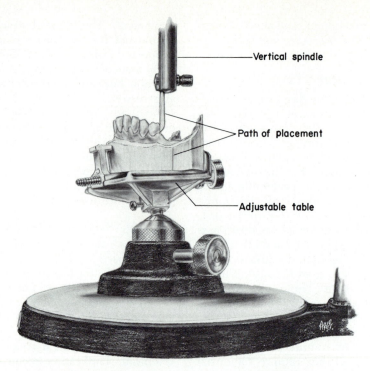

Vertical spindle

Path of placement

Adjustable table

Fig. 6-5. Most essential parts of a dental surveyor (Ney Parallelometer), showing vertical spindle in relation to adjustable table.

an understanding of direct retainers, an introduction of the dental cast surveyor is appropriate at this time. Surveying will be covered in detail in Chapter 10.

The cast surveyor (Fig. 6-5) is a simple enough instrument, but is most essential to planning partial denture treatment. Its main working parts are the vertical arm and the adjustable table that holds the cast in a fixed relation to the vertical arm. This represents that path of placement that the partial denture will ultimately take in the mouth.

The adjustable table may be tilted in relation to the vertical arm of the surveyor until a path that best satisfies all the factors involved can be found. A cast in a horizontal relationship to the vertical arm represents a vertical path of placement; a cast in a tilted relationship represents a path of placement toward the side of the cast that is tilted upward. The vertical arm, when brought in contact with a tooth surface, will indicate the areas available for retention and those

available for support, as well as the existence of tooth and other tissue interference to the path of placement.

When the surveyor blade contacts a tooth on the cast at its greatest convexity, a triangle is formed. The apex of the triangle is at the point of contact of the surveyor blade with the tooth, and the base is the area of the cast representing the gingival tissues (Fig. 10-18). The apical angle is called the angle of cervical convergence (Fig. 6-6). This angle may be measured as described in Chapter 10, or it may be estimated by observing the triangle of light visible between the tooth and the surveyor blade. For this reason a wide surveyor blade rather than a small cylindric tool is used so that the triangle of light may be more easily seen.

The following factors determine the amount of retention a clasp is capable of generating:
1. Size of the angle of cervical convergence
2. How far into the angle of cervical convergence the clasp terminal is placed

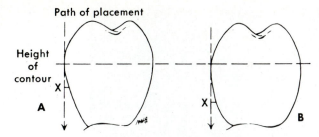

Fig. 6-6. Angle of cervical convergence on two teeth presenting dissimilar contours. Greater angle of cervical convergence on tooth **A** necessitates placement of clasp terminus, *X*, nearer the height of contour than when lesser angle exists, as in **B.** It is apparent that uniform clasp retention depends on degree of tooth undercut rather than on distance below the height of contour at which clasp terminus is placed.

3. Flexibility of the clasp arm, which is the product of—
   a. Its length, measured from its point of origin to its terminal end
   b. Its relative diameter, regardless of its cross-sectional form
   c. Its cross-sectional form or shape, that is, whether it is round, half-round, or some other form
   d. The material of which the clasp is made, that is, whether it is made of a cast gold alloy, cast chrome alloy, wrought gold alloy, or wrought chrome alloy (each alloy has its own characteristics in both cast and wrought form)

To be retentive a tooth must have a height of contour cervical to which the surface converges. Although most any single tooth when surveyed will have a height of contour or an area of greatest convexity, areas of cervical convergence may not exist when the tooth is viewed in relation to a given path of placement. Also, certain areas of cervical convergence may not be available for the placement of retentive clasps because of their proximity to gingival tissues.

This is best illustrated by mounting a spherical object such as an egg on the adjustable table of a dental surveyor (Fig. 6-7, *A*). The egg now represents the cast of a dental arch or, more correctly, one tooth of a dental arch. The egg is first placed perpendicular to the base of the surveyor and surveyed to determine the height of

convexity. The vertical arm of the surveyor represents the path of placement that a denture would take and, conversely, its path of removal.

With a carbon marker a circumferential line is drawn on the egg at its greatest circumference. This line, which Kennedy called the height of contour, is its greatest convexity. Cummer spoke of it as the guideline, since it is used as a guide in the placement of retentive and nonretentive clasps. To this, DeVan added the terms **suprabulge,** denoting the surfaces sloping superiorly, and **infrabulge,** denoting the surfaces sloping inferiorly. Prothero proposed that the height of convexity of a tooth be considered as the common base of two cones, the apex of one cone being somewhere above the occlusal surface, and the apex of the other being somewhere below the cervical circumference of the tooth.

Any areas cervical to the height of contour may be used for the placement of retentive clasp arms, whereas areas occlusal to the height of contour may be used for the placement of nonretentive reciprocating, or stabilizing components. Obviously only flexible components may be placed gingivally to the height of contour, because if rigid elements were to be so placed, the undercut areas would be areas of interference to placement and removal rather than areas of retention.

With the original guidelines on the egg, the egg is now tilted from the perpendicular to an angular relation with the base of the surveyor (Fig. 6-7, *B*). Its relation to the vertical arm of the surveyor has now been changed, just as a change in the position of a dental cast would bring about a different relationship with the surveyor. The vertical arm of the surveyor still represents the path of placement, but its relation to the egg is totally different.

Again, the carbon marker is used to delineate the greatest convexity or the height of contour. It will be seen that areas which were formerly infrabulge are now suprabulge, and vice versa. A retentive clasp arm placed below the height of contour in the original position may now be either excessively retentive or totally nonretentive, whereas a nonretentive reciprocal arm located above the height of contour in the first position now may be located in an area of undercut.

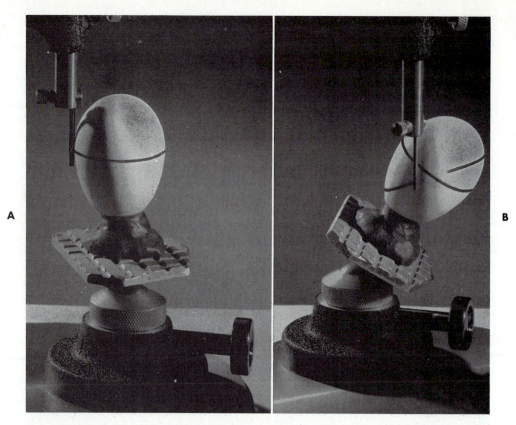

Fig. 6-7. A, When an egg is placed with its long axis parallel to surveying tool, height of contour is found at its greatest circumference. Similarly, height of contour may be identified on a single tooth when its long axis is placed parallel to surveying tool. Rigid parts of partial denture framework may be located in suprabulge areas above height of contour, whereas only flexible portions of clasp retainers may be placed in infrabulge areas below. Those infrabulge surfaces that will be crossed by rigid parts of partial denture framework must be eliminated either during mouth preparations or by blockout. **B,** If same egg is tilted in relation to vertical spindle of surveyor, areas formerly infrabulge are now found to be suprabulge and will accommodate nonretentive denture components. At the same time, however, areas formerly suprabulge or only slightly infrabulge are found to be so severely undercut that design and location of clasp retainers must be changed. Unfortunately, no single tooth in a partially edentulous arch may govern relation of cast to surveyor and thus the path of placement of partial denture. A compromise position must be found that, following mouth preparations, will satisfy all four factors: (1) no interference to placement, (2) effective location of retentive components, (3) most esthetic placement of all component parts, and (4) existence of guiding planes that will assure a definite path of placement and removal. (Courtesy J. M. Ney Co., Hartford, Conn.)

The location and degree of a tooth undercut available for retention is therefore relative to the path of placement and removal of the partial denture; at the same time, nonretentive areas on which rigid components of the clasp may be placed exist for a given path of placement only.

When the theory of clasp retention is applied to the abutment teeth in a dental arch, each tooth may be considered as an entity as far as the design of retentive and reciprocating components is concerned. This is possible because its relationship to the rest of the arch and to the design of the rest of the prosthesis has been considered previously in selecting the most suitable path of placement. Once the relation of the cast to the surveyor has been established, the height of contour on each abutment tooth becomes fixed, and the clasp design for each may be considered separately.

Clasp retention is based on the resistance of metal to deformation. For a clasp to be retentive, it must be placed in an undercut area of the tooth, where it is forced to deform when a vertical dislodging force is applied. It is this resistance to deformation that generates retention (Fig. 6-8). Such resistance is proportionate to the flexibility of the clasp arm.

It should be clearly understood that a retentive undercut exists only in relation to a given path of placement and removal, for if the path of escapement of the retentive clasp is parallel to the path of removal of the prosthesis, no retentive undercut exists (Fig. 6-9).

If conditions are found that are not favorable for the particular path of placement being considered, the conditions produced by a different path of placement should be studied. The cast is merely tilted in relation to the vertical arm until the most suitable path is found. Then mouth preparations are planned with a definite path of placement in mind.

The path of placement also must take into consideration the presence of tissue undercuts that will interfere with the placement of major connectors, the location of vertical minor connectors, the origin of bar clasp arms, and the denture bases.

A positive path of placement and removal is made possible by the contact of rigid parts of the denture framework with parallel tooth surfaces, which act as guiding planes. It is also made possible, to some extent, by simultaneous tooth contact on either side of the dental arch as the prosthesis is placed and removed. If some degree of parallelism does not exist during placement and removal, trauma to the teeth and supporting structures, as well as strain on the denture parts, is inevitable. This ultimately results in damage either to the teeth and their periodontal support, or to the denture itself, or both. Therefore, without guiding planes, clasp retention will either be detrimental or practically non-existent. If clasp retention is only frictional, be-

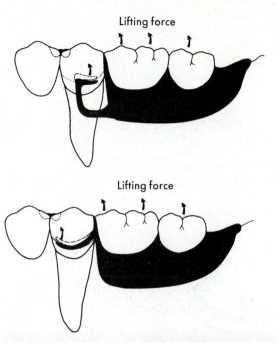

Fig. 6-8. Retention is provided primarily by flexible portion of clasp assembly. Retentive terminals are ideally located in measured undercuts in gingival third of abutment crowns. When force acts to dislodge restoration in occlusal direction, retentive arm is forced to deform as it passes from undercut location over height of contour. Amount of retention provided by clasp arm is determined by its length, diameter, taper, cross-sectional form, contour, type of alloy, and location and depth of undercut engaged.

cause of an **active** relationship of the clasp to the teeth, orthodontic movement or damage to periodontal tissues or both will result. **Instead a clasp should bear a passive relationship to the teeth except when a dislodging force is applied.**

Relative uniformity of retention

The size of the angle of convergence will determine how far into that angle a given clasp arm will be placed. Disregarding, for the time being, variations in clasp flexibility, relative uniformity of retention will depend on the location of the clasp terminal—not in relation to the height of contour, but in relation to the angle of cervical convergence.

The retention on all principal abutments (of which there will be two in Class I and Class II situations and three or more in Class III situa-

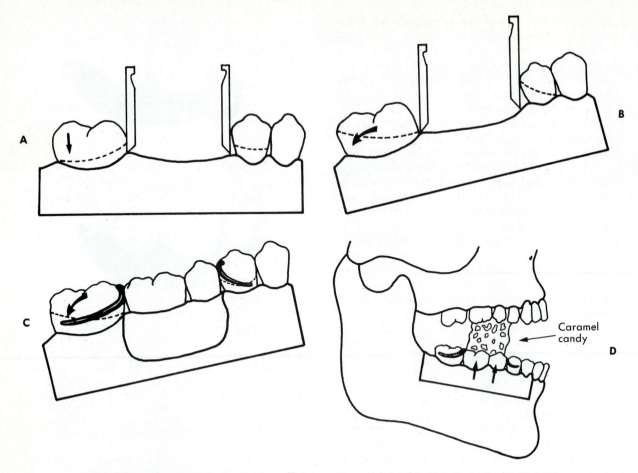

Fig. 6-9. A, Retentive areas are not sufficient to resist reasonable dislodging force when cast is surveyed at its most advantageous position (occlusal plane parallel to surveyor table). **B,** Tilting cast still creates functionally ineffective tooth contours, which are present only in relation to surveying rod and do not exist when compared to most advantageous position. **C,** Clasps are in ineffective retentive areas at this tilt. **D,** Retentive areas are not in path of displacement when restoration is subjected to dislodging forces in occlusal direction.

tions) should be as nearly equal as possible. Whereas esthetic placement of clasp arms is desirable, it may not be possible to place all clasp arms in the same occlusocervical relationship because of variations in tooth contours. The only exceptions are when retentive surfaces may be made similar by altering tooth contours or when two cast restorations are made with similar contours.

Instead the retentive clasp arms must be located so that they lie in the same approximate degree of undercut on each abutment tooth. In Fig. 6-6 this is at point *X* on both teeth, *A* and *B*, despite the variation in the distance below the height of contour. Should both clasp arms be placed equidistantly below the height of contour, the higher location on tooth *B* would have too little retention, whereas the lower location on tooth *A* would be too retentive.

The measurement of the degree of undercut by mechanical means is therefore most important. Although experience with undercut gauges is most important, the student should graduate with a thorough comprehension of all the factors influencing clasp retention and be able to apply them intelligently.

Flexibility of clasp arms

The following factors influence the flexibility of a clasp arm.

Length of clasp arm. The longer the clasp arm, the more flexible it will be, all other factors being equal. The length of a circumferential clasp arm is **measured from the point at which a uniform taper begins.** The retentive circumferential clasp arm should be tapered uniformly from its point of origin. The length of this uniform taper is the full length of the clasp arm (Fig. 6-10).

The length of a bar clasp arm also is measured from the point at which a uniform taper begins. Generally the taper of a bar clasp arm should begin at its point of origin from a metal base or at the point at which it emerges from a resin base (Fig. 6-11). While a bar clasp arm will usually be longer than a circumferential clasp arm, its flexibility will be less because its half-round form lies in several planes, which prevents its flexibility from being proportionate to its total length. Table 6-2 gives an approximate depth of undercut that may be used for the cast gold retentive clasp arms of the circumferential and bar-type clasps. Based on a proportional limit of 60,000 psi and on the assumption that the clasp

arm is properly tapered, the clasp arm should be able to flex repeatedly within the limits stated without hardening or rupturing because of fatigue. It has been estimated that alternate stress applications of the fatigue type are placed on a retainer arm during mastication and other force-inducing functions about 300,000 times a year. Table 6-3 provides the same data for chromium-cobalt alloys.

Diameter of clasp arm. The greater the average diameter of a clasp arm, the less flexible it will be, all other factors being equal. If its taper is absolutely uniform, the average diameter will be at a point midway between its origin and its terminal end. If its taper is not uniform, a point of flexure and therefore a point of weakness will exist that will then be the determining factor in its flexibility regardless of the average diameter of its entire length.

Cross-sectional form of clasp arm. Flexibility may exist in any form, but it is limited to only one direction in the case of the half-round form. The only universally flexible form is the round form, which is practically impossible to obtain by casting and polishing.

Since all cast clasps are essentially half round in form, they may flex away from the tooth, but edgewise flexing (and edgewise adjustment) is limited. For this reason cast retentive clasp arms are more acceptable in tooth-borne partial den-

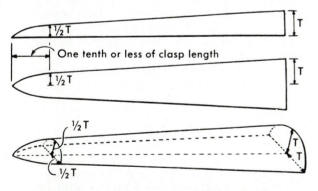

Fig. 6-10. Retentive cast clasp arm should be tapered uniformly from its point of attachment at clasp body to its tip. Dimensions at tip are about half those at point of attachment. Clasp arm so tapered is approximately twice as flexible as one without any taper. *T* is clasp thickness. (Courtesy J. F. Jelenko & Co., Inc., New York, N.Y.)

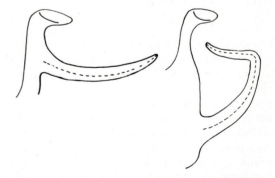

Fig. 6-11. Length of cast retentive clasp arm is measured along center portion of arm until it either joins clasp body (circumferential) or until it becomes part of denture base or is embedded in the base (bar-type clasp).

Table 6-2. *Permissible flexibilities of retentive, cast circumferential and bar-type clasp arms of type IV gold alloys**

Circumferential		Bar-type	
Length (inches)	Flexibility (inches)	Length (inches)	Flexibility (inches)
0 to 0.3	0.01	0 to 0.7	0.01
0.3 to 0.6	0.02	0.7 to 0.9	0.02
0.6 to 0.8	0.03	0.9 to 1.0	0.03

*Based on the approximate dimensions of Jelenko "preformed" plastic patterns, J.F. Jelenko & Co., Inc., New York, N.Y.

Table 6-3. *Permissible flexibilities of retentive, cast circumferential and bar-type clasp arms for chromium-cobalt alloys**

Circumferential		Bar-type	
Length (inches)	Flexibility (inches)	Length (inches)	Flexibility (inches)
0 to 0.3	0.004	0 to 0.7	0.004
0.3 to 0.6	0.008	0.7 to 0.9	0.008
0.6 to 0.8	0.012	0.9 to 1.0	0.012

*Based on the approximate dimensions of Jelenko "preformed" plastic patterns, J.F. Jelenko & Co., Inc., New York, N.Y.

tures in which they are called on to flex only during placement and removal of the prosthesis. A retentive clasp arm on an abutment adjacent to a distal extension base must not only flex during placement and removal but also must be capable of flexing during functional movement of the distal extension base. It must have either universal flexibility to avoid transmission of tipping stresses to the abutment tooth or be capable of disengaging the undercut when vertical forces directed against the denture are toward the residual ridge. A round clasp form is the only circumferential clasp form that may be safely used to engage a tooth undercut on the side of an abutment tooth **away** from the distal extension base. **The location of the undercut is perhaps the most important single factor in selecting a clasp for use with distal extension partial dentures.**

Material used for clasp arm. Whereas all cast alloys used in partial denture construction possess flexibility, their flexibility is proportionate to their bulk. If this were not true, other components of the partial denture could not have the necessary rigidity. The only disadvantages of cast gold partial dentures are that their bulk must be increased to obtain needed rigidity at the expense of added weight, and their cost. It cannot be denied that greater rigidity with less bulk is possible through the use of chromium alloys.

Although cast gold alloys may have greater resiliency than do cast chromium alloys, the fact remains that the structural nature of the cast clasp does not approach the flexibility and adjustability of the wrought-wire clasp. Having been formed by being drawn into a wire, the wrought-wire clasp arm has toughness exceeding that of a cast clasp arm. The tensile strength of a wrought structure is at least 25% greater than that of the cast alloy from which it was made. It may therefore be used in smaller diameters to provide greater flexibility without fatigue and ultimate fracture.

Reciprocal-stabilizing cast clasp arm

A reciprocal-stabilizing clasp arm should be rigid. Therefore it is shaped somewhat differently than is the cast retentive clasp arm, which must be flexible. Its average diameter must be greater than the average diameter of the opposing retentive arm to increase desired rigidity. Whereas a cast retentive arm is tapered in two dimensions as illustrated in Fig. 6-10, a reciprocal arm should be tapered in one dimension only, as is viewed in Fig. 6-12. To achieve such a form for the arm, freehand waxing of patterns is required.

CRITERIA FOR SELECTING A GIVEN CLASP DESIGN

In selecting a particular clasp arm for a given situation, its function and limitations must be carefully evaluated. **The dentist should not expect the technician to make the decision as to which clasp design is to be used. The choice of clasp design must be both biologically and mechanically sound, based on the diagnosis and**

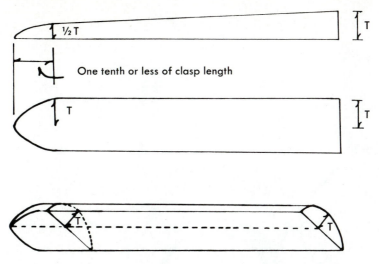

Fig. 6-12. Reciprocal arm of direct retainer assembly should be rigid. Arm tapered both lengthwise and widthwise is more flexible than arm of the same dimensions tapered only lengthwise.

treatment plan previously established. Extracoronal direct retainers should be considered as a combination of components of a removable partial denture framework designed and located to perform the specific functions of support, stabilization and reciprocation, and retention. It matters not whether the direct retainer assembly components are physically attached directly to each other or originate from major and minor connectors of the framework (Fig. 6-13). If attention was directed to the components of the direct retainer assembly itself and to the function each component contributes to the restoration, then designing a direct retainer for a particular situation is reduced to simple rationalization.

The advantages of any particular clasp design should lie in an affirmative answer to most or all of the following questions:

1. Is is flexible enough for the purpose for which it is being used? (On an abutment adjacent to a distal extension base, will tipping and torque be avoided?)
2. Does the clasp arm cover a minimum of tooth surface?
3. Will the clasp arm be as inconspicuous as possible?
4. Will tooth dimension be increased, which would relatively increase the width of the occlusal table?
5. Is the clasp design applicable to malposed or rotated abutment teeth?
6. Can it be used despite the presence of tissue undercuts?
7. Can the clasp terminal be adjusted to increase or decrease retention?
8. Will adequate stabilization be provided to resist horizontal and rotational movements?
9. Will rigidity be provided where it is needed?
10. Is the clasp arm likely to become distorted or broken? If so, can it be replaced?

With this background the various types of clasps will be considered. **The choice of a clasp is like the choice of a tool to be used in a given situation. Knowing what types are available and being familiar with their various advantages and limitations permits selection of a clasp design that best meets the needs of the individual situation.**

Although there are some rather complex designs for clasp arms, they may all be classified as falling into one of two categories. One is the

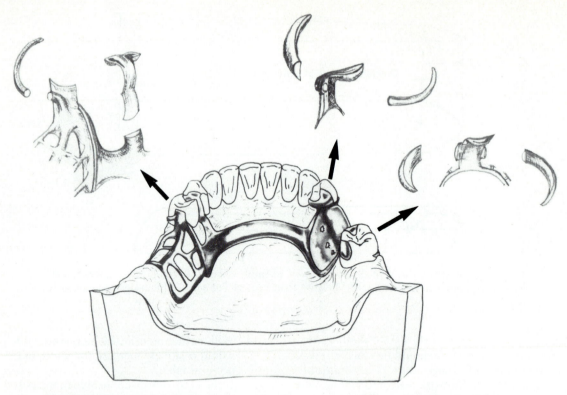

Fig. 6-13. Choice and definitive location of each component of direct retainer assembly must be based on preserving health of periodontal attachment in spite of rotational tendencies of distal extension denture. Knowledge of characteristics of each component of collective assemblies for a particular arch and rationalized rotational tendencies of denture simplifies design of removable restorations.

circumferential clasp arm, which approaches the retentive undercut from an occlusal direction. The other is the **bar clasp arm,** which approaches the retentive undercut from a cervical direction.

A clasp assembly may be a combination of cast circumferential and bar clasp arms and wrought-wire retentive arms in one of several possible combinations as illustrated in buccal and lingual views in Fig. 6-14.

No confusion should exist between the choice of clasp arm and the purpose for which it is used. Either type of cast clasp arm may be made tapered and retentive or rigid and nonretentive, depending on whether it is used for retention, stabilizing, or reciprocation. A clasp assembly should consist of (1) one or more minor connectors from which the clasp components originate,

(2) a principal rest, (3) a retentive arm engaging a tooth undercut only at its terminus, and (4) a nonretentive arm or other component on the opposite side of the tooth for reciprocation and stabilization against horizontal movement of the prosthesis. Rigidity of this clasp arm is essential to its purpose. An auxiliary occlusal rest may be used rather than a reciprocal clasp arm if it is located to accomplish the same purpose (Fig. 6-15). The addition of a lingual apron to a cast reciprocal clasp arm neither alters its primary purpose nor the need for proper location to accomplish that purpose.

BASIC PRINCIPLES OF CLASP DESIGN

Any clasp assembly must satisfy the basic principle of clasp design, which is that **more than 180 degrees of the greatest circumference of**

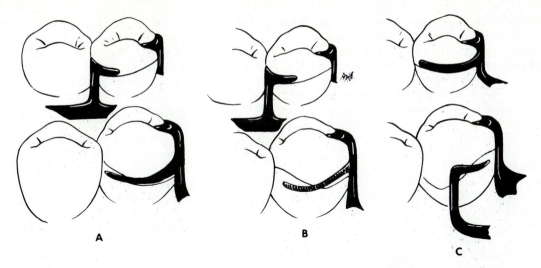

Fig. 6-14. Clasp assembly (mirrow views), including rest, may be combination of circumferential and bar clasp arms in one of several possible combinations. These mirror views are for abutments bounding a modification space. **A,** Cast circumferential retentive clasp arm with nonretentive bar clasp arm on opposite side for stabilization and reciprocation. **B,** Tapered wrought-wire circumferential retentive clasp arm with nonretentive bar clasp arm on opposite side for stabilization and reciprocation. **C,** Retentive bar clasp arm with nonretentive cast circumferential clasp arm on opposite side for stabilization and reciprocation.

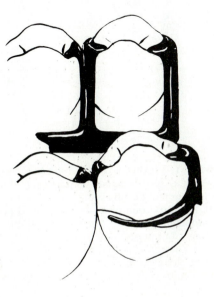

Fig. 6-15. Auxiliary occlusal rest (mirror view) may be used rather than reciprocal clasp arm without violating any principle of clasp design. Its greatest disadvantages are that second rest seat must be prepared and that enclosed tissue space results. Auxiliary occlusal rest is also sometimes used to prevent slippage when principal occlusal rest seat cannot be inclined apically from marginal ridge. Closure of interproximal space most often requires rests on adjacent teeth to avoid wedging effect when force is placed on denture.

the crown of the tooth must be included, passing from diverging axial surfaces to converging axial surfaces (Fig. 6-16). This may be in the form of continuous contact when circumferential clasp arms are used, or broken contact when bar clasp arms are used. **At least three areas of tooth contact must be embracing more than one half the tooth circumference.** These are the occlusal rest area, the retentive terminal area, and the reciprocal terminal area.

Other principles to be considered in the design of a clasp are as follows:

1. The occlusal rest must be designed so that movement of the clasp arms cervically is prevented.

2. Each retentive terminal should be opposed by a reciprocal arm or element capable of resisting any orthodontic pressures exerted by the retentive arm. Reciprocal and stabilizing elements must be rigidly connected bilaterally if reciprocation to the retentive elements is to be realized (Fig. 6-17).

3. Unless guiding planes will positively control the path of removal, retentive clasps should be bilaterally opposed; that is, buccal retention on one side of the arch should be opposed by buccal retention on the other, or lingual on one side opposed by lingual on the other. In Class II situations the third abutment may have either buccal or lingual retention. In Class III situations, retention may be either bilaterally or diametrically opposed.

4. The path of escapement of each retentive clasp terminal must be other than parallel to the path of removal of the prosthesis.

5. Amount of retention always should be the minimum necessary to resist reasonable dislodging forces.

6. **Clasp retainers on abutment teeth adjacent to distal extension bases should be designed so that they will avoid direct transmission of tipping and rotational forces to the abutment.** In effect, they must act as stressbreakers either by their design or by their construction. This is accomplished by proper location of the retentive terminal or by use of a more flexible clasp arm in relation to prospective rotation of the denture under varying directed forces.

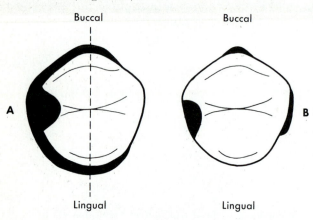

Fig. 6-16. **A,** Line drawn through illustration represents more than 180 degrees of greatest circumference of abutment from occlusal rest. Unless portions of lingual reciprocal arm and retentive buccal arm are extended beyond the line, clasp would not accomplish its intended purpose. If respective arms of retainer were not extended beyond the line, abutment could move away from retainer or removable partial denture could move away from abutment. **B,** Bar-type clasp assembly engagement of more than 180 degrees of circumference of abutment is realized by minor connector for occlusal rest, minor connector contacting guiding plane on distal proximal surface, and retentive bar arm.

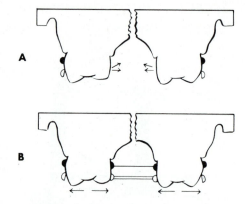

Fig. 6-17. **A,** Flexing action of retentive clasp arm initiates medially directed pressure on abutment teeth as its retentive tip springs over height of contour. **B,** Reciprocation to medially directed pressure is counteracted either by lingually placed clasp arms contacting abutments simultaneously with buccal arms and engaging same degree of undercut or by reciprocal elements of framework contacting lingual guiding planes when buccal arms begin to flex.

7. **Ideally, reciprocal elements of the clasp assembly should be located at the junction of the gingival and middle thirds of the crowns of abutment teeth. The terminal end of the retentive arm is optimally placed in the gingival third of the crown** (Figs. 6-18 to 6-20). These locations will permit the abutment teeth to better resist horizontal and torquing forces than they could if the retentive and reciprocal elements were located nearer the occlusal or incisal surfaces. As a metaphor, remember that a fencepost is more easily loosened by applying horizontal forces near its top than by applying the same forces nearer ground level.

The reciprocal clasp arm has three functions:

1. The reciprocal clasp arm should provide reciprocation against the action of the retentive arm. This is particularly important if the retentive arm is accidentally distorted toward the tooth, where it would become an active orthodontic force. The retentive clasp arm should be passive until a dislodging force is applied.

During placement and removal, reciprocation is most needed as the retentive arm flexes over the height of contour. Unfortunately the reciprocal clasp arm does not usually come into contact with the tooth until the denture is fully seated and the retentive clasp arm has again become passive, unless the abutment tooth has been specifically contoured. A momentary tipping force

is thus applied to the abutment during each placement and removal. This may not be a damaging force, since it is transient, so long as the force does not exceed the normal elasticity of the periodontal attachments. True reciprocation during placement and removal is usually possible only through the use of crown surfaces made parallel to the path of placement. The use of a ledge on a cast restoration permits the paralleling of the surfaces to be contacted by the reciprocal arm in such a manner that true reciprocation is made possible. This will be discussed in Chapter 13.

2. The reciprocal clasp arm should be located so that the denture is stabilized against horizontal movement. This is possible only through the use of rigid clasp arms, rigid minor connectors,

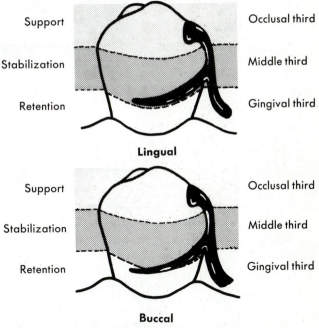

Fig. 6-19. Circumferential clasp on mandibular premolar (mirror view). *Support* is provided by occlusal rest; *stabilization* is provided by occlusal rest, proximal minor connector, lingual clasp arm, and rigid portion of buccal retentive clasp arm occlusal to height of contour; *retention* is realized by retentive terminal of buccal clasp arm; *reciprocation* is provided by nonflexible lingual clasp arm. Assembly engages more than 180 degrees of abutment's circumference.

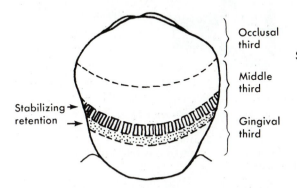

Fig. 6-18. Simple mechanical laws demonstrate that the nearer reciprocal-stabilizing and retentive elements of direct retainer assemblies are located to horizontal axis of rotation of abutment, the less likely that physiologic tolerance of periodontal ligament will be exceeded. Horizontal axis of rotation of abutment tooth is located somewhere in its root.

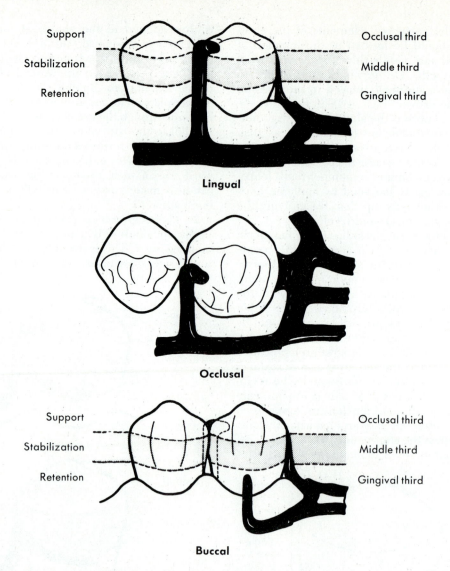

Fig. 6-20. Bar-type clasp on mandibular premolar. **Support** is provided by occlusal rest; **stabilization** is provided by occlusal rest and mesial and distal minor connectors; **retention** is provided by buccal I bar; **reciprocation** is obtained through location of minor connectors. Engagement of more than 180 degrees of circumference of the abutment is accomplished by proper location of components contacting axial surfaces.

and a rigid major connector. Horizontal forces applied on one side of the dental arch are resisted by the stabilizing components on the opposite side. These are not only the reciprocal clasp arms but also all rigid components contacting axial tooth surfaces. Obviously the great-

er the number of such components, within reason, the greater will be the distribution of horizontal stresses.

3. The reciprocal clasp arm may act to a minor degree as an indirect retainer. This is only true when it rests on a suprabulge surface of an abut-

ment tooth lying anterior to the fulcrum line. Lifting of a distal extension base away from the tissues is thus resisted by a rigid arm, which is not easily displaced cervically. The effectiveness of such an indirect retainer is limited by its proximity to the fulcrum line, which gives it a relatively poor leverage advantage, and by the fact that slippage along tooth inclines is always possible. The latter may be prevented by the use of a ledge on a cast restoration, but enamel surfaces are not ordinarily so prepared.

Circumferential clasp

Although a thorough knowledge of the principles of clasp design should lead to a logical application of those principles, it is better that some of the more common clasp designs be considered individually. The circumferential clasp will be considered first as an all-cast clasp.

The circumferential clasp is usually the most logical clasp to use with all tooth-supported partial dentures because of its retentive and stabilizing ability. Only when the retentive undercut may be approached better with a bar clasp arm or when esthetics will be enhanced should the latter be used (Fig. 6-21). The circumferential clasp arm does have the following disadvantages:

1. More tooth surface is covered than with a bar clasp arm because of its occlusal direction of approach.

2. On some tooth surfaces, particularly the buccal surface of mandibular teeth and the lingual surfaces of maxillary teeth, its occlusal approach may increase the width of the occlusal surface of the tooth.

3. In the mandibular arch more metal may be displayed than with a bar clasp arm.

4. As with all cast clasps, its half-round form prevents edgewise adjustment to increase or decrease retention. Adjustments in the retention afforded by a clasp arm should be made by moving a clasp terminal cervically into the angle of cervical convergence or occlusally into a lesser area of undercut. Tightening a clasp against the tooth or loosening it away from the tooth increases or decreases frictional resistance and does not affect the retentive potential of the clasp. **True adjustment is, therefore, impossible with most cast clasps.**

Despite its disadvantages the cast circumferential clasp arm may be used effectively, and many of these disadvantages may be minimized by proper design. Adequate mouth preparation will permit its point of origin to be placed far enough below the occlusal surface to avoid poor esthetics and increased tooth dimension (Fig.

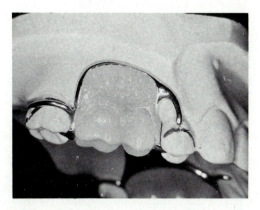

Fig. 6-21. Example of the two types of cast clasps in use. Molar abutment is engaged by circumferential clasp originating occlusal to height of contour, whereas premolar abutment is engaged by bar clasp originating from base gingival to height of contour. However, only terminal tip of this clasp is placed in measured undercut.

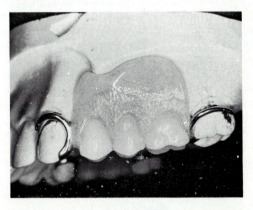

Fig. 6-22. Cast circumferential retentive clasp arms properly designed. They originate on or occlusally to height of contour, which they then cross in their terminal third, and engage retentive undercuts progressively as their taper decreases and their flexibility increases.

6-22). Although some of the other disadvantages listed imply that the bar-type clasp may be preferable, the circumferential type clasp is actually superior to a bar clasp arm that is improperly used or poorly designed. Experience has shown that the possible advantages of the bar clasp arm are too often negated by faulty application and design, whereas the circumferential clasp arm is less easily misused.

The basic form of the circumferential type clasp is a buccal and lingual arm originating from a common body (Fig. 6-23). **This clasp is used improperly when two retentive clasp arms originate from the body and occlusal rest areas and approach bilateral retentive areas on the side of the tooth away from the point of origin.** The correct form of this clasp has only one retentive clasp arm, opposed by a nonretentive reciprocal arm on the opposite side. A **common error** is to use this clasp improperly by making both clasp terminals retentive. This is not only unnecessary but also disregards the need for reciprocation and bilateral stabilization. Other common errors in the design of circumferential clasps are illustrated in Fig. 6-24.

Ring clasp. The circumferential type clasp may be used in several forms. One is the **ring-type clasp,** which encircles nearly all of a tooth from its point of origin (Fig. 6-25). It is used when a proximal undercut cannot be approached by other means. For example, when a mesiolingual undercut on a lower molar abutment cannot be approached directly because of its proximity to the occlusal rest area, yet cannot be approached with a bar clasp arm because of lingual inclination of the tooth, the ring clasp encircling the tooth allows the undercut to be approached from the distal aspect of the tooth.

The clasp should never be used as an unsupported ring (Fig. 6-26) because if it is free to open and close as a ring, it cannot provide either

reciprocation or stabilization. Instead the ring-type clasp should always be used with a supporting strut on the nonretentive side, with or without an auxiliary occlusal rest on the opposite marginal ridge. The advantage of an auxiliary rest is that further movement of a mesially inclined tooth is prevented by the presence of a distal rest. In any event the supporting strut should be regarded as being a minor connector from which the flexible retentive arm originates.

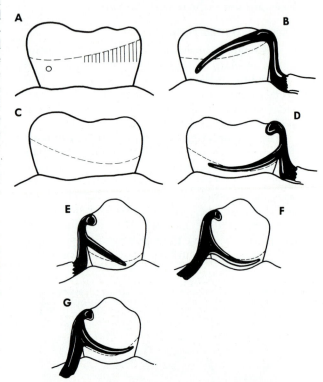

Fig. 6-24. Improper application of circumferential clasp design. **A,** Tooth with undesirable height of contour in its occlusal third. **B,** Unsuitable contour and location of retentive clasp arm on unmodified abutment. **C,** More favorable height of contour achieved by modification of abutment. **D,** Retentive clasp arm properly designed and located on modified abutment. **E,** Unsuitable contour and location of retentive arm in relation to height of contour (straight arm configuration provides poor approach to retentive area and is less resistant to dislodging force). **F,** Terminal portion of retentive clasp arm located too close to gingival margin. **G,** Clasp arm that is properly designed and located.

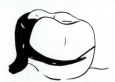

Fig. 6-23. Cast circumferential retentive clasp arm.

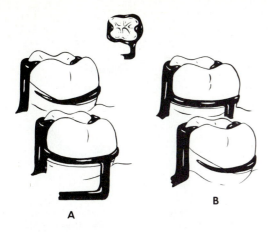

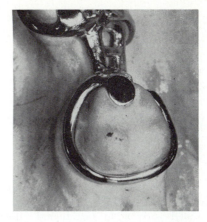

Fig. 6-25. Ring clasp(s) encircling nearly all of tooth from its point of origin. **A,** Clasp originates on mesiobuccal surface and encircles tooth to engage mesiolingual undercut. **B,** Clasp originates on mesiolingual surface and encircles tooth to engage mesiobuccal undercut. In either case supporting strut is used on nonretentive side (drawn both as direct view of near side of tooth and as mirror view of opposite side).

Fig. 6-26. Improperly designed clasp lacking necessary support. Such a clasp lacks any reciprocating or stabilizing action, since entire circumference of clasp is free to open and close. Instead, supporting strut should always be added on nonretentive side of abutment tooth, which then becomes, in effect, a minor connector from which tapered and flexible retentive clasp arm originates.

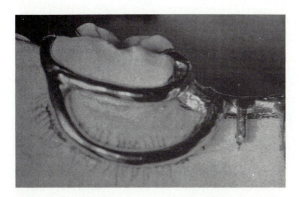

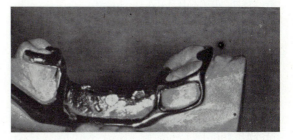

Fig. 6-28. Ring clasp engaging mesiobuccal undercut on mesially inclined lower right molar requires supporting bar on lingual surface to limit flexure to only retentive portion of clasp.

Fig. 6-27. Buccal strut supporting mesially originating ring clasp. Flexible retentive arm begins at distal occlusal rest and engages mesiolingual undercut. Despite its resemblance to bar-type clasp, this is a circumferential clasp by reason of its point of origin, the strut being actually an auxiliary minor connector.

Reciprocation then comes from the rigid portion of the clasp lying between the supporting strut and the principal occlusal rest (Figs. 6-27 and 6-28).

The ring-type clasp should be used on protected abutments whenever possible because it covers such a large area of tooth surface. Esthetics usually need not be considered on such a posteriorly located tooth.

A ring-type clasp may be used in reverse on an abutment located anterior to a tooth-bounded edentulous space (Fig. 6-29). Although potentially an effective clasp, this clasp covers an excessive amount of tooth surface and is esthetically objectionable. The only justification for its use is when a distobuccal or distolingual undercut cannot be approached directly from the oc-

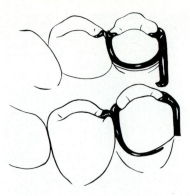

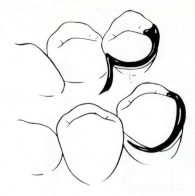

Fig. 6-29. Ring clasp may be used in reverse on abutment located anterior to toothbound edentulous space.

Fig. 6-30. Back-action circumferential clasp used on premolar abutment anterior to edentulous space. It is difficult to justify its use.

clusal rest area, yet tissue undercuts prevent its approach from a gingival direction with a bar clasp arm.

Back-action clasp. The **back-action clasp** is a modification of the ring clasp, with all of its disadvantages and no apparent advantages (Fig. 6-30). **It is difficult to ever justify its use.** The undercut can usually be approached just as well using a conventional circumferential clasp, with less tooth coverage and less display of metal. With the circumferential clasp the proximal tooth surface can be used as a guiding plane, as it should be, and the occlusal rest can have the rigid support it requires. An occlusal rest always should be attached to some rigid minor connector and should never be supported by a clasp arm alone. If the occlusal rest is part of a flexible assembly, it cannot function adequately as an occlusal rest. **Unfortunately the back-action clasp is still being used, despite the fact that it is biologically and mechanically unsound.**

Embrasure clasp. In the fabrication of an unmodified Class II or Class III partial denture there are no edentulous spaces on the opposite side of the arch to aid in clasping. Mechanically this is a disadvantage. However, when the teeth are sound and retentive areas are available or when multiple restorations are justified, clasping is accomplished by means of an **embrasure clasp** (Figs. 6-31 and 6-32).

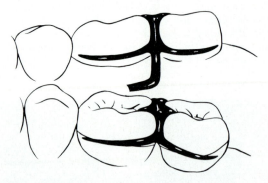

Fig. 6-31. Embrasure clasp is used where no edentulous space exists. Although in this drawing both retentive clasp arms are located on buccal surface and nonretentive arms on lingual surface, retention and reciprocation can be reversed on both teeth or on either tooth, depending on respective contours of the teeth. However, if second molar is sound and suitable stabilizing and retentive areas can be found, circumferential clasp may be used originating on distal surface of abutment.

Sufficient space must be provided between the abutment teeth in their occlusal third to make room for the common body of the embrasure clasp (Fig. 6-33), yet the contact area should not be eliminated entirely. Since vulnerable areas of the teeth are involved, abutment protection with inlays or crowns is indi-

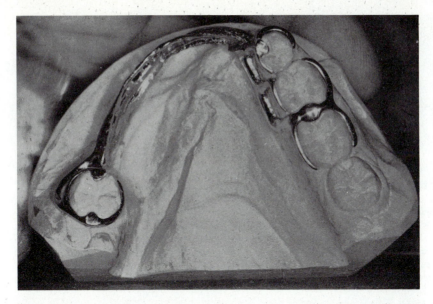

Fig. 6-32. Multiple clasping in surgically mutilated mouth. On the right are embrasure clasp, bar clasp arm, and conventional circumferential clasp engaging lingual undercuts on three abutment teeth. On the left is well-designed ring clasp engaging lingual undercut, with supporting strut on buccal surface and auxiliary occlusal rest to prevent mesial tipping. Note rigid design of major connector.

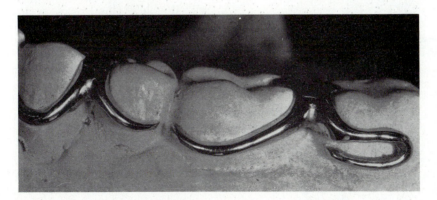

Fig. 6-33. Embrasure and hairpin circumferential retentive clasp arms. The terminus of each engages suitable retentive undercut. Use of hairpin-type clasp on second molar is made necessary by the fact that the only available undercut lies directly below point of origin of clasp arm.

cated in almost every instance. The decision to use unprotected abutments must be made at the time of oral examination and should be based on the age of the patient, caries index, and oral hygiene as well as on whether existing tooth contours are favorable. Preparation of adjacent, contacting, uncrowned abutments to receive any type of embrasure clasp of adequate interproximal bulk is difficult, especially when apposed by natural teeth.

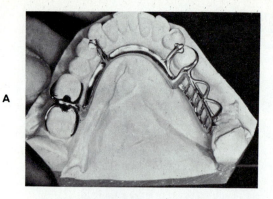 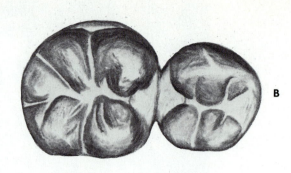

Fig. 6-34. A, Example of use of embrasure clasp for a Class II partially edentulous arch. Embrasure clasp on two left molar abutments was used in the absence of posterior modification space. **B,** Occlusal and proximal surfaces of adjacent molar and premolar prepared for embrasure clasp. Note that rest seat preparations are extended both buccally and lingually to accommodate retentive and reciprocal clasp arms. Adequate preparation confined to enamel can rarely be accomplished for such a clasp, especially when clasped teeth are opposed by natural teeth.

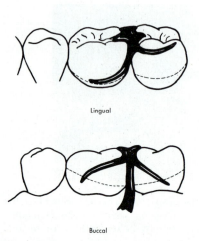

Fig. 6-35. Improper application of embrasure clasp design (mirror view). Failure to locate retentive and reciprocating-stabilizing arms in most advantageous positions (proper one third of crowns) is quite evident.

The embrasure clasp always should be used with double occlusal rests, even when definite proximal shoulders can be established (Fig. 6-34). This is to avoid interproximal wedging by the prothesis, which could cause separation of the abutment teeth and result in food impaction and clasp displacement. In addition to providing support, occlusal rests also serve to shunt food away from contact areas. For this reason occlusal rests should always be used whenever food impaction is possible.

Embrasure clasps should have two retentive clasp arms and two reciprocal clasp arms, either bilaterally or diagonally opposed. An auxiliary occlusal rest or a bar clasp arm can be substituted for a circumferential reciprocal arm as long as definite reciprocation and stabilization result. A lingually placed retentive bar clasp arm may be substituted if a rigid circumferential clasp arm is placed on the buccal surface for reciprocation, provided lingual retention is utilized on the opposite side of the arch. Common errors in the design of embrasure-type clasps are illustrated in Fig. 6-35.

• • •

Other modifications of the cast circumferential clasp are the multiple clasp, the half-and-half clasp, and the reverse-action clasp.

Multiple clasp. The **multiple clasp** is simply two opposing circumferential clasps joined at the terminal end of the two reciprocal arms (Fig. 6-36). It is used when additional retention is needed, usually on tooth-borne partial dentures. It may be used for multiple clasping in instances in which the partial denture replaces an entire half of the dental arch. It may be used rather than an embrasure clasp when the only available retentive areas are adjacent to each other. Its disadvantage is that two embrasure approaches are necessary rather than a single common embrasure for both clasps.

Half-and-half clasp. The **half-and-half clasp** consists of a circumferential retentive arm arising from one direction and a reciprocal arm arising from another (Fig. 6-37). Since the second arm must arise from a second minor connector, this arm is actually a bar clasp used with or without an auxiliary occlusal rest. Reciprocation arising from a second minor connector can usually be accomplished with a short bar or with an auxiliary occlusal rest, thereby avoiding so much tooth coverage. Thus it is apparent that there is little justification for the use of the half-and-half clasp in bilateral dentures. Its design was originally intended to provide dual retention, a principle that should be applied only to unilateral denture design.

Reverse-action clasp. The **reverse-action** or **hairpin clasp arm** is designed to permit engaging a proximal undercut from an occlusal approach (Fig. 6-38). Other methods of accomplishing the same result are with a ring clasp originating on the opposite side of the tooth or with a bar clasp arm originating from a gingival direction. However, when a proximal undercut must be used on a posterior abutment and when tissue undercuts or high tissue attachments prevent the use of a bar clasp arm, the reverse-action clasp may be used successfully. Although the ring clasp may be preferable, lingual undercuts may prevent the placement of a supporting strut without tongue interference. In this limited situation the hairpin clasp arm serves adequately, despite its several disadvan-

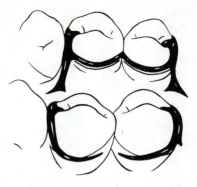

Fig. 6-36. Multiple clasp is actually two opposing circumferential clasps joined at terminal end of two reciprocal arms (mirror view).

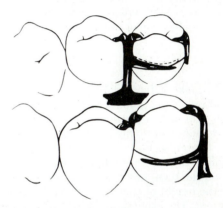

Fig. 6-37. Half-and-half clasp consists of one circumferential retentive arm arising from distal aspect and a second circumferential arm arising from mesial aspect on the opposite side, with or without secondary occlusal rest. Broken line illustrates nonretentive reciprocal clasp arm used without secondary occlusal rest (mirror view).

tages. The clasp covers considerable tooth surface and may trap debris; its occlusal origin may increase the functional load on the tooth, and its flexibility is limited. Esthetics usually need not be considered when the clasp is used on a posterior abutment, but the hairpin clasp arm does have the additional disadvantage of displaying too much metal for use on an anterior abutment.

Properly designed, the reverse-action clasp

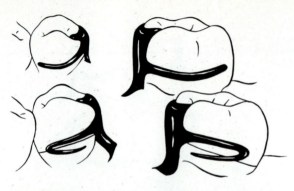

Fig. 6-38. Reverse-action or hairpin clasp arm may be used on abutments of tooth-borne denture when proximal undercut lies below point of origin of clasp (mirror view). It may be esthetically objectionable and covers considerable tooth surface and should be used only when a bar-type retentive arm is contraindicated because of a tissue undercut cervical to gingival margin.

should make a hairpin turn to engage an undercut below the point of origin (Fig. 6-38). The upper arm of this clasp should be considered a minor connector giving rise to the tapered lower arm. Therefore only the lower arm should be flexible; with the retentive portion beginning beyond the turn, only the lower arm should flex over the height of contour to engage a retentive undercut. The clasp should be designed and fabricated with this in mind.

These are the various types of cast circumferential clasps. As mentioned previously, they may be used in combination with bar clasp arms as long as differentiation is made by their location and bulk between retention and reciprocation. Circumferential and bar clasp arms may be made either flexible (retentive) or rigid (reciprocal) in any combination as long as each retentive clasp arm is opposed by a rigid reciprocal arm.

The use of many of the less desirable clasp forms can be avoided by changing the crown forms of the abutments with full restorations. In fabricating abutment coverage, tooth contours should be established that will permit the use of the most desirable clasp forms rather than reproduce a form that makes necessary the use of less desirable clasp designs.

Bar clasp

The term **bar clasp arm** is generally preferred over the less descriptive term **Roach clasp arm.** Reduced to its simplest terms, the bar clasp arm arises from the denture framework or a metal base and approaches the retentive undercut from a gingival direction (Fig. 6-21).

The bar clasp arm has been classified by the shape of the retentive terminal. Thus it has been identified as a T, modified T, I, Y, or almost any letter clasp arm. All have the same characteristics in common: they originate from the framework or base and approach the undercut from a gingival direction. **The form the terminal takes is of little significance as long as it is mechanically and functionally effective, covers as little tooth surface as possible, and displays as little metal as possible.**

The T and Y clasp arms are the most frequently misused. It is unlikely that the full area of a T or Y terminal is ever necessary for adequate clasp retention. Whereas the larger area of contact would provide greater frictional resistance, this is not true clasp retention, and only that portion engaging an undercut area should be considered retentive. Only one terminal of such a clasp arm is placed in an undercut area. The remainder of the clasp arm may be superfluous unless it is needed as part of the clasp assembly to encircle the abutment tooth more than 180 degrees of its greatest circumference, passing from diverging axial surfaces to converging axial surfaces. If the bar clasp arm is made to be flexible for retentive purposes, any suprabulge portion of the clasp will provide only limited stabilization, since it is also part of the flexible arm. Therefore in many instances the suprabulge portion of a T or Y clasp arm may be dispensed with, and the clasp terminal placed in an undercut. The terminal of the bar clasp should be designed to be biologically and mechanically sound rather than to conform to any alphabetical connotation.

A current concept of bar clasp design is the RPI system (rest, proximal plate, I-bar). There are a variety of philosophies on its application. Basically, however, the retainer consists of a **mesiocclusal rest** with the minor connector placed into the mesiolingual embrasure, but not contacting the adjacent tooth (Fig. 6-39, *A*). A distal

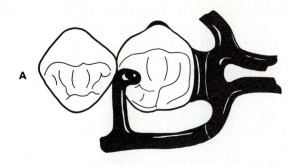

Fig. 6-39. Bar-type clasp assembly. **A,** Occlusal view. Component parts (proximal plate minor connector, rest with minor connector, and retentive arm) tripod abutment to prevent its migration. **B,** Proximal plate minor connector extends just far enough lingually so that together with mesial minor connector lingual migration of abutment is prevented. **C,** On narrow or tapered abutments (mandibular first premolars), proximal plate should be designed to be as narrow as possible but still sufficiently wide to prevent lingual migration. **D,** Only one terminal of retentive arm engaged undercut in gingival third of abutment.

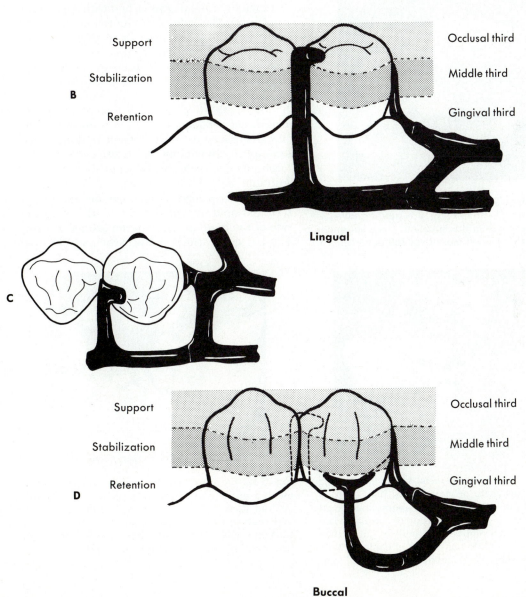

guiding plane, extending from the marginal ridge to the junction of the middle and gingival thirds of the abutment, is prepared to receive a **proximal plate** (Fig. 6-39, *B*). The buccolingual width of the guiding plane is determined by the contour of the tooth (Fig. 6-39, *C* and *D*). The proximal plate, in conjunction with the minor connector supporting the rest, provides the stabilizing and reciprocal aspects of the clasp as-

sembly. The **I-bar** should be located in the gingival third of the buccal or labial surface of the abutment in 0.01 inch undercut (Fig. 6-39, *C*). The whole arm of the I-bar should be tapered to its terminus with no more than 2 mm of its tip contacting the abutment. An approach arm must be located at least 4 mm from gingival margins and even more if possible.

In most situations the bar clasp arm can be used with tooth-borne partial dentures or tooth-borne modification areas or when an undercut that logically can be approached with a bar clasp arm lies on the side of an abutment tooth adjacent to a distal extension base (Figs. 6-40 to 6-44). If a tissue undercut prevents such use of a bar clasp arm, a mesially originating ring clasp, a cast, or a wrought-wire reverse-action clasp may be used. Preparation of adjacent abutments (natural teeth) to receive any type of interproximal direct retainer, traversing from lingual to buccal surfaces, is most difficult to adequately accomplish. Inevitably the relative size of the "occlusal table" is increased, contributing to undesirable and additional functional loading.

A bar clasp arm should not be used on a terminal abutment if the undercut lies on the side of the tooth away from the extension base. The bar clasp arm is not a particularly flexible

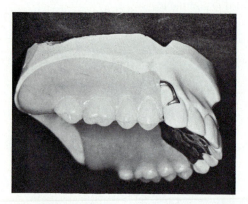

Fig. 6-40. Bar clasp arm properly used on terminal abutment. Mesial extension or T is neither advantageous nor desirable in this situation, since abutment tooth was encompassed more than 180 degrees.

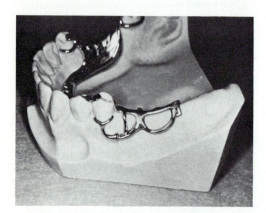

Fig. 6-41. Bar clasp arm on distal abutment must be made light enough to be flexible and may be used only when it can engage proximal undercut adjacent to extension base. Mesial T portion of clasp arm had to be placed to encompass abutment by more than 180 degrees. It is placed on height of contour. Note finishing line where clasp and denture base will join.

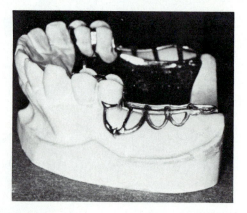

Fig. 6-42. Bar clasp arm on maxillary terminal abutment. Note uniform taper from point where it will emerge from resin base and that it engages tooth undercut on **side adjacent** to distal extension base. Butt-type joint for finishing line between direct retainer and acrylic resin base is provided.

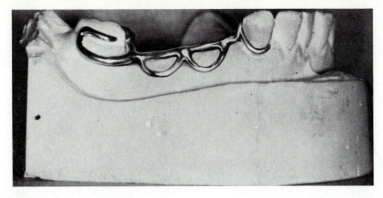

Fig. 6-43. Bar clasp arm on lower molar abutment engaging mesiobuccal undercut. Note proper use of parallel proximal guiding planes.

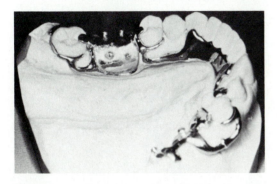

Fig. 6-44. Bar clasps used for both retention and re- ciprocation. Bar-type retainer on right second pre- molar engages distobuccal undercut. Bar-type config- uration on lingual aspect of the molar is used for re- ciprocation and stabilization and does not engage undercut.

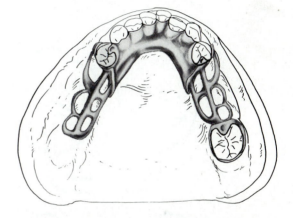

Fig. 6-45. Bar retainer is used on anterior abutment of modification space, and its terminus engages dis- tobuccal undercut. Denture will rotate around ter- minal abutments when force is directed toward basal seat on left. Such rotation will impart force on right premolar directed superiorly and anteriorly. How- ever, this direction of force is resisted in great part by mesial contact with canine. Direct retainer on right premolar engaging mesiobuccal undercut would tend to force tooth superiorly and posteriorly.

clasp arm because of the effects of its half-round form and its several planes of origin. Although the cast circumferential clasp arm can be made more flexible than can the bar clasp arm, the combination clasp is much preferred for use on terminal abutments when torque and tipping are possible because of engaging an undercut away from the distal extension base. Situations often exist in which a bar clasp arm may be used to advantage without jeopardizing a terminal abut- ment. A bar clasp arm swinging distally into the undercut is a logical choice, since movement of the abutment as the distal extension base moves tissueward is prevented by the distal location of the clasp terminal.

The specific indications for using a bar clasp arm are (1) when a small degree of undercut (0.25 mm) exists in the cervical third of the abut- ment tooth, which may be approached from a gingival direction, and (2) on abutment teeth when they support tooth-borne partial dentures or tooth-borne modification areas (Fig. 6-45). Thus use of the bar clasp arm is contraindicated when a deep cervical undercut exists or when a

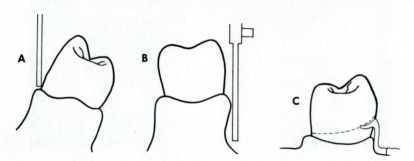

Fig. 6-46. Contraindications for selection of bar-type clasps. **A,** Severe buccal or lingual tilts of abutment teeth. **B,** Severe tissue undercuts. **C,** Shallow buccal or labial vestibules.

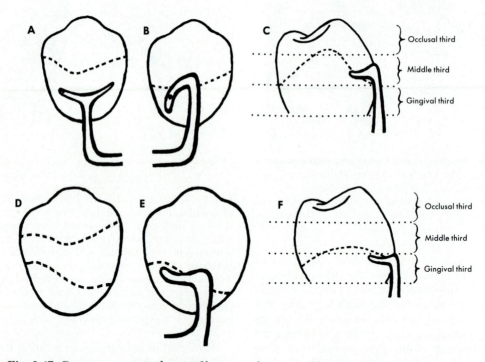

Fig. 6-47. Common errors in design of bar-type clasp assemblies. **A,** Survey line is unsuitable for bar clasp. **B,** Retentive portion of bar clasp arm improperly contoured to resist dislodging force in occlusal direction. **C,** Retentive tip not located in gingival third of abutment. **D,** Contour of abutment correctly altered to receive bar clasp. **E** and **F,** Correct position of bar clasp assembly.

severe tissue undercut exists, either of which must be bridged by excessive blockout. When severe tooth and tissue undercuts exist, a bar clasp arm usually is an annoyance to tongue and cheek and also traps food debris.

Other limiting factors in the selection of a bar clasp assembly include a shallow vestibule or an excessive buccal or lingual tilt of the abutment tooth (Fig. 6-46). Some common errors in the design of bar-type clasps are illustrated in Fig. 6-47.

There are several other types of bar clasps, one of which is the **infrabulge clasp.** It is designed so that the bar arm arises from the border of the denture base, either as an extension of a cast base or attached to the border of a resin base (Fig. 6-48). It is made more flexible than the usual bar clasp arm in that the portion of the cast base that gives rise to the clasp arm is separated from the clasp arm itself, either by a saw cut or by being cast against a separating shim

of matrix metal, which is later removed with acid. It may be made more flexible through the use of wrought wire, which either is attached to a metal base by soldering or is embedded in the border of a resin base.

Some of the advantages attributed to the infrabulge clasp are (1) its interproximal location, which may be used to esthetic advantage, (2) increased retention without tipping action on the abutment, and (3) less chance of accidental distortion resulting from its proximity to the denture border. The wearer should be meticulous in the care of a denture so made, not only for reasons of oral hygiene but also to prevent cariogenic debris from being held against tooth surfaces.

Combination clasp

The combination clasp consists of a wrought-wire retentive clasp arm and a cast reciprocal clasp arm (Fig. 6-49). Although the latter may

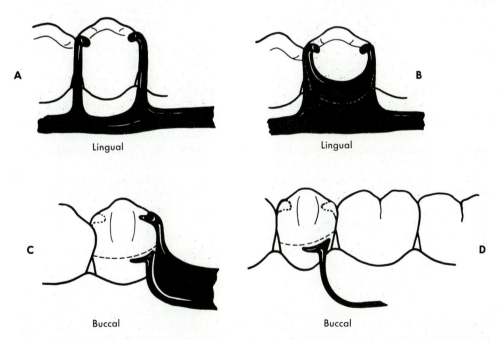

Fig. 6-48. Infrabulge clasp designed by M.M. DeVan (mirror view). **A** and **B,** Lingual aspect may be open or plated. DeVan recommended that two occlusal rests be used on each abutment. **C,** Clasp arm arises from border of metal base and is separated by saw cut or by having been cast against a metal shim, which is later removed. Wrought-wire retentive arm may be soldered to metal base to accomplish same purpose. **D,** Clasp arm is attached to buccal flange of acrylic resin denture base with autopolymerizing acrylic resin. This is usually a wrought-wire arm.

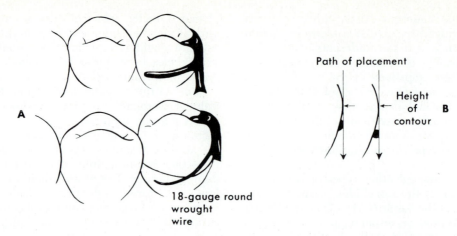

18-gauge round
wrought
wire

Path of placement

Height
of
contour

Fig. 6-49. A, Combination clasp consists of cast reciprocal arm and tapered, round wrought-wire retentive clasp arm. The latter is either cast to, or soldered to, cast framework. This design is recommended for anterior abutment of posterior modification space in Class II partially edentulous arch, where only a mesiobuccal undercut exists, to minimize the effects of first-class lever system. **B,** In addition to advantages of flexibility, adjustability, and appearance, wrought-wire retentive arm makes only line contact with abutment tooth, rather than broader contact of cast clasp.

be in the form of a bar clasp arm, it is usually a circumferential arm. The retentive arm is almost always circumferential, but it also may be used in the manner of a bar, originating gingivally from the denture base.

The advantages of the combination clasp lie in the **flexibility,** the **adjustability,** and the **appearance** of the wrought-wire retentive arm. It is used when maximum flexibility is desirable, such as on an abutment tooth adjacent to a distal extension base or on a particularly weak abutment when a bar-type direct retainer is contraindicated. It may be used for its adjustability when precise retentive requirements are unpredictable and later adjustment to increase or decrease retention may be necessary. A third justification for its use is its esthetic advantage over cast clasps. Being wrought in structure, it may be used in smaller diameters than may a cast clasp, with less danger of fracture. Since it is round, light is reflected in such a manner that the display of metal is less noticeable than with the broader surfaces of a cast clasp.

The most common use of the combination clasp is on an abutment tooth adjacent to a distal extension base where only a mesiogingival undercut exists in the abutment or where a gross

tissue undercut contraindicates a bar-type retainer. When a distal undercut exists that may be approached with a properly designed bar clasp arm or with a ring clasp (despite its several disadvantages), a cast clasp can be located so that it will not cause abutment tipping as the distal extension base moves tissueward. **When the undercut is on the side of the abutment away from the extension base, the tapered wrought-wire retentive arm offers greater flexibility than does the cast clasp arm and therefore better dissipates functional stresses. For this reason the combination clasp is preferred** (Fig. 6-50, *D*).

The combination clasp has two disadvantages: (1) the extra steps in fabrication, particularly when high-fusing chromium alloys are used, and (2) the fact that it may be distorted by careless handling on the part of the patient. The disadvantages of the wrought-wire clasp are offset by its several advantages, which are (1) its flexibility, (2) its adjustability, (3) its esthetic advantage over other retentive circumferential clasp arms, (4) the fact that a minimum of tooth surface is covered because of its line contact with the tooth rather than having the surface contact of a cast clasp arm, and (5) the fact that fatigue failures

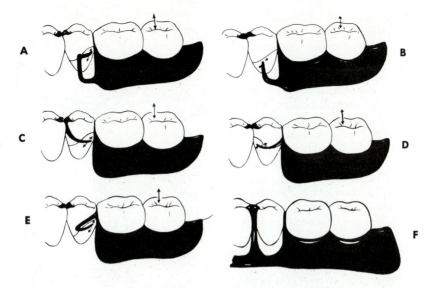

Fig. 6-50. Five types of extracoronal direct retainer assemblies that may be used on abutment adjacent to distal extension base to avoid or minimize the effects of cantilever design. Arrows indicate general direction of movement of retentive tips of retainer arms when denture base rotates toward and away from edentulous ridge. **A,** Distobuccal undercut engaged by one-half T-type bar clasp. Portion of clasp arm on and above height of contour will afford some stabilization against horizontal rotation of denture base. **B,** I bar placed in undercut at middle (anteroposteriorly) of buccal surface. This retainer contacts tooth only at its tip. Note that guiding plane on distal aspect of abutment is contacted by metal of denture framework and that mesial rest is used. **C,** Interproximal ring clasp engaging distobuccal undercut. Bar-type retainer cannot be used because of tissue undercuts inferior to buccal surface of abutment. **D,** Round, uniformly tapered 18-gauge wrought-wire circumferential retainer arm engaging mesiobuccal undercut. A wrought-wire arm, instead of a cast arm, must be used in this situation because of ability of wrought wire to flex omnidirectionally. Cast half-round retainer arm would not flex edgewise, resulting in excessive stress on tooth when rotation of denture base occurs. **E,** Hairpin clasp may be used when undercut lies cervical to origin of retainer arm. Both hairpin and interproximal ring clasps may be used to engage distobuccal undercut on terminal abutment of distal extension denture. However, distobuccal undercut on terminal abutment should be engaged by bar-type clasp in the absence of gross buccal tissue undercut cervical to terminal abutment. Hairpin and interproximal ring clasps are least desirable of clasping situations illustrated here. **F,** Lingual view shows use of double occlusal rests, connected to lingual bar by minor connector in illustrated designs. This design eliminates need for lingual clasp arm, places fulcrum line anteriorly to make better use of residual ridge for support, and provides stabilization against horizontal rotation of denture base.

in service are less likely to occur with the tapered wrought-wire retentive arm than with the cast, half-round retentive arm.

The disadvantages listed previously should not prevent its use regardless of the type of alloy being used for the cast framework. Technical problems are minimized by selecting the best wrought wire for this purpose and then either casting to it or soldering it to the cast framework. Selection of wrought wire, attachment of it to the framework, and subsequent laboratory procedures to maintain its optimal physical properties are presented in Chapter 11.

The patient may be taught to avoid distortion of the wrought wire by explaining that the fingernail should always be applied to its point of origin, where it is held rigid by the casting, rather than to the flexible terminal end. Frequently, lingual retention may be used rather than buccal retention, especially on a mandibular abutment, so that the wrought-wire arm is never touched by the patient during removal of the denture. Instead removal may be accomplished by lifting against the cast reciprocal arm located on the buccal side of the tooth. However, this negates the esthetic advantage of the wrought-wire clasp arm, and esthetics may be given preference when the choice must be made between buccal and lingual retention. In most cases, however, retention must be used where it is possible to create it and the clasp designed accordingly.

Lingual retention in conjunction with internal rests. The internal rest is covered in Chapter 5. It is emphasized that the internal rest is not used as a retainer but that its near-vertical walls provide for reciprocation against a lingually placed retentive clasp arm. For this reason visible clasp arms may be eliminated, thus meeting one of the principal objections to the extracoronal retainer.

Such a retentive clasp arm, terminating in an existing or prepared infrabulge area on the abutment tooth, may be of any acceptable design. It is usually a circumferential arm arising from the body of the denture framework at the rest area. It should be wrought, because the advantages of adjustability and flexibility make the wrought clasp arm preferable. It may be cast-to with gold or low fusing chromium-cobalt alloy or it may be assembled by being soldered to one of the higher fusing chromium-cobalt alloys. In any event, future adjustment or repair is facilitated.

The use of lingual extracoronal retention avoids much of the cost of the internal attachment yet disposes of a visible clasp arm when esthetics must be considered. Frequently it is employed with a tooth-supported partial denture only on the anterior abutments and, when esthetics is not a consideration, the posterior abutments are clasped in the conventional manner. (See Fig. 5-13.)

One of the dentist's prime considerations in clasp selection is the control of stress transferred to the abutment teeth when the patient exerts

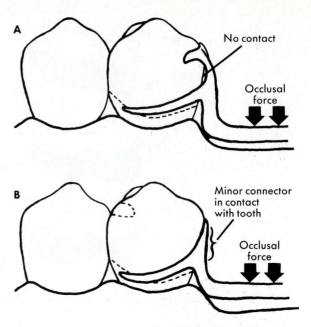

Fig. 6-51. **A,** Minor connector supporting distal rest does not contact prepared guiding plane, resulting in uncontrolled stress to abutment tooth. **B,** Minor connector contacts prepared guiding plane and directs stresses around arch through proximal contacts.

an occluding force on the artificial teeth. The location and design of rests, the clasp arms, and the position of minor connectors as they relate to guiding planes are key factors in controlling transfer of stress to abutments. Errors in the design of a clasp assembly can result in uncontrolled stress to abutment teeth and their supporting tissues. Some common errors and their corrections are illustrated in Figs. 6-51 and 6-52.

The choice of clasp designs should be based on biologic as well as mechanical principles. The dentist responsible for the treatment being rendered must be able to justify the clasp design used for each abutment tooth in keeping with these principles.

OTHER TYPES OF RETAINERS

Numerous other types of retainers for partial dentures have been devised that cannot be classified as being primarily of the intracoronal or

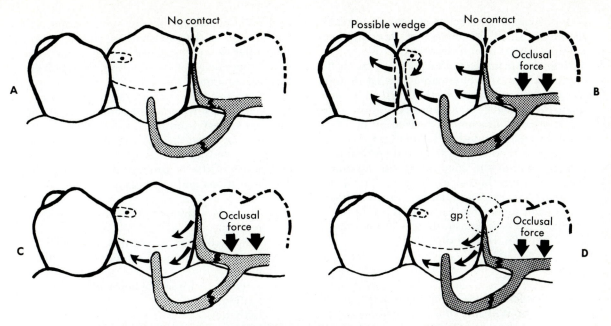

Fig. 6-52. A, Clasp assembly designed so that vertical occlusal force results in proximal plate moving cervically and out of contact with guiding plane as illustrated in **B.** This lack of contact may contribute to possible wedging effect. **C,** Extending contact of proximal plate on prepared guiding plane or as in **D,** eliminating space between artificial tooth and guiding plane (gp) will direct stresses around arch through proximal contacts.

extracoronal type. Neither can they be classified as relying primarily on frictional resistance or placement of an element in an undercut to prevent displacement of the denture. However, all these use some type of locking device, located either intracoronally or extracoronally, for providing retention without visible clasp retention. Although the motivation behind the development of other types of retainers has usually been a desire to eliminate visible clasp retainers, the desire to minimize torque and tipping stresses on the abutment teeth has also been given consideration.

All of the few retainers that will be discussed herein have merit, and much credit is due those who have developed specific devices and techniques for the retaining of partial dentures. Unfortunately not all can be included without devoting considerable space to the history and development of partial denture retaining devices. Also the use of patented retaining devices and other techniques falls in the same limited category as the internal attachment prosthesis and

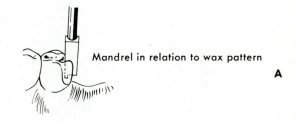

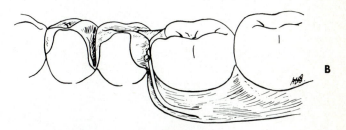

Fig. 6-53. Neurohr spring-lock attachment. **A,** Tapered mandrel used in surveyor to form vertical rest. **B,** Spring wire lock soldered to denture base, engaging depression in abutment tooth casting.

is, for economic and technical reasons, available to only a small percentage of those patients needing partial denture service.

Neurohr spring-lock attachment. One of the earlier attempts at eliminating partial denture clasps while at the same time providing adequate extracoronal retention was the spring-wire lock system of attachment devised by Dr. F.G. Neurohr and patented in 1930 (Fig. 6-53). The Neurohr method employs tapered vertical rests retained within the contours of the abutment tooth. A single buccal clasp arm, with a ball terminus, engages an undercut in the abutment casting and retains the partial denture in place. Occlusal stress is transmitted to the abutment tooth in a near vertical direction.

• • •

Dr. Franklin Smith's technique makes use of the Neurohr-Williams shoe in a manner similar to the Neurohr spring-lock attachment (Fig. 6-54). A single, short retentive clasp arm of 20-gauge wrought wire engages a small distobuccal,

horizontal groove in the abutment casting. The lateral walls of the rest shoe are parallel and as such offer some resistance to horizontal rotational tendencies of the denture. Additionally, this attachment permits some vertical rotation of the denture bases toward the residual ridges. It will also resist rotary displacement of the denture bases away from the residual ridges.

Smith has listed the following indications, advantages, contraindications, and disadvantages for his use of the Neurohr-Williams rest shoe. The indications and advantages claimed are as follows:

1. Stress-breaking action in respect to distal rotation
2. Lowered leverage point of applied force
3. Multiple options of retentive area placement
4. Internal reciprocal action and indirect retention
5. Esthetics
6. Stability, simplicity (in form)
7. Amenability to tilted teeth where "draw" is a problem with conventional approaches

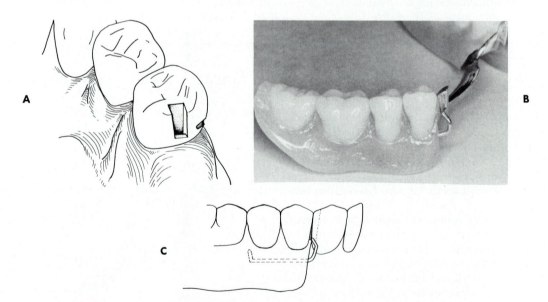

Fig. 6-54. **A,** Premolar abutment crown containing preformed rest seat. Groove one-half the depth of No. 557 bur is prepared at height of gingival seat of female portion. **B,** Retentive arm is fabricated from 20-gauge wrought wire. **C,** Assembled unit (schematic). Retentive arm is passive until dislodging force is applied to denture. (**B** courtesy Dr. Franklin Smith.)

8. Amenability to anterior abutments

The contraindications and disadvantages are as follows:

1. Anticipation of possible tooth (abutment) migration in an anterior direction
2. Preclusion where poor retentive qualities of an abutment casting are anticipated (for example, short or tapered crowns)
3. Any problem of inadequate crown length to retain the casting or house the intracoronal receptable (for example, short crown, deep impinging vertical overlap, large pulps)
4. Time, cost, and complexity of total procedure

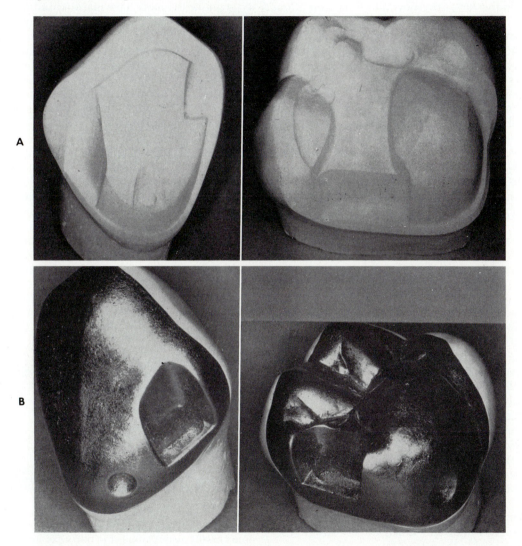

Fig. 6-55. A, Preparations for canine and molar abutment teeth on which dowel rest attachments will be constructed. **B,** Dowel rest attachments constructed on canine and molar abutment teeth. Note tapered nonlocking rest seat and dimple recessed in lingual surface, which will be engaged by corresponding boss on retentive arm of denture framework. (From Harris, F.N.: J. Prosthet. Dent. **5:**43-48, 1955.)

Dowel rest attachment. Dr. Morris J. Thompson and others have developed what is called the **dowel rest attachment** (Figs. 6-55 to 6-57). A boxlike rest seat is machined in the abutment casting for support of the partial denture, and a dimple is provided on the lingual surface of the abutment casting for retention. This dimple is engaged by a boss on a lingual arm on the denture framework, thereby affording retention without the use of a visible clasp arm. The lingual arm is an extension of the major connector, separated from it by a saw cut in the completed casting.

This attachment is most applicable to maxillary partial dentures, where the saw cut may be made in the palatal major connector. A stainless steel shim may be used rather than a saw cut to provide the necessary separation, which is then removed from the casting with acid. Flexibility of the retentive arm will be in proportion to its length as determined by the distance the separation is carried into the major connector.

The advantages that are given for this attachment are (1) no contact of the prosthesis with tooth structure, (2) stress-breaking effect resulting from the flexibility of the lingual arm engaging the dimple on the abutment casting, (3) hygienic contours, and (4) no visible clasp arms. One of the most obvious disadvantages of this type of attachment is the lack of other than minimum stabilization against horizontal movement of the partial denture. Abutment torque is avoided by making the rest seat free of any locking effect; but by so doing, since the only external arm is a flexible one, stabilization against horizontal movement may be minimal. Thus, as with many stressbreaker designs, the edentulous ridge is called on to resist horizontal movement of the prosthesis when only slightly aided by two opposing parallel walls and not by any rigid components located on the abutment teeth. The addition of anteriorly placed indirect retainers, one on each lingual side of the arch, seemingly would add much to the dowel rest denture.

A dowel rest attachment may be used in conjunction with a fixed partial denture (Fig. 6-58). It would not be a complicated procedure, provided the fixed restoration was fabricated in conjunction with the removable restoration. However, it is doubted that adequate preparation of the rest seat could be accomplished intraorally on an existing pontic. The attachment may also be used in the pontic involving only the lingual and lingual occlusal aspects of the pontic.

Internal attachments of the locking or dovetail type unquestionably have many advantages over the clasp-type denture for tooth-borne situations. It is, however, questionable whether the locking type of internal attachments for distal extension removable partial dentures are indicated, with or without stressbreakers and with or without splinted abutments, because of inherent excessive leverages most often associated with these attachments.

The nonlocking type of internal attachments, in conjunction with sound prosthodontic principles, can be advantagously used in many instances in Class I and II partially edentulous situations. However, unless the cross-arch axis of rotation is common to the bilaterally placed attachments, torque on the abutments may be experienced (Fig. 6-59). Excellent textbooks devoted to the use of manufactured intracoronal and extracoronal retainer systems are available. For this reason, this text concerns itself primarily with the extracoronal type of direct retainer assemblies (clasps).

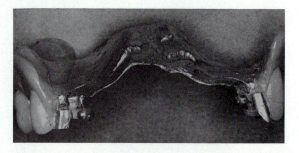

Fig. 6-56. Maxillary partial denture framework with nonlocking rest and lingual retentive arm originating from palatal major connector but separated from it with fine saw cut. Note boss on spring arm, which engages corresponding dimple in abutment restoration. (From Harris, F.N.: J. Prosthet. Dent. **5**:43-48, 1955.)

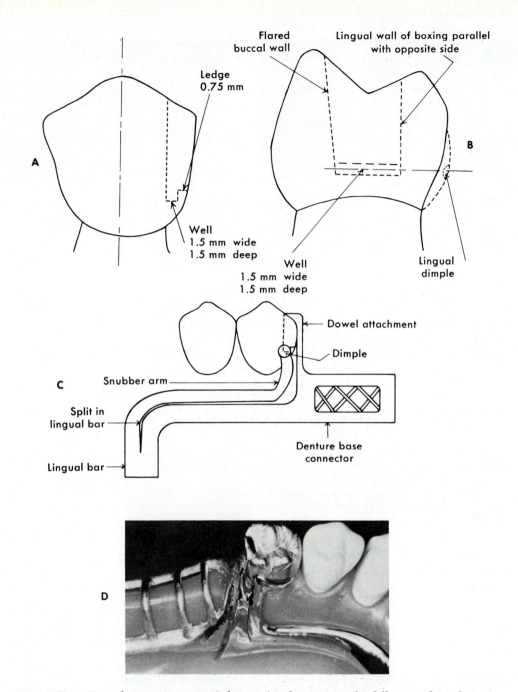

Fig. 6-57. **A,** Dowel rest preparation (schematic) in lower premolar full crown (buccal view). **B,** Proximal view (schematic) of dowel rest preparation and lingual dimple in lower left premolar full crown. **C,** Lingual view (schematic) of dowel rest attachment. Spring arm terminating in boss that engages dimple in abutment crown is separated from major connector by saw cut, or split lingual bar is cast around metal shim, which is later eliminated with acid. **D,** Removable partial denture framework incorporating construction specifications illustrated in **A, B,** and **C.** (**A** to **C** courtesy Dr. R.C. Van Dam; **D** courtesy Dr. L.E. Knowles.)

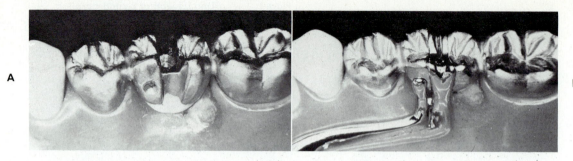

Fig. 6-58. A, Dowel rest preparation in pontic of fixed partial denture. Preparation provides for "snubber" arm on buccal surface of pontic to facilitate removal of denture by patient. **B,** Denture is in its resting position. Note that occlusal surface of pontic has been restored by the framework. (Courtesy Dr. L.E. Knowles.)

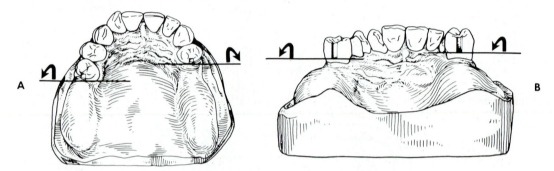

Fig. 6-59. A, Axes of rotation, although parallel, are not common because one axis is located anterior to other axis. **B,** When one nonlocking internal attachment is elevated farther from residual ridge than its cross-arch counterpart, the axes of rotation do not fall on a common line; thus some torquing of abutments should be anticipated. However, in many instances the effect produced by this situation will not exceed physiologic tolerance of supporting structures of abutments—all other torquing factors being equal.

SELF-ASSESSMENT AIDS

1. The framework of a removable partial denture must furnish **support, stabilization against horizontal (off vertical) movement, and mechanical retention.** How is mechanical retention accomplished?
2. What factor other than mechanical retention contributes to resistance of the denture to dislodging forces?
3. What is the function of a direct retainer (clasp)?
4. There are basically two types of direct retainers. Can you draw and label their component parts in correct positions on an abutment tooth?
5. Describe the principles by which the extracoronal direct retainer and the intracoronal retainer provide retention for the removable partial denture.
6. What is meant by the "height of contour" of an abutment tooth?
7. Draw a diagram of an abutment tooth and illustrate the angle of cervical convergence.
8. A direct retainer is an assembly of three components that perform individual function: (1) support, by a rest; (2) stabilization-reciprocation, by a clasp arm or other component; and (3) a retentive element. Do these elements necessarily have to arise from a common source?
9. Flexibility is permitted for only one component of a clasp assembly. Which one?
10. The amount of retention that a direct retainer is capable of generating depends on three factors. Can you visualize what these factors are?
11. The retentive arm of a direct retainer must be

flexible to engage an undercut in its terminal portion. Flexibility of the arm is a product of four physical and composition factors. Do you know what these important factors are?

12. Retention on all principal abutments should be as nearly equal as possible. To obtain this, which is the more important factor—the relation of the tip of the retentive arm to the height of contour or its depth in the angle of cervical convergence?

13. Can you describe the proportionate tapers of a cast, half-round retentive arm?

14. Can you describe the taper of a cast, half-round reciprocal-stabilizing arm of a direct retainer assembly? For what reason must there be a difference in form between a retentive arm and a reciprocal-stabilizing arm?

15. Name the two basic types of retentive clasp arms.

16. If a circumferential clasp arm approaches the retentive undercut from an occlusal direction, from which direction does a bar clasp arm approach the undercut?

17. A clasp assembly may be a combination of cast circumferential and bar clasp arms and wrought-wire retentive arms in one of several combinations. True or false?

18. A bar clasp arm is tapered in exactly the same way that a cast, half-round circumferential retentive clasp arm is tapered, differing only in configuration. Which arm is the more flexible if the two different arms are the same length? Why?

19. Permissible flexibilities of retentive cast circumferential and bar-type clasp arms based on length have been given in Table 6-1 in this chapter. Can a 0.7-inch bar-type arm be safely placed in the same depth of undercut that a 0.7-inch circumferential arm can? Based on the information contained in Tables 6-2 and 6-3, can you explain the differences between permissible flexibilities of duplicate retentive clasp arms made from a Type IV gold alloy and a chromium-cobalt alloy?

20. Cast clasp arms are essentially half-round in form, permitting flexing in only one direction. Which direction is this?

21. Wrought wire, 18-gauge round, is often used as a circumferential clasp arm. Its round form will permit flexing in what directions?

22. We speak of a reciprocal clasp arm. Can you explain what is meant by reciprocation and describe the condition that must be met for true reciprocation to occur?

23. A basic principle of direct retainer (clasp) design is that the retentive and reciprocal arms must encompass more than 180 degrees of the greatest circumference of the tooth, passing from diverging to converging axial surfaces. What would probably happen if a clasp designed otherwise was used?

24. Simple mechanical laws (of levers) demonstrate that the closer a direct retainer assembly is located to the tipping axis of the tooth, the less likely that the periodontal ligament will be taxed from rotation tendencies of the denture. Can you draw the coronal portion of an abutment, divide the enamel crown into thirds, and locate retentive, reciprocal, and stabilizing components optimally?

25. Clasp retainers on abutment teeth adjacent to distal extension bases should be designed so that they will avoid direct transmission of tipping and rotational forces to the abutment. Is this statement true or false?

26. The location of a usable undercut is perhaps the most important single factor in selecting a clasp for use with distal extension partial dentures. True or false?

27. There are many types and configurations of clasps. This can be most confusing, especially to the student dentist. However, if you will simply remember the three components necessary for a clasp assembly and their functions, locate the components to assure proper function, know that a distal extension denture will rotate under forces, and design accordingly, always thinking kindness to the periodontium, your difficulties in choosing the correct retainer will be minimized.

28. Under what circumstances may circumferential embrasure clasps be used? What are some real disadvantages of this type of retainer, including preparation of abutment teeth?

29. Give the indications for using a cast circumferential direct retainer.

30. What observations would lead you to select a bar-type clasp?

31. What is a combination clasp and what are the indications for its use?

32. State three advantages of the combination clasp.

33. Selection of wrought wire, attachment of it to the framework, and quality control in its use are discussed at the end of Chapter 11. You should have a thorough knowledge of the information presented there. It will assist you in decision making and maintaining quality control.

34. Nonlocking internal attachments we have used were discussed at the end of this chapter. Several good texts are available on manufactured intracoronal and extracoronal attachments. Self-assessment aids on internal attachments are not included in this text.

35. Can you visualize and name the most essential parts of a dental surveyor?

36. There are six factors that determine the amount of retention a clasp is capable of generating. One of these is the type of metal from which it is made. Can you name the other five?
37. How does **tilting** the cast affect the selected areas available for clasp retention?
38. The provisions for support and retention are two of the six basic principles of design of an extra-coronal retainer. What are the other four?
39. Can you visualize and draw four common errors in the design of a circumferential retainer? A bar-type retainer?
40. Would you agree that the single most important factor in selecting a type of direct retainer for a distal extension partial denture is the location of the undercut?

7 INDIRECT RETAINERS

Denture rotation about an axis
Factors influencing effectiveness of indirect
   retainers
Auxiliary functions of indirect retainers
Forms of indirect retainers
   Auxiliary occlusal rest
   Canine extensions from occlusal rests
   Canine rests
   Continuous bar retainers and linguoplates
   Modification areas
   Rugae support
   Direct-indirect retention

Movement of the base of an entirely tooth-borne partial denture **toward** the edentulous ridge is prevented primarily by rests placed on the abutment teeth located at each end of each edentulous space. Presuming that the denture framework is rigid and the rests are properly placed, occlusal forces are transmitted directly to the abutment teeth through the rests placed on those teeth. Movement of the base **away** from the edentulous ridge is prevented by the activation of the otherwise passive direct retainers on the same abutment teeth. Horizontal movement of the partial denture and longitudinal rotational movement of the denture base are prevented by stabilizing components on the same abutment teeth plus any auxiliary abutments contacted for stabilization. Rotation of the tooth-borne partial denture is therefore relatively non-existent.

In contrast, all Class I and Class II partial dentures having one or more distal extension bases are not totally tooth supported; neither are they completely retained by bounding abutments. Any Class III or Class IV partial denture that does not have adequate abutment support falls into the same category. These latter may

derive some support from the edentulous ridge and therefore may have a composite support from both teeth and ridge tissues.

Movement of a distal extension base **toward** the ridge tissues will be proportionate to the quality of those tissues, the accuracy and extent of the denture base, and the total functional load applied. Movement of a distal extension base **away** from the ridge tissues will occur either as a rotational movement about an axis or as displacement of the entire denture. The forces that tend to displace any denture are also the forces that cause rotation of a distal extension partial denture.

DENTURE ROTATION ABOUT AN AXIS

Presuming that direct retainers are functioning to prevent total displacement, rotational movement will occur about some axis as the distal extension base or bases either move toward or away from the underlying tissues. This axis is an imaginary line passing through teeth and direct retainers, around which line the denture rotates slightly when subjected to various forces directed toward residual ridges. It is called the

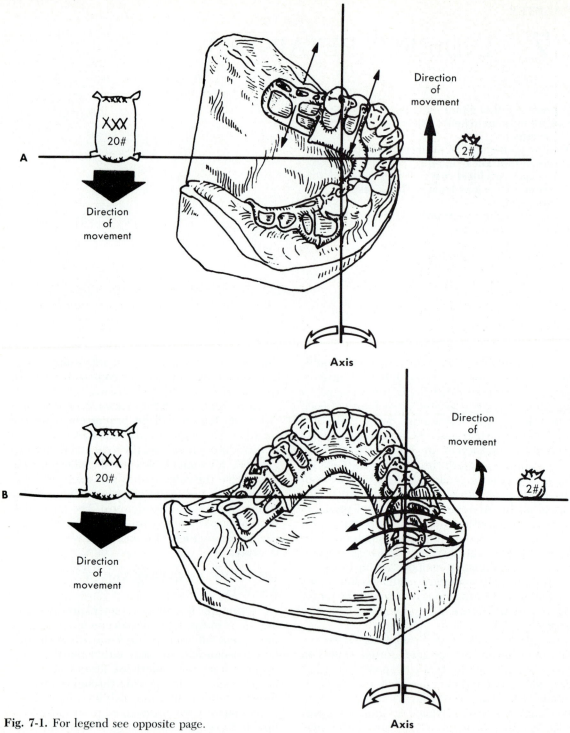

A

Direction of movement

Direction of movement

XXX 20#

2#

Axis

B

Direction of movement

Direction of movement

XXX 20#

2#

Axis

Fig. 7-1. For legend see opposite page.

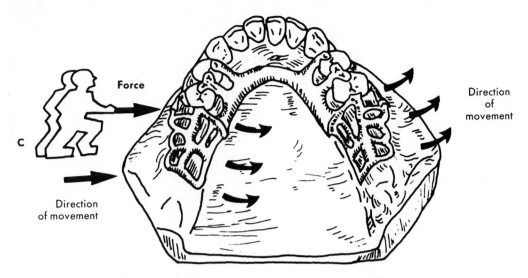

Fig. 7-1. Possible rotational movement of distal extension partial denture in function. **A,** On application of cervically directed force, rotation will occur around an imaginary line passing through second premolars. **B,** When cervically directed force is applied to one side only, rotation will occur around longitudinal axis formed by crest of residual ridge. **C,** Application of horizontal or off-vertical force results in rotation around an imaginary vertical axis. Vertical axes of rotation shift positions as direction and location of force applications change.

fulcrum line. More than one fulcrum line may be present for the same removable partial denture (Fig. 7-1).

The fulcrum line is identified on a Class I partial denture as passing through the rigid components of the direct retainer assemblies occlusal to the height of contour on the most posterior abutment on either side of the arch (Fig. 7-2, *A* and *B*). On a Class II partial denture the fulcrum line is always diagonal, passing through the abutment on the distal extension side and the most distal abutment on the other side (Fig. 7-2, *C*). If a modification area is present on that side, the additional abutment lying between the two principal abutments may be used for support of the indirect retainer if it is far enough removed from the fulcrum line (Fig. 7-2, *D*). In a Class IV partial denture the fulcrum line passes through the two abutments adjacent to the single edentulous space (Fig. 7-2, *E* and *F*). In a tooth- and tissue-supported Class III partial denture the fulcrum line is determined by considering the weaker abutment as nonexistent and that end of the base as being a distal extension (Fig. 7-2, *G* and *H*).

Movement of the denture base away from the tissues and about the fulcrum line is prevented by units of the partial denture framework that are located on definite rest seats on the opposite side of the fulcrum line from the distal extension base and the activation of the retentive element of the direct retainer assembly (Fig. 7-3). These anteriorly located components should be placed as far as possible from the distal extension base, affording the best possible leverage advantage against lifting of the distal extension base. Such units are called **indirect retainers.**

When the base(s) of an extension denture move away from the basal seat, an axis of rotation will pass through the most anteriorly located supporting elements of the denture framework, assuming that these anteriorly located elements are in their planned positions. In the absence of indirect retainers or components that function as indirect retainers, the axis of rotation will pass through the most posterior and bilaterally located tips of retainer arms engaging an undercut.

For the sake of clarity in discussing the location and functions of indirect retainers, fulcrum

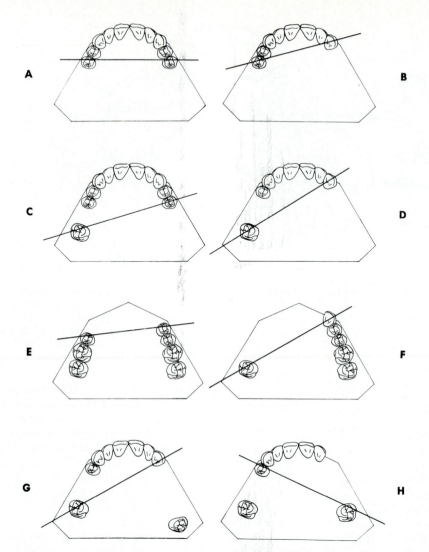

Fig. 7-2. Fulcrum line found in various types of partially edentulous arches, around which denture will probably rotate when bases are subjected to forces directed toward residual ridge. **A** and **B,** In Class I arch, fulcrum line passes through the most posterior abutments, provided some rigid component of framework is occlusal to abutments' heights of contour. **C,** In Class II arch, fulcrum line is diagonal, passing through abutment on distal extension side and the most posterior abutment on opposite side. **D,** If abutment tooth anterior to modification space lies far enough removed from fulcrum line, it may be used effectively for support of indirect retainer. **E** and **F,** In Class IV arch, fulcrum line passes through two abutments adjacent to single edentulous space. **G,** In Class III arch with posterior tooth on one side, which possibly will eventually be lost, fulcrum line is considered the same as though posterior tooth were not present. Thus its loss at some future date may not necessitate altering original design of the partial denture framework. **H,** In Class III arch with nonsupporting anterior teeth, adjacent edentulous area is considered to be tissue-supported end, with diagonal fulcrum line passing through two principal abutments as in Class II arch.

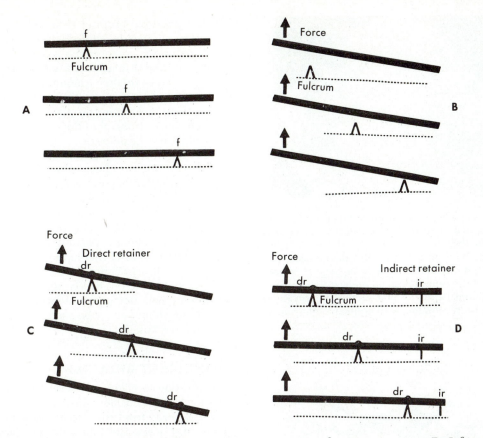

Fig. 7-3. Indirect retainer principle. **A,** Beams are supported at various points. **B,** Lifting force will displace entire beam in absence of retainers. **C,** With direct retainers at fulcrum, lifting force will depress one end of beam and elevate other end. **D,** With both direct and indirect retainers functioning, lifting force will not displace beam.

line should be considered the axis about which the denture will rotate when the bases move toward the residual ridge.

An indirect retainer consists of one or more rests and the supporting minor connectors (Figs. 7-4 and 7-5). Although it is customary to identify the entire assembly as the indirect retainer, it should be remembered that it is the rest that is actually the indirect retainer united to the major connector by a minor connector. This is to avoid interpreting any contact with tooth inclines as being part of the indirect retainer. **An indirect retainer should be placed as far from the distal extension base as possible in a prepared rest** seat on a tooth capable of supporting its function.

Whereas the most effective location of an indirect retainer is frequently in the vicinity of an incisor tooth, that tooth may not be strong enough to support an indirect retainer and may have steep inclines that cannot be favorably altered to support a rest. In such a case the nearest canine tooth or the mesial occlusal surface of the first premolar may be the best location, despite the fact that it is not as far removed from the fulcrum line. Whenever possible, two indirect retainers closer to the fulcrum line are then used to compensate for the compromise in distance.

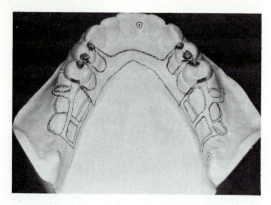

Fig. 7-4. Planning location for indirect retainers for Class I partial denture. The greatest distance from axis of rotation (fulcrum line) would fall on incisor teeth, which are ill-suited to provide adequate support without tooth movement or slippage of retainer or both. Dual occlusal rests on prepared rest seats at mesial marginal ridge of first premolars provide effective indirect retention with optimal tooth support.

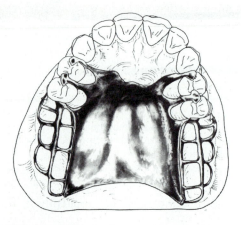

Fig. 7-5. Example of indirect retention used in conjunction with palatal plate–type major connector. Indirect retainers are located on first premolars. A secondary function of auxiliary occlusal rest assemblies is to prevent settling of anterior portion of major connector and to provide stabilization against horizontal rotation.

FACTORS INFLUENCING EFFECTIVENESS OF INDIRECT RETAINERS

The factors influencing the effectiveness of an indirect retainer are as follows:

1. Effectiveness of the direct retainers. Un-

less the principal occlusal rests are reasonably held in their seats by the retentive arms of the direct retainers, rotation about an axis will not occur, but total displacement will occur. Therefore an indirect retainer cannot activate the direct retainer to prevent lifting of the distal extension base away from the tissues.

2. Distance from the fulcrum line. Three areas must be considered:
   a. Length of the distal extension base
   b. Location of the fulcrum line
   c. How far beyond the fulcrum line the indirect retainer is placed

3. Rigidity of the connectors supporting the indirect retainer. All connectors must be rigid if the indirect retainer is to function as intended.

4. Effectiveness of the supporting tooth surface. The indirect retainer must be placed on a definite rest seat on which slippage or tooth movement will not occur. Tooth inclines and weak teeth should never be used for the support of indirect retainers.

AUXILIARY FUNCTIONS OF INDIRECT RETAINERS

In addition to effectively activating the direct retainer to prevent movement of a distal extension base away from the tissues, an indirect retainer may serve the following auxiliary functions:

1. It tends to reduce anteroposterior tilting leverages on the principal abutments. This is particularly important when an isolated tooth is being used as an abutment, a situation that should be avoided whenever possible. Ordinarily, proximal contact with the adjacent tooth prevents such tilting of an abutment as the base lifts away from the tissues.

2. Contact of its minor connector with axial tooth surfaces aids in stabilization against horizontal movement of the denture. Such tooth surfaces, when made parallel to the path of placement, may also act as auxiliary guiding planes.

3. Anterior teeth supporting indirect retainers are splinted against lingual movement.

4. It may act as an auxiliary rest to support a portion of the major connector. For example, a lingual bar may be supported against settling into the tissues by the indirect retainer acting as an auxiliary rest. One must be able to differentiate between an auxiliary rest placed for sup-

port for a major connector, one placed for indirect retention, and one serving a dual purpose. Some auxiliary rests are added solely to provide rest support to a segment of the denture and should not be confused with indirect retention.

5. It may provide the first visual indications for the need to reline an extension base partial denture. Deficiencies in basal seat support are manifested by the dislodgement of indirect retainers from their prepared rest seats when the denture base is depressed.

FORMS OF INDIRECT RETAINERS

The indirect retainer may take any one of several forms. All are effective in proportion to their **support** and the **distance from the fulcrum line.**

Auxiliary occlusal rest

The most frequently used indirect retainer is an auxiliary occlusal rest located on an occlusal surface as far away from the distal extension base as possible. In a mandibular Class I arch this is usually on the mesial marginal ridge of the first premolar on each side (Fig. 7-4). The longest perpendicular to the fulcrum line would be in the vicinity of the central incisors, which are too weak and have lingual surfaces that are too per-

pendicular to support a rest. Bilateral rests on the first premolars are quite effective, even though located closer to the axis of rotation.

The same principle applies to any maxillary Class I partial denture when indirect retainers are used. Bilateral rests on the mesial marginal ridge of the first premolars are generally used in preference to rests on incisor teeth (Fig. 7-5). Not only are they effective without jeopardizing the weaker single-rooted teeth, but also interference with the tongue is far less when the minor connector can be placed in the embrasure between canine and premolar rather than anterior to the canine teeth.

Indirect retainers for Class II partial dentures are usually placed on the marginal ridge of the first premolar tooth on the opposite side of the arch from the distal extension base (Fig. 7-6). Bilateral rests are seldom indicated except when an auxiliary occlusal rest is needed for support of the major connector or when the prognosis of the distal abutment is poor and provision is being considered for later conversion.

Canine extensions from occlusal rests

Occasionally a finger extension from a premolar rest is placed on the prepared lingual slope of the adjacent canine tooth (Fig. 7-7). Such an extension is used to effect indirect retention by increasing the distance of a resisting element from the fulcrum line. This is particu-

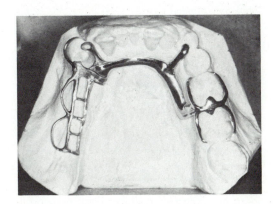

Fig. 7-6. Mandibular Class II design using embrasure clasp on nonedentulous side. Indirect retainer on distal marginal ridge of rotated first premolar is favorably located in relation to fulcrum line. Note use of wrought-wire retentive clasp arm on buccal surface of left first premolar. Bar-type retainer could not be used because of presence of gross tissue undercut (buccal) below first premolar and absence of usable undercut on its distobuccal surface.

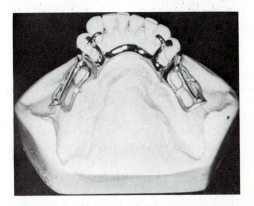

Fig. 7-7. Mandibular Class I design using canine extensions from occlusal rests as indirect retainers. Canine extensions must be placed in prepared rest seats so that resistance will be directed as nearly as possible along long axes of canine abutments.

larly applicable when a first premolar must serve as a primary abutment. The distance anterior to the fulcrum line is only the distance between the mesial occlusal rest and the anterior terminal of the finger extension. In this instance, although the extension rests on a prepared surface, it is used in conjunction with a terminal rest on the mesial marginal ridge of the premolar tooth. Tipping leverage on the canine tooth is predominantly avoided. **Even when not used as indirect retainers, canine extensions, continuous bar retainers, and linguoplates should never be used without terminal rests because of the resultant forces effective when they are placed on inclined planes alone.**

Canine rests

When the mesial marginal ridge of the first premolar is too close to the fulcrum line or when the teeth are lapped so that the fulcrum line is not accessible, a rest on the adjacent canine tooth may be used. Such a rest may be made more effective by placing the minor connector in the embrasure anterior to the canine, either curving back onto a prepared lingual rest seat or extending to a mesioincisal rest. The same types of canine rests as those previously outlined, which are the lingual or incisal rests, may be used. (See Chapter 5.)

Continuous bar retainers and linguoplates

Technically, continuous bar retainers and linguoplates are not indirect retainers, since they rest on unprepared lingual inclines of anterior teeth. The indirect retainers are actually the terminal rests at either end in the form of auxiliary occlusal rests or canine rests.

In Class I and Class II partial dentures a continuous bar retainer or linguoplate may extend the effectiveness of the indirect retainer if used with a terminal rest at each end. In tooth-borne partial dentures they are placed for other reasons but always with terminal rests. (See Chapter 4.)

In Class I and Class II partial dentures especially, a continuous bar retainer or the superior border of the linguoplate should never be placed above the middle third of the teeth so that orthodontic movement during the rotation of a distal extension denture is avoided. This is not so important when the six anterior teeth are in nearly a straight line, but when the arch is narrow and tapering, a continuous bar retainer or linguoplate on anterior teeth extends well beyond the terminal rests, and orthodontic movement of those teeth is more likely. Whereas these are intended primarily to stabilize weak anterior teeth, they may have the opposite effect if not used with discretion.

Modification areas

Occasionally the occlusal rest on a secondary abutment in a Class II partial denture may be used also as an indirect retainer. This will depend on how far from the fulcrum line the secondary abutment is located.

The primary abutments in a Class II, modification 1, partial denture are the abutment adjacent to the distal extension base and the most distal abutment on the tooth-borne side. The fulcrum line is a diagonal axis between the two terminal abutments (Fig. 7-8).

The anterior abutment on the tooth-borne side is a secondary abutment, serving to support and retain one end of the tooth-borne segment, as well as adding horizontal stabilization to the denture. If the modification space were not present, as in an unmodified Class II arch, auxiliary

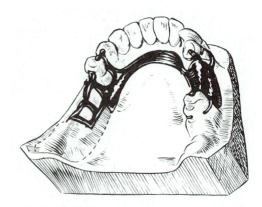

Fig. 7-8. Class II, modification 1, removable partial denture framework. Fulcrum line, when denture base is displaced toward residual ridge, runs from left second premolar to right second molar. When forces tend to displace denture away from its basal seat, supportive element of direct retainer assembly on right first premolar "acts" as indirect retainer.

occlusal rests and stabilizing components would still be essential to the design of the denture (Fig. 7-9). However, the presence of a modification space conveniently provides an abutment tooth for retention, stabilization, and support.

If the occlusal rest on the secondary abutment lies far enough from the fulcrum line, it may serve adequately as an indirect retainer. Its dual function then is tooth support for one end of the modification area and support for an indirect retainer. The most typical example is a distal occlusal rest on a first premolar when a second premolar and first molar are missing and the second molar serves as one of the primary abutments. The longest perpendicular to the fulcrum line falls in the vicinity of the first premolar, making the location of the indirect retainer nearly ideal.

On the other hand, if only one tooth, such as a first molar, is missing on the modification side, the occlusal rest on the second premolar abutment is too close to the fulcrum line to be effective. In such a case an auxiliary occlusal rest on the mesial marginal ridge of the first premolar is needed, both for indirect retention and for support for an otherwise unsupported major connector.

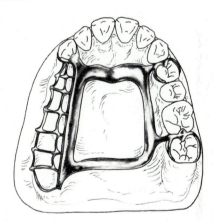

Fig. 7-9. Class II maxillary removable partial denture framework design. Fulcrum line runs from patient's right canine to left second molar. Forces that tend to unseat denture from its basal seat will be resisted by activation of retentive elements on canine and molar, using supportive elements on first premolar as terminus of resistance arm.

Support for a modification area extending anteriorly to a canine abutment is obtained by any one of the accepted canine rest forms, as previously outlined. In this situation the canine tooth provides nearly ideal indirect retention and support for the major connector as well.

Rugae support

Some authorities consider coverage of the rugae area of the maxillary arch as a means of indirect retention, since the rugae area is firm and usually well situated to provide indirect retention for a Class I denture. Although it is true that broad coverage over the rugae area can conceivably provide some support, the facts remain that tissue support is less effective than positive tooth support and that rugae coverage is undesirable if it can be avoided.

The use of rugae support for indirect retention is usually part of a palatal horseshoe design. Since posterior retention is usually inadequate in this situation, the requirements for indirect retention are probably greater than can be satisfied by tissue support alone.

Direct-indirect retention

In the mandibular arch, retention from the distal extension base alone is usually inadequate to prevent lifting of the base away from the tissues. In the maxillary arch, where only anterior teeth remain, full palatal coverage is usually necessary. In fact, with any Class I partial denture extending distally from the first premolar teeth, except when a maxillary torus prevents its use, palatal coverage may be used to advantage. While complete coverage may be in the form of a resin base, the added retention and lesser bulk of the cast metal palate makes the latter preferable. (See Chapter 4.) However, in the absence of full palatal coverage an indirect retainer should be used with other designs of major palatal connectors for the Class I removable partial denture.

SELF-ASSESSMENT AIDS

1. What elements prevent movement of the base(s) of a tooth-borne denture toward the basal seats?
2. Support of a distal extension removable partial denture is shared by abutment teeth and residual ridges. The quality of support furnished by the

residual ridges is proportionate to at least three factors. Can you name them?

3. Movement of a distal extension base away from basal seats will occur as a rotational movement or _____?

4. What is the difference between fulcrum line and axis of rotation?

5. Can you identify the fulcrum line on a Class I arch? Class II, modification 1? Class IV?

6. Define the term **indirect retainer.**

7. What components of a removable partial denture framework usually make an indirect retainer?

8. From the standpoint of leverage advantage, where should an indirect retainer be located?

9. An indirect retainer performs one major function and four auxiliary functions. Can you state these five functions?

10. The effectiveness of an indirect retainer is influenced by four factors. What are they?

11. What are the probable sequelae of trying to use a continuous bar retainer or linguoplate to serve the purpose of an indirect retainer?

12. In a Class II, modification 1 arch, especially if the modification is a long edentulous space, what component may act as an indirect retainer?

13. Discuss the inadequacy of using coverage of rugae to act as support for indirect retention.

14. Each design of the extension type removable partial denture should include an indirect retainer or some component that will act as an indirect retainer. True or false?

15. Bilaterally placed indirect retainers contribute to stability of the Class I restoration to a greater extent than does a single indirect retainer. True or false?

CHAPTER

8 DENTURE BASE CONSIDERATIONS

FUNCTIONS OF DENTURE BASES

The denture base supports artificial teeth and effects the transfer of occlusal forces to supporting oral structures (Fig. 8-1).

Although its primary purpose is related to masticatory function, the denture base also may add to the cosmetic effect of the replacement, particularly when modern techniques for tinting and the reproducing of natural looking contours are used. Most of the modern techniques for creating naturalness in complete denture bases are applicable equally well to partial denture bases.

Still another function of the denture base is the stimulation, by massage, of the underlying tissues of the residual ridge. Some vertical movement occurs with any denture base, even those supported entirely by abutment teeth, because of the physiologic movement of those teeth under function. It is clearly evident that oral tissues placed under functional stress within their physiologic tolerance maintain their form and tone better than similar tissues suffering from disuse. The term **disuse atrophy** is applicable to both periodontal tissues and the tissues of a residual ridge.

Tooth-supported partial denture base

Denture bases differ in functional purpose and may differ in the material of which they are made. In a tooth-borne prosthesis the denture base is primarily a span between two abutments supporting artificial occlusal surfaces. Thus occlusal forces are transferred directly to the abutment teeth through rests. Also, the denture base and the supplied teeth serve to prevent horizontal migration of the teeth in the partially edentulous arch and vertical migration of teeth in the opposing arch.

When only posterior teeth are being replaced, esthetics is usually a secondary consideration. On the other hand, when anterior teeth are replaced, esthetics may be of primary importance. Except for esthetic considerations, the tooth-borne partial denture base is essentially a framework supporting occlusal surfaces. Theoretically, occlusal surfaces alone would accomplish masticatory efficiency and maintain the relative position of the natural teeth. However, they would lack desirable esthetics, create undesirable food traps, and deprive the tissues of the stimulation by massage that they would receive from an accurate denture base. The reasons then

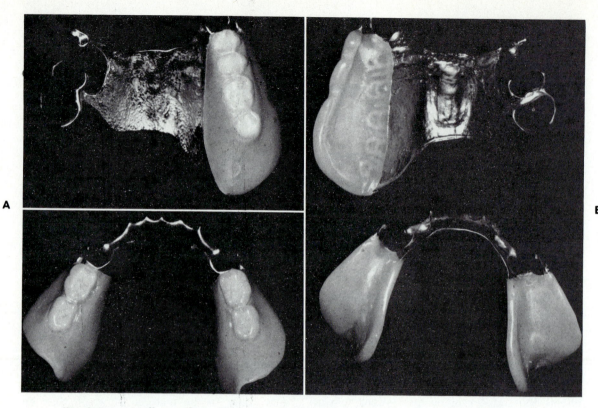

Fig. 8-1. A, Maxillary and mandibular distal extension removable partial dentures with acrylic resin denture bases. Posterior artificial teeth are attached to bases. **B,** Tissue sides of restorations in **A.** Bases are extended within limits of physiologic activity of surrounding oral structures.

for providing more than only the necessary support for occlusal surfaces in a tooth-borne denture are (1) esthetics, (2) cleanliness, and (3) stimulation of underlying tissues.

Distal extension partial denture base

In a distal extension partial denture the denture bases other than those in tooth-supported modifications must contribute to the support of the denture. Close to the terminal abutment only a framework supporting occlusal surfaces is necessary. However, farther from the abutment the support from the underlying ridge tissues becomes increasingly important. Maximum support from the residual ridge may be obtained only by using broad, accurate denture bases, which spread the occlusal load equitably over

the entire area available for such support. The space available for a denture base is controlled by the structures surrounding the space and their movement during function. Maximum support for the denture base therefore can be accomplished only by using knowledge of the limiting anatomic structures, knowledge of the histologic nature of the basal seat areas, accuracy of the impression, and accuracy of the denture base (Fig. 8-2). A principle as old as the snowshoe is that broad coverage furnishes the best support with the least load per unit area. Therefore support should be the primary consideration in selecting, designing, and fabricating a distal extension partial denture base. Of secondary importance but to be considered nevertheless are esthetics, stimulation of the un-

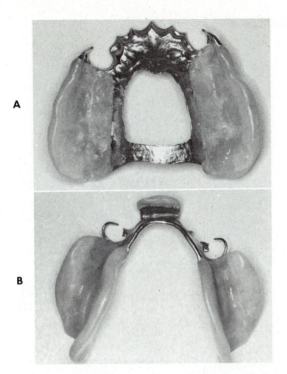

Fig. 8-2. A, Maxillary bilateral distal extension removable partial denture with acrylic resin denture bases. Bases are extended buccally within physiologic tolerance of border structures, and they cover tuberosities being extended into pterygomaxillary notches. **B,** Manidbular bilateral distal extension removable partial denture with acrylic resin denture bases. As in **A,** bases are fully extended. Lingual flanges are extended into retromylohyoid fossae. Impression procedure used established buccal shelves as primary stress-bearing areas of basal seats.

derlying tissues, and oral cleanliness. Methods we have used to accomplish maximum support of the restoration through its base(s) are presented in Chapter 14.

In addition to their difference in functional purposes, denture bases vary in material of construction. This is related to their function because of the need for future relining in one instance and usually not in another.

Since the tooth-supported base has an abutment tooth at each end on which a rest has been placed, future relining or rebasing may not be necessary to reestablish support. Relining is necessary only when tissue changes have occurred

beneath the tooth-borne base to the point that poor esthetics and accumulation of debris result. For these reasons alone, tooth-borne bases made soon after extractions should be constructed of a material that permits later relining. Such materials are the denture resins, the most common of which are copolymer and methyl methacrylate resins.

METHODS OF ATTACHING DENTURE BASES

Resin bases are attached to the partial denture framework by means of a minor connector designed so that a space exists between it and the underlying tissues of the residual ridge (Fig. 8-3). Relief of at least a 20-gauge thickness over the basal seat areas of the master cast is used to create a raised platform on the investment cast on which the pattern for the retentive frame is formed. Thus after casting, the portion of the retentive framework to which the resin base will be attached will stand away from the tissue surface sufficiently to permit a flow of resin base material beneath the surface.

The retentive framework for the base should be embedded in the base material with sufficient thickness of resin (1.5 mm) to allow for relieving if this becomes necessary during denture adjustment over tender areas or during relining procedures. Thickness is also necessary to avoid weakness and subsequent fracture of the resin base material surrounding the metal framework.

The use of plastic mesh patterns in forming the retentive framework is generally less satisfactory than a more open framework (Fig. 8-4). Less weakening of the resin by the embedded framework results from the use of the more open form. Pieces of 12- or 14-gauge half-round wax and 18-gauge round wax are therefore used to form a ladderlike framework rather than the finer latticework of the mesh pattern. The precise design of the retentive framework, other than that it should be located both buccally and lingually, is not so important as its effective rigidity and strength when embedded in the resin base—free of interference with future adjustment and with arrangement of artificial teeth and open enough to avoid weakening any portion of the attached resin (Fig. 8-5). Designing the retentive framework for a denture base by

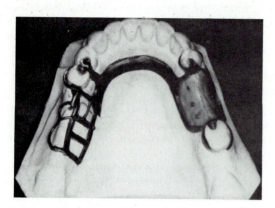

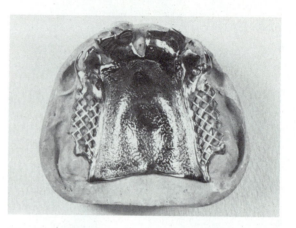

Fig. 8-3. Mandibular Class II, modification 1, design wax pattern developed on investment cast. Adequate provision is made for attaching major connector to resin base on edentulous side by way of ladderlike minor connector and butt-type joint. Cast base will be used for modification space. Note finishing lines on cast base pattern and "nail-head" minor connectors for retention of acrylic resin supporting prosthetically supplied teeth.

Fig. 8-4. Minor connectors to attach acrylic resin denture bases to this framework were made using plastic mesh pattern. Although rigid and possessing adequate strength, bulk of connector itself may contribute to weakening of acrylic resin base. A more open type of minor connector as illustrated in Fig. 8-6 seems preferable.

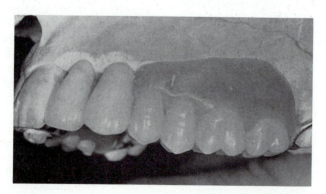

Fig. 8-5. Replaced lateral incisor and canine are abutted to residual ridge for better esthetics. Occasionally first premolar is treated similarly, depending on how visible this tooth is. Retentive framework for resin base must be designed so that interference with proper placement and arrangement of artificial teeth will not be encountered.

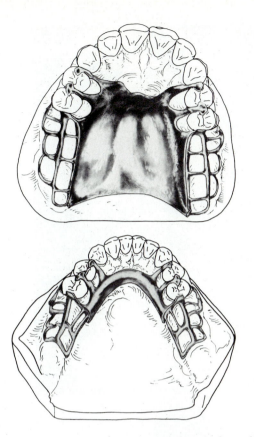

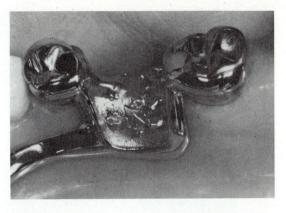

Fig. 8-7. Metal base was developed as integral part of framework for this tooth-borne restoration. Framework was cast in one piece. Note small "nail-heads" distributed over cast base as retaining mechanism for acrylic resin supporting artificial replacement tooth. Note also elevated and undercut borders of cast base.

Fig. 8-6. Note that minor connectors by which acrylic resin denture bases will be attached to framework are open, ladderlike configurations extending on both buccal and lingual surfaces. This not only provides excellent attachment of acrylic resin bases but also minimizes warping of bases resulting from the release of inherent strains in compression-molded acrylic resin.

having elements both buccal and lingual to the residual ridge not only will strengthen the resin base but also will minimize distortion of the base created by the release of inherent strains in the acrylic resin base during use or storage of the restoration (Fig. 8-6).

Metal bases are usually cast as integral parts of the partial denture framework (Fig. 8-7). Mandibular metal bases may also be assembled and attached to the framework with acrylic resin (Fig. 8-8).

IDEAL DENTURE BASE

The requirements for an ideal denture base are as follows:
1. Accuracy of adaptation to the tissues, with low volume change
2. Dense, nonirritating surface capable of receiving and maintaining a good finish
3. Thermal conductivity
4. Low specific gravity; lightness in the mouth
5. Sufficient strength; resistance to fracture or distortion
6. Self-cleansing factor, or easily kept clean
7. Esthetic acceptability
8. Potential for future relining
9. Low initial cost

Such an ideal denture base material does not exist; nor is it likely to be developed in the near future. However, any denture base—whether of resin or metal and regardless of the method of fabrication—should come as close to this ideal as possible.

ADVANTAGES OF METAL BASES

Except for those edentulous ridges with recent extractions, metal is preferred to resin for tooth-supported bases because of the several ad-

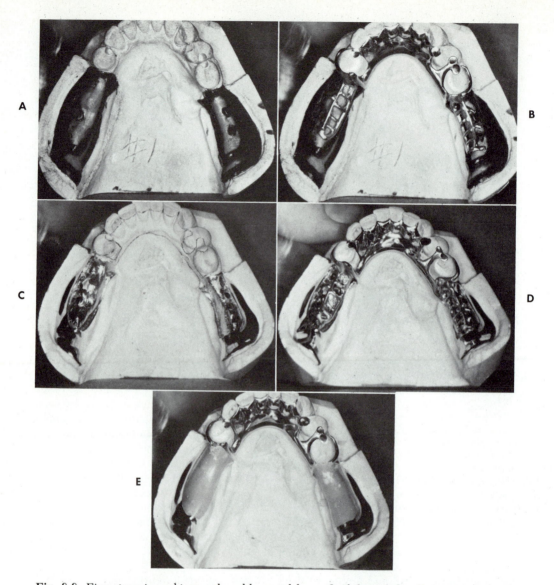

Fig. 8-8. Five steps in making replaceable metal bases for bilateral distal extension partial denture. **A,** Wax patterns for metal bases are formed on investment cast duplicate of corrected master cast. **B,** Original metal framework is placed over wax pattern, and the two are relieved or re-formed as needed to eliminate interference and to provide retention and finishing lines for resin attachment. **C,** Cast bases are returned to master cast. **D,** Three pieces are assembled on master cast. This should be done in laboratory, at which time any remaining interference is eliminated. **E,** Pieces have been assembled with self-curing acrylic resin. Final jaw relations may now be established on this assembled denture, or this may be deferred until patient and tissues have become accustomed to wearing prosthesis for a period of time before adding artificial teeth to denture base.

vantages of the metal base. Its principal disadvantage is that it can be relined only with difficulty, if at all. Nevertheless the stimulation that it gives to the underlying tissues is so beneficial that it probably prevents some alveolar atrophy that would otherwise occur under a resin base and thereby prolongs the health of the tissues that it contacts. Some of the advantages of a metal base are discussed in the following paragraphs.

Accuracy and permanence of form

Cast metal bases, whether of gold or chrome alloys, not only may be cast more accurately than denture resins but also maintain their accuracy of form without change in the mouth. Internal strains that may be released later to cause distortion are not present. Although some resins and some processing techniques are superior to others in accuracy and permanence of form, modern cast alloys are generally superior in this respect. Evidence of this fact is that an additional posterior palatal seal may be eliminated entirely when a cast palate is used for a complete denture, as compared with the need for a definite attempt in this regard when the palate is made of resin. Distortion of a resin base is manifest in the maxillary denture by a distortion away from the palate in the midline and toward the tuberosities on the buccal flanges. The greater the curvature of the tissues, the greater is this distortion. Similar distortions occur in a mandibular denture but are less easily detected. Accurate metal castings are not subject to distortion by the release of internal strains as are most denture resins.

Because of its accuracy, the metal base provides an intimacy of contact that contributes considerably to the retention of a denture prosthesis. Sometimes called **interfacial surface tension,** direct retention from a cast denture base is significant in proportion to the area involved. This has been previously mentioned as an important factor in both direct and direct-indirect retention of maxillary restorations. Such intimacy of contact is not possible with resin bases.

Permanence of form of the cast base is also assured because of its resistance to abrasion from denture cleaning agents. Cleanliness of the denture base should be stressed; however, constant brushing of the tissue side of the resin denture base, if effective, inevitably causes some loss of accuracy by abrasion. Intimacy of contact, which is never as great with a resin base as with a metal base, is therefore jeopardized further by cleaning habits. The metal bases, particularly the harder chrome alloys, withstand repeated cleaning without significant changes in surface accuracy.

Comparative tissue response

Clinical observations have demonstrated that the inherent cleanliness of the cast metal base contributes to the health of oral tissues when compared to an acrylic resin base. Perhaps some of the reasons for this are the greater density and the bacteriostatic activity contributed by ionization and oxidation of the metal base. Resin bases tend to accumulate mucinous deposits containing food particles, as well as calcareous deposits. Unfavorable tissue reaction to decomposing food particles and bacterial enzymes and to mechanical irritation from calculus results if the denture is not kept mechanically clean. Although calculus, which must be removed periodically, does precipitate on a cast metal base, other deposits do not accumulate as they do on a resin base. For this reason a metal base is naturally cleaner than is a resin base.

Thermal conductivity

Temperature changes are transmitted through the metal base to the underlying tissues, thereby helping to maintain the health of those tissues. Freedom of interchange of temperature between the tissues covered and the surrounding external influences (temperature of liquid and solid foods and inspired air) contributes much to the patient's acceptance of a denture and may help avoid the feeling of the presence of a foreign body. Conversely, denture resins have insulating properties that prevent interchange of temperature between the inside and the outside of the denture base.

Weight and bulk

Metal alloy may be cast much thinner than resin and still have adequate strength and rigidity. Still less weight and bulk are possible when the denture bases are made of chrome alloys.

Cast gold must be given slightly more bulk to provide the same amount of rigidity but may still be made with less thickness than resin materials.

There are times, however, when both weight and thickness may be used to advantage in denture bases. In the mandibular arch, weight of the denture may be an asset in regard to retention, and for this reason a cast gold base may be preferred. On the other hand, extreme loss of residual alveolar bone may make it necessary to add fullness to the denture base to restore normal facial contours and to fill out the buccal vestibule with a denture contour that will prevent food from being lost in the cheek and from working beneath the denture. In such situations a resin base may be preferred to the thinner metal base.

In the maxillary arch a resin base may be preferred to the thinner metal base to provide fullness when needed, such as in buccal flanges or to fill a maxillary buccal vestibule. Resin may also be preferred over the thinner metal base for esthetic reasons. In these instances the thinness of the metal base may be of no advantage, but in areas where the tongue and cheek need maximum room, thinness may be desirable.

Denture base contours for functional tongue and cheek contact can best be accomplished with resin. Whereas metal bases are usually made thin to minimize bulk and weight, resin bases may be contoured to provide ideal polished surfaces that contribute to the retention of the denture, restore facial contours, and avoid the accumulation of food at denture borders. Lingual surfaces usually are made concave except in the distal palatal area. Buccal surfaces are made convex at gingival margins, over root prominences, and at the border to fill the area recorded in the impression. Between the border and the gingival contours the base is made concave to aid in retention and to facilitate the food bolus's being returned to the occlusal table during mastication. Such contours prevent food from being lost in the cheek and from working under the denture. This cannot usually be accomplished with metal bases.

However, the advantages of a metal base need not necessarily be sacrificed for the sake of esthetics or desirable denture contours when the

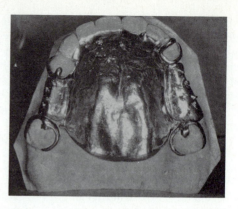

Fig. 8-9. Partial metal bases used with palatal plate and "pressed-on" anterior teeth. Attachment of artificial posterior teeth with resin is accomplished by diagonal spurs and lingual undercut finishing line. Visible buccal flange will be of resin, yet without sacrificing most advantages of metal base. Support anteriorly is provided by a mesioincisal rest on canine and by lingual rests on all remaining anterior teeth.

use of such a base is otherwise indicated. Denture bases may be designed to provide almost total metallic coverage, yet have resin borders to avoid a display of metal and to add buccal fullness when needed (Fig. 8-9). The advantages of thermal conductivity are not necessarily lost by covering a portion of the metal base as long as other parts of the denture are exposed to effect temperature changes through conduction.

METHODS OF ATTACHING ARTIFICIAL TEETH

Selection of artificial teeth for form, color, and material must precede attachment to the denture. Selection of teeth is discussed in Chapters 10 and 16.

Artificial teeth may be attached to denture bases by several means. These means are (1) with acrylic resin, (2) cemented, (3) processed directly to metal, and (4) cast with the framework.

1. **Porcelain or resin artificial teeth attached with resin.** Artificial porcelain teeth are mechanically retained. The posterior teeth are retained by acrylic resin in their diatoric holes. The anterior porcelain teeth are retained by acrylic resin surrounding the lingually placed

retention pins. Artificial resin teeth are retained by a chemical union with the acrylic resin of the denture base that occurs during laboratory processing procedures.

Attachment of the resin to the metal base may be accomplished by nailhead retention, retention loops, or diagonal spurs placed at random. Attachment mechanisms should be placed so that they will not interfere with the placement of the teeth on the metal base (Fig. 8-9).

Any junction of resin with metal should be at an undercut finishing line or associated with some retentive undercut. Since only a mechanical attachment exists between metal and resin, every attempt should be made to avoid separation and seepage, which results in discoloration and uncleanliness. Denture odors are frequently caused by accretions at the junction of resin with metal when only a mechanical union exists. Separation occurring between resin and metal leads eventually to some loosening of the resin base.

2. **Porcelain or resin tube teeth and facings cemented directly to metal bases** (Fig. 8-10). Some disadvantages of this type of attachment are the difficulties in obtaining satisfactory occlusion, lack of adequate contours for functional tongue and cheek contact, and unesthetic display of metal at gingival margins. The latter is avoided when the tooth is butted directly to the ridge, but then the retention for the tooth frequently becomes inadequate.

A modification of this method is the attachment of ready-made resin teeth to the metal base with acrylic resin of the same shade. This is called **pressing on** a resin tooth and is not the same as using resin for cementation. It is particularly applicable to anterior replacements, since it is desirable to know in advance of making the casting that the shade and contours of the selected tooth will be acceptable (as was referred to in Fig. 8-9). After a labial index of the position of the teeth is made, the lingual portion of the tooth may be cut away or a posthole prepared in the tooth for retention on the casting. Subsequently the tooth is attached to the denture with acrylic resin of the same shade. Since this is done under pressure, the acrylic resin attachment is comparable to the manufactured tooth in hardness and strength.

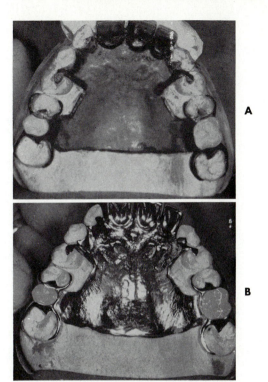

Fig. 8-10. Class III, modification 2, partial denture with palatal major connector supporting tubed teeth posteriorly and Steele's facings anteriorly. Design is actually anatomic replica palatal major connector extended anteriorly to support anterior replacements. Entire major connector is as thin as mechanically feasible and of uniform thickness, made possible by using anatomic replica pattern. Esthetics dictated the spacing between incisor teeth, which could not easily have been accomplished with fixed partial denture. Note also clearance lingual to premolar abutments. **A,** Wax and plastic pattern for this casting, with plaster index for positioning anterior Steele's facings. Backings are plastic waxed to anatomic replica palatal pattern. **B,** Completed casting.

Tube or side-groove teeth must be selected in advance of waxing the denture framework (Fig. 8-11). However, for best occlusal relationships, jaw relation records always should be made with the denture casting in the mouth. This problem may be solved by selecting tube teeth for width but with occlusal surfaces slightly higher than will be necessary. The teeth are ground to fit the ridge with sufficient clearance

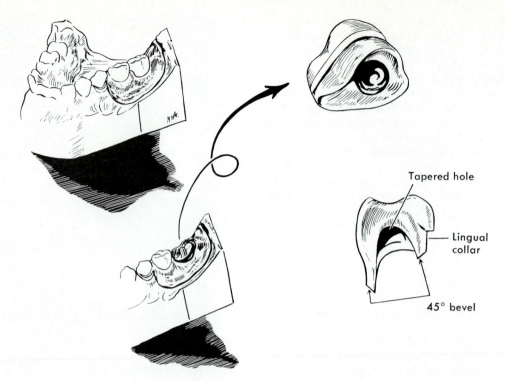

Fig. 8-11. Stock porcelain or resin tube tooth, or artificial tooth used as tube tooth, should be ground to accommodate cast coping as illustrated. Hole is drilled from underside of tooth, or if one is already present, it is made larger. Then tooth is ground to fit ridge with enough clearance for minimum thickness of metal. A 45-degree bevel is then formed around base of tooth, and finally a collar is created on lingual side, extending to interproximal area. Tooth is then lubricated and wax pattern for denture base formed around it.

beneath for a thin metal base and beveled to accommodate a boxing of metal. If a plastic tube tooth is used, the diatoric hole should be made slightly larger than provided. The casting is completed and tried in, occlusal relationships are recorded, and then the teeth are ground to harmonious occlusion with the opposing dentition. As will be discussed in Chapter 16, artificial posterior teeth on partial dentures should hardly ever be used unaltered but rather should be considered material from which occlusal forms may be created to function harmoniously with the remaining natural occlusion.

3. **Resin teeth processed directly to metal bases.** Modern cross-linked copolymers enable the dentist or technician to process acrylic resin teeth that have satisfactory hardness and abrasion resistance for many situations. Thus occlu-

sion may be created without resorting to the modification of ready-made artificial teeth (Fig. 8-12). Recesses in the denture pattern are either carved by hand or created around manufactured teeth that are used only to form the recess in the pattern. Occlusal relationships may be established either in the mouth on the denture framework or by the use of an articulator, and then the teeth are carved and processed in acrylic resin of the proper shade to fit the opposing occlusal record. Better attachment to the metal base than by cementation is thus possible. In addition, unusually long, short, wide, or narrow teeth may be created when necessary to fill spaces not easily filled by the limited selection of commercially available teeth.

Occlusion on resin teeth may be reestablished to compensate for wear or settling by repro-

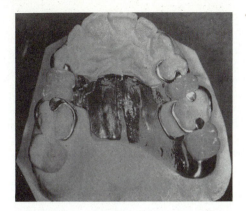

Fig. 8-12. Direct attachment of resin teeth to metal bases. These are waxed to fit space and opposing occlusion and processed to retention previously provided on metal framework. Occlusal surfaces of acrylic resin posterior teeth should be duplicated in cast inlay gold.

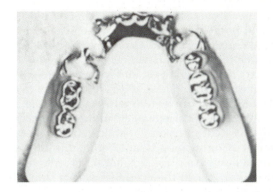

Fig. 8-13. Occlusal surfaces cast with inlay gold and attached to prosthetically supplied teeth.

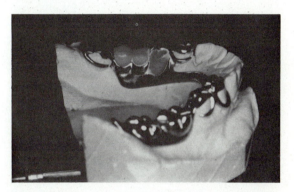

Fig. 8-14. Mandibular right first and second molars were cast as integral parts of framework. Interocclusal space limitation necessitated using metal rather than another form of artificial posterior teeth. Note overlays on premolar and molar abutments as part of framework to increase vertical dimension of occlusion.

cessing new acrylic occlusal surfaces at a later date when this becomes necessary. Distinction always should be made between the need for relining to reestablish occlusion (on a distal extension partial denture) or the need for rebuilding occlusal surfaces on an otherwise satisfactory base (on either a tooth-supported or a tooth- and tissue-supported partial denture).

Reestablishment of occlusion also may be accomplished by placing gold inlays on existing resin teeth. Although this may be done also on porcelain teeth, it is difficult to cut inlay recesses in porcelain teeth unless air abrasive methods are used. Therefore, if later additions to occlusal surfaces are anticipated, plastic teeth should be used, thereby facilitating the addition of new resin or cast gold surfaces (Fig. 8-13). A simple technique to fabricate cast gold occlusal surfaces and attach them to resin teeth is illustrated in Chapter 17.

4. **Metal teeth.** Occasionally a second molar tooth may be replaced as part of the partial denture casting (Fig. 8-14). This is usually done when space is too limited for the attachment of an artificial tooth and yet the addition of a second molar is desirable to prevent migration of an opposing second molar. Since the occlusal surface must be waxed before casting, perfect oc-

clusion is not possible. Since metal, particularly a chrome alloy, is abrasion resistant, the area of occlusal contact should be held to a minimum to avoid damage to the periodontium of the opposing tooth and the associated discomfort to the patient. Whereas occlusal adjustment on gold occlusal surfaces is readily accomplished, metal teeth made of chrome alloys are difficult to adjust and are objectionably hard for use as occlusal surfaces. Therefore they should be used only to fill a space and to prevent tooth migration and no more.

NEED FOR RELINING

The distal extension base differs from the tooth-borne base in several respects, one of which is that it must be made of a material that can be relined or rebased when it becomes necessary to reestablish tissue support for the distal extension base. Therefore resin denture base materials that can be relined are generally used.

Although satisfactory techniques for making distal extension partial denture bases of cast metal are available (Chapter 15), the fact that metal bases are difficult if not impossible to reline limits their use to stable ridges that will change little over a long period of time.

Loss of support for distal extension bases results from changes in residual ridge form over a period of time. These changes may not be readily visible; however, manifestations of this change can be assessed. One of these is a **loss of occlusion** between the distal extension denture base and the opposing dentition, increasing as the distance from the abutment increases (Fig. 8-15). This is proved by having the patient close on strips of 28-gauge green casting wax, or any similar wax tapping in **centric occlusion** only. Indentations in a wax strip of known thickness are quantitative, whereas marks made with articulating ribbon are only qualitative. In other

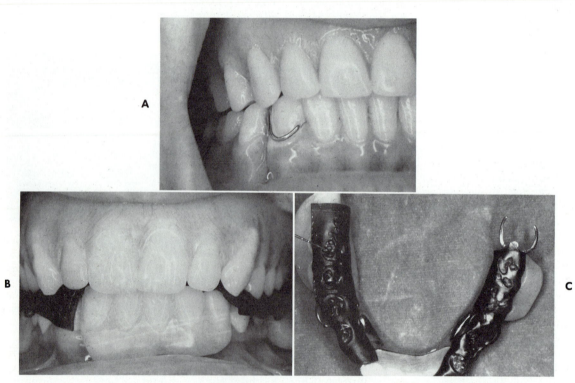

Fig. 8-15. A, Distal extension mandibular removable partial denture opposed by maxillary complete denture. There is no contact of opposing posterior teeth. Anterior teeth are in heavy contact at vertical dimension of occlusion. Unless corrected immediately, maxillary anterior portion of residual is destined to undergo rapid resorption. **B,** Another patient with mandibular Class II, modification 2, removable partial denture opposed by maxillary complete denture. Mandibular posterior teeth have been covered with strips of 28-gauge soft green wax, and patient has been assisted in tapping in centric relation. **C,** Mandibular denture is removed, and indentations in interposed wax strips are evaluated. Note relative absence of perforations in wax strips by opposing posterior teeth. Need for relining and correction of occlusal discrepancies is obvious, based on this record.

words, indentations in the wax may be interpreted as being light, medium, or heavy, whereas it is difficult if not impossible to interpret a mark made with articulating ribbon as being light or heavy. In fact, the heaviest occlusal contact may perforate paper articulating ribbon and make a lesser mark than areas of lighter contact. Therefore the use of any articulating ribbon is of limited value in checking occlusion intraorally. In making occlusal adjustments, articulating ribbon should be used only to indicate **where** to relieve after the **need for relief** has been established by using wax strips of known thickness. For this purpose, 28-gauge green or blue casting wax is generally used, although the thinner 30-gauge or the thicker 26-gauge wax may also be used for better evaluation of the clearance between areas not in contact.

Loss of support for a distal extension base will result in a loss of occlusal contact between the prosthetically supplied teeth and the opposing dentition and a return to heavy occlusal contact between the remaining natural teeth. Usually this is an indication that relining is needed to reestablish the original occlusion by reestablishing supporting contact with the residual ridge. It must be remembered, however, that occlusion on a distal extension base is sometimes

maintained at the expense of migration of the opposing natural teeth. In such a case, checking the occlusion alone will not show that settling of the extension base has occurred because changes in the supporting ridge may have also taken place.

A second manifestation of change also must be observable to justify relining. This second manifestation of change in the supporting ridge is evidence of rotation about the fulcrum line with the indirect retainers lifting from their seats as the distal extension base is pressed against the ridge tissues (Fig. 8-16). Originally, if the distal extension base was made to fit the supporting form of the residual ridge (Chapter 15), rotation about the fulcrum line is not visible. At the time the denture is initially placed, no teeter-totter should exist when alternating finger pressure is applied to the indirect retainer and the distal end of a distal extension base or bases. After changes in the ridge form, which cause some loss of support, rotation occurs about the fulcrum line when alternating finger pressure is applied. This is evidence of changes in the supporting ridge that must be compensated for by relining or rebasing.

If occlusal contact has been lost and rotation about the fulcrum line is evident, relining is

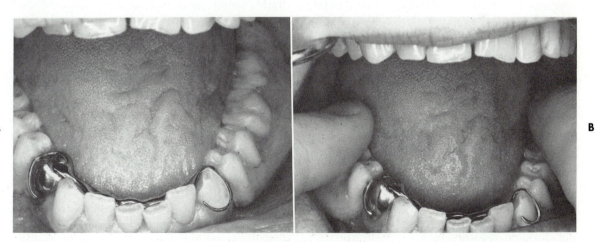

Fig. 8-16. A, Superior border of linguoplate major connector and rests appear to be in their planned relationships to remaining natural teeth in absence of occlusal load. **B,** Slight pressure on denture base activates direct retainers and elevates superior border of linguoplate, resulting in lack of planned contact. Denture bases should be relined to reestablish adequate base support by residual ridges.

indicated. On the other hand, if occlusal contact has been lost without any evidence of denture rotation and if stability of the denture base is otherwise satisfactory, reestablishing the occlusion is the remedy rather than relining. For the latter the original denture base may be used in much the same manner as the original trial base was used to record occlusal relation. Teeth may then be reoccluded to an opposing cast or to an occlusal template, using new teeth or cast gold occlusal surfaces. In any event new occlusion may be established on the existing bases. Relining in this instance would be the wrong solution to the problem.

Loss of support may also be assessed clinically by another method. A layer of rather free-flowing irreversible hydrocolloid is spread on the basal seat portion of the dried denture base(s), and the restoration is returned to the patient's mouth. Care is exercised to ensure that the framework is correctly seated (rests and indirect retainers in planned positions). The restoration is removed when the hydrocolloid has matured (set). Significant thicknesses of hydrocolloid remaining under the bases indicate a lack of intimate contact of the bases with the residual ridges, suggesting a need for relining.

More often, however, loss of occlusion is accompanied by settling of the denture base to the extent that rotation about the fulcrum line is manifest. Since relining is the only remedy short of making completely new bases, use of a resin base originally facilitates later relining. For this reason resin bases are generally preferred for distal extension partial dentures.

The question remains as to when, if ever, metal bases with their several advantages may be used for distal extension partial dentures. It is debatable as to what type of ridge will be the most likely to remain stable under functional loading without apparent change. Certainly the age and general health of the patient will influence the ability of a residual ridge to support function. Minimum and harmonious occlusion and the accuracy with which the base fits the underlying tissues will influence the amount of trauma that will occur under function. The absence of trauma plays a big part in the ability of the ridge to maintain its original form.

The best risk for the use of metal distal extension bases is a ridge that has supported a previous partial denture without having become narrowed or flat or consisting primarily of easily displaceable tissues. When such changes have occurred under a previous denture, further change may be anticipated because of the possibility that the oral tissues in question are not capable of supporting a denture base without retrogressive change. Despite every advantage in their favor, apparently there are some individuals whose ridges respond unfavorably to being called on to support any denture base.

In other instances, such as when a new partial denture is to be made because of the loss of additional teeth, the ridges may still be firm and healthy. Since the ridges have previously supported a denture base and have sustained occlusion, bony trabeculae will have become arranged to best support vertical and horizontal loading, cortical bone may have been formed, and tissues will have become favorable for continued support of a denture base.

Admittedly there are relatively few instances in which the need for future relining of a distal extension base need not be considered and metal bases may be used. There are, however, many instances that may be considered borderline. In these, metal bases may be used with full understanding on the part of the patient that a new or rebuilt denture may become necessary in the future if unforeseen tissue changes occur. A technique is given in Fig. 8-8 that permits replacing metal distal extension bases without having to remake the entire denture. This method should be seriously considered any time a distal extension partial denture is to be made with a metal base or bases.

For reasons previously outlined the possibility that tissues will remain healthier beneath a metal base than they will beneath a resin base may justify wider use of metal bases for distal extension partial dentures. Through careful treatment planning, better patient education of the problems involved in making a distal extension denture, and greater care in the fabrication of the denture bases, metal may be used to advantage in some situations in which resin bases are ordinarily used.

STRESSBREAKERS (STRESS EQUALIZERS)

The previous chapters on component parts of a partial denture have presumed absolute rigidity of all parts of the partial denture framework except the retentive arm of the direct retainer assembly. All vertical and horizontal forces applied to the supplied teeth are thus distributed throughout the supporting portions of the dental arch. Broad distribution of force is accomplished through the rigidity of the major and minor connectors. The effect of the stabilizing components is also made possible by the rigidity of the connectors.

In a distal extension restoration, strain on the abutment teeth is minimized through the use of functional basing, broad coverage, harmonious occlusion, and correct choice of direct retainers. Retentive clasp arms may be cast only if they engage undercuts on the abutment teeth in such a manner that tissue-ward movement of the extension base transmits only minimum leverage to the abutment. Otherwise, tapered wrought-wire retentive clasp arms should be used because of their greater flexibility. Because of its flexibility, the tapered, round wrought-wire clasp arm may be said to act somewhat as a stressbreaker between the denture base and the abutment tooth.

A concept of stress breaking exists, however, that insists on separating the action of the retaining elements from the movement of the distal extension base. Thus when the term **stressbreaker** is used, it is generally applied to a device that allows some movement between the denture base or its supporting framework and the direct retainers, whether they are intracoronal or extracoronal in design.

A stressbreaker is also sometimes referred to as a **stress equalizer.** The term **articulated prosthesis** is also frequently applied to a broken-stress partial denture.

Almost 50 years ago Kennedy wrote as follows:

Since the advent of the cast clasp and the removable bridge, a great number of men have advocated the use of "stress breakers" between their saddles and the clasps. These have been shown to be absolutely essential by dentists who have used cast clasps for partial dentures. They found that in a short time the teeth to which such clasps were attached loosened, and that this was due mainly to the rigidity of the clasp.

A well-designed round wire clasp is, in itself, a stress breaker, and allows sufficient saddle movement to prevent excessive strain upon the abutment teeth. . . .

In my hands, stress breakers used on partial dentures have permitted so much movement of the saddles, that they produce excessive soreness, and, after many trials, especially after patients have worn them for some time, I found that a greater number of abutment teeth were loosened than where we used the double bar, . . . the "continuous clasp" [what is now known as the secondary lingual bar or Kennedy bar]. It is only where we have too few teeth in the mouth that it is necessary to use some form of specially designed stress breaker between the clasps and saddles.

. . . Clasps should not be made so rigid that they hold the denture in place. We must depend on the inherent stability of the saddles to prevent strain on the teeth. . . . If there are only one or two teeth present, we would not expect these teeth to do the work of fourteen, without excessive strain being placed upon them, and it is in such conditions that some form of stress breaker becomes useful.*

Several partial denture textbooks have little to say about stressbreakers, as though to avoid a controversial subject. That the subject is controversial is evidenced by the rigid adherence to their use by some with apparent success, whereas properly designed rigid restorations are routinely used by others without harm to abutments. **It is only the improperly designed or ineffectively fabricated rigid restoration that has proved to be harmful to abutment teeth.** There is little question that some form of mechanical stressbreaker is preferable to a poorly designed and ineffectively fabricated rigid restoration!

It is interesting and significant to note that development and promotion of stressbreaker designs in this country have been largely through the efforts of the commercial dental laboratory. In most instances this has been caused by the failure of the dentist to furnish the laboratory with a master cast that provides for adequate

---

*From Kennedy, E.: Partial denture construction, Brooklyn, 1942, Denture Items of Interest Publishing Co., Inc.

denture base support. If the dentist is not inclined to employ carefully contoured abutment retainers that permit the use of proper clasp designs and is not willing to take the steps necessary to provide maximum support for tissue-supported denture bases, then probably one of the stressbreaker designs offered by the commercial dental laboratory should be used if the dentist insists on including removable partial prosthodontics in his or her practice.

Types of stressbreakers

Stressbreakers may be divided into two groups. In the first are those having a movable joint between the direct retainer and the denture base (Figs. 8-17 and 8-18). In this group fall the hinges, sleeves and cylinders, and ball-and-socket devices (some of which are spring loaded). Being placed between the direct retainer and the denture base, they may permit both vertical movement and hinge action of the distal extension base. This serves to prevent some direct transmission of tipping forces to the abutment teeth as the base moves tissue-ward under function.

Examples of this group are the various hinges, the Swiss-made Dalbo attachment, the Crismani attachment, the C & M 637 attachment, and the ASC 52 attachment (Fig. 8-19). Most of these attachments are prefabricated, but the laboratory may use dual-casting techniques for fabricating the attachment. Because of the rapid wear likely to occur with gold, such attachments are usually made of a harder alloy and therefore are usually machine made.

The articulated partial denture designs constitute the second group and include those designs having a flexible connection between the direct retainer and the denture base. These include the use of wrought-wire connectors, divided major connectors, and other flexible devices for permitting movement of the distal ex-

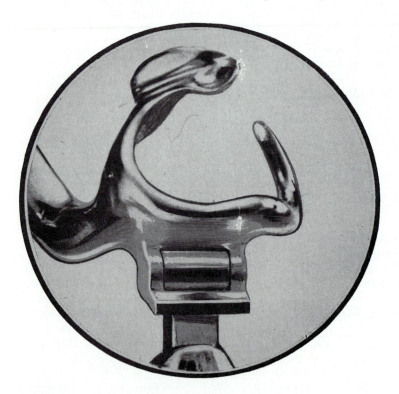

Fig. 8-17. D-E hinge-type stressbreaker using vertical stop to limit movement of denture base away from tissues. Trunnion design of stressbreaker also prevents lateral movement. (Courtesy Austenal, Inc., Chicago, Ill.)

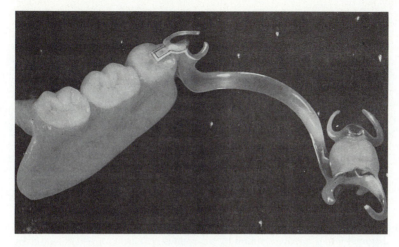

Fig. 8-18. Kennedy Class II, modification 1, partial denture using hinge stressbreaker of Baca design. Hinge and vertical movements are permitted by fact that action is protected by metal sleeve. (Courtesy Ticonium Division of CMP Industries, Inc., Albany, N.Y.)

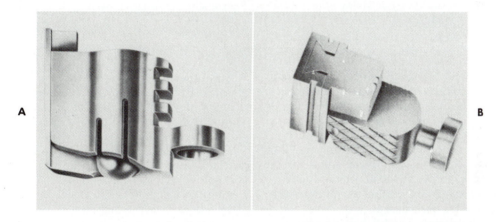

Fig. 8-19. A, Dalbo extracoronal retainer. Limited vertical and hinge movements of denture base is permitted by sleeve and spring design of retainer. **B,** Crismani intracoronal retainer design permits limited vertical movement of denture base.

tension base (Figs. 8-20 and 8-21). Included also in this group are those using a movable joint between two major connectors. These are generally fabricated by the laboratory with a dual-casting technique. The earliest of such connectors were double lingual bars of wrought metal, one supporting the clasps and other components and the other supporting and connecting the distal extension bases. The two bars were usually but not always united at the midline by binding with fine wire and soldering.

The double bar principle is still used in the form of split major connectors. Instead of using wrought metal, a single cast connector is made flexible by separating a portion of its length. This may be done by making a saw cut part way through a gold casting with a jeweler's saw or by casting to a thin shim; this is then removed, leaving a separation. Although mica and other materials have been used for this purpose, stainless steel is generally used (0.02 band material), which is then removed by acid. The nature of

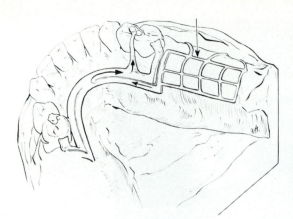

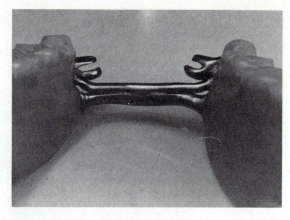

Fig. 8-20. Stressbreaking effect of split bar major connector. Vertical and diagonal forces (arrow) applied to tissue-supported base must pass anteriorly along lower bar and then back along more rigid upper bar to reach abutment tooth. Thus tipping forces that would otherwise be transmitted directly to abutment tooth are supposedly dissipated by flexibility of lower bar and distance traveled.

Fig. 8-21. Early type of stress equalizer. The direct retainers (clasps) are connected by 16-gauge round wrought wire. Inferiorly placed cast major connector joins denture bases. Heavy wrought wire and cast major connector are joined with solder at midline only. Need for indirect retention still exists even though stress equalizer is used.

chromium-cobalt alloys permits making one casting first and then waxing and casting the second part to the first without union. This facilitates making split bars and movable joints with fine precision and nearly imperceptible junction lines. In any event, the resulting flexibility of the major connector acts to prevent some direct transmission of forces to the abutment tooth.

A design using a dual-casting technique is the Ticonium hidden-lock design (Fig. 8-22). This is a two-piece casting. The top half, which is the major connector supporting the direct retainers and other rigid components, is cast first, and the bottom half, which is the connector between the denture bases, is cast to the major connector. The latter is completely independent of the first except that it is locked in by a circle-type retention, prepared in the wax pattern.

The hidden-lock is created by mechanical means, and the split between the two connectors is made possible by the thin oxide shell that forms during the making of the two sections. What appears to be a conventional lingual bar or linguoplate actually is two bars connected by a movable joint at the midline.

Still other devices permit disassembly of the denture by the patient for cleaning. All mechanical devices that are free to move in the mouth collect debris and become unclean; therefore disassembly is a desirable feature whether done daily by the patient or periodically by the dentist (some hinged devices have small screws that may be removed for cleaning or adjusting the action of the device).

In addition to the trapping of debris, some split connectors used as stressbreakers have been known to pinch the underlying soft tissues or the tongue as they open and close under function. Furthermore, such flexible connectors, especially those made of cast alloys, become fatigued through repeated flexing, resulting in permanent distortion of the denture framework and possible ultimate failure through fracture.

Regardless of their design, most all stressbreakers effectively dissipate vertical stresses, which is the purpose for which they are used. At the same time their flexibility or mechanical movement may eliminate the horizontal stability at the distal extension base that is inherent in a rigid partial denture design. The effectiveness

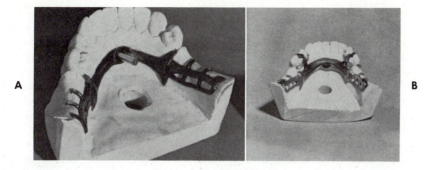

Fig. 8-22. Ticonium hidden-lock partial denture. **A,** Lower half of framework, consisting of lower half of lingual bar and denture base retainer, is cast first with bi-bevel circle formed in wax pattern by waxing around lightly oiled mandrel, which is removed to provide perfect circle within wax. This half is cast as illustrated. **B,** On second investment cast, original bar is replaced and remainder of framework is waxed to it. This portion consists of clasps, indirect retainers, and remainder of bar. Hidden-lock and split bar are made possible because of thin oxide shell that forms during second casting, leaving an almost imperceptible junction line between two sections. Hinge movement occurs at circle in midline. (Courtesy Ticonium Co., Albany, N.Y.)

of minor connectors, stabilizing components, occlusal rests, and indirect retainers is either lost or dissipated by the action of the stressbreakers. **As a result, consideration of the abutments is at the expense of the tissues of the residual ridge.** This is evidenced by the fact that the stress-broken denture will often require relief on the tissue side of the buccal flange. Since horizontal stresses cannot be resisted by rigid stabilizing components elsewhere in the arch, the residual ridge is forced to bear those horizontal forces alone. This and the added cost are the most obvious disadvantages to the use of stressbreakers in distal extension partial denture designs.

Advantages of stressbreakers

Some of the claimed advantages of stressbreakers by those who use them may be listed as follows:

1. Since the horizontal forces acting on the abutment teeth are minimized, the alveolar support of these teeth is preserved.

2. By careful choice of the type of flexible connector, it is possible to obtain a balance of stress between the abutment teeth and the residual ridge.

3. Intermittent pressure of the denture bases massages the mucosa, thus providing physiologic stimulation, which prevents bone resorption and eliminates the need for relining.

4. If relining is needed but not done, the abutment teeth are not damaged as quickly.

5. Splinting of weak teeth by the denture is made possible despite the movement of a distal extension base.

Disadvantages of stressbreakers

Some of the disadvantages of the stress-breaking principle are as follows:

1. The broken-stress denture is usually more difficult to construct and therefore more costly.

2. Vertical and horizontal forces are concentrated on the residual ridge, resulting in increased ridge resorption. Many stressbreaker designs are not well stabilized against horizontal forces. Proponents of broken-stress dentures claim that this is avoided by the intermittent massage, which stimulates and promotes better health of the residual ridge.

3. If relining is not done when needed, excessive resorption of the residual ridge may result. This is offset to some extent by the fact that such a denture base is no longer in occlusion

and that therefore resorption may not be progressive.

4. The effectiveness of indirect retainers is reduced or eliminated altogether.

5. The more complicated the prosthesis, the less it may be tolerated by the patient. Spaces between components are sometimes opened up in function, thus trapping food and occasionally the tissues of the mouth.

6. Flexible connectors may be bent and distorted by careless handling. Even a slightly distorted connector may bring more stress to bear on the abutment rather than less.

7. Repair and maintenance of any stressbreaker is difficult, costly, and frequently required.

Advantages of a rigid design

Some of the advantages of the rigid partial denture design may be listed as follows:

1. Mechanically the framework is easier and less costly to make.

2. Equitable distribution of stress between abutments and the residual ridge(s) is possible with a rigid design.

3. The need for relining the rigid prosthesis is less frequent, since the residual ridge does not have to carry the functional load unaided.

4. Indirect retainers and other rigid components may act to prevent rotational movement of the denture and will provide horizontal stabilization that is not possible when stressbreakers are used.

5. By reducing the number of flexible or movable parts, there is less danger of distortion by careless handling on the part of the patient.

Disadvantages of a rigid design

Some of the possible disadvantages of the rigid denture design are as follows:

1. Objectionable torque will be applied to the abutment teeth if abutment retainers are not passive and correctly designed.

2. Rigid continuous clasping may be hazardous when stressbreakers are not used.

3. Locking-type (dovetail) intracoronal retainers may not be used at all without stressbreakers on distal extension dentures because they are locked within the abutment, and tipping forces would be transmitted directly to the abutment tooth. Even when used in conjunction with multiple splinting of abutments, coupled with a minimum of occlusion on the distal extension denture base, locking-type retainers are still risky.

4. The use of tapered wrought-wire retentive clasp arms as stressbreakers may present some technical difficulties, particularly when high-fusing chrome alloys are used. Wrought wire may be crystalized by improper application of heat during casting or soldering operations, resulting in early fracture. Use of the type II wire will minimize problems associated with the application of heat. It also may be distorted by careless handling, leading to excessive or insufficient retention, or ultimate fracture caused by repeated adjustment.

5. If relining is not done when needed, the abutment tooth may be loosened and suffer permanent periodontal damage because of the repeated application of torque and tipping stresses.

The student is referred to two textbooks that describe in detail the use of stressbreakers and articulated partial denture designs: (1) *Precision Attachments in Dentistry*, ed. 3, by H.W. Preiskel and (2) *Theory and Practice of Precision Attachment Removable Partial Dentures*, by J.L. Baker and R.J. Goodkind.

SELF-ASSESSMENT AIDS

1. What is a denture base?
2. What is meant by the term **basal seat?**
3. Is the primary purpose of a denture base related to masticatory function?
4. To what extent may the denture base contribute to the factor of appearance?
5. Are the functions of tooth-supported and extension type bases somewhat different?
6. What are the functions of a tooth-supported partial denture base?
7. Describe the functions of a distal extension denture base.
8. The space available for a denture base is controlled by the structures surrounding the space and their movements during function. True or false?
9. We hear of the term **snowshoe effect** in designing denture bases. What does this mean to you?
10. By what means is an acrylic resin base attached to a framework?

11. A ladderlike minor connector is employed to attach an acrylic resin base to frameworks. Should this minor connector be rigid or flexible?
12. Is it important that a minor connector for an extension type acrylic resin base be located on both the buccal and lingual sides of the residual ridge? Can you defend your answer?
13. Is an open ladder type of design for connecting an acrylic resin base to a major connector preferred to a close "meshwork" design? Why?
14. Can you give a rule of thumb for the distal extent of a minor connector attaching the resin base to the major connector?
15. Quite obviously the minor connector for resin bases must be embedded totally in the resin base. What thickness of acrylic resin is necessary between the residual ridge and minor connector to allow adjustment of the base if it should become necessary?
16. Nine requirements for an ideal denture base are given in this chapter. Can you think of six of them?
17. Metal bases have distinct advantages over resin bases, such as thermal conductivity and accuracy and permanence of form. Do they have any other advantages?
18. What are the indications and contraindications for metal bases?
19. Can denture base contours for functional cheek and tongue contact best be accomplished with resin or metal?
20. Relining of extension bases becomes necessary to reestablish support of the base. Could this be a factor in selecting the material for a denture base?
21. How can it be determined when a denture base requires relining?
22. What is meant by the word stressbreaker in removable partial prosthodontics?
23. By what means can the action of the retaining elements be separated from movements of the extension base?
24. Stressbreakers may be divided into two broad groups. Can you give a couple of examples of each group?
25. What is meant by a dual-casting technique, and how is it accomplished?
26. Most designs of stressbreakers will rather effectively dissipate vertical forces to terminal abutments. However, this occurs at the expense of what supporting entity?
27. Contrast stressbreaker and rigid designs by giving advantages and disadvantages of each.

9 PRINCIPLES OF REMOVABLE PARTIAL DENTURE DESIGN

Biomechanical considerations
Other factors influencing design
Differentation between two main types of
 removable partial dentures
Essentials of partial denture design
Components of partial dentures
Additional considerations influencing design

BIOMECHANICAL CONSIDERATIONS

As Maxwell stated, "Common observation clearly indicates that the ability of living things to tolerate force is largely dependent upon the magnitude or intensity of the force." The supporting structures for removable partial dentures (abutment teeth and residual ridges) are "living things" and are subjected to forces. In consideration of maintaining the health of these structures, the dentist must also consider direction, duration, and frequency of force application as well as magnitude of the force.

In the final analysis it is bone that provides the support for a removable restoration, that is, alveolar bone by way of the periodontal ligament and bone of the residual ridge through its soft tissue covering. If potentially destructive forces can be minimized, then the physiologic tolerances of the supporting structures need not be tested. To a great extent the forces accruing through a removable restoration can be widely distributed, directed, and minimized by the selection, the design, and the location of components of the removable partial denture and by developing a harmonious occlusion.

Unquestionably the design of removable partial dentures requires a consideration of mechanics as well as biologic considerations. It is not required that a dentist be a mechanical genius to apply certain fundamental principles to minimize or distribute potentially destructive forces by rational design of a restoration. Imbued in most dentists, just through the maturing process, is an appreciation—perhaps unrecognized—for the application of mechanical laws. For example, the lid of a paint can is more easily pried off with a screwdriver than it is with a half dollar! The longer the handle, the less effort (force) it takes. We are then applying the mechanics of levers. By the same token a lever system built into a distal extension removable restoration can magnify, so to speak, the applied force to the terminal abutments, which is most undesirable.

Tylman correctly stated, "Great caution and reserve are essential whenever an attempt is made to interpret biological phenomena entirely by mathematical computation." However, an understanding of certain things mechanical and of simple machines should enhance our rationalization of the design of removable partial dentures to accomplish an objective of preservation of oral structures. A removable partial denture can be, and often is, unknowingly designed as a destructive machine.

Machines may be classified into two general

categories: simple and complex. Complex machines are combinations of many simple machines. There are six simple machines: lever, wedge, screw, wheel and axle, pulley, and inclined plane (Fig. 9-1). Of the simple machines the lever and the inclined plane most deserve our consideration in designing removable partial dentures—a consideration based on **avoiding** lever and inclined plane designs to the greatest extent possible.

In its simplest form a lever is a rigid bar supported somewhere along its length. It may rest on the support or may be supported from above.

The support point of the lever is called the fulcrum, and the lever can move around the fulcrum (Fig. 9-2). There are three types of levers: first, second, and third class (Fig. 9-3). The potential of a lever system to relatively magnify a force is illustrated in Fig. 9-4.

An extension-type removable partial denture will rotate when a force is placed on the denture base. It will rotate in relation to the three cranial planes because of differences in the support characteristics of the abutment teeth and the soft tissues covering the residual ridge (Fig. 9-5). Even though the gross movement may be small, there still exists the potential for detrimental, leverlike imposed forces to accrue on abutment teeth, depending on design of the prosthesis, especially when servicing of the prosthesis is neglected over a long period of time.

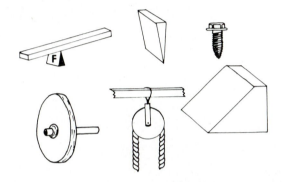

Fig. 9-1. Scientists today recognize six simple machines: lever, wedge, screw, wheel and axle, pulley, and inclined plane (F = fulcrum).

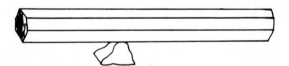

Fig. 9-2. Lever is simply rigid bar supported somewhere between its two ends. It can be used to move objects by application of force (weight) much less than weight of object being moved.

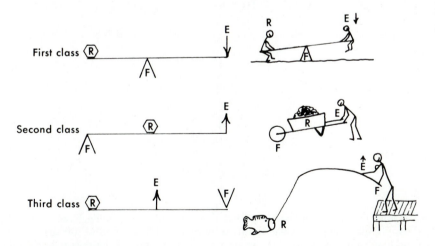

Fig. 9-3. There are three classes of levers. Classification is based on location of fulcrum, F; resistance, R; and direction of effort (force), E. Examples of each class are illustrated on right.

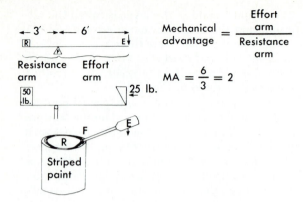

$$\text{Mechanical advantage} = \frac{\text{Effort arm}}{\text{Resistance arm}}$$

$$MA = \frac{6}{3} = 2$$

Fig. 9-4. Length of lever from fulcrum, *F*, to resistance, *R*, is called resistance arm. That portion of lever from fulcrum to point of application of force, *E*, is called effort arm. Whenever effort arm is longer than resistance arm, mechanical advantage is in favor of effort arm, proportional to difference in length of the two arms. In other words, when effort arm is twice the length of resistance arm, 25-pound weight on effort arm will balance 50-pound weight at end of resistance arm.

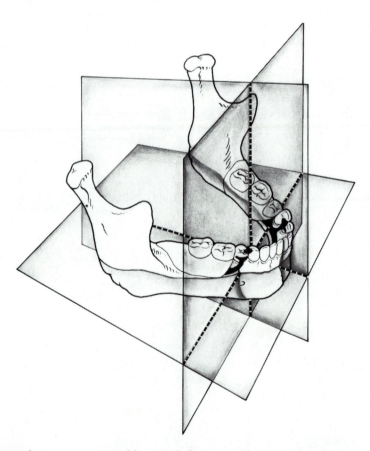

Fig. 9-5. Distal extension removable partial denture will rotate when force is directed on denture base. Differences in displaceability of periodontal ligament and soft tissues covering residual ridge permit this rotation. It would seem that rotation of denture is in combination of directions rather than unidirectional. In other words, distal extension denture can pitch, roll, and yaw.

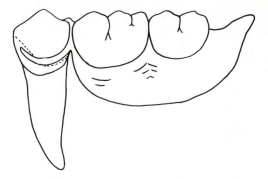

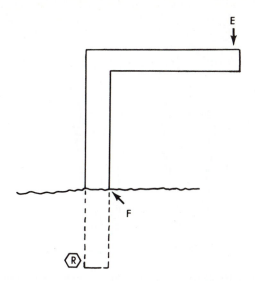

Fig. 9-6. Cantilever can be described as rigid beam supported at one end. When force is directed against unsupported end of beam, cantilever can act as first-class lever. Mechanical advantage in this illustration is in favor of effort arm, so to speak.

Fig. 9-7. Design often seen for distal extension removable partial denture. **Cast** circumferential direct retainer engages mesiobuccal undercut and is supported by distocclusal rest. Only difference in this design and locking-type internal attachment on distal aspect of premolar is in firmness of attachment to abutment. **This is a cantilever design**, and it may impart detrimental first-class lever force to abutment.

A cantilever is a beam supported only at one end and can act as a first-class lever (Fig. 9-6). A cantilever design should be avoided (Fig. 9-7). Examples of other leverlike designs as well as suggestions for alternative designs to avoid or to minimize their destructive potential are illustrated in Figs. 9-8 and 9-9.

A tooth is apparently better able to tolerate vertically directed forces than off-vertical or near horizontal forces. This characteristic is observed clinically and was substantiated many years ago by the work of Box and Synge of Toronto. It seems rational that more periodontal fibers are activated to resist the application of vertical forces to teeth than are activated to resist the application of off-vertical forces (Fig. 9-10).

Again, a distal extension removable partial denture rotates when forces are applied. Since it can be assumed that this rotation must create predominantly off-vertical forces, location of stabilizing and retentive components in relation to the horizontal axis of rotation of the abutment becomes extremely important. In other words an abutment tooth will better tolerate off-vertical forces if these forces accrue as near as pos-

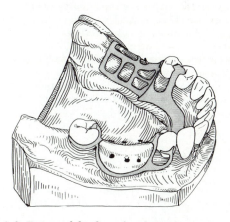

Fig. 9-8. Potential for first-class lever action exists in this Class II, modification 1, removable partial denture framework. If cast circumferential direct retainer with a mesiobuccal undercut on right first premolar were used, force placed on denture base could impart upward and posteriorly moving force on premolar, probably resulting in loss of contact between premolar and canine, with its soon-following sequelae. As designed with bar-type retainer, force during rotation of denture would be more anteriorly directed, thus maintaining contact. Other alternatives to first premolar design of direct retainer would be tapered wrought-wire retentive arm that uses mesiobuccal undercut or just has buccal stabilizing arm above height of contour or uses I-bar retentive arm on buccal surface.

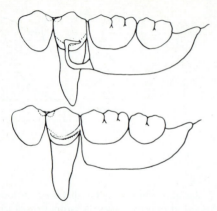

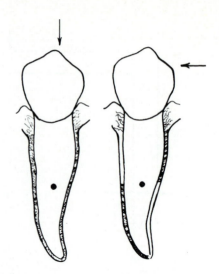

Fig. 9-9. Upper illustration uses bar-type retainer, minor connector contacting guiding plane on distal surface of premolar, and mesio-occlusal rest, thus eliminating cantilever or first-class lever force when denture rotates toward residual ridge. I-bar–type retentive arm could also be used. Lower figure uses tapered wrought-wire retentive arm, minor connector contacting guiding plane on distal surface of premolar, and mesio-occlusal rest. This design is applicable when distobuccal undercut (anteriorly tilted terminal abutments) cannot be found or created or when tissue undercut contraindicates placing bar-type retentive arm. It is a compromise; however, this design would probably be much more kind to periodontal ligament than would cast, half-round retentive arm.

Fig. 9-10. More periodontal fibers are apparently activated to resist forces directed vertically on tooth than are activated to resist horizontally (off-vertical) directed force. Horizontal axis of rotation, ●, is located somewhere in root of tooth.

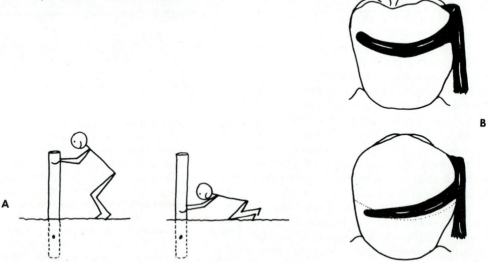

Fig. 9-11. A, Fencepost is more readily removed by application of force near its top than by applying same force nearer ground level. **B,** Retentive and reciprocal components (mirror view) of this direct retainer assembly are located much nearer occlusal surface than they should be. This is similar to left-hand figure in **A.**

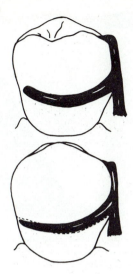

Fig. 9-12. Abutment has been contoured to allow rather favorable location of retentive and reciprocal-stabilizing components (mirror view). This is similar to right-hand figure in Fig. 9-11, *A*.

sible to the horizontal axis of rotation of the abutment (Fig. 9-11). The axial surface contours of abutment teeth must usually be altered to locate components of direct retainer assemblies more favorably in relation to the abutment's horizontal axis (Fig. 9-12).

OTHER FACTORS INFLUENCING DESIGN

As a direct result of examination and diagnosis the design of the removable partial denture must originate on the diagnostic cast so that all mouth preparations may be planned and performed with a specific design in mind. This will be influenced by many factors, some of which follow:

1. Which arch is to be restored and if both, their relationship to one another including
   a. occlusal relationship of remaining teeth
   b. orientation of the occlusal plane
   c. space available for restoration of missing teeth
   d. arch integrity
   e. tooth morphology
2. Type of major connector indicated, based on existing and correctable situations.
3. Whether the denture will be entirely tooth borne. If one or more distal extension bases are involved, the following must be considered:
   a. Need for indirect retention
   b. Clasp designs that will best minimize the forces applied to the abutment teeth during function
   c. Need for later rebasing, which will influence the type of base material used
   d. Secondary impression method to be used
4. Materials to be used, both for the framework and for the bases.
5. Type of replacement teeth to be used. This may be influenced by the opposing dentition.
6. Need for abutment restorations, which may influence the type of clasp arms to be used and their specific design.
7. Patient's past experience with a removable partial denture and the reasons for making a new denture. If, for example, a lingual bar has been objectionable, was it because of design, fit, or the patient's inability to accept it? Frequently an appraisal of these factors alone justifies the use of a contoured linguoplate rather than a lingual bar. If an anterior palatal bar has proved objectionable, was it because of bulk, location, or flexibility or tissue irritation? A design using a thin palatal major connector located more posteriorly may be preferable to an anterior bar or palatal U-shaped design located anteriorly.
8. Response of oral structures to previous stress, periodontal condition of the remaining teeth, the mount of abutment support remaining, and the need for splinting. This may be accomplished either by means of fixed restorations or by the design of the denture framework.
9. Method to be used for replacing single teeth or missing anterior teeth. The decision to use fixed restorations for these spaces rather than replacing them with the removable partial denture must be made at the time of treatment planning (Fig. 9-13). Such a decision will necessarily influence the design of the denture framework.

DIFFERENTIATION BETWEEN TWO MAIN TYPES OF REMOVABLE PARTIAL DENTURES

It is clear that two distinctly different types of removable partial dentures exist. Certain points of difference are present between the

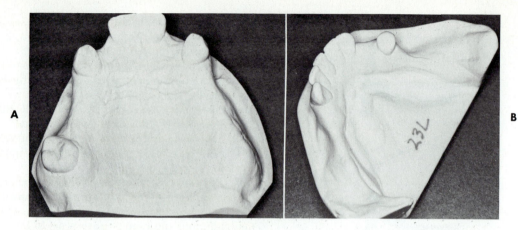

Fig. 9-13. **A,** Diagnostic cast of partially edentulous maxillary arch. Ideally, missing lateral incisors should be restored with fixed partial dentures. By so doing, not only will design of removable partial denture be simplified but canines will be spared some leverages created by rotation of denture in use. Prognosis for canines and central incisors will be greatly enhanced. **B,** Lone standing premolar in this mandibular arch should be splinted to right central and right lateral incisors, with fixed partial denture replacing missing canine. If it is used as lone standing abutment for removable restoration, first-class lever or cantilever forces cannot be avoided regardless of design.

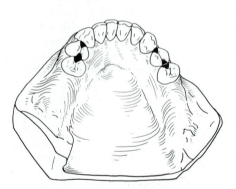

Fig. 9-14. Kennedy Class I partially edentulous arch. Major support for denture bases must come from residual ridges, tooth support from occlusal rests being effective only at anterior portion of each base.

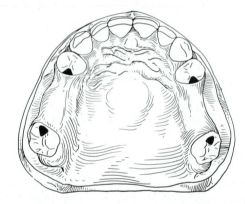

Fig. 9-15. Kennedy Class III, modification 1, partially edentulous arch, which provides total tooth support for prosthesis. Removable partial denture made for this arch is totally supported by rests on properly prepared occlusal rest seats on four abutment teeth.

Class I and Class II types of partial dentures on the one hand and the Class III type of partial denture on the other. The first consideration is **the manner in which each is supported.** The Class I type and the distal extension side of the Class II type derive their support to a great extent from the tissues underlying the base and only to a limited degree from the abutment teeth

(Fig. 9-14), whereas the Class III type derives all its support from the abutment teeth at each end of the edentulous space (Fig. 9-15).

Second, for reasons directly related to the manner of support, the **method of impression registration** required for each type will vary.

Third, the **need for some kind of indirect retention** exists in the distal extension type of partial denture, whereas in the tooth-borne, Class III type there is no extension base that can lift away from the supporting tissues because of the action of sticky foods and movements of the tissues of the mouth against borders of the denture. This is because each end of each denture base is secured by a direct retainer on an abutment tooth unless anterior teeth are replaced by the denture. Therefore the tooth-borne partial denture does not rotate about a fulcrum as does the distal extension partial denture.

Fourth, the manner in which the distal extension type of partial denture is supported often necessitates the **use of a base material that can be relined** to compensate for tissue changes. Acrylic resin is generally used as a base material for distal extension bases. The Class III partial denture, on the other hand, being entirely tooth supported, does not require relining except when it is advisable to eliminate an unhygienic, unesthetic, or uncomfortable condition resulting from loss of tissue contact. Metal bases therefore are more frequently used in tooth-borne restorations, since relining is not as likely to be necessary with them.

Differences in support. The distal extension partial denture derives its major support from the residual ridge with its fibrous connective tissue covering. Some areas of this residual ridge are firm, with limited displaceability, whereas other areas are displaceable, depending on the thickness and structural character of the tissues overlying the residual alveolar bone. The movement of the base under function determines the occlusal efficiency of the partial denture and also the degree to which the abutment teeth are subjected to torque and tipping stresses.

Impression registration. An impression registration for the construction of a partial denture must fulfill the following two requirements:

1. The anatomic form and the relationship of the remaining teeth in the dental arch, as well as the surrounding soft tissues, must be recorded accurately so that the denture will not exert pressure on those structures beyond their physiologic limits and so that its retentive and stabilizing components may be properly placed. Some impression material that can be removed from undercut areas without permanent distortion must be used to fulfill this requirement. The elastic impression materials such as revers-

ible hydrocolloid agar or irreversible hydrocolloid alginate, mercaptan rubber base (Thiokol), and silicone impression materials are therefore used for this purpose.

2. The supporting form of the soft tissues underlying the distal extension base of the partial denture should be recorded so that firm areas are used as primary stress-bearing areas and readily displaceable tissues are not overloaded. Only in this way can maximum support of the partial denture base be obtained. An impression material capable of displacing tissue sufficiently to register the supporting form of the ridge will fulfill this second requirement. One of the fluid mouth-temperature waxes or any of the readily flowing materials (rubber base, zinc oxide–eugenol impression paste, or silicone impression material [provided an individual, corrected tray is used]) may be employed for registering the supporting form.

No single impression material can satisfactorily fulfill both of the previously mentioned requirements. The compromise by recording just the anatomic form of both teeth and supporting tissues can result only in inadequate support for the distal extension base of the partial denture.

Differences in clasp design. A fifth point of difference between the two main types of partial dentures lies in their **requirements for direct retention.**

Direct retainers may be classified as being either intracoronal or extracoronal. The clasp-type partial denture, using the extracoronal direct retainer, is probably used a hundred times more frequently than is the intracoronal, or internal attachment, partial denture. This is not necessarily an indication of increasing preference for the clasp denture, nor is it a reflection on the excellence of the internal attachment denture. The fact remains, however, that although the internal attachment was devised more than forty-five years ago, for economic and other reasons the clasp denture is the more widely used. The clasp-type denture permits the rendering of a physiologically sound partial denture service to the greatest number of patients in keeping with the ability of the majority of patients to pay for such service.

The tooth-borne partial denture, being totally supported by abutment teeth, is retained and stabilized by a clasp at each end of each endentulous space. The only requirement of such clasps is that they flex sufficiently during placement and removal of the denture to pass over the height of contour of the teeth in approaching or escaping from an undercut area. While in its terminal position on the tooth, a retentive clasp should be passive and should not be called on to flex except when engaging the undercut area of the tooth for resisting a vertical dislodging force.

Cast retentive arms are generally used for this purpose. These may be either of the circumferential type, arising from the body of the clasp and approaching the undercut from an occlusal direction, or of the bar type, arising from the base of the denture and approaching the undercut area from a gingival direction. A modification of the latter type is the infrabulge clasp. Each of these two types of cast clasps has its advantages and disadvantages.

The direct retainer adjacent to a distal extension base must perform still another function in addition to that of resisting vertical displacement. Because of the lack of tooth support distally, the denture base will move tissueward under function proportionate to the quality of the supporting tissues, the accuracy of the impression registration, the accuracy of the denture base, and the total occlusal load applied. Because of this tissueward movement, those elements of the circumferential clasp that lie in a mesial undercut area must be able to flex sufficiently to dissipate stresses, which otherwise would be transmitted directly to the abutment tooth as leverage. On the other hand, a bar-type retainer placed to take advantage of a distal undercut moves farther into the undercut and does not overly stress the abutment tooth.

The cast circumferential clasp cannot effectively act to dissipate this stress for two reasons. First, the material itself can have only a limited flexibility, or else other parts of the casting (which must be rigid, such as lingual and palatal bars) would also tend to be flexible. The material employed being the same, the only variable factors are the bulk and diameter used in each component part. Second, and probably more important, the cast circumferential clasp is of necessity made half-round in shape. Since edgewise flexing is negligible, the clasp can flex in only one direction and therefore cannot ef-

fectively dissipate, by flexing, the torque stresses placed on it. For this reason some torque is inevitably transmitted to the abutment tooth and is magnified by the length of the lever arm.

Immediately there come to mind the stressbreakers, which are often incorporated into the partial denture design for this reason. Some dentists strongly believe that a stressbreaker is the best means of preventing leverage from being transmitted to the abutment teeth. Others believe just as strongly that a wrought-wire or bar-type retentive arm more effectively accomplishes this purpose with greater simplicity and ease of application. It cannot be denied that a retentive clasp arm made of wrought wire can flex more readily in all directions than can the cast half-round clasp arm and thereby more effectively dissipate those stresses that would otherwise be transmitted to the abutment tooth. The advantages and disadvantages of stressbreakers have been considered in detail in Chapter 8.

Only the retentive arm of the circumferential clasp, however, should be made of wrought metal. Reciprocation and stabilization against lateral movement must be obtained through the use of the rigid cast elements that make up the remainder of the clasp. This is called a combination clasp, being a combination of both cast and wrought materials incorporated into one direct retainer. It is frequently used on the terminal abutment for the distal extension partial denture and is indicated where a mesiobuccal but no distobuccal undercut exists or can be made, or where a gross tissue undercut, cervical and buccal to the abutment tooth, exists. It must always be remembered that the factor of length contributes to the flexibility of clasp arms. A short wrought-wire arm can be a destructive element because of its reduced ability to flex compared with a longer wrought-wire arm. However, in addition to its greater flexibility compared with the cast circumferential clasp, the combination clasp has further advantages of adjustability, minimal tooth contact, and better esthetics, which justifies its occasional use in tooth-borne designs also.

ESSENTIALS OF PARTIAL DENTURE DESIGN

The design of the partial denture framework should be carefully planned and outlined on an

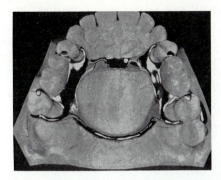

Fig. 9-16. Removable partial denture in maxillary Class III arch. Design consists of anterior and posterior palatal strap major connectors, resin-supported artificial teeth, and bar clasp arms throughout. (From McCracken, W.L.: J. Prosthet. Dent. **8:** 71-84, 1958.)

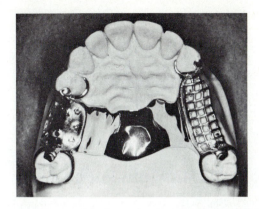

Fig. 9-17. Removable partial denture framework in maxillary Class III arch. Design consists of single palatal major connector, bar and circumferential clasp arms, and means to attach resin-supported artificial teeth.

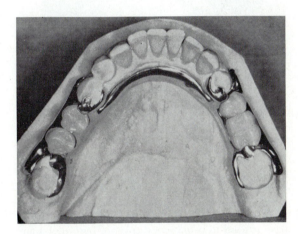

Fig. 9-18. Removable partial denture in mandibular Class III arch. Design consists of lingual bar major connector, metal bases and tube teeth, and bar clasp arms. Note mesially inclined left third molar with onlay-type reciprocal clasp arm. (From McCracken, W.L.: J. Prosthet. Dent. **8:**71-84, 1958.)

accurate diagnostic cast. After optimum health of oral tissues has been achieved and abutments have been modified to provide for rests, favorable location of framework components, and guiding planes, the master cast is made and carefully surveyed to determine the location of undercut areas that are either to be blocked out or used for retention. The design should provide for occlusal rests and rigid reciprocal arms on all abutment teeth to assure vertical and horizontal stability of the partial denture.

The design must include provision for adequate indirect retention that will function to counteract any lifting of the distal extension base away from the tissues. The indirect retainers should be placed in relation to a line drawn through the two principal abutments, which is the axis of rotation, or the **fulcrum line.** The indirect retainer may be in the form of an auxiliary occlusal rest, a continuous bar retainer in combination with terminal rests, a linguoplate with terminal rests, or an incisal rest on an anterior tooth. The indirect retainer should be placed as far as possible from this fulcrum line and should not terminate on a tooth incline, such as the lingual surface of an anterior tooth.

Some retentive elements for the attachment of the resin bases must be provided to complete the partial denture framework.

Class III removable partial denture (Figs. 9-16 to 9-21). The Kennedy Class III removable partial denture, being entirely tooth supported, may be made entirely to fit the anatomic form

of the teeth and surrounding structures. It does not require an impression of the functional form of the ridge tissues nor does it require indirect retention. Cast clasps of either the circumferential or the bar type may be used, or the combination clasp may be used if preferred. Unless a need for later relining is anticipated, as in the case of recently extracted teeth, the denture

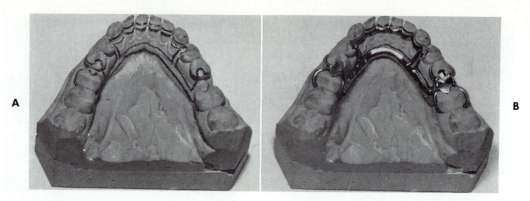

Fig. 9-19. A, Carefully designed tooth-borne framework outlined on master cast, in this particular instance to support anterior teeth in mouth of musician being traumatized by constant trumpet playing. Note positive lingual rest seats on canines. **B,** Cast framework as returned from laboratory, following precisely design prescribed by dentist.

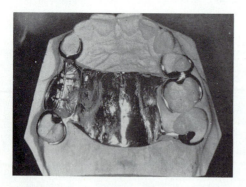

Fig. 9-20. Maxillary Class III partial denture framework designed for maximum periodontal support. Posterior occlusal rest and clasp arm on nonedentulous side are added for stabilization and to prevent settling of major connector at that point. Partial metal base is used to avoid any display of base metal anteriorly.

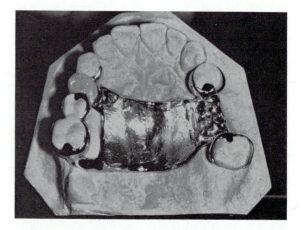

Fig. 9-21. Maxillary Class III, modification 1, partial denture designed as periodontal splint. Full crowns on patient's right premolar and molar are splinted together with continuous lingual ledges. Patient's left premolar is full crown with lingual ledge. Left molar abutment is unrestored but altered somewhat by recontouring. All gold guiding plane surfaces, lingual and proximal, were machined parallel to path of placement. Unilateral fixed partial dentures would not provide bilateral stabilization needed for this patient.

base may be made of metal, which has several advantages.

The Class III partial denture can frequently be used as a valuable aid to periodontal treatment because of its stabilizing influence on the remaining teeth (Fig. 9-20).

Class I, bilateral, distal extension partial dentures. The Class I, bilateral, distal extension partial denture is as completely unlike the Class III type as any two dental restorations could be. Since it derives its principal support from the tissues underlying its base, a Class I partial denture made to anatomic ridge form cannot have uniform and adequate support. Yet, unfortunately, many Class I mandibular partial dentures are being made from a single hydrocolloid impression. In such situations both the abut-

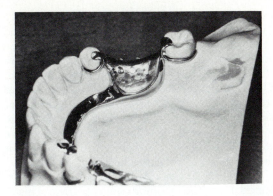

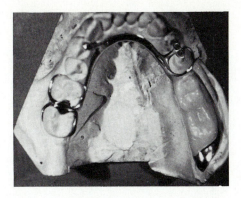

Fig. 9-22. Mandibular Class II, modification 1, partial denture framework for resin distal extension base and cast base on tooth-borne modification space. Bar-type retainers engage distobuccal undercuts on premolar abutments.

Fig. 9-23. Mandibular Class II partial denture with metal distal extension base. Acrylic resin attachment of prosthetically supplied teeth to metal base is with suitable mechanical retention (nail-heads, loops, or spurs, plus undercut finishing line). Embrasure clasps are used on nonedentulous side, with indirect retainer located favorably in relation to fulcrum line. Because of tissue undercut cervical to buccal surface of right second premolar and lack of distobuccal undercut, wrought-wire (tapered) retainer arm was used.

ment teeth and the residual ridges suffer because the occlusal load placed on the remaining teeth is inevitably made greater by the lack of adequate posterior support.

Many dentists, recognizing the need for some type of impression registration that will record the supporting form of the residual ridge, attempt to record this form with a metallic oxide, rubber base, or silicone impression material. Such materials actually only record the anatomic form of the ridge, except when special design of the impression trays permits placement of tissues overlying primary stress-bearing areas. Others prefer to place a base that was made to fit the anatomic form of the ridge under some pressure at the time that it is related to the remaining teeth, thus obtaining functional support. Any impression record will be influenced by the consistency of the impression material and the amount of hydraulic pressure exerted by its confinement within the impression tray. Still others, believing that a properly compounded mouth-temperature wax will displace only those tissues that are incapable of providing support to the denture base, use a wax secondary impression to record the supporting, or functional, form of the edentulous ridge.

Class II partial dentures (Figs. 9-22 and 9-23). The Kennedy Class II partial denture actually may be a combination of both tissue-borne and tooth-borne restorations. The distal exten-

sion base must have adequate tissue support, whereas tooth-borne bases elsewhere in the arch may be made to fit the anatomic form of the underlying ridge. Indirect retention must be provided for, but occasionally the anterior abutment on the tooth-borne side will serve to satisfy this requirement. If additional indirect retention is needed, provisions must be made for it.

Cast clasps are generally used on the tooth-borne side, whereas some clasp design must be used on the abutment tooth adjacent to the distal extension, which will prevent the application of torque to that tooth. The use of a cast circumferential clasp engaging a mesiobuccal undercut on the anterior abutment of the tooth-borne modification space is questioned as being sound. A Class II, modification 1 (posterior space), situation can result in a Class I leverlike design of the denture. It seems rational in this instance to use a bar-type retainer engaging a distobuccal undercut (Fig. 9-24). Should the bar-type retainer be contraindicated because of a gross tissue undercut or the existence of only a mesiobuccal undercut on the anterior abutment, then a combination direct retainer should be used having the retentive arm made of tapered

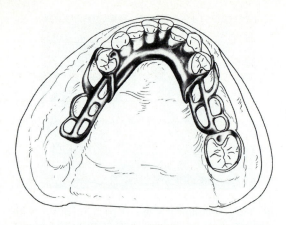

Fig. 9-24. Mandibular Class II, modification 1, partially edentulous arch. Note that bar-type retentive arms are used on both premolar abutments, engaging distobuccal undercuts at their terminal ends. Lever-like forces may not be as readily imparted to right premolar, contrasted with cast circumferential direct retainer engaging mesiobuccal undercut.

wrought wire. **A thorough understanding of the advantages and disadvantages of various clasp designs is necessary in determining the type of direct retainer that is to be used for each abutment tooth.**

The steps in the completion of the Class II partial denture follow closely those of the Class I partial denture, except that the distal extension base is usually made of a resin material, whereas the base for any tooth-borne areas is frequently made of metal. This is permissible because the residual ridge beneath tooth-borne bases is not called on to provide support for the denture, and later rebasing is not as likely to be necessary.

COMPONENTS OF PARTIAL DENTURES

All partial dentures have two things in common: (1) they must be supported by oral structures and (2) they must be retained against reasonable dislodging forces.

In the Class III partial denture three components are necessary: the connectors, the retainers, and the stabilizing components.

The partial denture that does not have the advantage of tooth support at each end of each edentulous space still must have support, but in this instance the support comes from both the teeth and the underlying ridge tissues rather than from the teeth alone. This is a composite support, and the prosthesis must be fabricated so that the resilient support provided by the edentulous ridge is coordinated with the more stable support offered by the abutment teeth. The three essentials—connectors, retainers, and stabilizing components—must be even more carefully designed and executed because of the movement of tissue-supported denture base areas. In addition, provision must be made for three other essentials, as follows:

1. The best possible support must be obtained from the resilient ridge tissues. This is accomplished by the impression technique more than by the partial denture design, although the amount of area covered by the partial denture is a contributing factor in such support.

2. The method of direct retention must take into account the inevitable tissueward movement of the distal extension base(s) under the stresses of mastication and occlusion. Direct retainers must be designed so that some flexing under an occlusal load will occur, resulting in the direct transmission of this load, instead of leverage, to the abutment teeth.

3. The partial denture having one or more distal extension denture bases must be designed so that movement of the unsupported and unretained end away from the tissues will be prevented or minimized. This is often referred to as indirect retention and is best described in relation to an axis of rotation through the rest areas of the principal abutments. However, retention from the partial denture base itself frequently can be made to prevent this movement of the denture base away from the tissues and, in such instances, may be discussed as direct-indirect retention.

The support of the partial denture by the abutment teeth is dependent on the alveolar support of those teeth, the rigidity of the partial denture framework, and the design of the occlusal rests. Through clinical and roentgenographic interpretation the dentist may evaluate the abutment teeth and decide whether they will provide adequate support. In some instances the splinting of two or more teeth is advisable, either by fixed partial dentures or by soldering two or more individual restorations together. In other instances a tooth may be deemed too weak to be used as an abutment, and extraction is indicated in favor of obtaining better support from an adjacent tooth.

Having decided on the abutments, the dentist is responsible for the preparation of the abutment teeth, for the design of cast restorations, and for the form of the occlusal rest seats. These may be prepared either in sound tooth enamel or in the cast restorations. The technician cannot be blamed for inadequate occlusal rest support. On the other hand, the technician is solely to blame if he extends the casting beyond or fails to include the total prepared area. If a definite occlusal rest seat is faithfully recorded in the master cast and delineated in the penciled design, no excuse can be made for poor occlusal rest form on the partial denture if the dentist has sufficiently reduced the marginal ridge area of the rest seat to avoid interference from opposing teeth.

Major connectors. A major connector should be properly located in relation to gingival and moving tissues and should be designed to be rigid. Rigidity in a major connector is necessary to provide proper distribution of forces to and from the supporting components.

A lingual bar connector should be tapered superiorly with a half-pear shape in cross section and should be relieved sufficiently but not excessively over the underlying tissues when such relief is indicated. The addition of a continuous bar retainer or a lingual apron does not alter the basic design of the lingual bar. These are added solely for support, stabilization, rigidity, and protection of the anterior teeth and specifically are neither connectors nor indirect retainers. The finished inferior border of either a lingual bar or a linguoplate should be gently rounded to avoid irritation to subadjacent tissues when the restoration moves even slightly in function.

The use of a linguoplate is indicated when the lower anterior teeth are weakened by periodontal disease. It is also indicated in Class I partially edentulous arches wherein the need for additional resistance to horizontal rotation of the denture is occasioned by excessively resorbed residual ridges. Still another indication is in those situations in which the floor of the mouth so closely approximates the lingual gingiva of anterior teeth that an adequately inflexible lingual bar cannot be positioned without impinging the gingival tissues.

Experience with the linguoplate has shown that with good oral hygiene the underlying tissues remain healthy and there are no harmful effects to the tissues from the metallic coverage per se. However, adequate relief must be provided whenever a metal component crosses the gingival margins and the adjacent gingivae. Excessive relief should be avoided because tissues tend to fill a void, resulting in the overgrowth of abnormal tissue. The amount of relief used, therefore, should be only the minimum necessary to avoid gingival impingement.

It does not seem that there are many advantages to be found in the use of the continuous bar retainer versus the linguoplate. In rare instances, when a linguoplate would be visible through multiple interproximal embrasures, the continuous bar retainer may be preferred for esthetic reasons only. In other instances, when a single diastema exists, a linguoplate may be cut out in this area to avoid display of metal, without sacrificing its use when otherwise indicated.

Rigidity of a palatal major connector is just as important and its location and design just as critical as for a lingual bar. A U-shaped palatal connector is rarely justified except to avoid an inoperable palatal torus that extends to the junction of the hard and soft palates. Neither can the routine use of a narrow, single palatal bar be justified. The combination anterior-posterior palatal strap–type major connector is mechanically and biologically sound if it is located so that it does not impinge on tissues. The broad, anatomic palatal major connector is frequently preferred because of its rigidity, better acceptance by the patient, and greater stability without tissue damage. In addition, this type of connector may provide direct-indirect retention that may sometimes, but rarely, eliminate the need for separate indirect retainers.

Direct retainers for tooth-borne partial dentures. Retainers for tooth-borne partial dentures have only two functions, and these are to retain the prosthesis against reasonable dislodging forces without damage to the abutment teeth and to aid in resisting any tendency of the denture to be displaced in a horizontal plane. There can be no movement of the prosthesis tissue-ward because each terminus is supported by a rest. There can be no movement away from the tissues, and therefore no rotation about a fulcrum, because each terminus is secured by a direct retainer.

Any type of direct retainer is acceptable as long as the abutment tooth is not jeopardized by its presence. Intracoronal (frictional) retainers are ideal for tooth-borne restorations and offer esthetic advantages not possible with extracoronal (clasp) retainers. Nevertheless the circumferential and bar-type clasp retainers are mechanically effective and are more economically constructed than are intracoronal retainers. Therefore they are more universally used.

Vulnerable areas on the abutment teeth must be protected by restorations with either type of retainer. The clasp retainer must not impinge on gingival tissues. The clasp must not exert excessive torque on the abutment tooth during placement and removal. It must be located the least distance into the tooth undercut for adequate retention, and it must be designed with a minimum of bulk and tooth contact.

The bar clasp arm should be used only when the area for retention lies close to the gingival margin of the tooth and little tissue blockout is necessary. If the clasp must be placed high occlusally or if an objectionable space would exist beneath the bar clasp arm because of blockout of tissue undercuts, the bar clasp arm should not be used. In the event of an excessive tissue undercut, consideration should be given to recontouring the abutment and using some type of circumferential direct retainer.

Direct retainers for distal extension partial dentures. Retainers for distal extension partial dentures, while retaining the prosthesis, must also be able to flex or disengage when the denture base moves tissueward under function. Thus the retainer may act as a stressbreaker. Mechanical stressbreakers accomplish the same thing, but they do so at the expense of horizontal stabilization. When some kind of mechanical stressbreaker is used, the denture flange must be able to act to prevent horizontal movement. Clasp designs that allow for flexing of the retentive clasp arm may accomplish the same purpose as that of mechanical stressbreakers, without

sacrificing horizontal stabilization and generally with less complicated techniques.

In evaluating the ability of a clasp arm to act as a stressbreaker, one must realize that flexing in one plane is not enough. The clasp arm must be freely flexible in any direction, as dictated by the stresses applied. Bulky, half-round clasp arms cannot do this and neither can a bar clasp engaging an undercut on the side of the tooth away from the denture base. Round, tapered clasp forms offer advantages of greater and more universal flexibility, less tooth contact, and better esthetics. **Either the combination circumferential clasp with its tapered wrought-wire retentive arm or the carefully located and properly designed bar clasp should be used on all abutment teeth adjacent to extension denture bases.**

Stabilizing components. Stabilizing components of the partial denture framework are those rigid components that assist in stabilizing the denture against horizontal movement. The purpose of all stabilizing components should be to distribute stresses equally to all supporting teeth without overworking any one tooth.

All minor connectors that contact vertical tooth surfaces (and all reciprocal clasp arms) act as stabilizing components. It is necessary that minor connectors have sufficient bulk to be rigid and yet that they present as little bulk to the tongue as possible. This means that they should be confined to interdental embrasures whenever possible. When minor connectors are located on vertical tooth surfaces, it is best that these surfaces be parallel to the path of placement. When cast restorations are used, these surfaces of the wax patterns should be made parallel on the surveyor before casting.

Reciprocal clasp arms also must be rigid, and they must be placed occlusally to the height of contour of the abutment teeth, where they will be nonretentive. By their rigidity, these clasp arms reciprocate the opposing retentive clasp, and they also prevent horizontal movement of the prosthesis under functional stresses. For a reciprocal clasp arm to be placed favorably, some reduction of the tooth surfaces involved is frequently necessary to increase the suprabulge area.

When crown restorations are used, a lingual

reciprocal clasp arm may be inset into the tooth contour by providing a ledge on the crown on which the clasp arm may rest. This permits the use of a wider clasp arm and restores a more nearly normal tooth contour, at the same time maintaining its strength and rigidity.

Guiding planes. The term **guiding planes** is defined as two or more parallel, vertical surfaces of abutment teeth, so shaped as to direct a prosthesis during placement and removal. After the most favorable path of placement has been ascertained, axial surfaces of abutment teeth are found, or are prepared, parallel to the path of placement and therefore become parallel to each other. Guiding planes may be contacted by various components of the restoration—the body of an extracoronal direct retainer, the stabilizing arm of a direct retainer, the minor connector portion of an indirect retainer—or by a minor connector specifically designed to contact the guiding plane surface.

The functions of guiding plane surfaces are as follows: (1) **to provide for one path of placement and removal of the restoration** (to eliminate detrimental strain to abutment teeth and framework components during placement and removal); (2) **to ensure the intended actions of reciprocal, stabilizing, and retentive components** (to provide retention against dislodgement of the restoration when the dislodging force is directed other than parallel to the path of removal, and also to provide stabilization against horizontal rotation of the denture); (3) **to eliminate gross food traps between abutment teeth and components of the denture.**

Guiding plane surfaces should be found or created so that they are as nearly parallel to the long axes of abutment teeth as possible. Establishing guiding planes on several abutment teeth (preferably more than two teeth), located at widely separated positions in the dental arch, provides for a more effective use of these surfaces. The effectiveness of guiding plane surfaces is also enhanced if these surfaces lie in more than one common axial surface of the abutment teeth (Fig. 9-25).

As a rule of thumb, proximal guiding plane surfaces should be about **two thirds** as wide as the distance between the tips of adjacent buccal and lingual cusps and should extend vertically

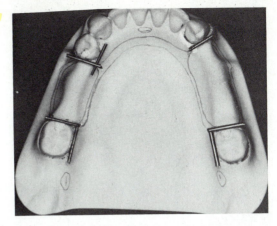

Fig. 9-25. Prospective guiding plane surfaces are indicated by wires placed on abutment teeth. All these surfaces, when used, can be made vertically parallel to path of placement. However by including guiding plane surfaces, which are divergent cross-arch, resistance to horizontal rotation of denture is enhanced.

about **two thirds** the length of the "enamel crown" portion of the tooth from the marginal ridge cervically. In preparing guiding plane surfaces, care must be exercised to avoid creating buccal or lingual line angles (Fig. 9-26). Assuming that the stabilizing or retentive arm of a direct retainer may originate in the guiding plane region, a line angle preparation would weaken either or both components of the clasp assembly.

A guiding plane should generally be located on the abutment surface adjacent to an edentulous area. However, excess torquing is inevitable if guiding planes squarely facing each other on a lone standing abutment adjacent to an extension area are used (Fig. 9-27).

Ridge support. Support for the tooth-borne denture or the tooth-borne modification space comes entirely from the abutment teeth by means of rests. Support for the distal extension denture base comes primarily from the soft tissues overlying the residual alveolar bone. In the latter, rest support is effective only at the abutment end of the denture base.

The effectiveness of tissue support depends on four things: (1) the quality of the residual ridge, (2) the total occlusal load applied, (3) the accuracy of the denture bases, and (4) the accuracy and type of impression registration.

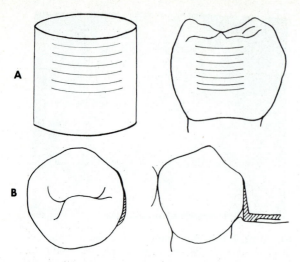

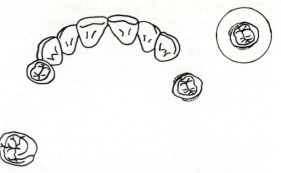

Fig. 9-27. Guiding planes squarely facing each other should not be prepared on lone standing abutment. Minor connectors of framework (hatched areas) would place undue strain on abutment when denture rotated vertically either superiorly or inferiorly. Such unfavorable leverage could be avoided by simply preparing guiding plane surfaces to slightly diverge in buccal direction (inset).

Fig. 9-26. **A,** Guiding plane surface should be like area on cylindric object. It should be continuous surface unbounded by even "rounded" line angles. **B,** Minor connector contacting guiding plane surface has same curvature as does that surface. From occlusal view it tapers buccally from thicker lingual portion, thus permitting closer contact of abutment tooth and prosthetically supplied tooth. Viewed from buccal aspect, minor connector contacts "enamel" crown of tooth on its proximal surface only about two thirds its length.

The quality of the residual ridge cannot be influenced, except to improve it by tissue conditioning, or to modify it by surgical intervention. Such modifications are frequently advisable but are less frequently done.

The total occlusal load applied to the residual ridge may be influenced by reducing the occlusal area. This is done by the use of fewer, narrower, and more effectively shaped artificial teeth (Fig. 9-28).

The accuracy of the denture base is influenced by the choice of materials and by the exactness of the processing techniques. Inaccurate and warped denture bases influence adversely the support of the partial denture. Materials and techniques that will assure the greatest dimensional stability should be selected.

The accuracy of the impression technique is entirely in the hands of the dentist. Maximum tissue coverage for support and the use of primary stress-bearing areas should be the primary

objectives in any partial denture impression technique. The manner in which this is accomplished should be based on a biologic comprehension of what happens beneath a distal extension denture base when an occlusal load is applied.

The distal extension partial denture is unique in that its support is derived both from abutment teeth, which are comparatively unyielding, and from soft tissues, which may be comparatively yielding under occlusal forces. Resilient tissues, being unable to provide support for the denture base comparable to that offered by the abutment teeth, are displaced by the occlusal load. Only the projections of the underlying residual bone remain to be traumatized by occlusal forces. This problem of support is further complicated by the fact that the patient has natural teeth remaining on which he may exert far greater force than he would were he completely edentulous. This fact is clearly evident from the damage often occurring to an edentulous ridge when it is opposed by a few remaining anterior teeth in the other arch, and especially when the opposing occlusion of anterior teeth has been arranged so that contact exists in both centric and eccentric positions.

Ridge tissues recorded in their resting, or nonfunctioning, form are incapable of providing

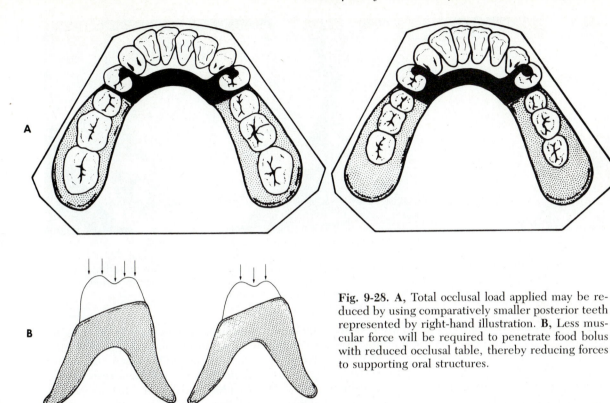

Fig. 9-28. A, Total occlusal load applied may be reduced by using comparatively smaller posterior teeth represented by right-hand illustration. **B,** Less muscular force will be required to penetrate food bolus with reduced occlusal table, thereby reducing forces to supporting oral structures.

the composite support needed for a denture that derives its support from both hard and soft tissue. Three factors must be considered in the acceptance of an impression technique for distal extension partial dentures: (1) the material should record the tissues covering the primary stress-bearing areas in their supporting form; (2) tissues within the basal seat area other than primary stress-bearing areas must be recorded in their anatomic form; and (3) the total area covered by the impression should be as great as possible, to distribute the load over as large an area as can be tolerated by the border tissues. This is an application of the principle of the snowshoe.

Anyone who has had the opportunity to compare two master casts for the same partially edentulous arch—one cast having the distal extension area recorded in its anatomic, or resting, form and the other cast having the distal extension area recorded in its functional form—has been impressed by the differences in the two

(Fig. 9-29). A denture base processed to the functional form is generally less irregular, and it has greater area coverage than does a denture base processed to the anatomic, or resting, form. Moreover, and of far greater significance, **a denture base made to anatomic form exhibits less stability under rotating forces than does a denture base processed to functional form** and thus fails to maintain its occlusal relation with the opposing teeth. By having the patient close onto strips of soft wax, it is evident that occlusion is maintained at a point of equilibrium over a longer period of time when the denture base has been made to the functional form. In contrast, evidence exists that there has been a rapid settling of the denture base when it has been made to the anatomic form, with an early return of the occlusion to natural tooth contact only. Such a denture not only fails to distribute the occlusal load equitably, but it also allows rotational movement, which is damaging to the abutment teeth and their investing structures.

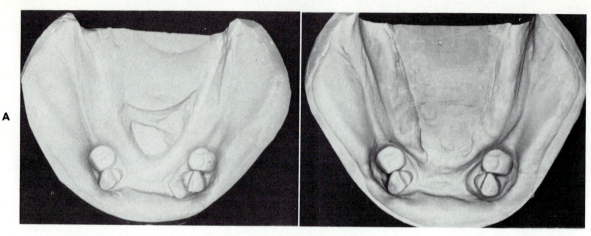

Fig. 9-29. A, Cast of partially edentulous arch representing anatomic form of residual ridges. Impression was made in stock tray using irreversible hydrocolloid. **B,** Impression recording the functional or supporting form of residual ridges was made in individualized impression tray, permitting placement of tissues and definitive border molding.

Indirect retainers. An indirect retainer must be placed as far anteriorly from the fulcrum line as adequate tooth support permits, if it is to function with the direct retainer to restrict movement of a distal extension base away from the basal seat tissues. It must be placed on a rest seat prepared in an abutment tooth that is capable of withstanding the forces placed on it. An indirect retainer cannot function effectively on an inclined tooth surface, nor can a single weak incisor tooth be used for this purpose. Either a canine or premolar tooth should be used for the support of an indirect retainer, and the rest seat must be prepared with as much care as is given any other rest seat. An incisal rest or a lingual rest may be used on an anterior tooth, provided a definite seat can be obtained either in sound enamel or on a cast restoration.

A second purpose that indirect retainers serve in partial denture design is that of support for major connectors. A long lingual bar or an anterior palatal major connector is thereby prevented from settling into the tissues. Even in the absence of a need for indirect retention, provision for such auxiliary support is sometimes indicated.

Contrary to common usage, a continuous bar retainer or a linguoplate does not in itself act as an indirect retainer. Since these are located on inclined tooth surfaces, they serve more as **an orthodontic appliance** than as support for the partial denture. When a linguoplate or a continuous bar retainer is used, terminal rests should always be provided at either end to stabilize the denture and to prevent orthodontic movement of the teeth contacted to the greatest extent possible. Such terminal rests may function also as the indirect retainers, but these would function equally well in that capacity without the continuous bar retainer or linguoplate.

ADDITIONAL CONSIDERATIONS INFLUENCING DESIGN

Every effort should be made by the dentist to gain the greatest support possible for removable restorations by using abutments bounding edentulous spaces. Not only will the residual ridges be relieved of some support contribution, but design of the framework may be greatly simplified. To this end, use of splint bars, internal clip attachments, and overlay abutments should be considered.

Use of a splint bar for denture support. In the Chapter 13 discussion of missing anterior teeth, mention is made of the fact that missing anterior teeth are best replaced with a fixed partial denture that also replaces posterior teeth elsewhere in the arch. The following is quoted

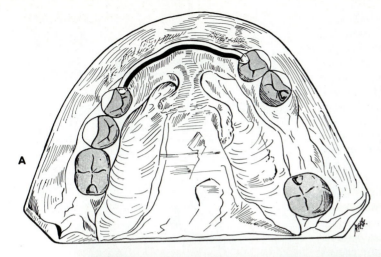

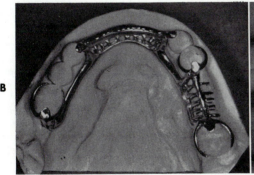

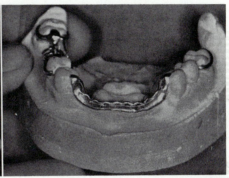

Fig. 9-30. A, Splint bar attached to double abutments on either side of arch. Although this may be made of hard gold alloy, its rigidity is better assured by making bar of chromium-cobalt alloy that fits into recesses prepared in abutment pieces, attaching it by electric soldering. **B** and **C,** Denture framework designed to fit and be supported by splint bar.

from that chapter: "From a biomechanical standpoint, . . . a removable partial denture should replace only the missing posterior teeth **after** the remainder of the arch has been made intact by fixed restorations."

Occasionally a situation is found in which, economics aside, it is necessary that several missing anterior teeth be replaced with the removable partial denture rather than by fixed restorations. This may be because of the length of the edentulous span, the loss of sufficient residual ridge by resorption, accident, or surgery, or the result of a situation in which too much vertical space prevents the use of a fixed partial denture or in which esthetic requirements can better be met through the use of teeth added to the denture framework. In such instances it is necessary that the best possible support for the replaced anterior teeth be provided. Ordinarily this is

done through the placement of occlusal or lingual rests, or both, on the adjacent natural teeth, but when the edentulous span is too large to assure adequate support from the adjacent teeth, another method must be used. This is included here only because it influences the design of the major connector that must then be used.

An anterior splint bar may be attached to the adjacent abutment teeth in such a manner that a fixed splint results, but with a smooth, contoured bar resting lightly on the gingival tissues to support the removable partial denture (Fig. 9-30, *A*). As with any fixed partial denture, the type of abutment retainers and the decision to use multiple abutments will depend on the length of the span and the stability of the teeth being used as abutments. Regardless of the type of abutment retainers used, the connecting bar must be cast separately and of a rigid alloy, or a commercially available bar may be used and attached to the abutments by soldering.

The length of the span influences the choice of size of a splint bar. Long spans require more rigid bars (10-gauge) than short spans (13-gauge). Rather then rely on soldered junctions alone, it is best that recesses be formed in the abutment pieces and that the connecting bar, which rests lightly on the tissues, be cast or made to fit into these recesses; they are then attached by soldering.

Because of the greater rigidity of the chromium-cobalt alloys, the splint bar is preferably cast in one of these materials and then attached to the gold abutment pieces by electric soldering. The complete assembly (abutment pieces and connecting bar) is then cemented permanently to the abutment teeth, the same as a fixed partial denture. The impression for the partial denture is then made, and a master cast obtained that accurately reproduces the contours of the tissue bar. The denture framework is then made to fit this bar by extending the major connector to cover and rest upon the splint bar. Either retention for the attachment of a resin base, or any other acceptable means of attaching the replaced anterior teeth, is incorporated into the denture design (Fig. 9-30, *B* and *C*.) In those situations wherein the removable restoration will be practically tooth supported, the splint bar may be curved to follow the crest of the residual ridge, as seen in Fig. 9-30, *A*. However, in a distal extension situation, because of the vertical rotation of the denture, caution must be exercised to form the splint bar so that excessive torque will not accrue to its supporting abutments (Fig. 9-31). The proximal contours of abutments adjacent to splint bars should be parallel to the path of placement. This serves two purposes: (1) it permits a desirable arrangement of artificial teeth and (2) it aids in resisting horizontal rotation of the restoration.

The splint bar must be positioned anteroposteriorly in relation to the residual ridge to allow a normal arrangement of artificial teeth. The resulting partial denture will have the esthetic and other advantages of removable anterior replacements but will have positive support from the underlying splint bar (Fig. 9-32).

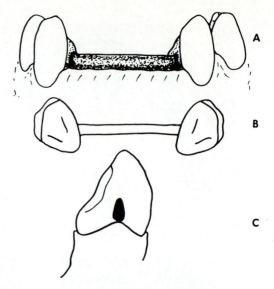

Fig. 9-31. A, Insofar as possible, "incisal" portion of splint bar should be flat when viewed frontally. Provision must be made in construction and location of bar so that dental floss may be threaded underneath bar to allow proper cleaning by patient. **B,** As viewed from above, bar is in straight line between abutments. This is especially critical for distal extension dentures to avoid excess torque on abutments as denture rotates in function. **C,** Sagittal section through bar demonstrates rounded form of bar making point contact with residual ridge. Whole "tissue" surface of bar is easily accessible for cleaning with dental floss. Pear-shaped bar (in cross section) will permit rotation of removable partial denture without appreciable resistance or torque.

Internal clip attachment. The internal clip (or grip) attachment differs from the splint bar in that the internal clip attachment provides both support and retention at the connecting bar (Fig. 9-33).

The connecting bar is made of 11-gauge platinum alloy wire, and the female grip is made of 27-gauge plate metal. Rather than resting on the tissues of the residual ridge as does the splint bar, the wire bar is located slightly above the tissues. Retention is provided by the plate metal grip, which is contoured to fit the bar and is partially embedded by means of retention spurs or loops into the overlying resin denture base.

The internal clip attachment thus provides both support and retention for the anterior mod-

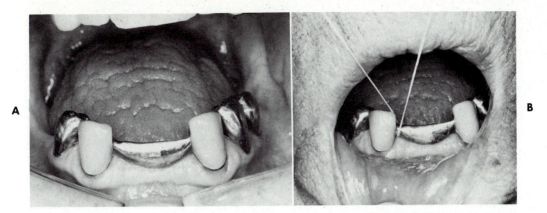

Fig. 9-32. A, Lower canines splinted together with splint bar. Longevity of these teeth is greatly enhanced by splinting. Tissue surfaces are minimally contacted by rounded form of lower portion of bar. Anterior and posterior slopes of splint bar must be compatible with path of placement of denture. **B,** Floss is used by patient to clean inferior portion of splint bar.

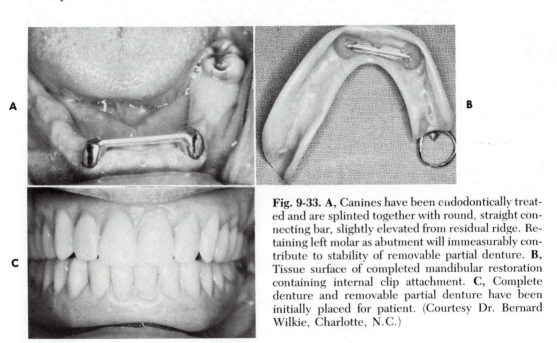

Fig. 9-33. A, Canines have been endodontically treated and are splinted together with round, straight connecting bar, slightly elevated from residual ridge. Retaining left molar as abutment will immeasurably contribute to stability of removable partial denture. **B,** Tissue surface of completed mandibular restoration containing internal clip attachment. **C,** Complete denture and removable partial denture have been initially placed for patient. (Courtesy Dr. Bernard Wilkie, Charlotte, N.C.)

ification area and may serve to eliminate both occlusal rests and retentive clasps on the adjacent abutment teeth.

Overlay abutment as support for a denture base. Every consideration should be directed to preventing the need for a distal extension removable partial denture. In many instances it is possible to salvage the roots and a portion of the crown of a badly broken down molar through endodontic treatment. A periodontally involved molar, otherwise indicated for extraction, may sometimes be salvaged by periodontal and endodontic treatment accompanied with reduction of the clinical crown almost level with gingival

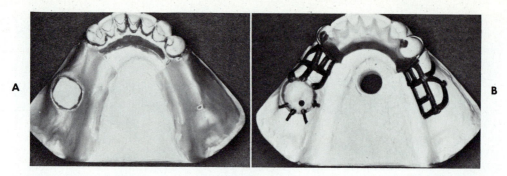

Fig. 9-34. A, Master cast has been prepared for duplicating in refractory investment to develop wax pattern for removable partial denture framework, supported by overlay abutment second molar. Molar could not be restored by conventional means. It was endodontically treated, and crown was reduced to slightly elevated dome shape. Pulp chamber was filled with silver amalgam alloy. **B,** Wax pattern has been developed on investment cast, and provision has been made to attach properly extended acrylic resin denture base. Bilateral distal extension denture has been avoided by planning overlay prosthesis.

tissues. An unopposed molar may have overly erupted to such an extent that restoring the tooth with a crown is inadequate to develop a harmonious occlusion. Then too, it is not unusual to encounter a molar that is so grossly tipped anteriorly that it cannot serve as an abutment unless the clinical crown is reduced drastically.

Such teeth as just described should be considered for possible support for an otherwise distal extension denture base. Endodontic treatment and preparation of the coronal portion of the tooth as a slightly elevated dome-shaped abutment often offer an alternative to a distal extension base (Fig. 9-34). The student is referred to the Selected Reading Resources section (textbooks; abutment retainers) for sources of information on overdenture abutments and overlay-type prostheses.

SELF-ASSESSMENT AIDS

1. Forces are transmitted to abutment teeth and residual ridges by removable partial dentures. One of the factors of a force is its magnitude. Can you recall the other three factors of a force that a dentist must consider in designing removable partial dentures?
2. The design of a removable restoration requires a consideration of mechanics as well as biologic considerations. True or false?
3. There are six simple machines recognized today. What are they?
4. Can a simple machine impart a greater force (effort) than the effort expended to activiate it?
5. Of the simple machines, which two are more likely to be encountered in the design of removable partial dentures?
6. What is a lever? A cantilever?
7. Can you name the three classes of levers and given an example of each?
8. Of the three classes of lever systems, which two are most likely to be encountered in removable partial prosthodontics?
9. Can you figure the mechanical advantage of a lever system, given dimensions of effort and resistance arms?
10. What class lever system is most likely to be encountered with a restoration on a Class II, modification 1, arch when a force is placed on the extension base?
11. What factor permits a distal extension denture to rotate when the denture base is forced toward the basal seat?
12. Is an abutment tooth better able to resist a force directed apically or directed horizontally? Why?
13. Where is the horizontal (tipping) axis of an abutment tooth located?
14. Where is the horizontal (tipping) axis of a fence post located?
15. If you had to shake a fence post out of the ground, where would you apply the force—at its top or at ground level?
16. Why should components of a direct retainer assembly be located as close to the tipping axis of a tooth as practical?

17. The text suggests at least nine factors that will influence the design of a removable partial denture. How many of these considerations can you jot down?

18. Do you feel that design of a denture is influence by the classification of the arch being restored?

19. There are really only two types of removable partial dentures. What are they?

20. Since there are two basic types of removable partial dentures, it is evident that a dentist must consider (1) the manner in which each is supported, (2) the method of impression registration, (3) the need or lack of need for indirect retention, and (4) the use of a base material that can be readily relined. Could you write a meaningful essay of 100 words or less about each of these listed considerations?

21. What is a guiding plane?

22. What are the functions of guiding plane surfaces contacted by minor connectors? There are at least three functions.

23. Should guiding planes prepared on enamel surfaces of abutment teeth be rounded or flat? Why?

24. Can you give a rule of thumb for the dimensions of proximal guiding planes?

25. Direct retainers for tooth-borne dentures differ in design from those employed in extension-type dentures to a great extent. What requirement, in relation to an undercut, exists for the direct retainer (clasp) on a terminal abutment of an extension denture when the denture base is forced in heavier contact with the residual ridge?

26. Name the component(s) of a removable partial denture that must be rigid. Name the component(s) in which flexibility is desirable.

27. Would you agree that a fixed partial denture, where indicated, should be the restoration of choice, in lieu of a removable partial denture?

28. What method should usually be used to replace single missing teeth or missing anterior teeth? Can you justify your answer?

29. You are confronted with a Class I arch in which all molars and first premolars are missing. Should you consider replacing the first premolars with fixed partial dentures rather than restoring the spaces with removable restoration? Why?

30. What is a splint bar?

31. Can you draw a splint bar from a frontal, horizontal, and sagittal view?

32. What purposes are served by using splint bars where indicated.

33. A decision has been made to use a splint bar from canine to canine. Will this decision influence the design of the framework?

34. For what reasons must a splint bar be convex, rather than concave, adjacent to the residual ridge?

35. Is a 13-gauge splint bar adequate for a span from canine to canine? Why or why not?

36. Do you know what an internal clip attachment is? Have you ever seen one?

37. The internal clip attachment must be used in conjunction with some type of bar supported by abutment teeth. What is the cross-sectional shape of such a bar? What advantages accrue from using such a design for a restoration?

38. You are confronted with a mandibular arch with only the six anterior teeth and two second molars remaining. The maxillary arch is edentulous. The anterior teeth are restorable individually and show no mobility or periodontal involvement. The molars, however, are grossly involved with caries; in fact most of the clinical crown is gone. They also show a Miller mobility classification of 1 and exhibit a 5 to 6 mm gingival crevicular depth. They can be treated peridontally and endodontically. In such a situation, if finances were not a factor, would you: (1) extract both molars? (2) prepare the molars for an overlay prosthesis? (3) extract all the mandibular teeth and treat the patient with complete dentures?

39. If you elected to prepare the molars mentioned in the preceding section for an overlay prosthesis, state your reasons for so doing in terms of benefits to the patient.

10 SURVEYING

Description of dental surveyor
Purposes of surveyor
Factors that determine path of placement and
    removal
Step-by-step procedures in surveying a
    diagnostic cast
Final path of placement

Recording relation of cast to surveyor
Surveying the master cast
Measuring retention
Blocking out the master cast
Relieving the master cast
Paralleled blockout, shaped blockout, arbitrary
    blockout, and relief

A dental surveyor has been defined as an instrument used to determine the relative parallelism of two or more surfaces of the teeth or other parts of the cast of a dental arch. **Therefore the primary purpose of surveying is to plan those modifications of oral structures necessary to fabricate a removable partial denture.**

Any one of several moderately priced surveyors on the market will adequately accomplish the procedures necessary to rationalize the design and construction of a partial denture. In addition, these surveyors may be used to parallel internal rests and intracoronal retainers. With handpiece holder added, they also may be used to machine internal rests and to parallel guiding plane surfaces of abutment restorations.

DESCRIPTION OF DENTAL SURVEYOR

Perhaps the most widely used surveyors are the Ney (Fig. 10-1) and the Jelenko (Fig. 10-2) surveyors. Both of these are precision-made instruments, but differ principally in that the Jelenko arm swivels, whereas the Ney arm is fixed. The technique for surveying and trimming blockout is therefore somewhat different. Other surveyors also differ in this respect, and the dentist may prefer one over another for this reason.

The principal parts of the Ney surveyor are as follows:

1. Platform on which the base is moved

2. Vertical arm that supports the superstructure
3. Horizontal arm from which the surveying tool suspends
4. Table to which the cast is attached
5. Base on which the table swivels
6. Paralleling tool or guideline marker (This tool contacts the convex surface to be studied in a tangential manner. The relative parallelism of one surface to another may thus be determined. By substituting a carbon marker, the height of contour then may be delineated on the surfaces of the abutment teeth and also on areas of interference requiring reduction on blockout.)
7. Mandrel for holding special tools (Fig. 10-3)

The principal parts of the Jelenko surveyor are essentially the same as those for the Ney surveyor except that by loosening the nut at the top of the vertical arm, the horizontal arm may be made to swivel. The objective of this feature, originally designed by Dr. Noble Wills, is to permit freedom of movement of the arm in a horizontal plane rather than to depend entirely on the horizontal movement of the cast. To some this is confusing because two horizontal movements must thus be coordinated. For those who prefer to move the cast only in a horizontal relationship to a fixed vertical arm, the nut may be tightened and the horizontal arm used in a

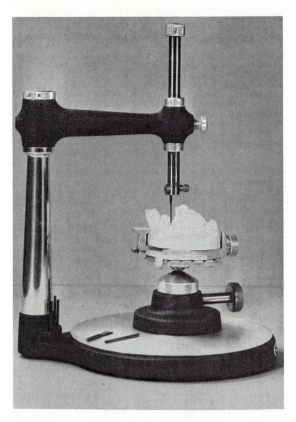

Fig. 10-1. Ney surveyor is widely used because of its simplicity and durability. Dental students should be required to own such a surveyor. By becoming familiar with and dependent on its use, they are more likely to continue using the surveyor in practice as necessary piece of equipment toward more adequate diagnosis, effective treatment planning, and performance of many other aspects of prosthodontic treatment. (Courtesy J.M. Ney Co., Hartford, Conn.)

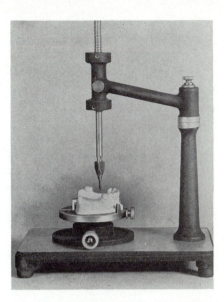

Fig. 10-2. Jelenko surveyor. Note spring-mounted paralleling tool and swivel at top of vertical arm. Horizontal arm may be fixed in any position by tightening nut at top of vertical arm. (Courtesy J.F. Jelenko & Co., Inc., New York, N.Y.)

fixed position. The jointed horizontal arm of the Williams surveyor (Fig. 10-4) differs from both the Ney and Jelenko surveyors. This feature permits the vertical arm to be moved to scribe the survey lines without moving the cast.

Another difference in the Ney and Jelenko surveyors is that the vertical arm on the Ney surveyor is retained by friction within a fixed bearing. The shaft may be moved up or down within this bearing, but remains in any vertical position until again moved. The shaft may be fixed in any vertical position desired by tight-

ening a set screw. In contrast, the vertical arm of the Jelenko surveyor is spring mounted and returns to the top position when released. It must be held down against spring tension while in use, which, to some, is a disadvantage. The spring may be removed, but the friction of the two bearings supporting the arm does not hold it in position as securely as does a bearing designed for that purpose. These minor differences in the two surveyors lead to personal preference, but do not detract from the effectiveness of either surveyor when properly used.

Since the shaft on the Ney surveyor is stable in any vertical position, yet may be moved vertically with ease, it lends itself well for use as a drill press when a handpiece holder is added (Fig. 10-5). The handpiece may thus be used to cut recesses in gold restorations with precision by using burs or carborundum points of various sizes in a dental handpiece.

Several other types of surveyors have been designed and are in use today. Many of these are more elaborate and costly, yet possess little advantage over the more simple type of surveyors.

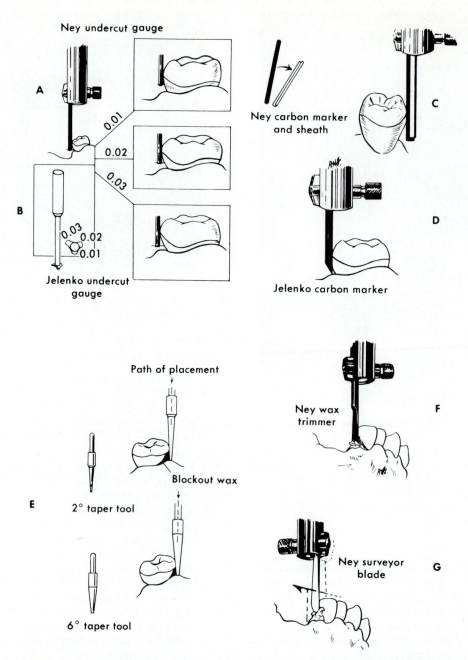

Fig. 10-3. Various tools that may be used with dental surveyor. **A,** Ney undercut gauges. **B,** Jelenko undercut gauge. **C,** Ney carbon marker with metal reinforcement sleeve. **D,** Jelenko carbon marker. **E,** Tapered tools, 2- and 6-degree, for trimming blockout when some nonparallelism is desired. **F,** Ney wax trimmer for paralleling blockout. **G,** Surveying blade being used for trimming blockout.

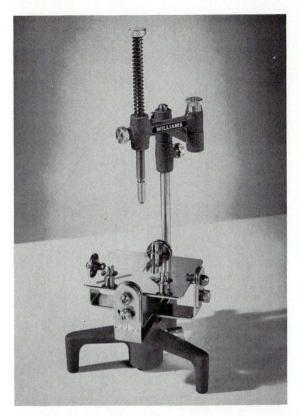

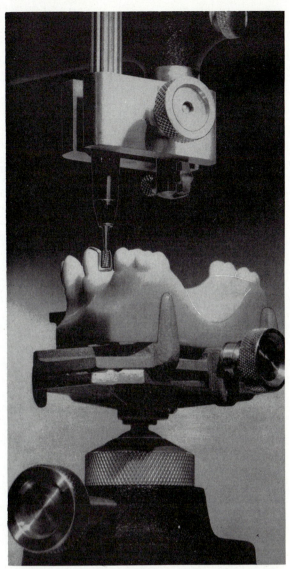

Fig. 10-4. Williams surveyor, which features Gimbal stage table that is adjustable to any desired anterior, posterior, or lateral tilt. Degree of inclination can be recorded for repositioning of cast at any time. Distinct advantage of this table over universal tilt table is that center of rotation always remains constant. Superstructure of this surveyor consists of jointed arm and spring-supported survey rod, all components of which can be locked in fixed position if desired. This surveyor is perhaps best suited for placement of internal attachments, rather than for cast analyzing and other purposes. (Courtesy Williams Gold Refining Co., Buffalo, N.Y.)

PURPOSES OF SURVEYOR

The surveyor may be used for surveying the diagnostic cast, recontouring abutment teeth on the diagnostic cast, contouring wax patterns, measuring a specific depth of undercut, surveying ceramic veneer crowns, placing intracoronal retainers, placing internal rests, machining cast restorations, and surveying and blocking out the master cast.

Fig. 10-5. Ney handpiece holder attached to vertical spindle of surveyor may be used as drill press to cut internal rests and recesses in wax patterns and gold castings and to establish lingual surfaces above ledge, which are parallel to path of placement in abutment restorations. (Courtesy J.M. Ney Co., Hartford, Conn.)

Surveying the diagnostic cast. Surveying the diagnostic cast is **essential** to effective diagnosis and treatment planning. The objectives are as follows:

1. To determine the most acceptable path of placement that will eliminate or minimize interference to placement and removal (Fig. 10-6). **The path of placement is the direction in which a restoration moves from the point of initial contact of its rigid parts with the supporting teeth to the terminal resting position, with rests seated and the denture base in contact with the tissues.** The **path of removal** is exactly the reverse, since it is the direction of restoration movement from its terminal resting position of the last contact of its rigid parts with the supporting teeth. When the restoration is properly designed to have positive guiding planes, the patient may place and remove the restoration with ease in only one direction because of the guiding influence of tooth surfaces made parallel to that path of placement.

2. To identify proximal tooth surfaces that are or can be made parallel so that they act as guiding planes during placement and removal.

3. To locate and measure areas of the teeth that may be used for retention.

4. To determine whether tooth and bony areas of interference will need to be eliminated either by extraction or by selecting a different path of placement.

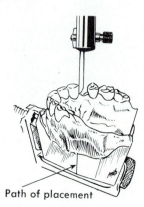

Path of placement

Fig. 10-6. Tilt of cast on adjustable table of surveyor in relation to vertical arm establishes path of placement and removal that partial denture will take. All mouth preparations must be made to conform to previously determined path of placement, which has been recorded by scoring base of cast or by tripoding.

5. To determine the most suitable path of placement that will permit locating retainers and artificial teeth to the best esthetic advantage.

6. To permit an accurate charting of the mouth preparations to be made. This includes the preparation of proximal tooth surfaces to provide guiding planes and the reduction of excessive tooth contours to eliminate interference and to permit a more acceptable location of reciprocal and retentive clasp arms. By marking these areas on the diagnostic cast with red pencil using an undercut gauge to estimate the amount of tooth structure that may safely (without exposing dentin) be removed, and then trimming the marked areas on the stone cast with the surveyor blade, the angulation and extent of tooth reduction may be established before preparing the teeth in the mouth (Fig. 10-7). With the diagnostic cast on the surveyor at the time of mouth preparations, reduction of tooth contours may thus be accomplished with acceptable accuracy.

7. To delineate the height of contour on abutment teeth and to locate areas of undesirable tooth undercut that are to be avoided, eliminated, or blocked out. This will include areas of the teeth to be contacted by rigid connectors, the location of nonretentive reciprocal and stabilizing arms, and the location of retentive clasp terminals.

8. To record the cast position in relation to the selected path of placement for future reference. This may be done by locating three dots or parallel lines on the cast, thus establishing the horizontal plane in relation to the vertical arm of the surveyor (Fig. 10-15).

Contouring wax patterns. The surveyor blade is used as a wax carver during this phase of mouth preparation so that the proposed path of placement may be maintained throughout the preparation of cast restorations for abutment teeth (Fig. 10-8).

All proximal surfaces of wax patterns adjacent to an edentulous area should be made parallel to the previously determined path of placement. Similarly, all other tooth contours that will be contacted by rigid connectors should be made parallel whenever possible. The surfaces of restorations on which reciprocal and stabilizing components will be placed should be contoured to permit their location well below occlusal surfaces and on nonretentive areas. Those surfaces

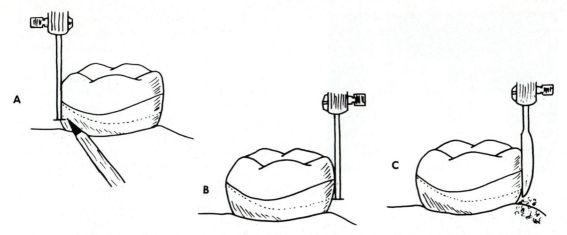

Fig. 10-7. A, Solid line represents height of contour on abutment at selected orientation of diagnostic cast to verticle spindle of surveyor. Dotted line represents desirable height of contour to optimally locate component of direct retainer assembly. A 0.01-inch (0.25 mm) undercut gauge is used to mark location of tip of retentive arm of direct retainer. **B,** By reducing axial contour of stone tooth only 0.01 inch, optimal height of contour can be achieved without exposing dentin. **C,** Stone tooth is trimmed with surveyor blade to desired height of contour. Trimmed area is marked in red pencil and serves as blueprint for similar recontouring in mouth. If we can safely assume that enamel is 1 mm thick in area of contemplated reduction, only 0.25 mm of enamel need be removed to achieve optimal height of contour.

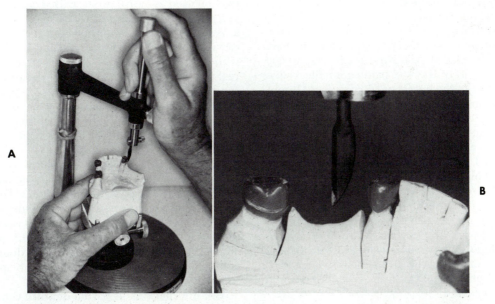

Fig. 10-8. A, Wax patterns have been carved to meet requirements of occlusion. **B,** After cast has been oriented to surveyor at predetermined path of placement, vertical surfaces of wax patterns are altered with surveyor blade to meet specific requirements for optimum placement of framework components.

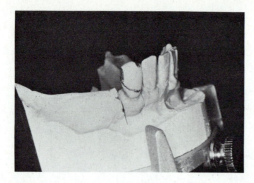

Fig. 10-9. Final glaze has not been placed on veneer crown. Cast has been reoriented to surveyor by indices or tripod marks on cast, and height of contour has been scribed on veneer crown. Alterations to surfaces to conform to ideal placement of components now can be performed by machining operation. Final glaze is placed on veneer crown only after necessary recontouring is accomplished.

of the restoration that are to provide retention for clasp arms should be contoured so that retentive clasps may be placed in the cervical third of the crown and to the best esthetic advantage. Generally a small amount of undercut (0.375 mm or less) is sufficient for retentive purposes.

Surveying ceramic veneer crowns. Ceramic veneer crowns are often used to restore abutment teeth on which extracoronal direct retainers will be placed. The surveyor is used to contour all areas of the wax pattern for the veneer crown except the buccal or labial surface. It must be remembered that one of the principal goals in using a porcelain veneer restoration is to develop an esthetic replica of a natural tooth. It is unlikely that the ceramic veneer portion can be fabricated exactly to the form required for the planned placement of retentive clasp arms without some reshaping with stones. Before the final glaze is accomplished, the abutment crowns should be returned to the surveyor on a full arch cast to assure the correct contour of the veneered portions or to locate those areas that need recontouring (Fig. 10-9). **The final glaze is accomplished only after the crowns have been recontoured.**

Placement of intracoronal retainers (internal attachments). In the placement of intracoronal retainers, the surveyor is used as follows:

1. To select a path of placement in relation to the long axes of the abutment teeth that will avoid areas of interference elsewhere in the arch
2. To cut recesses in the stone teeth on the diagnostic cast for estimating the proximity of the recess to the pulp (in conjunction with roentgenographic information as to pulp size and location), and to facilitate the fabrication of metal or resin jigs to guide the preparations of the recesses in the mouth
3. To carve recesses in wax patterns, to place internal attachment trays in wax patterns, or to cut recesses in the gold casting with the handpiece holder, whichever method is preferred
4. To place the keyway portion of the attachment in the casting before investing and soldering, each keyway located parallel to the other keyways elsewhere in the arch

The student is referred to the Selected Reading Resources section of the textbook for sources of information on intracoronal retainers (internal attachments).

Placement of internal rest seats. The surveyor may be used as a drill press, with a dental handpiece attached to the vertical arm by means of a handpiece holder. Internal rest seats may be carved in the wax patterns and further refined with the handpiece after casting, or the entire rest seat may be cut in the cast restoration with the handpiece. It is best that the outline form of the rest seat be carved first in wax and merely refined on the casting with the handpiece.

An internal rest differs from an internal attachment in that some portion of the cast prosthesis is waxed and cast to fit into the rest seat rather than a matched key and keyway attachment being used (Figs. 5-11 and 5-12). The former is usually nonretentive but provides a definite seat for a removable restoration or a cantilever rest for a broken-stress fixed partial denture. When used with fixed partial dentures, nonparallel abutment pieces may thus be placed separately.

The internal rest in partial denture construction provides a positive occlusal support that is more favorably located in relation to the rotational axis of the abutment tooth than is the conventional spoon-shaped occlusal rest. It also provides horizontal stabilization through the parallelism of the vertical walls, thereby serving the same purpose as stabilizing and reciprocal arms placed extracoronally. Because of the movement of a distal extension base, more torque may be applied to the abutment tooth by an interlocking type of rest, and for this reason its use in conjunction with a distal extension partial denture is contraindicated. The ball-and-socket, spoon-shaped occlusal, or noninterlocking rest should be used in distal extension partial denture designs. The use of the dovetailed or interlocking internal rest should be limited to tooth-borne removable restorations, except when it is used in conjunction with some kind of stressbreaker between the abutment pieces and the movable base. The use of stressbreakers has been considered in Chapter 8.

Internal rest seats may be made in the form of a nonretentive box, a retentive box fashioned after the internal attachment, or a semiretentive box. In the latter the walls are usually parallel and nonretentive, but a recess in the floor of the box prevents proximal movement of the male portion. Internal rest seats are cut with dental burs of various sizes and shapes. Tapered or cylindric fissure burs are used to form the vertical walls, and small round burs are used to cut recesses in the floor of the rest seat.

Machining cast restorations. With handpiece holder attached (Fig. 10-5), axial surfaces of cast and ceramic restorations may be refined by machining with a suitable cylindric carborundum point. Proximal surfaces of crowns and inlays, which will serve as guiding planes, and vertical surfaces above crown ledges may be improved by machining, but only if the relationship of one crown to another is correct. Unless the seating of removable dies is accurate and held in place with additional stone or plaster, cast restorations should first be tried in the mouth and then transferred, by means of a plaster index impression, to a reinforced stone cast for machining purposes. The new cast is then positioned on the surveyor, conforming to the path of placement of the partial denture, and vertical surfaces are machined with a true running cylindric carborundum point.

Whereas machined parallelism may be con-

sidered ideal and beyond the realm of everyday application, its merits more than justify the additional steps required to accomplish it. When such parallelism is accomplished and reproduced in a master cast, it is essential that subsequent laboratory steps be directed toward the use of these parallel guiding plane surfaces.

Surveying the master cast. Since surveying the master cast follows mouth preparations, the path of placement, the location of retentive areas, and the location of remaining interference must be known before proceeding with the final design of the denture framework. The objectives are as follows:

1. To select the most suitable path of placement by following mouth preparations that satisfy the requirements of **guiding planes, retention, noninterference,** and **esthetics.**

2. To permit measurement of retentive areas and to identify the location of clasp terminals in proportion to the flexibility of the clasp arm being used. Flexibility will depend on many factors: (a) the alloy used for the clasp, (b) the design and type of the clasp, (c) whether its form is round or half-round, (d) whether it is of cast or wrought material, and (e) the length of the clasp arm from its point of origin to its terminal end. Retention will then depend on (a) the flexibility of the clasp arm, (b) the magnitude of the tooth undercut, and (c) the depth the clasp terminal is placed into this undercut.

3. To locate areas of undesirable remaining undercut that will be crossed by rigid parts of the restoration during placement and removal. These must be eliminated by blockout.

4. To trim blockout material parallel to the path of placement prior to duplication (Fig. 10-10).

• • •

The partial denture must be designed so that (1) it will not stress abutment teeth beyond their physiologic tolerance, (2) it can be easily placed and removed by the patient, (3) it will be retained against reasonable dislodging forces, and (4) it will not create an unfavorable appearance. It is necessary that the diagnostic cast be surveyed with these principles in mind. Mouth preparation should therefore be planned in accordance with certain factors that will influence the path of placement and removal.

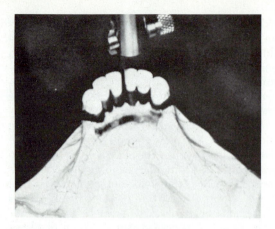

Fig. 10-10. Only terminal portion of retentive direct retainer arm of metal framework may be located in undercut. All other areas of involved teeth should be blocked out parallel to path of placement. Lingual interproximal spaces presenting undercuts must be blocked out parallel to path of placement when linguoplate has been planned as major connector. The small carbon steel diagnostic stylus, warmed slightly with alcohol torch, simplifies this block-out procedure.

FACTORS THAT DETERMINE PATH OF PLACEMENT AND REMOVAL

The factors that will determine the path of placement and removal are guiding planes, retentive areas, interference, and esthetics.

Guiding planes. Proximal tooth surfaces that bear a parallel relationship to one another must either be found or be created to act as guiding planes during placement and removal of the denture. Guiding planes may be compared to the valve guides in an engine and act to assure a definite path of placement as the rigid parts of the prosthesis contact parallel tooth surfaces.

Guiding planes are necessary to assure the passage of the rigid parts of the prosthesis past existing areas of interference. Thus the denture can be easily placed and removed by the patient without strain on the teeth contacted or on the denture itself and without damage to the underlying soft tissues.

Guiding planes are also necessary to assure predictable clasp retention. For a clasp to be retentive, its retentive arm must be forced to flex. Hence, guiding planes are necessary to give

a positive direction to the movement of the restoration to and from its terminal position.

Retentive areas. Retentive areas must exist for a given path of placement, and must be contacted by retentive clasp arms that are forced to flex over a convex surface during placement and removal. Satisfactory clasp retention is no more than the resistance of metal to deformation. For a clasp to be retentive, its path of escapement must be other than parallel to the path of removal of the denture itself; otherwise it would not be forced to flex and thereby generate the resistance known as retention. Clasp retention is therefore dependent on the existence of a definite path of placement and removal.

Although desirable, retention at each principal abutment does not necessarily have to be balanced in relation to the tooth on the opposite side of the arch, that is, exactly equal and opposite in magnitude and relative location. This is, of course, assuming that positive reciprocation to retentive elements is present (which must be cross-arch). **Retention should be sufficient only to resist reasonable dislodging forces.** In other words, it should be the minimum acceptable for adequate retention against reasonable dislodging forces.

Fairly even retention may be obtained by one of two means. One is to change the path of placement to increase or decrease the angle of cervical convergence of opposing retentive surfaces of abutment teeth. The other is to alter the flexibility of the clasp arm by changing its design, its size and length, or the material of which it is made.

Interference. The prosthesis must be designed so that it may be placed and removed without encountering tooth or soft tissue interference. A path of placement may be selected that encounters interference only if the interference can be eliminated during mouth preparations or on the master cast by a reasonable amount of blockout. Interference may be eliminated during mouth preparations by surgery, extraction, modifying interfering tooth surfaces, or altering tooth contours with cast restorations.

Generally, interference that **cannot** be eliminated for one reason or another will take precedence over the factors of retention and guiding planes. Sometimes certain areas can be made

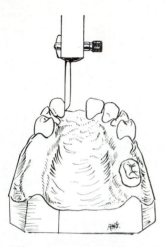

Fig. 10-11. When anterior teeth must be replaced with partial denture, vertical path of placement may be necessary to avoid excessively altering abutment teeth and supplied teeth.

noninterfering only by selecting a different path of placement at the expense of existing retentive areas and guiding planes. These must then be modified with restorations that are in harmony with the path dictated by the existing interference. On the other hand, if areas of interference **can** be eliminated by various reasonable means, they should be. By so doing, the axial contours of existing abutments may frequently be used with little alteration.

Esthetics. By one path of placement the most esthetic location of artificial teeth is made possible, and less clasp metal and base material may be displayed.

The location of retentive areas may influence the path of placement selected, and therefore retentive areas always should be selected with the most esthetic location of clasps in mind. When restorations are to be made for other reasons, they should be contoured to permit the least display of clasp metal. Generally, less metal will be displayed if the retentive clasp is placed at a more distogingival area of tooth surface, made possible either by the path of placement selected or by the contour of cast restorations.

Esthetics also may dictate the choice of path selected when missing anterior teeth must be replaced with the partial denture. In such situations a more vertical path of placement is nec-

essary so that neither the artificial teeth nor the adjacent natural teeth will have to be modified excessively (Fig. 10-11). In this instance esthetics may take precedence over other factors. This necessitates the preparation of abutment teeth to eliminate interferences and to provide guiding planes and retention in **harmony with** that path of placement dictated by esthetic factors.

Esthetics ordinarily should not be the primary factor in partial denture design. **Therefore the replacement of missing anterior teeth should be accomplished by means of fixed restorations whenever possible, rather than permit their replacement to influence the mechanical and functional effectiveness of the partial denture.** Since the primary consideration should be the preservation of the remaining oral tissues, esthetics should not be allowed to jeopardize the success of the partial denture.

STEP-BY-STEP PROCEDURES IN SURVEYING A DIAGNOSTIC CAST

Attach the cast to the adjustable surveyor table by means of the clamp provided. Position the adjustable table so that the occlusal surfaces of the teeth are approximately parallel to the platform (Fig. 10-12). (This is only a tentative, but practical, way to start considering the factors that influence the path of placement and removal.)

Guiding planes. Determine the relative parallelism of proximal tooth surfaces by contacting proximal tooth surfaces with the surveyor blade or diagnostic stylus. Alter the cast position anteroposteriorly until the proximal surfaces are in a parallel relation to one another, or near enough that they can be made parallel by recontouring. This will determine the **anterior-posterior tilt** of the cast in relation to the vertical arm of the surveyor (Fig. 10-13). Although the surveyor table is universally adjustable, it should be thought of as having only two axes, thus allowing only anterior-posterior and lateral tilting.

In making a choice between having contact with a proximal surface at the cervical area only or contact at the marginal ridge only, the latter is preferred because a plane may then be established by recontouring (Fig. 10-14). It is obvious that when only gingival contact exists, a cast restoration is the only means of establishing a

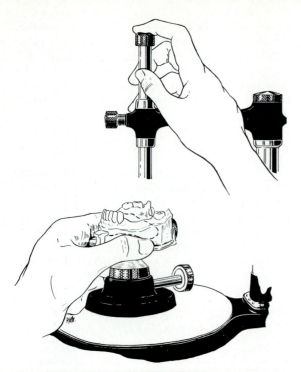

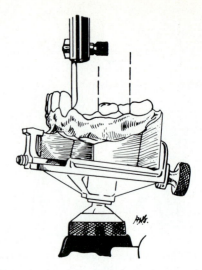

Fig. 10-13. Relative parallelism of proximal tooth surfaces will determine anterior-posterior tilt of cast in relation to vertical arm of surveyor.

Fig. 10-12. Recommended method for manipulating dental surveyor. Right hand is braced on horizontal arm of surveyor, and fingers are used, as illustrated, to raise and lower vertical shaft in its spindle. Left hand holding cast on adjustable table slides horizontally on platform in relation to vertical arm. Right hand must be used also to loosen and tighten tilting mechanism as suitable anterior-posterior and lateral tilt of cast in relation to surveyor is being determined.

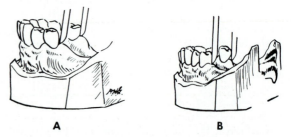

A   **B**

Fig. 10-14. In selecting most desirable anterior-posterior tilt of cast in relation to surveyor blade, choice must be made between positions illustrated in **A** and **B**. In **A**, distal surface of left premolar abutment would have to be extended by means of a cast restoration. In **B**, right premolar could be altered slightly to provide acceptably parallel guiding plane. Unless cast restorations are necessary for other reasons, tilt shown in **B** is almost always preferred.

guiding plane. Therefore if a tilt that does not provide proximal contact is accepted, the proximal surface must be established with some kind of restoration. In making a choice between having a good guiding plane on one proximal surface and none on another as against having a good plane on one and recontouring the other, the latter is preferred, and the need for such alteration is indicated on the diagnostic cast with red pencil. This holds true only when cast restorations are not otherwise necessary.

The end result of selecting a suitable anterior-posterior tilt should be **to provide the greatest combined areas of parallel proximal surfaces that may act as guiding planes.** Other axial surfaces of abutment teeth may also be used as guiding planes. However, this is realized most often by having the stabilizing component of the direct retainer assembly contacting in its entirety the axial surface of the abutment, which has been found or made parallel to the path of placement (Figs. 13-7 to 13-9). Therefore a lateral tilt of the cast to the vertical arm of the surveyor must also be considered as well as the anterior-posterior tilt to use guiding planes.

Retentive areas. By contacting buccal and lingual surfaces of abutment teeth with the surveyor blade, the amount of retention existing below their height of convexity may be determined. This is best accomplished by directing a small source of light toward the cast from the side away from the dentist. The **angle of cervical convergence** is best observed as a triangle of light between the surveyor blade and the apical portion of the tooth surface being studied.

Alter the cast position by tilting it laterally until not grossly different retentive areas exist on the principal abutment teeth. If only two abutment teeth are involved, as in a Kennedy Class I partially edentulous arch, they are both principal abutments. However, if four abutment teeth are involved, as in a Kennedy Class III, modification 1, arch, they are all principal abutments, and retentive areas should be located on all four. But if three abutment teeth are involved, as in Kennedy Class II, modification 1, arch, the posterior abutment on the tooth-borne side and the abutment on the distal extension side are considered to be the principal abutments, and retention is somewhat equalized accordingly. The third abutment may be considered to be secondary, and less retention is expected from it than from the other two. An exception is when the posterior abutment on the tooth-borne side has a poor prognosis and the denture is designed to ultimately be a Class I. In such a situation the two stronger abutments are considered to be principal abutments.

In tilting the cast laterally to establish reasonable uniformity of retention, it is necessary that the table be rotated about an imaginary longitudinal axis without disturbing the anterior-posterior tilt previously established. The resulting position is one that provides or makes possible parallel guiding planes and provides for acceptable retention on the abutment teeth. Note that possible interference to this tentative path of placement has not, as yet, been taken into consideration.

Interference. If a mandibular cast is being surveyed, check the lingual surfaces that will be crossed by a lingual bar major connector during placement and removal. Bony prominences and lingually inclined premolar teeth are the most common causes of interference to a lingual bar connector.

If the interference is bilateral, surgery or recontouring of lingual tooth surfaces, or both, may be unavoidable. If it is only unilateral, a change in the lateral tilt may be necessary to avoid an area of tooth or tissue interference. In changing the path of placement to avoid interference, previously established guiding planes and an ideal location for retentive elements may be lost. Then the decision must be made whether to remove the existing interference by whatever means necessary or to resort to restorations on the abutment teeth, thereby changing the proximal and retentive areas to conform to the new path of placement.

In like manner, bony undercuts that will offer interference to the seating of denture bases must be studied and the decision made to remove them surgically, to change the path of placement at the expense of guiding planes and retention, or to design denture bases to avoid such undercut areas. The latter may be done by shortening buccal and labial flanges and distolingual extension of denture bases. **However, it should be remembered that the maximum area available for support of the denture base should be used whenever possible.**

Interference to major connectors rarely exists in the maxillary arch. Areas of interference are usually found on bucally inclined posterior teeth and those bony areas on the buccal aspect of edentulous spaces. As with the mandibular cast, the decision must be made whether to eliminate them, to change the path of placement at the expense of guiding planes and retention, or to design the connectors and bases to avoid them.

Other areas of possible interference to be studied are those surfaces of abutment teeth that will support or be crossed by minor connectors and clasp arms. While interference to vertical minor connectors may be blocked out, doing so may cause discomfort to the patient's tongue and may create objectionable spaces, which could result in the trapping of food. Also it is desirable that tooth surfaces contacted by vertical connectors be used as auxiliary guiding planes whenever possible. Too much relief is perhaps better than too little because of the possibility of irritation to soft tissues, but it is always better that the relief be placed intentionally rather than as a blockout of interference. If possible, a minor connector should pass vertically along a tooth surface that is either parallel to the path of placement (which is considered ideal) or tapered occlusally. If tooth undercuts that would necessitate the use of an objectionable amount of blockout exist, they may be eliminated or minimized by slight changes in the path of placement or eliminated during mouth preparations. The need for such alteration should be indicated on the diagnostic cast in red pencil after final acceptance of a path of placement.

Tooth surfaces on which reciprocal and stabilizing clasp arms will be placed should be studied to see if sufficient areas exist above the height of convexity for the placement of these components. The addition of a clasp arm to the occlusal third of an abutment tooth adds to its occlusal dimension and therefore to the occlusal loading of that tooth. **Nonretentive and stabilizing clasp arms are best located between the middle third and gingival third of the crown rather than on the occlusal third.**

Areas of interference to more ideal placement of clasp arms usually can be eliminated by reshaping tooth surfaces during mouth preparations, and this is indicated on the diagnostic cast. Gross areas of interference to the placement of clasps may necessitate minor changes in the path of placement or changes in the clasp design. For example, a bar clasp arm originating mesially from the major connector to provide reciprocation and stabilization might be substituted for a distally originating circumferential arm.

Areas of interference frequently overlooked are the distal line angles of premolar abutment teeth and the mesial line angles of molar abutments. These areas frequently offer interference to the origin of circumferential clasp arms. If not detected at the time of initial survey, they are not included in the plan for mouth preparations. When such an undercut exists, three alternatives may be considered:

1. It may be blocked out the same as any other area of interference. This is by far the least satisfactory method because the origin of the clasp must then stand away from the tooth in proportion to the amount of blockout used. Although this is perhaps less objectionable than its being placed occlusally, it may be objectionable to the tongue and the cheek and may create a food trap.

2. It may be circumvented by approaching the retentive area from a gingival direction with a bar clasp arm. This is frequently a satisfactory solution to the problem if other contraindications to the use of a bar clasp arm are not present, such as a severe tissue undercut or a retentive area that is too high on the tooth.

3. It may be eliminated by reducing the tooth contour during mouth preparation. This permits the use of a circumferential clasp arm originating well below the occlusal surface in a satisfactory manner. If the tooth is to be modified during mouth preparations, it should be indicated on the diagnostic cast with red pencil.

When the retentive area is located objectionably high on the abutment tooth or the undercut is too severe, interference may also exist on tooth surfaces that are to support retentive clasps. Such areas of extreme or high convexity must be considered as areas of interference and should be reduced accordingly. These areas are likewise indicated on the diagnostic cast for reduction during mouth preparations.

Esthetics. The path of placement thus established must yet be considered from the standpoint of esthetics, both as to the location of clasps and as to the arrangement of artificial teeth.

Clasp designs that will provide satisfactory esthetics for any given path of placement usually may be selected. In some instances gingivally placed bar clasp arms may be used to advantage; in others circumferential clasp arms located cervically may be used. This is especially true when other abutment teeth located more posteriorly may bear the major responsibility for retention. In still other instances a tapered wrought-wire retentive clasp arm may be placed to better esthetic advantage than a cast clasp arm. The location of clasp arms for esthetic reasons does not ordinarily justify altering the path of placement at the expense of mechanical factors. It should, however, be considered concurrently with other factors, and if a choice between two paths of equal merit permits a more **esthetic placement** of clasp arms by one path than the other, that path **should be given preference.**

When anterior replacements are involved, the

choice of path is limited to a more vertical one for reasons previously stated. In this instance alone esthetics must be given primary consideration, even at the expense of altering the path of placement and making all other factors conform. This factor should be remembered when considering the other three factors, so that compromises can be made at the time other factors are being considered.

FINAL PATH OF PLACEMENT

The final path of placement will be the anterior-posterior and lateral position of the cast, in relation to the vertical arm of the surveyor, that best satisfies all four factors, that is, **guiding planes, retention, interference,** and **esthetics.**

All proposed mouth changes should be indicated on the diagnostic cast in red pencil, with the exception of restorations to be done. These may also be indicated on an accompanying chart if desired. Extractions and surgery are given priority to allow for healing. The remaining red marks represent the actual modifications of the remaining teeth to be done, which consists of the preparation of proximal surfaces, the reduction of buccal and lingual surfaces, and, last, the preparation of rest seats. **Except when they are placed in the wax pattern for a cast restoration, the preparation of rest seats should always be deferred until all other mouth preparations have been completed.**

The actual location of rests will be determined by the proposed design of the denture framework. Therefore the tentative design should be sketched on the diagnostic cast in pencil after the path of placement has been decided on. This is done not only to locate rest areas, but also to record graphically the plan of treatment before mouth preparations. **In the intervening time between patient visits, other partial denture restorations may have been considered. The dentist should have the plan of treatment readily available at each succeeding appointment to avoid confusion and to be a reminder as to what is to be done and in what sequence.**

The plan for treatment should include (1) the diagnostic cast with the mouth preparations and the denture design marked on it, (2) a chart showing the proposed design and the planned treatment for each abutment, (3) a working chart showing the total treatment involved that will permit a quick review and a checkoff of each step as the work progresses, and (4) a record of the fee quoted for each phase of treatment that can be checked off as it is recorded on the patient's permanent record.

Red pencil marks on the diagnostic cast are used to indicate the location of areas to be modified, as well as the location of rests. Although it is not necessary that rest areas be prepared on the diagnostic cast, it is advisable for the beginning student to have done so before proceeding to alter the abutment teeth. This applies equally to crown and inlay preparations on abutment teeth. It is advisable, however, for even the most experienced dentist to have trimmed the stone teeth with the surveyor blade wherever tooth reduction is to be done. This identifies not only the **amount** to be removed in a given area, but also the **plane** in which the tooth is to be prepared. For example, a proximal surface may need to be recontoured in only the upper third or the middle third to establish a guiding plane that will be parallel to the path of placement. This is not usually parallel to the long axis of the tooth, and if the rotary instrument is laid against the side of the tooth, the existing surface angle will be maintained, rather than establishing a new plane that is parallel to the path of placement.

The surveyor blade, representing the path of placement, may be used to advantage to trim the surface of the abutment tooth whenever a red mark appears. The resulting surface represents the amount of tooth to be removed in the mouth and indicates the angle at which the handpiece must be held. The cut surface on the stone tooth is not again marked with red pencil, but is **outlined** in red pencil to positively locate the area to be prepared.

RECORDING RELATION OF CAST TO SURVEYOR

Some method of recording the relation of the cast to the vertical arm of the surveyor must be used so that it may be returned to the surveyor for future reference, especially during mouth preparations. The same applies to the need for returning any working cast to the surveyor for shaping wax patterns, trimming blockout on the master cast, or locating clasp arms in relation to undercut areas.

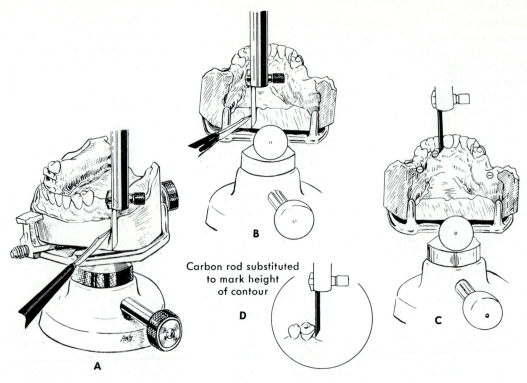

Carbon rod substituted
to mark height
of contour

Fig. 10-15. A and **B**, Path of placement having been determined, base of cast is scored to record its relation to surveyor for future repositioning. **C**, Alternate method to record relation of cast to surveyor is known as **tripoding**. Carbon marker is placed in vertical arm of surveyor, and arm is adjusted to height by which cast can be contacted in three divergent locations. Vertical arm is locked in position, and cast is brought into contact with tip of carbon marker. Three resultant marks are encircled with colored lead pencil for ease of identification. Reorientation of cast to surveyor is accomplished by tilting cast until plane created by three marks is at right angle to vertical arm of surveyor. **D**, Height of contour is then delineated by carbon marker.

Obviously the trimmed base will vary with each cast; therefore recording the position of the surveyor table is of no value. If it were, calibrations could be incorporated on the surveyor table, which would allow the same position to be reestablished. Instead, the position of each cast must be established separately, and any positional record applies only to that cast.

Of several methods, two seem to be the most convenient and accurate. One method is to place three widely divergent dots on the tissue surface of the cast with the tip of a carbon marker, having the vertical arm of the surveyor in a locked position. Preferably these dots should not be placed on areas of the cast involved in the framework design. Then the dots should be encircled with a colored pencil for easy identification. On returning the cast to the surveyor, it may be tilted until the tip of the surveyor blade or diagnostic stylus again contacts the three dots in the same plane. This will produce the original position of the cast and therefore the original path of placement. This is known as **tripoding** the cast (Fig. 10-15). Some dentists prefer to make tiny pits in the cast at the location of the tripoding dots to preserve the orientation of the cast and to transfer this relationship to the refractory cast.

A second method is to score two sides and the dorsal aspect of the base of the cast with a sharp instrument held against the surveyor blade (Fig. 10-15). By tilting the cast until all three lines are again parallel to the surveyor blade, the original cast position can be reestablished. Fortunately the scratch lines will be reproduced in any duplication, thereby permitting any duplicate cast to be related to the surveyor in a similar manner. Whereas a diagnostic cast and a master cast cannot be made interchangeable, a refractory cast, being a duplicate of the master cast, can be repositioned on the surveyor at any time. The technician must be cautioned not to trim the sides of the cast on the cast trimmer and thereby lose the reference marks for repositioning.

SURVEYING THE MASTER CAST

The master cast must be surveyed as a new cast, but the prepared proximal guiding plane surfaces will indicate the correct anterior-posterior tilt. Some compromises may be necessary, but the amount of guiding plane surface remaining after blockout should be the maximum for each tooth. Areas above the point of contact with the surveyor blade are not considered to be part of the guiding plane area and neither are gingival undercut areas, which will be blocked out.

The lateral tilt will be the position that provides equal retentive areas on all principal abutments in relation to the planned clasp design. Factors of flexibility, including the need for extra flexibility on distal extension abutments, must be considered in deciding what will provide equal retention on all abutment teeth. For example, cast circumferential or cast bar retention on the tooth-borne side of a Class II design will be balanced against the 18-gauge wrought-wire retention on a distal abutment only if the more rigid cast clasp engages a lesser undercut that the wrought-wire clasp arm. Therefore the degree of undercut alone does not assure relatively equal retention unless clasp arms of equal length, diameter, form, and material are used.

Gross interference will have been eliminated during mouth preparation. Thus for a given path of placement providing guiding planes and balanced retention, any remaining interference must be eliminated with blockout. If mouth

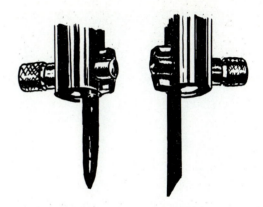

Fig. 10-16. Worn carbon marker (left) should be discarded because it will invariably misleadingly mark other than true height of contour for given orientation of cast to vertical spindle of surveyor. Unworn carbon (right) with angled end is preferable for marking heights of contour on abutment teeth and performing survey of soft tissue areas.

preparations have been adequately planned and executed, the undercuts remaining to be blocked out should be minimal.

The base of the cast is now scored, or the cast is tripoded as described previously. The surveyor blade or diagnostic stylus then may be replaced with a carbon marker, and the height of convexity of each abutment tooth and soft tissue contours may be delineated. Similarly, any areas of interference to the rigid parts of the framework during seating and removal should be indicated with the carbon marker to locate areas to be blocked out or relieved.

Carbon markers that become the slightest bit worn from use should be discarded. A worn (tapered) carbon marker will indicate heights of contour more occlusally located than they actually exist. The carbon marker must be parallel to the vertical spindle of the surveyor (Fig. 10-16).

MEASURING RETENTION

The surveyor is used with the master cast for two purposes: (1) to delineate the height of convexity of the abutment teeth both to locate clasp arms and to identify the location and magnitude of retentive undercuts and (2) to trim blockout of any remaining interference to placement and removal of the denture. The areas involved are

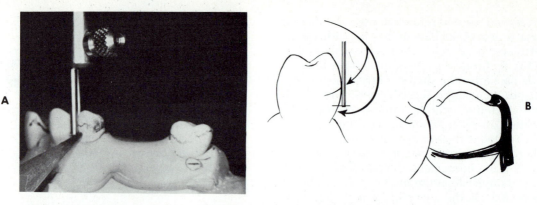

Fig. 10-17. A, Undercut gauge will measure depth of undercut below height of contour. Tip of I-bar–type direct retainer will be placed at area being marked. Depth to which retentive clasp arm can be placed depends not only on its length, taper, diameter, and alloy from which it is made but also on type of clasp. Circumferential clasp arm is more flexible than is bar-type clasp arm of same length (Chapter 6). **B,** Specific measurement of undercut gingiva to height of contour may be ascertained by use of undercut gauge attached to surveyor. Simultaneous contact of shank of undercut gauge at height of contour and contact of lip of specific undercut gauge on tooth in infrabulge area establishes definitive degree and location of undercut. Therefore tip of retentive arm of direct retainer may be placed in "planned depth of undercut."

those that will be crossed by rigid parts of the denture framework.

The exact undercut that retentive clasp terminals will occupy must be measured and marked on the master cast (Fig. 10-17, *A* and *B*). Undercuts may be measured with an undercut gauge, such as those provided with the Ney and Jelenko surveyors. The amount of undercut is measured in hundredths of an inch, the gauges allowing measurements up to 0.03 inch. Theoretically the amount of undercut used may vary with the clasp to be used up to a full 0.03 inch. However, undercuts of 0.01 inch are often adequate for retention by cast retainers, an amount that can be measured with practical accuracy, whereas tapered wrought-wire retention may safely use up to 0.02 inch without inducing undesirable torque on the abutment tooth, **provided the wire retentive arm is long enough (at least 8 mm). The use of 0.03 inch is rarely, if ever, justified with any clasp.** When greater retention is required, such as when abutment teeth remain on only one side of the arch, multiple abutments should be used rather than increasing the retention on any one tooth.

When a source of light is directed toward the tooth being surveyed, a triangle of light is visible. This triangle is bounded by the surface of the abutment tooth on one side and the blade of the surveyor on the other, the apex being the point of contact at the height of convexity and the base of the triangle being the gingival tissues (Fig. 10-18). Retention will be determined by (1) the magnitude of the angle of cervical convergence below the point of convexity, (2) the depth at which the clasp terminal is placed in the angle, and (3) the flexibility of the clasp arm. The intelligent application of various clasp designs and their relative flexibility is of greater importance than the ability to measure an undercut with precise accuracy.

The final design may now be drawn on the master cast with a fine crayon pencil, preferably one that will not come off during duplication. Graphite is usually lifted in duplication, but some crayon pencil marks will withstand duplication without blurring or transfer.* Sizing or spraying the master cast to protect such pencil

*Such as the Dixon Thinex pencil.

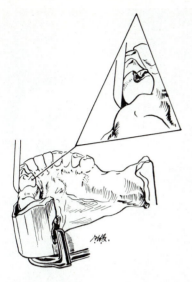

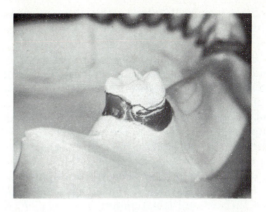

Fig. 10-18. Tooth undercut is best viewed against good source of light passing through triangle, which is bounded by surface of abutment tooth, surveyor blade, and gingival tissues.

Fig. 10-19. Wax ledge on buccal surface of molar abutment will be duplicated in refractory cast for exact placement of clasp pattern. Note that ledge has been carved slightly below penciled outline of clasp arm. This will allow gingival edge of clasp arm to be polished and still remain in its planned relationship to tooth when denture is seated. It should also be noted that wax ledge definitively establishes planned placement of direct retainer tip into measured undercut.

marks is usually not advisable unless done with extreme care to avoid obliterating the surface detail.

BLOCKING OUT THE MASTER CAST

After the establishment of the path of placement and the location of undercut areas on the master cast, any undercut areas that will be crossed by rigid parts of the denture (which is every part of the denture framework but the retentive clasp terminals) must be eliminated by blockout.

In the broader sense the term **blockout** includes not only the areas crossed by the denture framework during seating and removal, but also (1) those areas not involved that are blocked out for convenience, (2) ledges on which clasp patterns are to be placed, (3) relief beneath connectors to avoid tissue impingement, and (4) relief to provide for later attachment of the denture base to the framework.

Ledges or shelves (shaped blockout) for locating clasp patterns may or may not be used (Fig. 10-19). However, this should not be confused with the actual blocking out of undercut areas that would offer interference to the place-

ment of the denture framework. Only the latter is made on the surveyor, with the surveyor blade or diagnostic stylus being used as a paralleling device.

Blockout material may be purchased, or it may be made according to the following formula:

Melt and mix together:
4½ sheets of baseplate wax
4½ sticks of temporary gutta percha stopping
3 sticks of sticky wax
½ tsp. kaolin
Add ½ tube lipstick for color.

Some of the ready-made blockout materials contain a mixture of wax and clay. Hard inlay wax also may be used satisfactorily as a blockout material. It is easily applied and is easily trimmed with the surveyor blade. Trimming is facilitated by slightly warming the surveyor blade with an alcohol torch. Whereas it is true that any wax will melt more readily than a wax-clay mixture if the temperature of the duplicating material is too high, it should be presumed that the duplicating material will not be used at such an elevated temperature. If the temperature of the duplicating material is high enough to damage a wax blockout, other distortions resulting in an inaccurate duplication will also be likely.

Paralleled blockout is necessary cervical to guiding plane surfaces and over all undercut areas that will be crossed by major or minor connectors. Other areas that are to be blocked out for convenience and to avoid difficulties in duplication should be blocked out with hard baseplate wax or an oil-base modeling clay (artist's modeling clay). **A modeling clay that is water soluble should not be used when duplication procedures are involved.** Such areas are the labial surfaces and labial undercuts not involved in the denture design and the sublingual and distolingual areas beyond the limits of the denture design. These are blocked out arbitrarily with hard baseplate wax or clay, but since they have no relation to the path of placement, they do not require the use of the surveyor.

Areas to be crossed by rigid connectors, on the other hand, should be trimmed with the surveyor blade or some other surveyor tool parallel to the path of placement (Fig. 10-20). This imposes a considerable responsibility on the technician. If the blockout is not sufficiently trimmed to expose guiding plane surfaces, the effect of these guiding planes, which were carefully established by the dentist, will be nullified. If, on the other hand, the technician is overzealous in paralleling the blockout, the stone cast may be abraded by heavy contact with the surveyor blade. Although the resulting cast framework would seat back onto the master cast without interference, interference to placement in the mouth would result. This would neces-

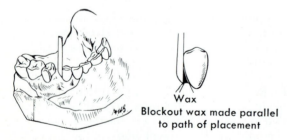

Fig. 10-20. All guiding plane areas must be parallel to path of placement, and all other areas that will be contacted by rigid parts of denture framework must at least be free of undercut if not parallel.

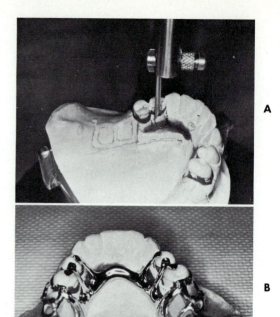

Fig. 10-21. Relationship of parallel blockout and relief to partial denture framework. **A,** Interproximal spaces to be occupied by minor connectors are blocked out parallel to path of placement. In like manner, tissue undercuts intimate to lingual bar and minor connectors are blocked out **parallel** to path of placement rather than using arbitrary blockout. Arbitrary blockout in lingual bar region creates unnecessary spaces for entrapment of food. Guiding planes have been prepared on distal aspect of second premolar abutments. Blockout of tissue surface inferior to buccal surface of right second premolar is required. Since this slight undercut coincided with placement of bar-type direct retainer arm, it was blocked out **parallel** to path of placement to avoid damaging tissue when denture rotated or when restoration was being removed or placed. Edentulous ridges have been covered with 20-gauge sheet wax to provide space for denture base to totally enclose denture base minor connector. A 20-gauge sheet-wax relief is preferable if residual ridges have undergone excessive vertical resorption and space available to place artificial teeth is adequate. **B,** Finished removable partial denture framework accurately fits blocked out master cast. Adjustment of framework by grinding to fit master cast or mouth is practically eliminated when blockout of cast has been meticulously carried out.

sitate relieving the casting at the chair, which is not only an embarrassing and time-consuming operation, but also one that may have the effect of obliterating guiding plane surfaces.

RELIEVING THE MASTER CAST

Tissue undercuts that must be blocked out are paralleled in much the same manner as tooth undercuts. The difference between **blockout** and **relief** must be clearly understood (Figs. 10-21 and 10-22). For example, tissue undercuts that would offer interference to the seating of a lingual bar connector are blocked out with blockout wax and trimmed parallel to the path of placement. This does not in itself necessarily afford relief to avoid tissue impingement. In addition to such blockout, a relief of varying thickness must sometimes be used, depending on the location of the connector, the relative slope of the alveolar ridge, and the predictable effect of denture rotation. It must be assumed that indirect retainers, as such, or indirect retention is provided in the design of the denture to prevent

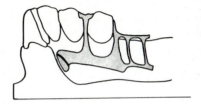

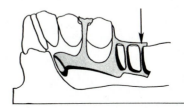

Fig. 10-23. Sagittal section of cast and denture framework. Lingual alveolar ridge slopes inferiorly and posteriorly (upper figure). When force is directed to displace denture base downward, lingual bar rotates upward but does not impinge on soft tissue of alveolar ridge (lower figure). Therefore in such instances adequate relief to avoid impingement is gained when tissue side of lingual bar is highly polished during finishing process.

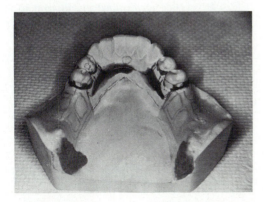

Fig. 10-22. Relief and blockout of master cast before duplication. All undercuts involved in denture design (except tips of retentive clasp arms) have been blocked out **parallel** to path of placement. Residual ridges have been relieved with 20-gauge sheet wax. Small wax window has been created adjacent to distogingival surface of each posterior abutment. Framework will occupy this space and will definitively establish most anterior extent of denture bases in these regions. Severe undercuts in retromylohyoid regions of cast have been arbitrarily blocked out to prevent possible distortion of duplicating mold when master cast is removed.

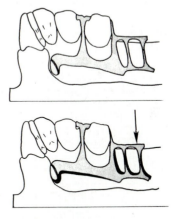

Fig. 10-24. Undercut alveolar ridge was blocked out parallel to path of placement in fabricating lingual bar (upper figure). Application of vertical force to create rotation of lingual bar upward will cause impingement of lingual tissue on alveolar ridge (lower figure). To avoid impingement in these instances, master cast should not only be blocked out parallel to path of placement, but an additional relief of 32-gauge sheet wax should also be used in blocking out cast in such undercut areas.

Table 10-1. *Differentiations between parallel blockout, shaped blockout, arbitrary blockout, and relief*

Site	Material	Thickness
Paralleled blockout		
Proximal tooth surfaces to be used as guiding planes	Hard baseplate wax or blockout material	Only undercut remaining gingival to contact of surveyor blade with tooth surface
Beneath all minor connectors	Hard baseplate wax or blockout material	Only undercut remaining gingival to contact of surveyor blade with tooth surface
Tissue undercuts to be crossed by rigid connectors	Hard baseplate wax or blockout material	Only undercut remaining below contact of surveyor blade with surface of cast
Tissue undercuts to be crossed by origin of bar clasps	Hard baseplate wax or blockout material	Only undercut remaining below contact of surveyor blade with surface of cast
Deep interproximal spaces to be covered by minor connectors or linguoplates	Hard baseplate wax or blockout material	Only undercut remaining below contact of surveyor blade with surface of cast
Beneath bar clasp arms to gingival crevice	Hard baseplate wax or blockout material	Only undercut area involved in attachment of clasp arm to minor connector
Shaped blockout		
On buccal and lingual surfaces to locate plastic or wax patterns for clasp arms	Hard baseplate wax	Ledges for location of reciprocal clasp arms to follow height of convexity so that they may be placed as cervical as possible without becoming retentive Ledges for location of retentive clasp arms to be placed as cervical as tooth contour permits; point of origin of clasp to be occlusal or incisal to height of convexity, crossing survey line at terminal fourth, and to include undercut area previously selected in keeping with flexibility of clasp type being used
Arbitrary blockout		
All gingival crevices	Hard baseplate wax	Enough to just eliminate gingival crevice
Gross tissue undercuts situated below areas involved in design of denture framework	Hard baseplate wax or oil-base clay	Leveled arbitrarily with wax spatula
Tissue undercuts distal to cast framework	Hard baseplate wax or oil-base clay	Smoothed arbitrarily with wax spatula
Labial and buccal tooth and tissue undercuts not involved in denture design	Hard baseplate wax or oil-base clay	Filled and tapered with spatula to within upper third of crown
Relief		
Beneath lingual bar connectors or the bar portion of linguoplates when indicated (see text)	Adhesive wax sealed to cast; should be wider than major connector to be placed on it	32-gauge wax if slope of lingual alveolar ridge is parallel to path of placement 32-gauge wax after parallel blockout of undercuts if slope of lingual alveolar ridge is undercut to path of placement
Areas in which major connectors will contact thin tissue, such as hard areas so frequently found on lingual of mandibular ridges and elevated median palatal raphes	Hard baseplate wax	Thin layer flowed on with hot wax spatula; however, if maxillary torus must be covered, the thickness of the relief must represent the difference in the degree of displacement of the tissues covering the torus and the tissues covering the residual ridges
Beneath framework extensions onto ridge areas for attachment of resin bases	Adhesive wax, well adapted and sealed to cast beyond involved area	20-gauge wax

rotation of the lingual bar inferiorly. A vertical downward rotation of the denture bases around posterior abutments places the bar increasingly farther from the lingual aspect of the alveolar ridge when this surface slopes inferiorly and posteriorly (Fig. 10-23). Adequate relief of soft tissues adjacent to the lingual bar is obtained by the initial finishing and polishing of the framework in these instances. However, excessive upward vertical rotation of a lingual bar will impinge lingual tissues if the alveolar ridge is nearly vertical or undercut to the path of placement (Fig. 10-24). The region of the cast involving the proposed placement of the lingual bar should, in this situation, be first relieved by parallel blockout and then by a 32-gauge wax strip. Low-fusing casting wax such as Kerr's green casting wax should not be used for this purpose, for it is too easily thinned during adapting and may be affected by the temperature of the duplicating material. Pink casting wax should be used, but it is difficult to adapt uniformly. A pressure-sensitive adhesive-coated casting wax is preferable because it adapts readily and adheres to the cast surface. Any wax, even the adhesive type, should be sealed all around its borders with a hot spatula to prevent its lifting when the cast is moistened before or during duplication.

Horizontal rotational tendencies of mandibular distal extension denture probably account for many of the tissue irritations seen adjacent to a lingual mandibular major connector. These irritations can usually be avoided by blocking out all undercuts adjacent to the bar parallel to the path of placement and then including adequate stabilizing components in the design of the framework to resist horizontal rotation. Judicious relief of the tissue side of the lingual bar with rubber wheels at the site of the irritation will most often correct the discrepancy, all other factors being equal. Under no circumstances should the rigidity of the major connector be jeopardized by grinding any portion of it.

Still other areas requiring relief are the gingival crossings and gingival crevices. All gingival areas should be protected from possible impingement resulting from rotation of the denture framework, and all gingival crevices should be bridged by the denture framework. Hard inlay wax may be used to block out gingival crevices (Fig. 10-21).

PARALLELED BLOCKOUT, SHAPED BLOCKOUT, ARBITRARY BLOCKOUT, AND RELIEF

Table 10-1 differentiates between **paralleled blockout, shaped blockout, arbitrary blockout,** and **relief.** The same factors apply to both the maxillary and mandibular arches, except that relief is ordinarily not used beneath palatal major connectors, as it is with mandibular lingual bar connectors, except when maxillary tori cannot be circumvented or when resistive median palatal raphes are encountered.

SELF-ASSESSMENT AIDS

1. How would you define a dental cast surveyor?
2. What are the basic parts of a surveyor?
3. Do you recall the term **height of contour** and can you relate it to a direct retainer assembly?
4. Since no component of a removable partial denture may engage an undercut except a portion of the retentive arm of a direct retainer, then both desirable and undesirable undercuts must be known in designing a restoration. True or false?
5. When planning the design of a partial denture, there are four factors that must be considered in determining the path of placement and removal. Two of these factors are retention and esthetics. Can you name the other two factors?
6. With the diagnostic cast securely clamped to the adjustable table and the diagnostic stylus in the vertical spindle, what orientation of the occlusal plane to the base of the surveyor is recommended as a provisional study position?
7. You are considering a design for a Class III, modification 1, arch. Which directional tilt of the cast will indicate the greatest area of parallel proximal surfaces to act as guiding planes—anterior-posterior or lateral?
8. Suppose, in the above situation, that the diagnostic stylus touches only gingival areas of the proximal surfaces. What are your options to obtain guiding plane surfaces?
9. When possible retentive areas are being ascertained, the cast is tilted laterally. How do you avoid changing the established anterior-posterior tilt of the cast?
10. Uniformity of retention bilaterally is desirable. In what manner does the angle of cervical convergence contribute to obtaining uniform retention?
11. What are the most common causes of interference to the placement of a mandibular major connector?
12. Why should soft tissue contours be surveyed as well as teeth?

13. What advantages accrue in having the tip of the carbon marker touch gingival areas intermittently when marking the heights of contour of abutment teeth?

14. After the diagnostic cast has been surveyed, how can you record the relationship of the cast to the vertical spindle of the surveyor in three dimensions?

15. What is the disadvantage of using a carbon marker that is even only slightly worn?

16. What is an undercut gauge? How can it be used to measure the depth of undercut in the angle of cervical convergence?

17. Heights of contour in many instances will be more optimally located for direct retainer assemblies if axial surfaces are recontoured. How may an undercut gauge assist in determining whether they can be recontoured without exposing dentin?

18. Diagnostic casts are quite often altered during design on the surveyor or in other uses. Why is it a good idea to have duplicate diagnostic casts?

19. The designed diagnostic cast can readily serve as a blueprint to accomplish like contouring of abutment teeth during mouth preparation procedures. How may the contoured areas on the diagnostic cast be indicated to avoid overlooking these areas when preparing them in the mouth?

20. After mouth preparation procedures are completed and a master cast has been made, it must be surveyed to definitively locate components. What are your guides to relate the cast to the surveyor?

21. The terminal portion of the retentive arm of a direct retainer should engage a planned and measured undercut. Using the same degree of undercut bilaterally will not necessarily assure relative equal retention. What factor other than the degree of undercut must be considered?

22. After the path of placement is established, undercut areas that will be crossed by rigid parts must be eliminated. Do you know how this is accomplished? With what materials?

23. By what means can the definitive locations of components of the framework be transferred from the master cast to the duplicate investment (cast) on which the pattern for the framework will be developed?

24. Can you explain the differences between shaped blockout, arbitrary blockout, relief of the master cast, and paralleled blockout?

25. Why should undercuts on the master cast not involved with the framework be blocked out?

26. How do you handle the blockout of gingival crevices that will be crossed by a component of the framework?

27. What relief of a mandibular master cast is required for the lingual aspect of the alveolar ridge that will be covered by a lingual bar or linguoplate when (1) the ridge slopes inferiorly and posteriorly, (2) the ridge is parallel to the path of placement, and (3) the ridge is undercut to the path of placement?

28. Why should a master cast be relieved at all?

29. What determines the amount of palatal relief required when a major connector must traverse the median palatal raphe in a Class I arch?

30. What are the requirements for relief on a master cast for minor connectors that will attach acrylic resin bases to the major connector?

31. What uses can you think of for a dental cast surveyor other than surveying casts for designs and preparation of master casts for duplication in a refractory investment?

32. How can a dental cast surveyor help you in developing optimal contour for crowns?

33. By what means can some dental cast surveyors be converted into a convenient drill press or machining tool?

34. Ceramometal restorations in many instances require machining before the final glazing procedures to make sure that contours as originally planned are accomplished. How can this be done?

35. Internal rests on crowns may be machined using the surveyor as a drill press, or they may be made by another method involving the dental cast surveyor. Do you know this other method?

36. Why would a dental cast surveyor be required to place some types of manufactured internal attachments?

37. What are some sequelae of marring a master cast during surveying or blockout procedures?

38. Can you think of an application for use of the dental cast surveyor in planning for a fixed partial denture?

11 DIAGNOSIS AND TREATMENT PLANNING

The purpose of dental treatment is to respond to a patient's needs. Each patient, however, is unique and as singular as a fingerprint. Treatment, therefore, must be highly individualized for the patient as well as the disease entity.

Meaningful treatment embodies three fundamentally different processes: (1) ascertaining a patient's needs, (2) developing a treatment plan relevant to these needs, and (3) executing the treatment.*

It should be emphasized that the dentist must be prepared to interpret and apply the concept of optimal services to patients whose individual circumstances—despite their needs—may dictate no treatment, limited treatment, or extensive treatment.

OBJECTIVES OF PROSTHODONTIC TREATMENT

The objectives of any prosthodontic treatment may be stated as (1) the elimination of disease, (2) the preservation of the health and relation-

ship of the teeth and the health of the remaining oral tissues, and (3) the selected replacement of lost teeth and the restoration of function in an esthetically pleasing manner.

Patients with missing teeth may specifically request their replacement, especially when anterior teeth are missing and the patients are concerned only with the cosmetic implications. On the other hand, they may seek diagnosis and advice, the result of which is frequently the recommendation that the missing teeth be replaced with either fixed or removable restorations. In many instances the patient is usually concerned only with the replacement of the missing teeth. The dentist's primary obligation to the patient is to emphasize the importance of restoring the total mouth to a state of health and of preserving the remaining teeth and surrounding tissues. Incident to this is the functional and esthetically acceptable replacement of missing teeth in a harmonious relation with the remaining teeth and surrounding structures.

In many instances restoration of lost function must be modified and minimized to avoid over-

---

*From Kabcenell, J.L.: Planning for individualized prosthetic treatment, J. Prosthet. Dent. 34:389-392, 1975.

loading the supporting structures. The prevention of tooth migration, the healthful stimulation of oral tissues, and the preservation of the remaining teeth are of greater importance. The extent to which lost masticatory function can be restored depends on the tissue tolerance of the individual, as influenced by age, general health, and the health of the oral tissues.

Diagnosis and treatment planning for oral rehabilitation must take into consideration some or all of the following procedures: the restoration of individual teeth, the restoration of harmonious occlusal relationships, the replacement of missing teeth by fixed restorations, and the replacement of other missing teeth by means of removable partial dentures. Therefore selection of the type, amount, and chronology of treatment should be ascertained before irreversible procedures are undertaken.

The treatment plan for the partial denture, which is too frequently the final step in an extensive and lengthy sequence of treatment, should precede earlier treatment so that abutment teeth and other areas in the mouth may be properly prepared to support and retain the partial denture. **This means that diagnostic casts for designing and planning partial denture treatment must be made before definitive treatment is undertaken.** The design drawn on the diagnostic cast, along with a detailed chart of mouth conditions and proposed treatment, is the master plan for the mouth preparations and the partial denture to follow.

Failures of partial dentures, other than structural defects, can usually be attributed to inadequate diagnosis, failure to properly evaluate the conditions present, and failure to prepare the patient and his mouth properly before construction of the master cast. The importance of the examination, the consideration of favorable and unfavorable aspects, and the importance of planning the elimination of unfavorable influences cannot be stressed too strongly.

ORAL EXAMINATION

A complete oral examination should precede any mouth rehabilitation procedures. An oral examination should be complete—not limited to only one arch. It should include, in addition to a visual and digital examination of the teeth and surrounding tissues with mouth mirror, explorer, and periodontal probe, a complete intraoral roentgenographic survey, a vitality test of critical teeth, **and an examination of casts correctly oriented on an adjustable articulator.**

During the examination the objective to be kept foremost in mind should be the consideration of the possibilities for maintaining the remaining oral structures in a state of health for the longest period of time. In addition to the elimination of infection, the primary objectives should be the prevention of tooth migration and the correction of traumatic influences. Second should be the consideration of the best method for restoring lost function within the limits of tissue tolerance of the patient. Third, and not before, the decision should be made as to how best to maintain or improve on the appearance of the mouth. As the first two objectives are satisfied, so will the requirement of a comfortable and esthetically pleasing restoration also be satisfied.

Sequence for oral examination. An oral examination should be accomplished in the following sequence:

1. **Visual examination.** Visual examination will reveal many of the signs of dental disease. Consideration of **caries susceptibility** is of primary importance. The number of restored teeth present, signs of recurrent caries, and evidence of decalcification should be noted. Only those patients with demonstrated good oral hygiene habits and low caries susceptibility may be considered good risks without resorting to such prophylactic measures as the crowning of abutment teeth.

Evidence of periodontal disease, inflammation of gingival areas, and the degree of gingival recession should be observed at the time of initial examination. In addition, the depths of periodontal pockets should be determined by instrumentation and the degree of mobility of the teeth by digital examination. Although evidence of periodontal disease is detectable visually, the **extent** of damage to the supporting structure by periodontal disease must be determined by roentgenographic interpretation and instrumentation.

The number of teeth remaining, the location of the edentulous areas, and the quality of the residual ridge will have a definite bearing on the proportionate amount of support that the partial denture will receive from the teeth and the edentulous ridges. Tissue contours may appear representative of a well-formed edentulous residual ridge. Palpation often indicates, however, that supporting bone has been resorbed and has been replaced by displaceable, fibrous connective tissue. Such a situation is common in maxillary tuberosity regions. The removable partial denture cannot be supported adequately by tissues that are easily displaced, and this tissue should be removed surgically, unless otherwise contraindicated, in preparing the mouth. A small but stable residual ridge is preferable to a larger unstable ridge to obtain support for the denture.

The presence of tori or other bony exostoses must be detected and an evaluation of their presence in relation to framework design must be made. Failure to palpate the tissue over the median palatal raphe to ascertain the difference in its displaceability as compared to the displaceability of the soft tissues covering the residual ridges will often lead to a "rocking," unstable, uncomfortable denture and dissatisfied patient. Adequate relief of palatal major connectors must be planned, and the amount of relief required is directly proportionate to the difference in displaceability of the tissues over the midline of the palate and the tissues covering the residual ridges.

During the examination not only must each arch be considered separately but also its occlusal relationship with the opposing arch. A situation that looks simple when the teeth are apart may be complicated when the teeth are in occlusion. For example, an extreme vertical overlap may complicate the attachment of anterior teeth to a maxillary denture. Extrusion of a tooth or teeth into an opposing edentulous area may complicate the replacement of teeth in the edentulous area, or it may create cuspal interference, which will complicate the location and design of clasp retainers and occlusal rests. When occlusal interference cannot be adequately determined by visual examination, the interposition of wax strips of varying thickness between the teeth may assist in determining the amount of interference or clearance present. Such findings subsequently will be evaluated further by a study of mounted diagnostic casts.

2. **Relief of pain and discomfort and placement of temporary restorations.** It is advisable not only to relieve discomfort arising from tooth defects but also to determine as early as possible the extent of caries and to arrest further caries activity until definitive treatment can be instituted. By restoring tooth contours with temporary restorations, the impression will not be torn on removal from the mouth, and a more accurate diagnostic cast may be obtained.

3. **Complete intraoral roentgenographic survey** (Fig. 11-1). The objectives of a roentgenographic examination are (a) to locate areas of infection and other pathosis that may be present; (b) to reveal the presence of root fragments, foreign objects, bone spicules, and irregular ridge

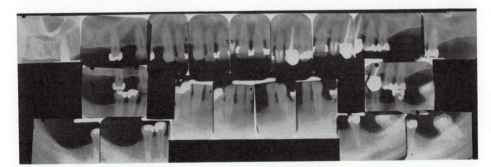

Fig. 11-1. Complete intraoral roentgenographic survey of remaining teeth and adjacent edentulous areas reveals much information vital to effective diagnosis and treatment planning. Response of bone to previous stress is of particular value in establishing prognosis of teeth that are to be used as abutments.

formations; (c) to reveal the presence and extent of caries and the relation of carious lesions to the pulp; (d) to permit evaluation of existing restorations as to evidence of recurrent caries, marginal leakage, and overhanging gingival margins; (e) to reveal the presence of root canal fillings and to permit their evaluation as to future prognosis (the design of the partial denture may hinge on the decision to retain or extract an endodontically treated tooth); (f) to permit an

PARTIAL DENTURE DIAGNOSIS AND TREATMENT RECORD

Patient:______________________________ Reg. No.__________

Student:______________________________ Date:__________

Pertinent Radiographic Findings:______________________________

	UPPER	LOWER
Kennedy Classification		
Initial	Class____, Mod.____	Class____, Mod.____
Final	Class____, Mod.____	Class____, Mod.____
Abutment Teeth		
Teeth to be Extracted and Reason		
Surgical Preparation of Ridges		
Abutment Restorations (Tooth No. & Type Restorations)		
Final Mouth Preparations:		
Guiding Planes		
Reduction of Tooth Contours		
Occlusal Rests		
Date above completed		
Impression Materials Used:		
For Master Cast		
For Correction of Supporting Ridges		
Denture Base Materials		
Tooth Selection		
Occlusal Registration; Methods Used		
Drawing of Partial Denture Design: Metal framework in blue, Resin bases or attachments in red, Wrought retentive clasp arms in red.	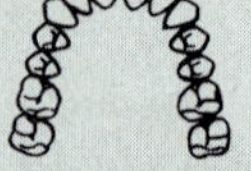 MAXILLARY OCCLUSAL VIEW	MANDIBULAR OCCLUSAL VIEW
Placement Date:		
Post-Placement Notes:		

Fig. 11-2. Diagnosis and treatment record chart for recording treatment plan and pertinent data.

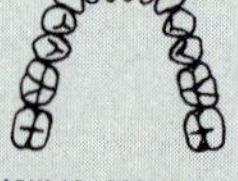

evaluation of periodontal conditions present and to establish the need and possibilities for treatment; and (g) to evaluate the alveolar support of abutment teeth— the number, the supporting length, and the morphology of their roots, the relative amount of alveolar bone loss suffered through pathogenic processes, and the amount of alveolar support remaining.

4. **A thorough and complete oral prophylaxis.** An adequate examination can be accomplished best with the teeth free of accumulated calculus and debris. Also, accurate diagnostic casts of the dental arches can be obtained only if the teeth are clean; otherwise the teeth reproduced on the diagnostic casts are not a true representation of tooth and gingival contours. Cursory examination may precede an oral prophylaxis, but a complete oral examination should be deferred until the teeth have been thoroughly cleaned.

5. **The exploration of teeth and investing structures.** These can be explored by instrumentation and visual means. This should include a determination of tooth mobility and an examination of occlusal relationships. At this time the presence of tori and other bony protuberances should be noted and their clinical significance evaluated. Also, history and diagnosis charts should be filled out at this time, as well as a simple working chart for future reference (Figs. 11-2 and 11-3). The latter does not become part of the patient's permanent record but registers the nature and sequence of treatment, and it can be used by the dentist as a checklist during treatment. A breakdown of the fee may be recorded on the back of this chart for easy reference if adjustments or substitutions become necessary by changes in the diagnosis as the work progresses.

6. **Vitality tests of remaining teeth.** Vitality tests of remaining teeth should be given particularly to teeth to be used as abutments and those having deep restorations or deep carious lesions. This may be done either by thermal or by electronic means, whichever the dentist has learned to interpret best.

7. **Determining the height of the floor of the mouth to locate inferior borders of lingual mandibular major connectors.** Mouth preparation procedures are influenced by a choice of the major connectors. This determination must pre-

cede altering contours of abutment teeth.

8. **Impressions for making accurate diagnostic casts.** The casts preferably will be articulated on a suitable instrument. The importance of accurate diagnostic casts and their use will be discussed later in this chapter.

The fee for examination, which should include the cost of the roentgenographic survey and the examination of articulated diagnostic casts, should be established before the examination and should not be related to the cost of treatment. It should be understood that the fee for examination is based on the time involved and the service rendered and that the material value of the roentgenographs and diagnostic casts is incidental to the effectiveness of the examination.

The examination record should always be available in the office for future consultation. If consultation with another dentist is requested, modern respect for the hazards of un-

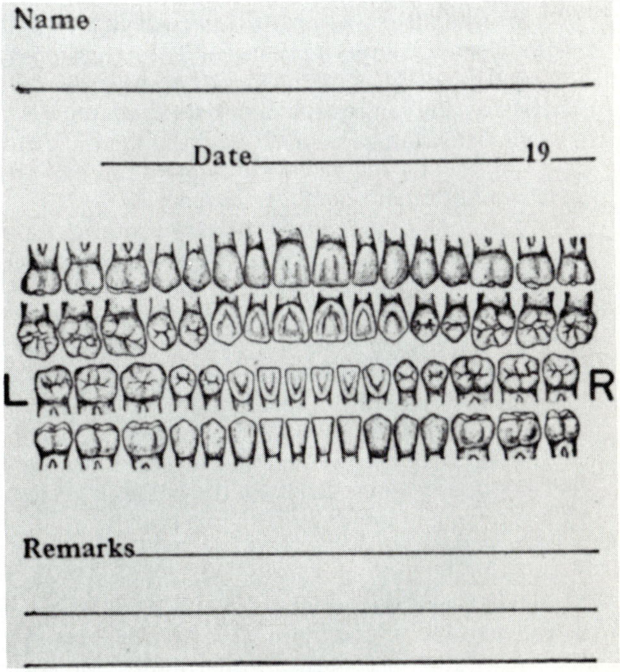

Fig. 11-3. Simple working chart. Restorations for individual teeth, crowns, and fixed partial dentures to be made may be marked on chart and checked off as completed during mouth preparations.

necessary radiation justifies the dentist loaning the roentgenograms for this purpose. However, duplicate films should be retained in the dentist's files.

DIAGNOSTIC CASTS

A diagnostic cast should be an **accurate** reproduction of the teeth and adjacent tissues. In a partially edentulous arch this must include the edentulous spaces, since these also must be evaluated in determining the type of denture base to be used and the extent of available denture-supporting area.

A diagnostic cast is usually made of dental stone because of its strength and the fact that it is less easily abraded than is dental plaster. Generally the improved dental stones (die stones) are not used for diagnostic casts because of their cost. Their greater resistance to abrasion does, however, justify their use for master casts.

The impression for the diagnostic cast is usually made with an irreversible hydrocolloid (alginate) in a perforated partial denture impression tray. The size of the arch will determine the size of the tray to be used. The tray should be sufficiently oversize to assure an optimum thickness of impression material to avoid distortion or tearing on removal from the mouth. The technique for the making of impressions will be covered in more detail in Chapter 14.

Purposes of diagnostic casts. Diagnostic casts serve several purposes as an aid to diagnosis and treatment planning. Some of these are as follows:

1. Diagnostic casts are used to supplement the oral examination by permitting a view of the occlusion from the lingual as well as from the buccal aspect. Analysis of the existing occlusion is made possible when opposing casts are occluded, as well as a study of the possibilities for improvement either by occlusal adjustment, occlusal reconstruction, or both. The degree of overclosure, the amount of interocclusal space needed, and the possibilities of interference to the location of rests also may be determined.

As stated previously, opportunites for improvement of the occlusal scheme, either by occlusal adjustment or occlusal reconstruction or both, are made possible by the use of mounted diagnostic casts. Such procedures often include

"diagnostic waxing" to determine the possibility of enhancing the occlusion before definitive treatment is begun (Fig. 11-4). In other words, diagnostic casts permit the dentist to "plan ahead" and avoid undesirable compromises in the treatment being given a patient.

2. Diagnostic casts are used to permit a topographic survey of the dental arch that is to be restored by means of a removable partial denture. The cast of the arch in question may be surveyed individually with a cast surveyor to determine the parallelism or lack of parallelism of tooth surfaces involved and to establish its influence on the design of the partial denture. The principal considerations in studying the parallelism of tooth and tissue surfaces of the dental arch are (a) proximal tooth surfaces, which can be made parallel to serve as guiding planes, (b) retentive and nonretentive areas of the abutment teeth, and (c) areas of interference to placement and removal. From such a survey a path of placement may be selected that will satisfy requirements for parallelism and retention to the best mechanical, functional, and esthetic advantage. Then mouth preparations may be planned accordingly.

3. Diagnostic casts are used to permit a logical and comprehensive presentation to the patient of his present and future restorative needs, as well as of the hazards of future neglect. Occluded and individual diagnostic casts can be used to point out to the patient (a) evidence of tooth migration and the existing results of such migration, (b) effects of further tooth migration, (c) loss of occlusal support and its consequences, (d) hazards of traumatic occlusal contacts, and (e) cariogenic and periodontal implications of further neglect.

Treatment planning actually may be accomplished with the patient present so that economic considerations may be discussed also. Such use of diagnostic casts permits a justification of the proposed fee through the patient's understanding of the problems involved and of the treatment needed. Inasmuch as mouth rehabilitation procedures are frequently protracted, there must be complete accord between dentist and patient before extensive treatment is begun, and financial arrangements must be consummated during the planning phase.

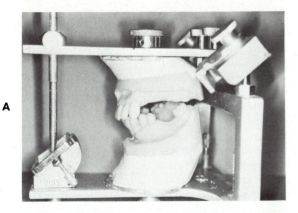

A

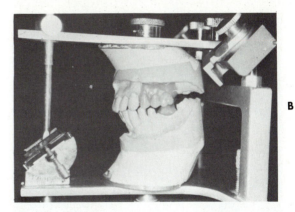

B

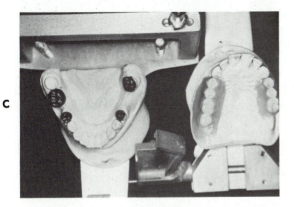

C

Fig. 11-4. A, Diagnostic casts have been mounted, and articulator has been adjusted by intraoral, eccentric, maxillomandibular records. **B,** Lower stone abutment teeth for prospective fixed partial dentures have been reduced so that diagnostic occlusal waxing may be performed. Maxillary artificial teeth have been arranged in conjunction with waxing of lower occlusal surfaces to satisfy demands of proposed occlusal scheme. **C,** Anterior stone teeth have also been altered to satisfy occlusal scheme. With such guides developed on diagnostic casts, similar oral preparatory procedures can be accomplished for predetermined end result. (**C** from Morris, A.L., and Bohannon, H.M., editors: Dental specialties in general practice, Philadelphia, 1969, W. B. Saunders Co.)

4. Individual impression trays may be fabricated on the diagnostic casts, or the diagnostic cast may be used in selecting and fitting a stock impression tray for the final impression. If wax blockout is to be used in the fabrication of individual trays, a duplicate cast made from an irreversible hydrocolloid (alginate) impression of the diagnostic cast should be used for this purpose. The diagnostic cast is too valuable for future reference to risk damage resulting from the making of an impression tray. On the other hand, if only a wet asbestos blockout is used, the diagnostic cast may be used without fear of damage.

Since essential areas will be known in advance of making the final impression, the tray must be selected or made with these in mind. These areas as recorded in the final impression may then be examined critically for possible artifacts.

5. Diagnostic casts may be used as a constant reference as the work progresses. Penciled marks indicating the type of restorations, the areas of tooth surfaces to be modified, the location of rests, and the design of the partial denture framework, as well as the path of placement and removal, all may be recorded on the diagnostic cast for future reference (Fig. 11-5). Then these steps may be checked off the work sheet as they are completed.

Areas of abutment teeth to be modified may first be changed on the diagnostic cast by trimming the stone cast with the surveyor blade. A record is thus made of the location and degree of modification to be done in the mouth. This must be done in relation to a definite path of placement. Any mouth preparations to be accomplished with new cast restorations require that wax patterns be shaped in accordance with

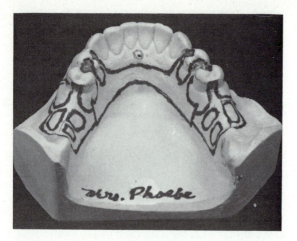

Fig. 11-5. Proposed mouth changes and design of partial denture framework are indicated in pencil on diagnostic cast in relation to previously determined path of placement.

a previously determined path of placement. Even so, the shaping of abutment teeth on the diagnostic cast serves as a guide to the form of the abutment pattern. This is particularly true if the contouring of wax patterns is to be delegated to the technician, as it may be in a busy practice.

6. **Unaltered diagnostic casts should become a permanent part of the patient's record because records of conditions existing before treatment are just as important as are preoperative roentgenograms. Therefore diagnostic casts should be duplicated, one cast serving as a permanent record and the other cast being used in situations that may require alterations to it.**

Mounting diagnostic casts. Although some diagnostic casts may be occluded by hand, occlusal analysis is much better accomplished when casts are mounted on an adjustable articulator. By definition an articulator is "a mechanical device that represents the temporomandibular joints and jaw members, to which maxillary and mandibular casts may be attached." Since the dominant influence on mandibular movement in a partially edentulous mouth is the cusps of the remaining teeth, an anatomic reproduction of condylar paths is probably not obtainable. Still, movement of the casts in relation to one another as

influenced by the cusps of the remaining teeth, when mounted at a reasonably accurate radius from the axis of condylar rotation, permits a relatively valid analysis of occlusal relations. This is much better than a simple hinge mounting.

It is probably still better that the casts be mounted in relation to the axis-orbital plane to permit better interpretation of the plane of occlusion in relation to the horizontal plane. Whereas it is true that an axis-orbital mounting has no functional value on a non-arcon instrument, since that plane ceases to exist when opposing casts are separated, the value of such a mounting lies in the orientation of the casts in occlusion. (An **arcon** articulator is one in which the condyles are attached to the lower member as they are in nature, the term being a derivation coined by Bergström from the words **articulation** and **condyle.** All the more widely used articulators such as the Hanau [H series], Dentatus, and improved Gysi have the condyles attached to the upper member and are therefore **non-arcon** instruments.)

Mounting maxillary cast to axis-orbital plane. The face-bow is a relatively simple device used to obtain a transfer record for orienting a maxillary cast on an articulating instrument. Originally the face-bow was used only to transfer a **radius** from condyle reference points so that a given point on the cast would be the same distance from the condyle as it is on the patient. The addition of an adjustable infraorbital pointer to the face-bow and the addition of an orbital plane indicator to the articulator make possible also the transfer of the **elevation** of the cast in relation to the axis-orbital plane. This permits the maxillary cast to be correctly oriented in the articulator space comparable to the relationship of the maxillae to the Frankfort horizontal on the patient. To accommodate a maxillary cast so oriented and still have room for the mandibular cast, the posts of the conventional articulator must be lengthened. The older Hanau model H articulator usually will not permit a face-bow transfer using an infraorbital pointer.

A face-bow may be used to transfer a comparable radius from arbitrary reference points, or it may be designed so that the transfer can be made from hinge axis points. The latter type of transfer requires that a hing-bow attached to the mandible be used initially to determine the hinge axis points, to which the face-bow is then adjusted for making the hinge axis transfer.

A face-bow transfer of the maxillary cast, which is oriented to the axis-orbital plane, to a suitable articulator is an uncomplicated procedure. Hanau series 158 and 96H-2 and the Dentatus model ARH will accept this transfer, since these models have the longer posts and orbital plane indicator necessary for such a transfer (Fig. 11-12). Both the Hanau face-bow models 164-2, 153, and 132-25M and the Dentatus face-bow type AEB incorporate the infraorbital pointer that permits transfer of the infraorbital plane to the articulator. Neither of these is a hinge axis bow but is used instead at an arbitrary point.

The location of this arbitrary point or axis has long been the subject of some controversy. Gysi and others have placed it 11 to 13 mm anterior to the upper one third of the tragus of the ear on a line extending from the upper margin of the external auditory meatus to the outer canthus of the eye (Fig. 11-6). Others have placed it 13 mm anterior to the posterior margin of the center of the tragus of the ear on a line extending to the corner of the eye. Bergström has located the arbitrary axis 10 mm anterior to the center of a spherical insert for the external auditory meatus and 7 mm below the Frankfort horizontal plane.

In a series of experiments reported by Beck it was shown that the arbitrary axis suggested by Bergström falls consistently closer to the kinematic axis than do the other two. It is desirable that an arbitrary axis be placed as close as is possible to the kinematic axis. Although most authorities agree that any of the three axes will permit a transfer of the maxillary cast with reasonable accuracy, it would seem that the Bergström point compares most favorably with the kinematic axis.

The lowest point on the inferior orbital margin is taken as the third point of reference for establishing the axis-orbital plane. Some authorities use the point on the lower margin of the bony orbit in line with the center of the pupil of the eye. For the sake of consistency the right infraorbital point is generally used and the face-bow assembled in this relationship. All three points (right and left axes and infraorbital point)

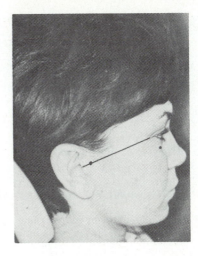

Fig. 11-6. Location of arbitrary axis 11 to 13 mm anterior to upper third of tragus of ear from line extending from upper margin of external auditory meatus to outer canthus of eye. Lowest point on inferior orbital margin is marked as third point of reference for establishing axis-orbital plane.

are marked on the face with an ink dot before making the transfer.

Casts are prepared for mounting on an articulator by placing three index grooves in the base of the cast. Two V-shaped grooves are placed in the posterior section of the cast and one groove in the anterior portion (Fig. 11-7).

An occlusion rim should be used in face-bow procedures involving the transfer of casts representative of the Classes I and II partially edentulous situations. Without occlusion rims, such casts cannot be located accurately in the imprints of the wax covering the face-bow fork. Tissues covering the residual ridges may be displaced grossly when the patient closes into the wax on the face-bow fork. Therefore the wax imprints of the soft tissues are not true negatives of the edentulous regions of the diagnostic casts.

The face-bow fork is covered with a roll of softened baseplate wax with the wax distributed equally on the top and on the underneath side of the face-bow fork. Then the fork should be pressed lightly on the diagnostic cast with the midline of the face-bow fork corresponding to the midline of the central incisors (Fig. 11-8). This will leave imprints of the occlusal and in-

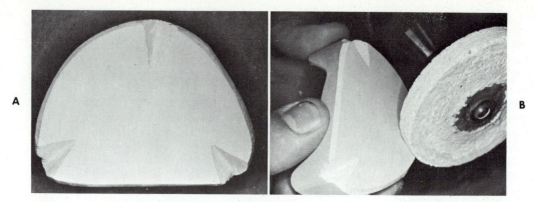

Fig. 11-7. A, Base of cast has been prepared for mounting. **B,** Triangular grooves can be conveniently and quickly cut in base of cast by using 3-inch stone mounted in laboratory lathe.

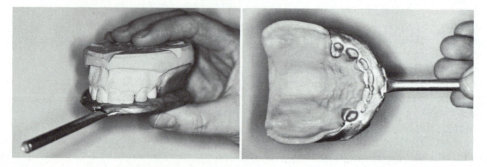

Fig. 11-8. Orienting face-bow fork to maxillary cast and occlusion rims will avoid displacing occlusion rim in mouth when patient closes to maintain face-bow fork in position. Face-bow fork illustrated here is Whip-Mix type. When offset type of face-bow fork (Hanau) is used, offset handle must be on patient's left.

cisal surfaces of the maxillary cast and occlusion rim on the softened baseplate wax and is an aid in correctly orienting the face-bow fork in the patient's mouth. The face-bow fork is placed in position in the mouth, and the patient is asked to close the lower teeth into the wax to stabilize it in position. It is removed from the mouth and chilled in cool water and then replaced in position in the patient's mouth. An alternative method of stabilizing the face-bow fork and recording bases is to enlist the assistance of the patient (Fig. 11-9).

With the face-bow fork in position, the face bow toggle is slipped over the anterior projection of the face-bow fork and positioned so that the calibrations on the shaft on either side read

the same as they rest lightly on the two dots located anterior to the external auditory meatuses. The calibrated shafts are then locked in this bilaterally equal position. The face-bow may have to be removed to accomplish this. It is then returned to position and locked to the face-bow fork while being held with equal contact over the dots on either side of the face. This accomplishes the **radius** aspect of the face-bow transfer.

With the infraorbital pointer on the extreme right side of the face-bow, it is angled toward the infraorbital point previously identified with an ink dot. It is then locked into position with its tip lightly touching the skin at the dot (Fig. 11-10). This establishes the **elevation** of the face-

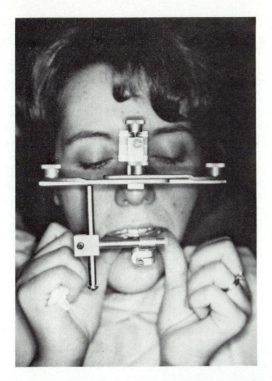

Fig. 11-9. Whip-Mix face-bow has been adjusted on patient, and toggles have been tightened. Patient assisted in stabilizing face-bow fork and occlusion rim by holding them securely in position with her thumbs while dentist adjusted and locked instrument in position.

bow in relation to the axis-orbital plane. Extreme care must be taken to avoid any slip that might damage the patient's eye.

With all elements tightened securely, the patient is asked to open, and the entire assembly is removed intact, rinsed with cold water, and set aside. The face-bow records not only the radius from the condyles to the incisal contacts of the upper central incisors but also the angular relationship of the occlusal plane to the axis-orbital plane.

The face-bow must be positioned on the articulator in the same axis-orbital relation as on the patient (Figs. 11-10 and 11-11). The calibrated condyle rods of the face-bow ordinarily will not fit the condyle shafts of the articulator unless the width between the condyles just happens to be the same. With a Hanau model C face-bow the calibrations must be reequalized when in position on the articulator. For example, they have read 74 (mm) on each side of the patient but must be adjusted to read 69 (mm) on each side of the articulator. With some later model articulators having adjustable condyle rods, these may instead be adjusted to fit the face-bow. It is necessary that the face-bow be centered in either case.

The third point of reference is the orbital plane indicator, which must be swung to the

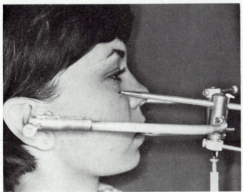

Fig. 11-10. Hanau S-M face-bow is positioned on face so that calibrations on shaft on either side read the same as they rest lightly on two dots located anterior to external auditory meatus. Infraorbital pointer is adjusted to rest lightly on infraorbital point previously marked on face.

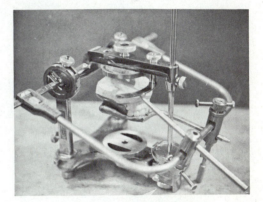

Fig. 11-11. Hanau face-bow model S-M attached to articulator before mounting of maxillary cast. Note elevation of face-bow with orbital plane indicator. Handle of offset face-bow fork must be on patient's left side; otherwise two face-bow toggles as used here would interfere with each other.

right so that it will be above the tip of the infraorbital pointer. The entire face-bow with maxillary cast in place must be raised until the tip of the pointer contacts the orbital plane indicator (Figs. 11-11 and 11-12). The elevation having thus been established, for all practical purposes the orbital plane indicator and pointer may now be removed because they may interfere with placing the mounting stone.

An auxiliary device called a **cast support** is available*; it is used to support the face-bow fork and the maxillary cast during the mounting operation (Fig. 11-12). With this device the weight of the cast and the mounting stone is supported separately from the face-bow, thus preventing possible downward movement resulting from their combined weight. The cast support is raised to supporting contact with the face-bow fork after the face-bow height has been adjusted

to the level of the orbital plane. Use of some type of cast support is highly recommended as an adjunct to face-bow mounting.

The keyed and lubricated maxillary cast is now attached to the upper arm of the articulator with the mounting stone, thus completing the face-bow transfer (Fig. 11-13). Not only will the face-bow have permitted the upper cast to be mounted with reasonable accuracy, but it also will have served as a convenient means of supporting the cast during mounting. The ease and speed with which a face-bow transfer can be effected makes ridiculous the frequently expressed objection to its use on the basis of time involved. Once mastered, its use becomes a great convenience rather than a time-consuming nuisance.

---

*Hanau Engineering Co., Buffalo, N.Y.

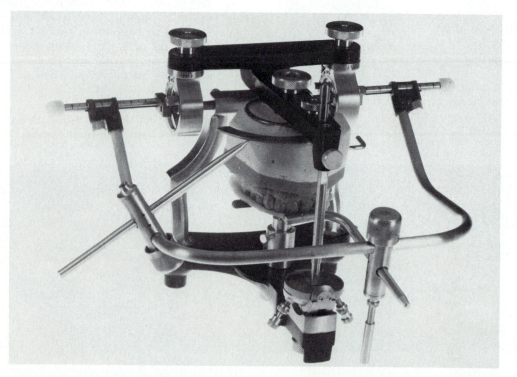

Fig. 11-12. Hanau Model 158-6 (X.P.R.) articulator with Model 159 combination ear piece/face-bow attached. Maxillary cast is secured to upper arm of articulator by split remounting plate. Cast support is attached to lower arm of articulator to support maxillary cast for mounting with stone. Orbital indicator and pointer can be used with procedures employing infraorbital notch as third point of reference during face-bow application and transfer.

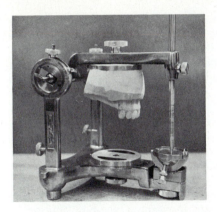

Fig. 11-13. Maxillary diagnostic cast mounted by face-bow transfer. Note that cast has been keyed before mounting and may be removed for repositioning on surveyor.

It is preferable that the maxillary cast be mounted while the patient is still present, thus eliminating a possible reappointment if the face-bow record is unacceptable for some reason. Not too infrequently the face-bow record has to be redone with the offset type face-bow fork repositioned to avoid interference with some part of the articulator.

An ear face-bow to orient the maxillary cast to an articulator is used by many dentists (Fig. 11-14). Its use, although described by Dalbey in 1914, had been rather limited until the early 1960s.

In an investigation by Teteruck and Lundeen it was demonstrated that by the ear face-bow method the maxillary cast could consistently be oriented more accurately to the hinge axis than

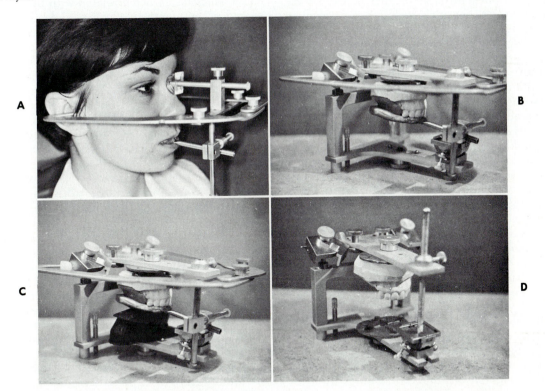

Fig. 11-14. A, Whip-Mix ear face-bow and face-bow fork are assembled on patient. **A nasion** relator forms anterior third point of reference in establishing **axis-orbital plane. B,** Face-bow assembly and cast are transferred to Whip-Mix articulator (an arcon instrument). **C,** Two wedge-shaped, rubber door stops are used to support face-bow fork and cast during mounting procedures. **D,** Mounting of maxillary cast is completed. Plane of occlusion as observed on articulator is same as that in mouth when Frankfort plane of patient is parallel to floor.

by the method using an arbitrary mark on the tragus-canthus line. The ear face-bow is a simple instrument to use, does not require measurements or marks on the face, consumes less time for its use, and is as accurate if not more so than are other arbitrary methods of face-bow transfer.

Jaw relationship records for diagnostic casts. One of the first critical decisions that must be made in a removable partial denture service involves the selection of the horizontal jaw relationship to which the removable partial denture will be constructed—centric relation or centric occlusion. All mouth preparation procedures depend on this analysis. Failure to make this decision correctly may result in the destruction of the residual ridges and supporting structures of the teeth.

Almost all dentists agree that deflective occlusal contacts in centric occlusion and eccentric positions must be corrected as a preventive measure. Not all dentists agree that centric relation and centric occlusion must be harmonious in the natural dentition. Apparently there are many dentitions that function satisfactorily with the opposing teeth maximally intercusped or interdigitated in an eccentric position without either diagnosable or subjective indications of temporomandibular joint dysfunction, muscle dysfunction, or disease of the supporting structures of the teeth. In many such situations no attempt should be made to alter the occlusion. It is not required to interfere with an occlusion simply because it does not completely conform to a relationship that is considered ideal.

If most natural posterior teeth remain and there is no evidence of temporomandibular joint disturbances, neuromuscular dysfunction, or periodontal disturbances related to occlusal factors, the proposed restoration may safely be constructed in centric occlusion (maximum interdigitation of remaining teeth). The proposed restoration, however, should be constructed so that centric occlusion is in harmony with centric relation when most natural centric stops are missing. By far the greater majority of removable partial dentures should be constructed in the horizontal jaw relationship of centric relation. In most instances in which edentulous spaces have not been restored the remaining posterior teeth will have assumed malaligned positions through drifting, tipping, or extrusion. Correction of the

natural occlusion to create a coincidence of centric relation and centric occlusion is indicated in such situations.

Regardless of the method employed in creating a harmonious functional occlusion, an evaluation of the existing relationships of the opposing natural teeth must be made. This evaluation is in addition to, and in conjunction with, other diagnostic procedures that contribute to an adequate diagnosis and treatment plan.

Diagnostic casts provide an opportunity to evaluate the relationship of remaining oral structures when correctly mounted on an adjustable articulator by using a face-bow transfer and interocclusal records. Diagnostic casts are mounted in centric relation (most retruded relation of the mandible to the maxillae) so that deflective occlusal contacts can be correlated with those observed in the mouth. Deflective contacts of opposing teeth are usually destructive to the supporting structures involved and should be eliminated. Diagnostic casts demonstrate the nature and location of such interfering tooth contacts and indicate the direction that must be followed for their correction. Necessary alteration of teeth to harmonize the occlusion can be performed initially on the mounted diagnostic casts to act as guides for similar necessary corrections in the mouth. In many instances the degree of alteration required will indicate the need for crowns or onlays to be fabricated or for the recontouring, repositioning, or the elimination of extruded teeth.

The maxillary cast is correctly oriented to the opening axis of the articulator by means of the face-bow transfer and becomes spatially related to the upper member of the articulator in the same relationship that the maxillae are related to the hinge axis and the Frankfort plane. Similarly, when a centric relation record is made at an established vertical dimension, the mandible is in its most retruded relation to the maxillae. Therefore when the maxillary cast is correctly oriented to the axis of the articulator, the mandibular cast automatically becomes correctly oriented to the opening axis, with an accurate centric relation record.

It is necessary to prove that the relationship of the mounted casts is correct. This can be done simply by making another interocclusal record, fitting the casts into the record, and checking to see that the condylar elements of the articulator are snug against the condylar housings. If this is not seen, it can be assumed that the original record was incorrect, the record was correct and the mounting procedure faulty, or the last record made was incorrect. Since centric relation is the only jaw position that can be routinely assumed by the patient, mountings in this position can be verified for correctness.

A straightforward protrusive record is made to adjust the horizontal condylar inclines on the articulator. Lateral eccentric records are made so that the lateral condylar inclinations can be properly adjusted. All interocclusal records should be made as near the vertical relation of occlusion as possible. Opposing teeth or occlusion rims must not be allowed to contact when the records are made. A contact of the inclined planes of opposing teeth will invalidate an interocclusal record.

In some instances a mounting of a duplicate diagnostic cast in centric occlusion also may be desirable to definitively study this relationship on the articulator. Since articulators only simulate jaw movements, it is not unreasonable to assume that the relationship of the casts mounted in centric relation may differ minutely in the centric occlusion seen on the articulator and observed in the mouth. When diagnostic casts are hand related by maximum intercuspation for purposes of mounting on an articulator, it is essential that three (preferably four) positive contacts of opposing posterior teeth are present, having molar contacts on each side of the arch. If occlusion rims are necessary to correctly orient casts on an articulator, centric relation should usually be the choice of the horizontal jaw relationship to which the removable partial denture will be constructed.

Materials and methods for recording centric relation. Materials available for recording centric relation are (1) wax, (2) modeling plastic, (3) quick-setting impression plaster, (4) metallic oxide impression paste, (5) polyether impression materials, and (6) silicone impression materials. Of these, wax is the least satisfactory material because it may not be uniformly softened when introduced into the mouth and because it does not remain rigid and dimensionally stable after removal.

Modeling plastic is a satisfactory record medium because it can be flamed and tempered until uniformly soft before it is placed into the mouth. After chilling, it is sufficiently stable to permit the mounting of casts with accuracy. For these reasons it is a satisfactory medium for recording occlusal relations for either complete or partial dentures. It also can be used with opposing natural teeth.

Impression plaster has advantages of softness when introduced and rigidity when set, which makes it a satisfactory material for recording jaw relations. Its use is highly recommended when occlusion rims are indicated to mount casts correctly or to adjust articulators with interocclusal eccentric records.

Impression paste offers many of the advantages of plaster, with less friability. Although not strong enough to be used alone, when supported by a gauze mesh it is a satisfactory recording medium. Also it may be used with occlusion rims.

After the paste sets, the frame is removed from the mouth and the buccal side of the gauze released where it was secured with sticky wax. The tube on the lingual side may then be slid off the lingual extension of the frame. The frame is not needed when mounting casts with this type of registration, since the tube alone lends sufficient support to the interocclusal record.

The mandibular cast should be mounted on the lower arm of the articulator with the articulator inverted (Fig. 11-15). The articulator is first locked in centric position, and the incisal pin is adjsuted so that the anterior distance between the upper and lower arms of the articulator will be increased 2 to 3 mm greater than the normal parallel relationship of the arms. This is done to compensate for the thickness of the interocclusal record so that the arms of the articulator will again be nearly parallel when the interocclusal record is removed and the opposing casts contact.

The base of the cast should be keyed and lightly lubricated for future removal. With the diagnostic casts accurately seated and secured in the occlusal record, the mandibular cast is affixed with stone to the lower member of the inverted articulator.

An articulator mounting thus made will have related the casts in centric relation. The dentist then can proceed to make an occlusal analysis

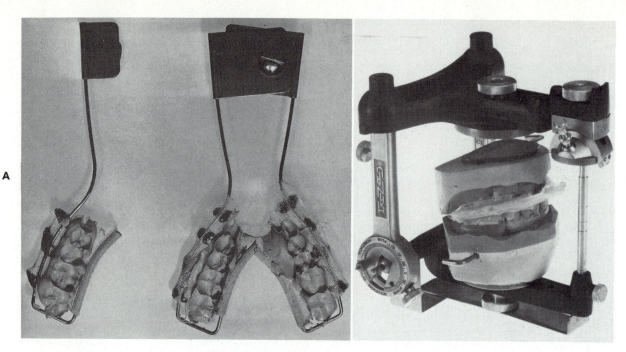

Fig. 11-15. **A,** Adjustable frame may be used either bilaterally or unilaterally but is always used bilaterally in removable partial denture procedure. Each gauze bib is made with tube that is slid over open lingual portion of frame and attached to its buccal portion with sticky wax. For bilateral use, frame must be adjusted to mouth or cast to avoid interference distal to last teeth in occlusion. Metallic oxide impression paste is applied to both sides of gauze, frame is oriented in mouth, and patient's lower jaw is closed into rehearsed horizontal jaw relation until paste hardens. After set record is removed from mouth, sticky wax is released from frame and tube is slid off frame. Gross excess and any sharp projections into interproximal spaces and into deep sulci are trimmed with sharp knife before record is placed between casts for mounting on articulator. **B,** Hanau model 96H2 articulator in inverted position on stand used as a stabilizing mechanism for mounting mandibular cast. Adjustable frame (see **A**) used to record centric relation is used to relate mandibular cast to previously mounted maxillary cast. Mandibular cast is attached to lower arm of articulator with stone.

by observing the influence of cusps in relation to one another after the articulator has been adjusted by using eccentric interocclusal records.

After an occlusal analysis has been made, the casts may be removed from their mounting for the purpose of surveying them individually and for other purposes as outlined previously. The indexed mounting ring record also should be retained throughout the course of treatment in the event that further study should be needed. It is advisable that the mounting be identified with the articulator used so that it may always be placed back onto the **same articulator**.

INTERPRETATION OF EXAMINATION DATA

As a result of the oral examination and diagnosis, certain data should be recorded, much of which are based on decisions that are the result of the diagnosis and reflect the patient's present and predictable health status. These are as follows:

Roentgenographic interpretation

Many of the reasons for roentgenographic interpretation during oral examination are outlined herein and are considered in greater detail in other texts. The aspects of such interpretation that are the most pertinent to partial denture construction are those relative to the prognosis of remaining teeth that may be used as abutments.

The quality of the alveolar support of an abutment tooth is of primary importance because the tooth will have to withstand greater stress loads when supporting a dental prosthesis. Abutment teeth providing total abutment support to the prosthesis, be it either fixed or removable, will have to withstand a greater load than before and especially greater horizontal forces. The latter may be minimized by establishing a harmonious occlusion and by distributing the horizontal forces among several teeth through the use of rigid connectors. Bilateral stabilization against horizontal forces is one of the attributes of a properly designed tooth-borne removable prosthesis. In many instances abutment teeth may be aided more than weakened by the presence of a bilaterally rigid partial denture.

In contrast, abutment teeth adjacent to distal extension bases are subjected not only to vertical and horizontal forces but to torque as well because of the movement of the tissue-supported base. Vertical support and stabilization against horizontal movement with rigid connectors are just as important as they are with a tooth-borne prosthesis, and the partial denture must be designed accordingly. In addition, the abutment tooth adjacent to the extension base will be subjected to torque in proportion to the design of the retainers, the size of the denture base, the tissue support received by the base, and the total occlusal load applied. With this in mind, each abutment tooth must be evaluated carefully as to the alveolar support present and the past reaction of that bone to occlusal stress.

Value of interpreting bone density. The quality and quantity of bone in any part of the body is often evaluated by roentgenographic means. A detailed treatise concerning the bone support of the abutment tooth should include many considerations not possible to include in this text because of space limitations. The reader should realize that subclinical variations in bone may exist but may not be observed because of the limitations inherent in technical methods and equipment.

Of importance to the prosthodontist when evaluating the quality and quantity of the alveolar bone are the height and the quality of the remaining bone. In estimating bone height, care must be taken to avoid interpretive errors resulting from angulation factors. Technically, when an exposure is being made, the central ray should be directed at right angles to both the tooth and the film. The most commonly used roentgenographic technique; that is, the short-cone technique, does not follow this principle; instead the ray is directed through the root of the tooth at a predetermined angle. This technique invariably causes the buccal bone to be projected higher on the crown than the lingual or palatal bone. Therefore in interpreting bone height, it is imperative to follow the line of the lamina dura from the apex toward the crown of the tooth until the opacity of the lamina materially decreases. At this point of opacity change a less dense bone extends farther toward the tooth crown. This additional amount of bone represents false bone height. Thus the true height of the bone is ordinarily where the lamina shows a marked decrease in opacity. At this point the trabecular pattern of bone superimposed on the tooth root is lost. The portion of the root between the cementoenamel junction and the true bone height has the appearance of being bare or devoid of covering.

Roentgenographic evaluation of bone quality is hazardous but is often necessary. It is essential to emphasize that changes in bone calcification up to 25% often cannot be recognized by ordinary roentgenographic means. Optimum bone qualities are ordinarily expressed by normal-sized interdental trabecular spaces that usually tend to decrease slightly in size as examination of the bone proceeds from the root apex toward the coronal portion. The normal interproximal crest is ordinarily shown by a relatively thin white line crossing from the lamina dura of one tooth to the lamina dura of the adjacent tooth. Considerable variation in the size of trabecular spaces may exist within the limits of normal, and the roentgenographic appearance of crestal alveolar bone may vary considerably, depending on its shape and the direction that the x-ray takes as it passes through the bone.

Normal bone usually responds favorably to ordinary stresses. Abnormal stresses, however, may create a reduction in the size of the trabecular pattern, particularly in that area of bone directly adjacent to the lamina dura of the affected tooth. This decrease in size of the trabecular pattern (that is, **so-called bone condensation**) is often regarded as a favorable bone response, indicative of an improvement in bone quality. This is not necessarily an accurate interpretation. Such bone changes usually indicate stresses that should be relieved because if the resistance of the patient decreases, the bone may exhibit a progressively less favorable response in future roentgenograms.

An increased thickness of the periodontal space ordinarily suggests varying degrees of tooth mobility. This should be evaluated clinically. Roentgenographic evidence coupled with clinical findings may suggest to the dentist the inadvisability of using such a tooth as an abutment. Furthermore, an irregular intercrestal bone surface should make the dentist suspicious of active bone deterioration.

It is essential that the dentist realize that roentgenographic evidence shows the **result** of changes that have taken place and may not necessarily represent the present condition. For example, periodontal disease may have progressed beyond the stage visibly demonstrated in the roentgenograms. As was pointed out earlier, roentgenographic changes are not observed until approximately 25% of the calcific content has been depleted. On the other hand, bone condensations probably do represent the present situation.

Roentgenographic findings should serve the dentist as an adjunct to clinical observations. Too often the roentgenographic appearance alone is used in arriving at a diagnosis. Roentgenographic interpretation also will serve an important function if used periodically **after** the prosthesis has been placed. Future bone changes of **any type** suggest traumatic interference from some source. The nature of such interference should be determined and corrective measures taken.

Index areas. Index areas are those areas of alveolar support that disclose the reaction of bone to additional stress. Favorable reaction to such stress may be taken as an indication of future reaction to an added stress load. Teeth that

have been subjected to abnormal loading because of the loss of adjacent teeth or that have withstood tipping forces in addition to occlusal loading may be better risks as abutment teeth than those that have not been called on to carry an extra occlusal load (Figs. 11-16 and 11-17). If occlusal harmony can be improved and unfavorable forces minimized by the reshaping of occlusal surfaces and the favorable distribution of occlusal loading, such teeth may be expected to support the prosthesis without difficulty. At the same time, other teeth, although not at present carrying an extra load, may be expected to react favorably because of the favorable reaction of alveolar bone to abnormal loading elsewhere in the same arch.

Such index areas are those around teeth that have been subjected to abnormal occlusal loading, that have been subjected to diagonal occlusal loading caused by tooth migration, and that have reacted to additional loading, such as around existing fixed partial denture abutments. The reaction of the bone to additional stresses in these areas may be either positive or negative, with evidence of a supporting trabecular pattern, a heavy cortical layer, and a dense lamina dura, or the reverse response. With the former the patient is said to have a **positive bone factor**, meaning the ability to build additional support wherever needed. With the latter the patient is said to have a **negative bone factor**, meaning inability to respond favorably to stress.

Alveolar lamina dura. The alveolar lamina dura is also considered in a roentgenographic interpretation of abutment teeth. The lamina dura is the thin layer of hard cortical bone that normally lines the sockets of all teeth. It affords attachment for the fibers of the periodontal membrane, and, as with all cortical bone, its function is to withstand mechanical strain. In a roentgenogram the lamina dura is shown as a **radiopaque** white line around the radiolucent dark line that represents the periodontal membrane.

When a tooth is in the process of being tipped, the center of rotation is not at the apex of the root but in the apical third. Resorption of bone occurs where there is pressure, and apposition occurs where there is tension. Therefore during the active tipping process the lamina dura is

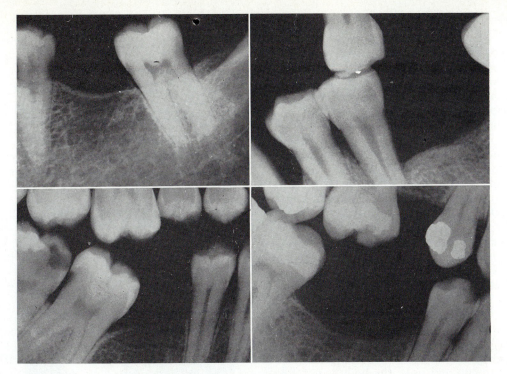

Fig. 11-16. Reaction of bone adjacent to teeth that have been subjected to abnormal stress serves as indication of probable reactions of that bone when such teeth are used as abutments for fixed or removable restorations. Such areas are called **index areas**.

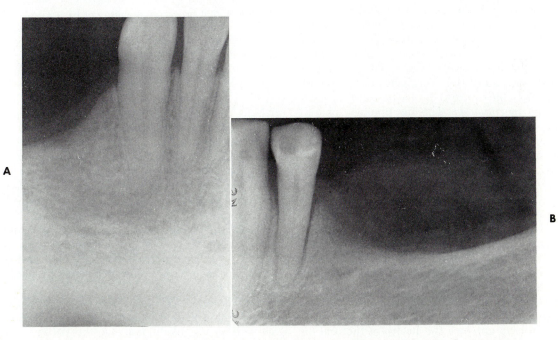

Fig. 11-17. A, Canine has provided support for distal extension partial denture for 10 years. There has obviously been positive bone response to increased stress generated by partial denture. **B,** Mandibular first premolar has provided support for distal extension denture for 3 years. Bone response to past additional stress has been unfavorable.

uneven, with evidence of both pressure and tension on the same side of the root. For example, in a mesially tipping lower molar the lamina dura will be thinner on the coronal mesial and apical distal aspects and thicker on the apical mesial and coronal distal aspects because the axis of rotation is not at the root apex but above it. When the tooth has been tipped into an edentulous space by some change in the occlusion and becomes set in its new position, the effects of leverage are discontinued. The lamina dura on the side to which the tooth is sloping becomes uniformly heavier, which is nature's reinforcement against abnormal stresses. The bone trabeculations are arranged at right angles to the heavier lamina dura.

Thus it is possible to say that for a given individual, nature is able to build support where it is needed and on this basis to predict future reaction elsewhere in the arch to additional loading of teeth used as abutments. However, since bone is approximately 30% organic, and this mostly protein, and since the body is not able to store a protein reserve in large amounts, any change in body health may be reflected in the patient's ability to maintain this support permanently. When systemic disease is associated with faulty protein metabolism and when the ability to repair is diminished, bone is resorbed and the lamina dura is disturbed. Therefore the loading of any abutment tooth must be kept to a minimum inasmuch as the patient's future health status and the eventualities of aging are unpredictable.

Root morphology. The morphologic characteristics of the roots determine to a great extent the ability of prospective abutment teeth to resist successfully additional rotational forces that may be placed on them. Teeth with multiple and divergent roots will resist stresses better than teeth with fused and conical roots, since the resultant forces are distributed through a greater number of periodontal fibers to a larger amount of supporting bone (Fig. 11-18).

Third molars. Unerupted third molars should be considered as prospective future abutments to eliminate the need for a distal extension removable partial denture (Fig. 11-19). The increased stability of a tooth-borne denture is most desirable to enhance the health of the oral environment.

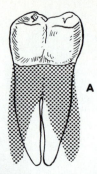

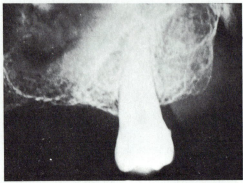

Fig. 11-18. **A,** Prognosis for abutment service is more favorable for molar with divergent roots (shaded) than for same tooth if its roots were fused and conical. **B,** Evidence that prospective abutment has conical and fused roots indicates necessity for formulating framework design that will minimize additional stresses placed on tooth by abutment service.

Periodontal considerations

Periodontal conditions present throughout the mouth in general and around abutment teeth in particular include the amount of alveolar support remaining and the past and predictable future reaction to additional occlusal stress. Evidence of tooth mobility should be noted as well as suggestions as to its cause and the corrective measures to be employed. This may involve simple correction of occlusal disharmony, or it may involve extensive periodontal treatment and in some instances splinting of periodontally weakened teeth.

Oral hygiene habits of the patient and the likelihood of patient cooperation in this regard, as well as the likelihood that the patient will return periodically for maintenance after recon-

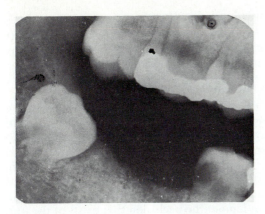

Fig. 11-19. First and second molars have been lost by this 18-year-old patient. Distal extension removable partial denture may be constructed until third molar erupts and is fully formed. Tooth-borne restoration can then be constructed.

struction are essential considerations. The teeth remaining will need attention no less after placement of a partial denture and perhaps even more so. Denture bases may need relining to compensate for changes in the supporting tissues. Therefore the patient must be willing to share with the dentist the responsibility for maintaining the health of the mouth after restorative treatment.

The most decisive evidence of oral hygiene habits is the condition of the mouth before the initial prophylaxis. Good or bad oral hygiene is basic to the patient's nature, and although it may be influenced somewhat by patient education, the long-range view must be taken. It is reasonably fair to assume that the patient will do little better in the long-term future than he has done in the past. In making decisions as to the method of treatment based on oral hygiene, **the future in years,** rather than in weeks and months, must be considered. Probably in this instance it is better not to give the patient the benefit of any doubt as to future oral hygiene habits. Rather, the benefit should come from protective measures where any doubt exists as to future oral hygiene habits.

Caries activity

Caries activity in the mouth, past and present, and the need for protective restorations must be considered. The decision to use full coverage is based on the age of the patient, evidence of caries activity, and the patient's oral hygiene habits. Occasionally three-quarter crowns may be used where buccal or lingual surfaces are completely sound, but intracoronal restoration (inlays) is seldom indicated in any mouth with evidence of past extensive caries or precarious areas of decalcification, erosion, or exposed cementum.

Prospective surgical preparation

Need for surgery or extractions must be evaluated. The same criteria apply to surgical intervention in the partially edentulous arch as in the completely edentulous arch. Grossly displaceable soft tissues covering basal seat areas and hyperplastic tissue should be removed to provide a firm denture foundation. Mandibular tori should be removed if they will interfere with the optimal location of a lingual bar connector or a favorable path of placement. Any other areas of bone prominence that will interfere with the path of placement should be removed also. The path of placement will be dictated primarily by the tooth guidance of the abutment teeth. Therefore some areas may present interference to the path of placement of the partial denture by reason of the fact that other unalterable factors such as retention and esthetics must take precedence in selecting that path.

Recent clinical research in preprosthetic surgical concepts has contributed significant developments to management of the compromised partially edentulous patient. Use of hydroxylapatite for ridge augmentation has proven to be a viable alternative method of improving ridge support for the denture base areas. Likewise, use of osseointegrated implants may provide a foundation for developing suitable abutment support for removable partial dentures. As in any surgical procedure, results are dependent on careful treatment planning and cautious surgical management.

Extraction of teeth may be indicated for one of the following three reasons:

1. If the tooth cannot be restored to a state of health, extraction may be unavoidable. Modern advancements in the treatment of periodontal disease and in restorative procedures, including endodontic therapy, have resulted in the saving of teeth that were once considered un-

treatable. **All avenues of treatment should be considered both from a prognostic and an economic standpoint before recommending extraction.**

2. A tooth may be removed if its absence will permit a more serviceable and less complicated partial denture design. Teeth in extreme malposition—lingually inclined mandibular teeth, buccally inclined maxillary teeth, and mesially inclined teeth posterior to an edentulous space—may be removed if an adjacent tooth is in good alignment and with good support is available for use as an abutment. Justification for extraction lies in the decision that a suitable crown, which will provide satisfactory contour and support, cannot be fabricated or that orthodontic treatment to realign the tooth is not feasible. An exception to the arbitrary removal of a malposed tooth is when by so doing a distal extension partial denture base would have to be made rather than the more desirable tooth-supported base through the use of the tooth in question. If alveolar support is adequate, a posterior abutment should be retained if at all possible in preference to a tissue-supported extension base.

Teeth deemed to have insufficient alveolar support may be extracted if their prognosis is poor and if other adjacent teeth may be used to better advantage as abutments. The decision to extract such a tooth should be based on the degree of mobility and other periodontal considerations and on the number, length, and shape of the roots contributing to its support.

3. A tooth may be extracted if it is so unesthetically located as to justify its removal to improve appearance. In this regard a veneer crown should be considered in preference to removal. If removal is advisable because of unesthetic tooth position, the biomechanical problems involved in replacing anterior teeth with a removable partial denture must be weighed against the problems involved in making an esthetically acceptable fixed restoration. Admittedly the removable replacement is frequently the more esthetic of the two, despite modern advancements in retainers and pontics. However, the mechanical disadvantage of the removable restoration frequently makes the fixed replacement of missing anterior teeth preferable.

Endodontic treatment

Need for **prospective or planned endodontic** treatment includes abutments for overlay type removable partial dentures.

Analysis of occlusal factors

From the occlusal analysis made from mounted diagnostic casts the dentist must decide whether it is best to accept and maintain the existing occlusion or to attempt to improve on it by means of occlusal adjustment and the restoration of occlusal surfaces. **It must be remembered that the partial denture can only supplement the occlusion that exists at the time the prosthesis is constructed.** The dominant force dictating the occlusal pattern will be the cuspal harmony or disharmony of the remaining teeth and their proprioreceptal influence on kinematic movement. At best the supplied teeth can only be made to harmonize with the cause and effect of the existing occlusion.

Improvements in the natural occlusion must be accomplished before the construction of the denture, not subsequent to it. The objective of occlusal reconstruction by any means should be occlusal harmony of the restored dentition in relation to the natural forces already present or established. Therefore one of the earliest decisions in planning reconstructive treatment must be whether to accept or reject the existing vertical dimension of occlusion and the occlusal contact relationships in centric and eccentric positions. If occlusal adjustment is indicated, cuspal analysis always should precede any corrective procedures in the mouth by selective grinding. On the other hand, if reconstruction is to be the means of correction, the manner and sequence should be outlined as part of the overall treatment plan.

Fixed restorations

There may be a need for fixed restorations rather than including them in the partial denture to the detriment of isolated abutment teeth. The advantage of splinting must be weighed against the total cost, with the weight of experience always in favor of using fixed restorations for tooth-bounded spaces. One of the least successful of partial denture designs is where multiple tooth-bounded areas are replaced with the partial dentures in conjunction with isolated abutment teeth and distal extension bases. Biomechanical considerations and the future health of the remaining teeth should be given preference over economic considerations where such a choice is possible.

Orthodontic treatment

Occasionally, orthodontic movement of malposed teeth followed by retention through the use of fixed restorations makes possible a better partial denture design mechanically and esthetically than could otherwise be used.

Need for determining type of mandibular major connector

As discussed in Chapter 4, one of the criteria for determining the use of the lingual bar or linguoplate is the height of the floor of the patient's mouth when the tongue is elevated. Since the inferior border of both the lingual bar and linguoplate are placed at the same vertical level and since subsequent mouth preparations depend in part on the selection of the mandibular major connector, determination of the type of major connector must be made during the oral examination. This determination is facilitated by measuring the height of the elevated floor of the patient's mouth in relation to lingual gingivae with a periodontal probe and recording the measurement for later transfer to diagnostic and master casts. It is most difficult to make a determination of the type of mandibular major connector to be used solely from a stone cast that may or may not accurately indicate the active range of movement of the floor of the patient's mouth. Too many mandibular major connectors are ruined, being made flexible because subsequent grinding of the inferior border is necessary to relieve impingement of the sensitive tissues of the floor of the mouth.

Need for reshaping remaining teeth

Many failures of partial dentures can be attributed to the fact that the teeth were not reshaped properly to receive clasp arms and occlusal rests before the impression for the master cast was made. Of particular importance are the paralleling of proximal tooth surfaces to act as guiding planes, the preparation of adequate rest

areas, and the reduction of unfavorable tooth contours. To neglect to plan such mouth preparations in advance is inexcusable.

The design of clasps is dependent on the location of the retentive, reciprocal, and supporting areas in relation to a definite path of placement and removal. Failure to reshape unfavorably inclined tooth surfaces and, if necessary, to place onlays and crowns with suitable contours not only complicates the design and location of clasp retainers but also frequently leads to failure of the partial denture because of poor clasp design.

A malaligned tooth or one that is inclined unfavorably may make it necessary to place certain parts of the clasp so that they interfere with the opposing teeth. Unparallel proximal tooth surfaces not only will fail to provide needed guiding planes during placement and removal but also will make excessive blockout necessary. This inevitably results in the connectors being placed so far out of contact with tooth surfaces that food traps are created. To pass lingually inclined lower teeth, clearance for a lingual bar major connector may have to be so great that a food trap will result when the restoration is fully seated, and the lingual bar will be located so that it will interfere with tongue comfort and function. These are only some of the objectionable consequences of inadequate mouth preparations.

Reduction of unfavorable tooth contours

Slight reduction of unfavorable tooth contours will greatly facilitate the design of the partial denture framework. The need for modification of tooth contours must be established during the diagnosis and treatment planning phase of partial denture service.

The amount of reduction of tooth contours should be kept to a minimum, and all modified tooth surfaces should not only be repolished after reduction but also should be subjected to fluoride treatment to lessen the incidence of caries. If it is not possible to produce the contour desired without perforating the enamel, inlays or crowns must be used. The age of the patient, caries activity evidenced elsewhere in the mouth, and apparent oral hygiene habits must be taken into consideration when deciding between reducing the enamel or modifying tooth contours with protective restorations.

Some of the areas frequently needing correction are the lingual surfaces of mandibular premoalrs, the mesial and lingual surfaces of mandibular molars, the distobuccal line angle of maxillary premolars, and the mesiobuccal line angle of maxillary molars. The actual degree of inclination of teeth in relation to the path of placement and the location of retentive and supportive areas are not readily interpretable during visual examination. These are established during a comprehensive survey of the diagnostic cast with a cast surveyor, which should follow the visual examination.

DIFFERENTIAL DIAGNOSIS: FIXED OR REMOVABLE PARTIAL DENTURES

Total oral rehabilitation is an objective in treating the partially edentulous patient. The replacement of missing teeth by means of fixed restorations is the method of preference; a removable restoration should be used only where a fixed restoration is contraindicated.

There are inherent risks in the use of unilateral removable partial dentures that cotraindicate their use when a fixed partial denture is indicated. Some of these risks are (1) possible aspiration, (2) lack of cross-arch stabilization, and (3) excessive stress to abutment teeth.

The dentist must follow the best procedure for the welfare of the patient who is always free to seek more than one opinion. Ultimately, the choice of treatment must meet the economic limitations and personal desires of the patient.

Indications for use of fixed restorations

Tooth-bounded edentulous regions. Generally any unilateral edentulous space bounded by teeth suitable for use as abutments should be restored with a fixed partial denture cemented to one or more abutment teeth at either end. The length of the span and the periodontal support of the abutment teeth will determine the number of abutments required.

Lack of parallelism of the abutment teeth may be counteracted with copings or locking recesses to provide parallel sectional placement. Sound abutment teeth make possible the use of more conservative retainers such as inlays rather than

full crowns. The age of the patient, evidence of caries activity, oral hygiene habits, and soundness of remaining tooth structure must be considered in any decision to use less-than-full coverage for abutment teeth.

There are two specific contraindications for the use of unilateral fixed restorations. One is a long edentulous span and abutment teeth that would not be able to withstand the trauma of horizontal and diagonal occlusal forces. The other is abutment teeth, weakened by periodontal disease, that would benefit from cross-arch stabilization. In either situation a bilateral removable restoration can be used more effectively to replace the missing teeth.

Modification spaces. A removable partial denture for a Class III arch is better supported and stabilized when a modification area on the opposite side of the arch is present. Such an edentulous area need not be restored by a fixed partial denture, since it may simplify the design of the removable partial denture (Fig. 11-20). Additional modification spaces, however, particularly those involving single missing teeth, are better restored separately by means of fixed dentures. Not only is a lone-standing abutment thus stabilized by the splinting effect of a fixed restoration, but also a possible teeter-totter effect of the denture is avoided, and the denture is

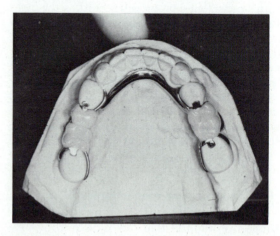

Fig. 11-20. Class III, modification 1, restoration. Modification space has been included in design of denture rather than restored with fixed partial denture. Design for removable restoration is greatly simplified, resulting in significantly enhanced stability.

made less complicated by not having to include other abutment teeth for the support and retention of an additional edentulous space or spaces.

When an edentulous space that is a modification of either a Class I or Class II arch exists anterior to a lone-standing abutment tooth, this tooth is subjected to trauma by the movements of a distal extension partial denture far in excess of its ability to withstand such stresses. The splinting of the lone abutment to the nearest tooth is mandatory. Splinting is best accomplished in such a situation by means of a fixed partial denture uniting the two teeth on either side of the edentulous space. **The abutment crowns should be contoured for support and retention of the partial denture,** and in addition, a means of supporting a stabilizing component on the anterior abutment of the fixed partial denture or on the occlusal surface of the pontic usually should be provided.

Anterior modification spaces. Usually any missing anterior teeth in a partially edentulous arch, except in a Kennedy Class IV arch in which only anterior teeth are missing, are best replaced by means of a fixed restoration. There are exceptions. Sometimes a better esthetic result is obtainable when the anterior replacements are supplied by the removable partial denture (Fig. 11-21). This is also true when ex-

cessive tissue and bone resorption necessitates the placement of pontics too far posteriorly for good esthetics and for an acceptable relation with the opposing teeth. However, in most instances, from a mechanical and biologic standpoint, anterior replacements are best accomplished with fixed restorations. The replacement of missing posterior teeth with a removable partial denture is then made much less complicated and gives more satisfactory results.

Nonreplacement of missing molars. Frequently the decision of whether to replace unilaterally missing molars must be made. To do so with a removable denture necessitates the making of a distal extension restoration with the major connector joining the edentulous side to retentive and stabilizing components located on the nonedentulous side of the arch. Leverage factors are always unfavorable, and the retainers that must be used on the nonedentulous side are frequently unsatisfactory. Several factors therefore will influence the decision to make a unilateral, distal extension partial denture.

First, the opposing teeth must be considered. If they are to be prevented from extrusion and migration, some opposing occlusion must be provided. This would influence the replacement of the missing molars far more than any improvement in masticating efficiency that might

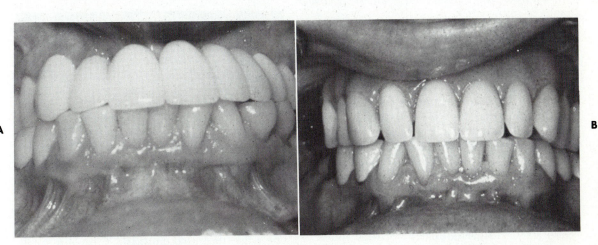

Fig. 11-21. A, Exceedingly long maxillary edentulous span restored with fixed partial denture. Note extreme labial inclinations of pontics resulting in lack of support for upper lip and compromised appearance. **B,** Appearance has been greatly improved by restoring edentulous span with removable restoration.

result. The replacement of missing molars on one side is seldom necessary for reasons of mastication alone.

Second, the future of a maxillary tuberosity must be considered. Left uncovered, the tuberosity frequently will seem to drop and increase in size. However, covering the tuberosity with a partial denture base, in combination with the stimulating effect of the intermittent occlusion provided, helps to maintain the normalcy of the tuberosity. This is of considerable importance in any future denture replacements. In such an instance it may be better to make a unilateral removable partial denture than to leave a maxillary tuberosity uncovered.

A third consideration is the condition of the opposing second molar. If this tooth is missing or can logically be ignored or eliminated, then only first molar occlusion need be supplied by using a cantilever-type fixed restoration. Occlusion need be only minimum to maintain occlusal relations between the natural first molar in the one arch and the prosthetic molar in the opposite arch. Such a pontic should be narrow buccolingually and need not occlude with more than one half to two thirds of the opposing tooth. Frequently such a restoration is the preferred method of treatment. However, unless three abutments are used to support a cantilever molar opposed by a natural molar, only limited success should be anticipated.

Indications for removable partial dentures

Although a removable partial denture should be considered only when a fixed restoration is contraindicated, there are several specific indications for the use of a removable restoration.

Distal extension situations. Except in situations in which the replacement of missing second (and third) molars is either inadvisable or unnecessary, or in which unilateral replacement of a missing first molar can be accomplished by means of a multiple abutment, cantilevered fixed restoration, replacement of missing posterior teeth without the assistance of a posterior abutment must be accomplished with a removable partial denture. The most common partially edentulous situations are the Kennedy Class I and Class II. With the latter an edentulous space

on the opposite side of the arch is often conveniently present, or can be effected, to aid in the required retention and stabilization of the partial denture. If no space is present, embrasure clasps or intracoronal retainers generally must be used. As previously stated, all other edentulous areas are best replaced with fixed partial dentures.

After recent extractions. The replacement of teeth after recent extractions cannot be accomplished satisfactorily with a fixed restoration. When relining will be required later or when a fixed restoration will be constructed later, a temporary removable partial denture must be used. If an all-resin denture is used rather than a more elaborate partial denture, the immediate cost to the patient is much less, and the resin denture lends itself best to future temporary modifications.

Tissue changes are inevitable following extractions. Tooth-bounded edentulous areas (as a result of extractions) are best initially restored with removable partial dentures. Relining of a tooth-supported resin denture base thus is made possible. It is usually done to improve esthetics, oral cleanliness, or patient comfort. Support for such a restoration is supplied by occlusal rests on the abutment teeth at each end of the edentulous space.

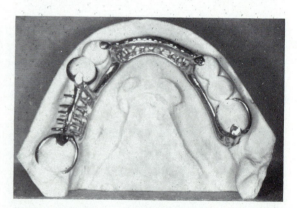

Fig. 11-22. Class III, modification 1, partially edentulous arch. Restoration of choice is removable denture rather than fixed prosthesis. Cross-arch stabilization is assured with rigid framework. Additional benefit is opportunity to arrange anterior teeth for optimal esthetics.

Long span. A long span may be totally tooth supported if the abutments and the means of transferring the support to the denture are adequate and if the denture framework is rigid (Fig. 11-22). There is little if any difference between the support afforded a removable partial denture and that afforded a fixed restoration by the adjacent abutment teeth. However, in the absence of cross-arch stabilization, the torque and leverage on the two abutment teeth would be excessive. Instead, a removable denture deriving retention, support, and stabilization from abutment teeth on the opposite side of the arch is indicated as the logical means of replacing the missing teeth.

Need for effect of bilateral stabilization. In a mouth weakened by periodontal disease, because of the lack of cross-arch stabilization, a fixed restoration may jeopardize the future of periodontally involved abutment teeth unless the splinting effect of multiple abutments is employed. The removable partial denture on the other hand may act as a periodontal splint through its effective cross-arch stabilizing of teeth weakened by periodontal disease. When abutment teeth throughout the arch are properly prepared and restored, the beneficial effect of a removable partial denture can be far greater than that of a unilateral fixed partial denture.

Excessive loss of residual bone. The pontic of a fixed partial denture must be related to the residual ridge in such a manner that the contact with the mucosa is gentle. Whenever excessive resorption has occurred, teeth supported by a

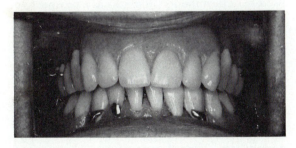

Fig. 11-23. In situations involving excessive residual ridge resorption, artificial teeth supported by denture base can often provide more esthetic and functional result than fixed partial denture.

denture base may be arranged in a more acceptable buccolingual position than is possible with a fixed partial denture.

Artificial teeth supported by a denture base can be located without regard to the crest of the residual ridge and more nearly in the position of the natural dentition for normal tongue and cheek contacts. This is particularly true of a maxillary denture (Fig. 11-23).

Anteriorly, loss of residual bone occurs from the labial aspect. Often the incisive papilla lies at the crest of the residual ridge. Since the central incisors are normally located anterior to this landmark, any other location of artificial central incisors is unnatural. An anterior fixed partial denture made for such a mouth will have pontics resting on the labial aspect of this resorbed ridge and will be too far lingual to provide desirable lip support. Frequently the only way the incisal edges of the pontics can be made to occlude with the opposing lower anterior teeth is to use a labial inclination that is excessive and unnatural, and both esthetics and lip support suffer thereby. Because the same condition exists with a removable partial denture in which the anterior teeth are abutted on the residual ridge, a labial flange must be used to permit the teeth to be located more nearly in their natural position.

The same method of treatment applies to the replacement of missing mandibular anterior teeth. Sometimes a mandibular anterior fixed partial denture is made six or more units in length, in which the remaining space necessitates either leaving out one anterior tooth or using the original number of teeth but with all of them too narrow for esthetics. In either instance the denture is nearly in a straight line because the pontics follow the form of the resorbed ridge. A removable partial denture will permit the location of the replaced teeth in a favorable relation to the lip and opposing dentition regardless of the shape of the residual ridge. When such a removable prosthesis is made, however, positive support must be obtained from the adjacent abutments.

Unusually sound abutment teeth. Sometimes the excuse for making a removable restoration is the wish to see sound teeth preserved in their natural state and not prepared for abutment re-

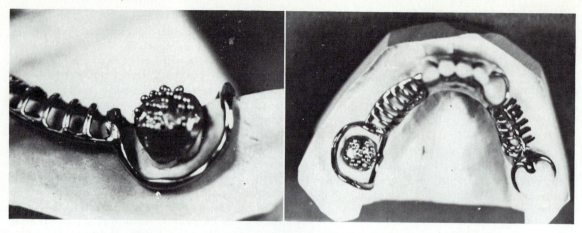

Fig. 11-24. A, Left second molar had guarded prognosis as abutment for removable partial denture. Framework was designed as for Class II modification arch using linguoplate major connector, bar-type retainer on left lateral incisor, and wrought-wire retentive arm on right canine. Telescoping crown was fabricated over coping on left second molar and will be retained by acrylic resin denture base. Subsequent loss of second molar would require only modification of denture base (relining to accomplish functional basing). **B,** Sagittal view of crown. Note cast retention beads on occlusal surface of the crown.

tainers. The reasons for the loss of the teeth being replaced must be considered. If loss is because of caries, then it is likely that caries will occur eventually in the abutment teeth. If the teeth were lost because of periodontal disease, then the periodontium of the remaining teeth must be evaluated. If the teeth were lost as a result of neglect of minimum caries and if the caries activity seems to be arrested, the use of existing tooth surfaces to support a removable restoration may be justified. If the oral hygiene habits of the patient are favorable and if the abutment teeth are sound with good periodontal support, unprotected abutments may be used to support and retain a removable restoration. When this condition exists, the dentist should not hesitate to reshape and modify existing enamel surfaces to provide proximal guiding planes, occlusal rest areas, optimum retentive areas, and surfaces on which nonretentive stabilizing components may be placed.

It is only in selected instances that the making of a removable prosthetic restoration on unprotected abutments can be justified.

Abutments with guarded prognoses. If the prognosis of an abutment tooth is questionable or if it becomes unfavorable while under treat-

ment, it might be possible to compensate for its impending loss by a change in denture design. The questionable or condemned tooth or teeth may then be included in the original design and if subsequently lost, the partial denture can be added to, remade, or replaced (Fig. 11-24). Many partial denture designs do not lend themselves well to later additions, although this eventuality should be considered in the design of the denture.

When the tooth in question will be used as an abutment, every diagnostic aid should be used to determine its prognosis as a prospective abutment. It is usually not so difficult to add a tooth or teeth to a partial denture as it is to add a retaining unit when the original abutment is lost and the next adjacent tooth must be used for that purpose.

It is sometimes possible to design a removable partial denture so that a single posterior abutment, about which there is some doubt, can be retained and used at one end of the tooth-supported base. Then if the posterior abutment is lost, it could be replaced by adding an extension base to the existing denture framework. Such an original design must include provisions for future indirect retention, flexible clasping of the

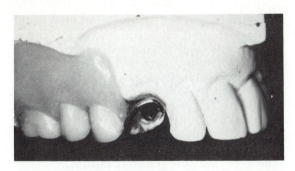

Fig. 11-25. Modifying partial denture design to accommodate loss of canine abutment would be extremely difficult (if not impossible). Problems related to new clasp assembly for lateral incisor as abutment are manifold. New restoration is indicated; however, present denture could be modified to serve in temporary capacity.

future abutment, and provision for establishing tissue support. Anterior abutments that are considered poor risks may not be so freely used because of the problems involved in adding a new abutment retainer when the original one is lost (Fig. 11-25). It is rational that such questionable teeth be condemned in favor of more suitable abutments, even though the original treatment plan must be modified accordingly.

Economic considerations. Economics should not be the sole criterion in arriving at a method of treatment. When, for economic reasons, complete treatment is out of the question and yet replacement of missing teeth is indicated, the restorative procedures dictated by these considerations must be described clearly to the patient as being of an interim nature and not representative of the best that modern dentistry has to offer. Ordinarily a prosthesis that is made to satisfy economic considerations alone is doomed to limited success, and both professional esteem and the patient suffer thereby.

CHOICE BETWEEN COMPLETE DENTURES AND REMOVABLE PARTIAL DENTURES

When the diagnosis preceding prosthodontic service is made, the probable length of service that can be expected from a partial denture must always be weighed against the patient's economic status. A decision may have to be made between a partial denture and a complete denture, in either arch or both. One patient may prefer complete dentures to the traumatic experience of complete oral rehabilitation, regardless of ability to pay. Others may be so determined to keep their own teeth that they will make great financial sacrifices if given a reasonable assurance of success of oral rehabilitation.

The value of listening to the patient during the examination and the diagnostic procedures should not be disregarded nor treated lightly. During the presentation of pertinent facts, time should be allowed for patients to express themselves freely as to their desires in retaining and restoring their natural teeth. At this time a treatment plan may be influenced or even drastically changed to conform to the expressed and implied wishes of the patient.

For example, there may be a reasonable possibility of saving teeth in both arches through the use of partial dentures. With only anterior teeth remaining, a partial denture can be made to replace the posterior teeth by using good abutment support and in the maxillary arch using full palatal coverage for retention and stability. If patients express a desire to retain their anterior teeth "at any cost" and if the remaining teeth are esthetically acceptable and functionally sound, the dentist should make every effort to provide successful treatment. On the other hand, complete dentures may best satisfy other patients' requirements because of economic or other reasons. If patients prefer a mandibular partial denture because of fear of difficulty in wearing a mandibular complete denture, then, all factors being acceptable, their wishes should be respected and treatment planned accordingly.

Still other patients, for economic or other reasons, may prefer to have complete dentures made for both arches rather than undergo complete rehabilitation of the partially edentulous arches. It is frequently unwise to insist on the latter course with such patients. **The professional obligation to present the facts and then do the best in accordance with the patients' expressed desires still applies.**

Other patients may wish to retain remaining teeth for an indefinite but relatively short period of time, with eventual complete dentures a foregone conclusion. In this instance the professional obligation may be to recommend interim partial dentures without extensive mouth preparations. Such dentures will aid in mastication and will provide esthetic replacements, at the same time serving as conditioning restorations, which will make the later transition to complete dentures somewhat easier. Such partial dentures should be designed and fabricated with care, but the total cost of partial denture service should be considerably less.

An expressed desire on the part of patients to retain only six mandibular anterior teeth must be considered carefully before being agreed to as the planned treatment. The advantages to the patients are obvious: they may retain six esthetically acceptable teeth; they do not become totally edentulous; and they have the advantage of direct retention that would not be possible if they were completely edentulous. Retaining even the mandibular canine teeth would accomplish the latter two objectives. These advantages cannot be denied. Yet the disadvantages, which are less obvious to patients, must also be considered and explained to them. These are mechanical and functional considerations; that is, the edentulous maxilla anteriorly is structurally not able to withstand the trauma of positive tooth contact against natural opposing teeth. The possible result is the loss of residual maxillary bone, loosening of the maxillary denture because of the tripping influence of the natural mandibular teeth, and the loss of basal foundation for the support of future prostheses. However, if the maxillary anteriors are arranged to contact in eccentric positions only and patients comply with periodic recall, these problems are certainly minimized. The presence of inflamed hyperplastic tissue is a frequent sequel to continued loss of support and denture movement.

The prevention of this sequence of events lies in the maintenance of positive occlusal support posteriorly and the continual elimination of traumatic influence from the remaining anterior teeth. Such support is sometimes impossible to maintain without frequent relining or remaking of the lower partial denture base. On the other hand, this may cause undesirable resorption of the posterior ridges because of overloading. The results in any event are undesirable, and the

patient must be made aware of the hazards involved.

Whereas some patients are able to wear a lower partial denture supported only by anterior teeth against a complete maxillary denture, the odds are that undesirable consequences will result unless the patient faithfully follows the instructions of the dentist. In no other situation in treatment planning is the general health of the patient and the quality of residual alveolar bone as critical as it is in this situation.

In addition to considering the age and health of patients and their ability to build bone in response to stress, it is well to consider why the teeth being replaced were extracted. In all probability any history of severe periodontal disease precludes the wearing of such combination dentures successfully. On the other hand, the loss of teeth because of caries or the premature loss of teeth that might have been saved justifies the conclusion that the residual bone is probably healthy and will be able to withstand stresses within reasonable limits. In such instances, combination dentures may be constructed if the patient is made aware of the need for periodic examination and is willing to make the transition to a complete lower denture on the first signs of serious damage to supporting structures.

The final treatment plan should represent the best possible course for the patient after consideration has been given to all physical, mental, mechanical, esthetic, and economic factors involved.

FACTORS IN SELECTING METAL ALLOYS FOR REMOVABLE PARTIAL DENTURE FRAMEWORKS

Practically all cast frameworks for removable partial dentures are made either from a gold alloy (Type IV) or from a chromium-cobalt alloy. The choice of the alloy from which the framework of a removable partial denture will be constructed is logically made during the treatment planning phase. Inherent differences in the physical properties of alloys presently available to the dental profession must be considered in making this choice. For example, mouth preparation procedures, especially the recontouring of abutment teeth for the optimum placement of retentive elements, depend to a large extent on the modulus of elasticity (stiffness) of a particular alloy.

Chromium-cobalt alloys are used many times more than the gold alloys in removable partial prosthodontics. The popularity of the chromium-cobalt alloys has been attributed to their low density (weight), high modulus of elasticity (stiffness), low material cost, and resistance to tarnish.

Use of the chromium-cobalt alloys in preference to the gold alloys continues to be somewhat controversial among members of the dental profession. This controversy stems in part from the necessity of using specialized equipment and techniques in the application of the chromium-cobalt alloys, which has restricted the fabrication of frameworks almost entirely to commercial dental laboratories.

Each of the alloys has advantages under certain conditions. The material considered capable of rendering the best overall service to the patient over a period of years is the one that should be used. The choice of alloy is based on several factors: (1) weighed advantages or disadvantages of the physical properties of the alloy, (2) the dimensional accuracy with which the alloy can be cast, (3) the availability of the alloy, (4) the versatility of the alloy, and (5) the individual clinical observation and experiences with alloys in respect to quality control and service to the patient.

The following are comparable characteristics of gold alloys and chromium-cobalt alloys: (1) each is well tolerated by oral tissues; (2) they are equally acceptable esthetically; (3) enamel abrasion by either alloy is insignificant on vertical tooth surfaces; (4) a low-fusing chrome-cobalt alloy or gold alloy can be cast to wrought wire, and wrought-wire components may be soldered to either gold or chrome-cobalt alloys (these characteristics are important in overcoming the objection by some dentists to the increased stiffness of chromium-cobalt alloys for the portions of direct retainers that must engage an undercut of the abutment tooth); (5) the accuracy obtainable in casting either alloy is clinically acceptable under strictly controlled investing and casting procedures; and (6) soldering procedures for the repair of frameworks can be performed on each alloy.

Comparative physical properties. Chromium-cobalt alloys generally have a lower **yield strength** than the gold alloys used for removable partial dentures (Table 11-1). Yield strength is the greatest amount of stress an alloy will withstand and still return to its original shape in an unweakened condition. Possessing a lower proportional limit, the chromium-cobalt alloys will deform permanently at lower loads than gold alloys. Therefore the dentist must design the chromium-cobalt framework so that the degree of deformation expected in a direct retainer is less than a comparable degree of deformation for a gold component.

The **modulus of elasticity** refers to stiffness of an alloy. Gold alloys have a modulus of elasticity

Table 11-1. *Mechanical properties of representative stellite alloys**

Properties	Stellite alloys†					Hardened partial denture gold alloys
	A	B	D	E	21	
Yield strength (psi)	64,500	61,000	56,000	62,400	82,300	65,000-90,000
Tensile strength (psi)	180,500	107,500	84,500	102,500	101,300	107,000-120,000
Elongation (%)	3.4	3.2	6.0	1.9	8.2	1.5-8.0
Modulus of elasticity (psi × 10^{-6})	28.0	29.5	27.5	28.5	36.0	13-15
Hardness (R[30N])‡	53.0	60.0	51.0	55.0	—	—

*From Peyton, F.A.: Dent. Clin. North Am., pp. 759-771, Nov. 1958.
†Data for lettered alloys from Taylor, D.F., Liebfritz, W.A., and Adler, A.G.: J. Am. Dent. Assoc. **56:**343-351, 1958; for Stellite No. 21 from Metals Handbook, 1948 ed., p. 579; for gold alloys from manufacturers property charts.
‡Rockwell 30N hardness scale.

approximately one half of that for chromium-cobalt alloys for similar uses. The greater stiffness of chromium-cobalt alloy is advantageous but at the same time offers disadvantages. Greater rigidity can be obtained with the chromium-cobalt alloy in reduced sections in which cross-arch stabilization is required, thereby eliminating an appreciable bulk of the framework. Its greater rigidity is also an advantage when the greatest undercut that can be found on an abutment tooth is in the nature of 0.005 inch. A gold retentive element would not be as efficient in retaining the restoration under such conditions as would the chromium-cobalt clasp arm.

A high yield strength and a low modulus of elasticity produce higher **flexibility.** The gold alloys are approximately twice as flexible as the chromium-cobalt alloys, which is a distinct advantage in the optimum location of retentive elements of the framework in many instances. The greater flexibility of the gold alloys usually permits location of the tips of retainer arms in the gingival third of the abutment tooth. As mentioned earlier, this problem, because of the stiffness of the chromium-cobalt alloys, can be overcome by including wrought-wire retentive elements in the framework.

The bulk of a retentive clasp arm for a removable partial denture is often reduced for greater flexibility when chromium-cobalt alloys are used as opposed to gold alloys. This, however, is inadvisable, since the grain size of the chromium-cobalt alloys is usually larger and is associated with a lower proportional limit, and so a decrease in the bulk of cast clasps increases the likelihood of fracture or permanent deformation. The retentive clasp arms for both alloys should be approximately the same size, but the depth of undercut used for retention must be reduced by one half when chromium-cobalt is the choice of alloys. Chromium-cobalt alloys are reported to work-harden more rapidly than gold alloys, and this, associated with coarse grain size, may lead to failure in service. When adjustments by bending are necessary, they must be executed with extreme caution and limited optimism.

Chromium-cobalt alloys have a lower **density** than gold alloys in comparable sections and are therefore about one half as heavy as the gold alloys. Weight of the alloy in most instances is not a valid criterion for selection of one metal over another, since after placement of a partial denture the patient seldom notices the weight of the restoration. The comparable lightness of the chromium-cobalt alloys, however, is an advantage when full palatal coverage is indicated for the bilateral distal extension denture. Weight is a factor that must be considered when the force of gravity must be overcome so that usually passive direct retainers will not be activated constantly to the detriment of abutment teeth.

The hardness of chromium-cobalt alloys offers a disadvantage when a component of the framework, such as a rest, is opposed by a natural tooth or one that has been restored. We have observed what is believed to be excessive wear of natural teeth opposed by some of the various chromium-cobalt alloys as contrasted to the Type IV gold alloys.

It has been observed that gold frameworks for removable partial dentures are more prone to produce uncomfortable galvanic shocks to abutment teeth restored with silver amalgam than frameworks made of chromium-cobalt alloy. This may not be a valid criterion for the selection of a particular alloy when the dentist has complete control over the choice of restorative materials. It may, however, be a consideration in some institutional dental services in which silver amalgam restorations must, of necessity, be placed rather than gold restorations.

Wrought wire: selection and quality control. Wrought-wire direct retainer arms may be attached to the restoration by embedding a portion of the wire in an acrylic resin denture base, by soldering to the fabricated framework, or by casting the framework to the wire. The physical (mechanical) properties of available wrought wires are most important considerations in selecting a proper wire for the desired method of attachment. These properties are yield strength or proportional limit, percentage elongation, tensile strength, and fusion temperature. After selection of the wire the procedures to which the wire is subjected in fabricating the restoration become critical in maintaining quality control for service, or putting it another way, improper laboratory procedures can diminish certain desirable physical properties of the wrought

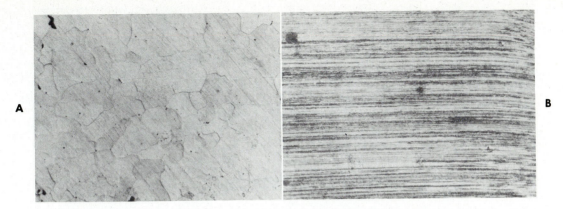

Fig. 11-26. A, Photomicrograph of Type IV gold alloy (×200). Grain structure appears in form of crystalline aggregate. **B,** Internal structure of gold wrought wire appears to be fibrous (×200). Original crystals have become entangled and elongated as result of being drawn from ingot.

structure so as to render it relatively useless for its intended purpose.

All alloys solidify in crystalline form when they cool from the molten state. The properties of wrought structures are different from cast structures in mechanical characteristics and in microstructure (Fig. 11-26). It is considered that many mechanical properties of the wrought structure are superior to those of the cast structure. Craig* has suggested that the tensile strength of the wrought structure is approximately 25% greater than that of the cast alloy from which it was made. The wrought structure's hardness and strength are also greater. This means that a wrought structure having a smaller cross-section than a cast structure may be used as a retainer arm (retentive) to perform the same function.

Craig has also suggested that a minimum yield strength of 60,000 psi is required for the retentive element of a direct retainer. A percentage elongation of less than 6% is indicative that a wrought wire may not be amenable to contouring without attendant undesirable changes in microstructure.

When wrought wire is heated, its physical properties and microstructure may be considerably altered depending on the temperature,

*Craig, R.G.: Restorative dental materials, ed. 6, St. Louis, 1980, The C.V. Mosby Co.

heating time, and cooling operation. In a cast-to process, wrought wire is subjected to a one-half hour heat-soaking period of burnout at 1250° F when a Type IV gold is used for the framework. When a low-fusing (2350° F) chromium-cobalt alloy (Ticonium) is selected for the framework, the burnout subjects the invested wire to a heat-soaking period of 2 hours at 1300° F. When wrought wire is soldered to frameworks by electric soldering, it is subjected to a momentary temperature of about 1500° F—of course depending on the solder used. The yield strength of both gold and base metal alloy (Ticonium) wrought wires can be drastically reduced simply by subjecting the wire to too much heat. If the heat is high enough and long enough, the fibrous microstructure of the wrought wire disappears and is replaced by a grain or crystalline microstructure. The process is known as recrystallization or grain growth and is a most undesirable occurrence in wrought-wire retainer arms (Fig. 11-27).

To avoid recrystallization of wrought wire, high fusing wires should be selected, and temperatures must be rigidly controlled when either using the cast-to or soldering methods. Each manufacturer of wrought forms for dental applications furnishes charts listing their products and the physical properties of each product. Two examples of such information are demonstrated in Fig. 11-28. The percentage of nobility metals

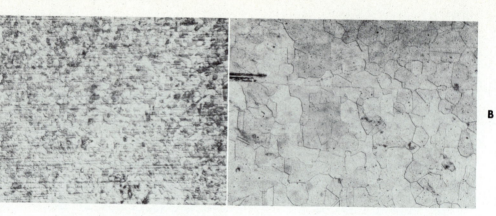

A   B

Fig. 11-27. A, Internal structure of gold wrought wire subjected to 1400° F for 1 hour (×200). Recrystallization has been initiated, although evidence of once fibrous structure of wire is still apparent. Useful strength (yield strength) of wire and other physical properties have been reduced because of recrystallization. **B,** Piece of wrought wire (from same specimen as in **A** and Fig. 11-24) subjected to 1500° F for 1 hour (×200). Grain growth has occurred, and useful physical properties of wire have been further reduced. Internal structure of this wire probably renders it unfit for adequate service as retentive portion of direct retainer assembly.

NEY WIRE PROPERTIES

ALLOY	Condition	Ultimate Tensile Strength Lbs/in.²	Kg/cm²	Proportional Limit Lbs/in.²	Kg/cm²	Elongation Percent 2 in. or 5.1 cm	Hardness BHN	HV	Fusion Temp. °F	°C	Density dwt./in.³	gm/cm³	Nobility Gold & Platinum Group Metals
ELASTIC #4*	S	117,500	8,260	86,500	6,080	15	190	215					
	H	173,000	12,160	131,000	9,170	7	270	305	1925	1050	164	15.6	79.5%
ELASTIC #12	S	125,000	8,790	88,000	6,190	20	175	200					
	H	178,000	12,510	135,000	9,490	15	275	310	2010	1150	127	12.1	61.0%
PALINEY #7**	S	120,000	8,440	89,000	6,260	24	180	205					
	H	180,000	12,650	148,000	10,400	9	280	315	1985	1085	125	11.9	55.0%
PALINEY #6**	S	110,000	7,730	63,500	4,460	24	150	170					
	H	170,000	11,950	127,000	8,930	15	270	305	1970	1075	115	10.9	45.0%
NEYLASTIC H.F.**	S	110,000	7,730	75,000	5,270	20	215	245					
	H	145,000	10,190	85,000	5,980	6	260	295	1830	1000	183	17.4	76.0%
GOLD COLOR ELASTIC*	S	120,000	8,440	73,000	5,130	14	200	225					
	H	165,000	11,600	135,000	9,490	1	290	330	1675	915	160	15.2	73.0%
DENTURE CLASP (GOLD COLOR)	S	100,000	7,030	52,000	3,660	22	160	180					
	H	157,000	11,040	122,000	8,580	1	265	300	1650	900	145	13.8	61.5%
PGP***		125,000	8,790	80,000	5,620	15	200	225	2790	1535	185	17.6	100%
P & I***		120,000	8,440	115,000	8,080	2	180	200	3250	1790	226	21.5	100%

* This product appears on The American Dental Association List of Certified Dental Material.
** This wire recommended for Crozat Technic.
*** This wire recommended for cast-to applications.

Fig. 11-28. Physical properties and nobility gold and platinum group metal content of various wires are furnished in chart form by manufacturers. Such information is necessary to select wrought wire for particular purpose and attachment method. (**A** courtesy J.M. Ney Company, Bloomfield, Conn.; **B,** courtesy J.F. Jelenko and Company, New Rochelle, N.Y.)

JELENKO GOLD WIRES		Solders Recommended	Hardness: Brinell D.P.H.	U. T. S. lbs./sq. in. (kg./cm.²)	% Elong. in 2 in. (5 cm.)	Yield Strength lbs./sq. in. (kg./cm.²)	No. of Cold Bends	Fusion Temperature (Approx.)
EXTRA HIGH FUSING (All Gold Alloys Can Be Cast To It, Including Jelenko "O")	† **NO. 12 WIRE** (Plat. Color)	Jelenko "O" Ortho Solder Can Be Used With All Others	Q 183 Q 200 H 204 H 225	88,500 (6,220) 103,000 (7,240)	11 9	66,500 (4,675) 70,000 (4,920)	6 5	2225°F. 1218°C.
HIGH FUSING (Can be Cast Against) For Clasps, Bars, Pins Including Jelenko "O"	**SUPER WIRE*** (Plat. Color)	Orthoflex H.F.	Q 200 Q 220 H 255 H 280	132,000 (9,280) 175,000 (12,303)	20 12	89,000 (6,260) 127,000 (8,930)	6.5 3.5	1845°F. 1007°C.
	THRIFT WIRE (Plat. Color)	Alboro H.F.	Q 200 Q 220 H 250 H 275	126,000 (8,860) 170,000 (11,950)	20 4	78,000 (5,485) 118,000 (8,295)	6.0 3.5	1890°F. 1032°C.
MEDIUM HIGH FUSING (Can Be Cast Against) For Clasps, Bars and Wrought Structures	**STANDARD WIRE** (Gold Color)	708 650 615	Q 165 Q 180 H 260 H 285	110,400 (7,760) 165,000 (11,600)	22 8	54,000 (3,795) 112,000 (7,875)	6.0 3.5	1735°F. 946°C.
MEDIUM FUSING (Not to be Cast Against) For Clasps, Bars and Dowels	**NO. 25 WIRE** (Gold Color)	650 615 585	Q 145 Q 160 H 230 H 250	93,200 (6,550) 147,000 (10,330)	26 9	53,000 (3,725) 112,000 (7,875)	6.0 3.5	1615°F. 879°C.
	NO. 2 WIRE (Gold Color)	650 615 585	Q 140 Q 155 H 250 H 275	95,000 (6,680) 155,000 (10,900)	27 5	48,000 (3,375) 110,000 (7,735)	5.0 1.5	1620°F. 882°C.
For PARALLEL PIN WORK	**PONTO WIRE** (Plat. Color)		230 250	136,000 (9,560)	20	105,000 (7,380)	5.5	2732°F. 1500°C.

† Hardens in a manner similar to Jelenko "O" Cast Gold. (After casting, slow cool from approximately 1800°F. (982°C.) in flask.) NOTE: Ponto wire is knurled. "Q" is quenched or softened and "H" is hardened. Heat treatment instructions included with each wire.

Jelenko Wires are immunized, Calor-Ohmically Heat Hardened, and furnished in straight 1 ft. (0.3m) lengths unless otherwise specified.

MADE IN THESE GAUGES
12 13 14 15 16 17 18 19 20 21 22 23 24 25 26

AVAILABLE IN THESE STYLES
Round Half Round Half Round "Bevelled"
Anterior Posterior Oval

Fig. 11-28, cont'd. For legend see opposite page.

is given. Additionally, most manufacturers designate those wires that may be cast-to.

ADA Specification No. 7 addresses itself to wrought gold wire both as to content and minimum physical properties. This specification recognizes two types of wire, namely a Type I (high precious metal alloy) and a Type II (low precious metal alloy). Table 11-2 compares the minimum mechanical properties. A knowledge of ADA Specification No. 7 and reference material furnished by dental manufacturers will enhance the proper selection of wrought wire for specific methods of attachment to the framework or removable restoration.

Our laboratory experiments involving soldering procedures and casting alloys to various gold alloy wrought wires under controlled conditions, indicate that gold wrought wires having a proportional limit of 70,000 psi in the semihardened condition, a fusion temperature above 1800° F, and a nobility gold and platinum group content of at least 61% are satisfactory for such operations. None of the wires tested having at least the above physical properties showed recrystallization in photomicrographs. All the gold wires, including the platinum, gold, and palladium type wire, were heat soaked for two hours at 1300° F in a refractory investment. The furnace in which this was carried out was accurately calibrated.

When a Type IV gold alloy was cast against the selected gold wrought wires and a PGP wrought wire, there was no evidence of recrystallization. A low-fusing chromium-cobalt alloy (Ticonium) was cast against the PGP wire without recrystallization occurring.

It was noted on examination of only heat-soaked invested wires that all wires appeared to be surface oxidized. Since such oxidation will likely prevent interface wetting of the wire and

cast alloy, mechanical retention of the wire in the cast framework should be provided. This can be accomplished simply by having the portion of the wrought wire embedded in the framework contoured to lie in two planes (Fig. 11-29).

Matching color gold solders may be used to solder wrought retainers to any type alloy framework by electric soldering. Recrystallization of gold wrought wires and PGP wire has been noted in specimens when a triple thick 19K gold solder with a melting temperature of 1675° F was used. However, a 650 fine gold solder with a melting temperature of 1420° to 1490° F produced no recrystallization of the wrought structures. Since color matching gold solders with a melting range of 1400 to 1500° F are available and can be used for soldering both gold alloys and gold to chromium-cobalt alloys and are entirely adequate for the job, it seems prudent to employ the lower-fusing solder.

Electric soldering is preferred to torch soldering to attach wrought wires to a framework because of the rapid localization of heat at the electrode. Triple thick, color-matching gold solder should be used. The additional bulk of triple thick solder will retard melting momentarily while the carbon electrode conducts heat to the area being soldered. Use of a flux is essential to prevent oxidation of the parts being joined and the solder itself. A borax type flux is recommended for soldering gold alloys to gold alloys. However, a fluoride type flux must be employed when chromium-cobalt alloys are soldered to alloys containing chromium. A fluoride type flux should also be used when a gold alloy is soldered to a chromium-cobalt alloy. Electric soldering for repair of removable partial dentures is described in Chapter 21.

Gold wrought wires are usually furnished in a semihardened condition by their manufacturer

Table 11-2. *Comparative specifications contained in ADA Specification No. 7*

	Type I	Type II
Content of metals of the gold, platinum group (minimum)	75%	65%
Minimum fusion temperature	1742° F	1898° F
Minimum yield point value (hardened or oven cooled)	125,000 psi	95,000 psi
Minimum elongation (hardened)	4%	2%
Minimum elongation (softened)	15%	15%

and may be safely contoured without annealing. Additionally the application of heat in the cast-to and soldering processes suggests that some annealing may occur. Therefore it is recommended that gold alloy wrought wires be given a hardening heat treatment after either being soldered or cast-to just before beginning final finishing procedures on the metal framework. A hardening heat treatment will increase the pro-

portional limit, tensile strength, and hardness of a wrought, cast-to or soldered gold wire. An acceptable hardening heat treatment for most gold alloys consists of placing the framework in a furnace at 840° F for about 5 minutes and then uniformly cooling the oven to 480° F in 30 minutes and immediately quenching the framework in water on removal from the furnace. It should be mentioned here that PGP wire and the base metal wrought wire (Ticonium) are not affected by the hardening heat treatment just mentioned.

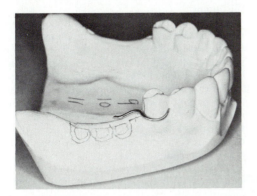

Fig. 11-29. Wrought-wire retainer arm has been contoured to design on duplicate stone cast of blocked-out master cast. It will be transferred to refractory cast and will become integral part of framework pattern and will be cast-to. Wire is contoured in two planes and will be mechanically retained in casting.

Regardless of the method of attaching the wrought wire retainer either by embedding, soldering, or cast-to, tapering the wrought arm seems most rational. A retainer arm is in essence a cantilever and can be made more serviceable and efficient by tapering. Tapering permits more uniform distribution of service stresses throughout the length of the arm, being readily demonstrated by photoelastic stress analysis. Uniform tapering of an 18-gauge, round wire arm can be accomplished, as illustrated in Fig. 11-30, before the retainer arm is contoured. The dimensions of the taper we prefer are illustrated in Fig. 11-31.

It should be mentioned here that our clinical experience with one base metal wrought wire suggests that it is applicable to the three differ-

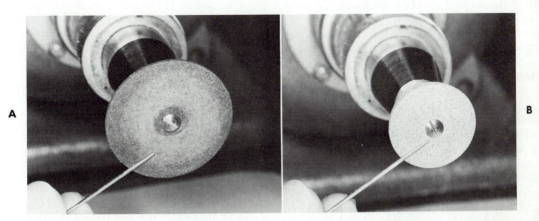

Fig. 11-30. A, Round, 18-gauge wrought wire is uniformly tapered to length of retainer arm contacting abutment. This is conveniently accomplished by rapidly spinning wire in angled contact with fast-running, abrasive cut-off disk in dental lathe. **B,** Tapered wire is polished by spinning wire in angled contact with fast-running, mildly abrasive rubber disk in dental lathe.

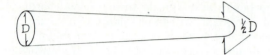

Fig. 11-31. Round, 18-gauge wrought wire for retentive component of direct retainer assembly (clasp) is uniformly tapered from its full diameter to one-half diameter at its terminus. Tapering should precede contouring wire for retainer arm.

ent methods of attaching wire retainers. This wrought wire is Ticonium 18-gauge round wire. Its composition consists primarily of cobalt, chrome, tungston, and nickel. Physical properties of the wire furnished by the manufacturers are tensile strength, 200,000 psi; yield strength, 133,000 psi; and percentage elongation, 19%.

Summary. In making a selection of materials it must be remembered that fundamentals do not change. These are inviolable. It is only methods, procedures, and substances—by which the dentist effects the best possible end result—that change. The responsibility of decision still rests with the dentist, who must **evaluate all factors** in relation to the **results** desired. In any instance therefore, the dentist must weigh the problems involved, compare and evaluate the characteristics of different potential materials, and then choose the road leading to the greatest possible service to the patient.

After the dentist makes a choice of alloys to be used in rendering a service to the patient, only those alloys that conform to the specifications set forth by the American Dental Association for the particular type of alloy should be prescribed.

It is to the lasting credit of those interested in biomaterials that continual research is being conducted to incorporate as many desirable characteristics in the chromium-cobalt alloys used in prosthodontics as possible. Efforts are being made to simplify casting procedures while obtaining greater accuracy and to make these alloys available to the profession at reasonable cost. There is little doubt in our minds but that a chromium-cobalt alloy will be developed, retaining the desirable characteristics that these alloys presently possess—plus many of the physical characteristics of Type IV gold alloys. Such an alloy could surely be made universally available to the dental profession and within the economy of all nations to use. Unfortunately this is not presently true of precious metal alloys.

SELF-ASSESSMENT AIDS

1. State in your own words the purpose of dental treatment.
2. Meaningful treatment of a patient embodies three fundamentally different processes. Can you name these processes in chronological order of accomplishment?
3. What are the objectives of a prosthodontic treatment for a partially edentulous patient?
4. Do you feel that ascertaining the past dental experiences of a patient you are treating for the first time would contribute to patient management?
5. Do you usually review the present health status of the patient before conducting an oral examination?
6. Diagnostic casts should be made before definitive treatment is undertaken. What two specific purposes would they serve?
7. It is not unusual for a patient to be primarily concerned with the cosmetic implications of a missing tooth. What are the obligations of the dentist to broaden the concern of total treatment?
8. A logical sequence of a thorough oral examination includes at least eight different procedures accomplished in order. Two of the eight procedures are a thorough prophylaxis and the placement of individual temporary restorations. Can you think of the other six factors?
9. For what reason should the definitive location of the inferior border of a mandibular major connector be ascertained as a part of an oral examination?
10. Rationalize the importance of the following areas that must be ascertained by radiographic interpretation:
    a. Quality of alveolar support of prospective abutment teeth
    b. Interpretation of relative bone density
    c. Increased width of the periodontal space
    d. Index areas
    e. Lamina dura
    f. Root morphology
    g. Unerupted third molars
11. What is a diagnostic cast?
12. Can you describe a diagnostic cast of a partially edentulous arch that may be considered a quality cast?
13. Diagnostic casts serve several purposes as aids in diagnosis and treatment planning. Can you think of six different uses for them?

14. Two sets of diagnostic casts (one a duplicate set) should be made for a patient requiring treatment. Why?

15. What can be gained from a study of accurately mounted diagnostic casts on a programmed, semiadjustable articulator?

16. The base of a diagnostic cast should be prepared in a certain way before any mounting on the articulator. Can you describe the preparation and tell why it is important?

17. What is a record base? An occlusion rim?

18. Are record bases usually necessary to correctly orient diagnostic casts of partially edentulous arches to an articulator? Why?

19. What four maxillomandibular records are necessary to orient casts to an arcon type articulator and to program the articulator?

20. What is meant by "proving the articulator," and how is it accomplished?

21. Can you name and describe the use of at least six different materials used for recording maxillomandibular relations?

22. In relation to occlusion, one of the earliest decisions to be made in diagnosis is whether to accept or reject the existing occlusion as demonstrated by the correctly oriented and articulated diagnostic casts. True or false?

23. Improvements in the natural occlusion must be accomplished before construction of the denture, not subsequent to it. True or false?

24. The decision-making process in planning the restoration of a partially edentulous mouth must include a differential diagnosis of fixed or removable restorations or a combination of both as a means of restoration. Usually, where indicated, a fixed restoration is preferred to a removable restoration. True or false?

25. What are the indications for the use of fixed restorations in (a) tooth-bounded edentulous regions, (b) posterior modification spaces, and (c) anterior modification spaces?

26. Although a removable partial denture should be considered as the means of treatment only when a fixed partial denture is contraindicated, there are several specific indications for the use of a removable restoration. Briefly discuss these indications related to (a) distal extension situations, (b) postextraction periods, (c) long tooth-bounded edentulous spans, (d) need for bilateral stabilization, (e) excessive loss of residual bone, (f) esthetics in the anterior region of the mouth, (g) abutments with guarded prognoses, and (h) economic considerations.

27. In many instances the dentist is confronted with the decision of treating the partially edentulous patient with removable partial dentures or complete dentures. Discuss the following factors that certainly have a bearing on the decision-making process: (a) economics, (b) patient preference or desires of patient, (c) age, (d) health, (e) present periodontal status, and (f) dental IQ or prospective IQ.

28. As a result of oral examination and diagnosis, certain data should be recorded, much of which is based on decisions that are the result of diagnosis, patient's attitudes, and economics. Some of these data are present and predictable health status, periodontal conditions present, oral hygiene habits, caries activity, need for extractions or surgery, need for fixed restorations, and need for orthodontic treatment. There are at least five more areas of treatment that should be recorded at this time. Can you think what they are?

29. Most frameworks for removable partial dentures today are made of some type of chromium-cobalt alloy rather than with an extra hard gold alloy. Four reasons are usually projected for this wide variation. What are they?

30. The choice of an alloy(s) is based on what factors?

31. Compare the physical properties of yield strength (proportional limit) and percentage elongation of chromium-cobalt alloy and partial denture gold alloy.

32. Which alloy is the stiffest in comparable sections—gold alloy or chromium-cobalt alloy? What are the advantages and disadvantages of comparable stiffness?

33. The retentive clasp arms for both chromium-cobalt and gold alloys should be dimensionally the same. Why or why not?

34. Many dentists prefer to use wrought-wire retentive arms in certain instances. Wrought wire may be attached to the denture by being cast-to, soldered, or embedded in the resin base. Does the method of attachment have a bearing on the selection of framework alloy and wrought wire? Why?

35. Excessive heat can alter the physical characteristics of any alloy. Discuss the precautions that must be taken in cast-to and soldering processes when wrought wire is used.

36. In the cast-to process using wrought wire, what phenomenon takes place that requires the portion of the wire covered by the casting alloy to be contoured in at least two planes for positive retention.

37. Discuss the choice of solders and soldering procedures for wrought wire.

38. How would you go about selecting a wrought wire for a specific application of the wire?

39. Why should certain alloys be given a hardening heat treatment? Can you describe a hardening heat treatment for alloys described as precious metal alloys?

40. A wrought wire consisting of only platinum, gold, and paladium (is) (is not) affected by a hardening heat treatment after being cast-to with a Type IV gold alloy.

41. There are inherent risks in the use of unilateral removable partial dentures. One is the risk of aspiration. What are some other risks?

42. Recent clinical research has contributed several significant developments to the management of compromised partially edentulous patients. Two of these developments are related to the field of implant prosthodontics. Name them?

12 PREPARATION OF MOUTH FOR REMOVABLE PARTIAL DENTURES

The preparation of the mouth is fundamental to a successful removable partial denture service. Thorough mouth preparation, perhaps more than any other single factor, contributes to the philosophy that the prescribed prosthesis must not only replace what is missing but, of perhaps even greater importance, must also preserve what is remaining.

Mouth preparation follows the preliminary diagnosis and the development of a tentative treatment plan. Final treatment planning may be deferred until the response to the preparatory procedures can be ascertained. In general, mouth preparation includes procedures in three categories: oral surgical preparation, periodontal preparation, and preparation of abutment teeth. The objectives of the procedures involved in all three areas are to return the mouth to optimum health and to eliminate any condition that would be detrimental to the success of the partial denture.

Naturally, mouth preparation must be accomplished before the impression procedures that will produce the master cast on which the denture will be constructed. Oral surgical and periodontal procedures should precede abutment tooth preparation and should be completed far enough in advance to allow for the necessary healing period. If at all possible, a period of **at least** 6 weeks, but preferably 3 months, should be provided between surgical and restorative dentistry procedures.

ORAL SURGICAL PREPARATION

As a rule, all surgical treatment for the removable partial denture patient should be completed as early as possible. By their very nature the surgical procedures generally indicated include the manipulation of both hard and soft tissues, which introduces the necessity for adequate healing time before the fabrication of the prosthesis. When possible, necessary endodontic surgery, periodontal surgery, and oral surgery should be planned so that they can be completed during the same time frame. The longer the interval between the surgery and the impression procedure, the more complete the healing and consequently the more stable the denture bearing area.

A variety of oral surgical techniques can prove beneficial to the clinician in preparing the patient for prosthetic replacements. However, it is not the purpose of this section to present the details of surgical correction. Rather, attention is called to some of the more common oral conditions or changes in which surgical intervention is indicated as an aid to denture design and construction and as an aid to the restoration's successful function in contributing further to the health and well-being of the patient. Additional information concerning the actual techniques employed is available in oral surgery texts and in articles of dental periodical literature. It is important to emphasize, however, that the dentist providing the partial denture treatment bears the responsibility for seeing that the necessary surgical procedures are accomplished. Measures to control apprehension, including the use of intravenous and inhalation agents, have made the most extensive surgery acceptable to patients. Whether the dentist chooses to perform these procedures himself or elects to refer the patient to someone else, perhaps more qualified, is immaterial. The important consideration is that the patient not be deprived of any treatment that would enhance the success of the partial denture.

Extractions. Planned extractions should occur early in the treatment regimen, but not before a careful and thorough evaluation of each remaining member of the dental arch is completed. Regardless of its condition, each tooth must be evaluated concerning its strategic importance and its potential contribution to the success of the removable partial denture. With the knowledge and technical capability available in dentistry today, **almost any tooth may be salvaged** if its retention is sufficiently important to warrant the procedures necessary. On the other hand, heroic attempts to salvage seriously involved teeth or those of doubtful nature whose retention would contribute little if anything, even if successfully treated and maintained, are contraindicated. The extraction of **nonstrategic** teeth that present complications or those whose presence may be detrimental to the design of the partial denture thus becomes not an admission of defeat but a valuable asset to treatment and an integral part of the overall treatment plan.

Removal of residual roots. Generally all retained roots or root fragments should be re-

moved. This is particularly true if they are in close proximity to the tissue surface or, of course, if there is evidence of associated pathology. Residual roots adjacent to abutment teeth may contribute to the progression of periodontal pockets and compromise the results to be expected from subsequent periodontal therapy. The removal of root tips can be accomplished from the facial or palatal surfaces without resulting in a reduction of alveolar ridge height or endangering adjacent teeth (Fig. 12-1).

Impacted teeth. All impacted teeth should be considered for removal. This applies equally to impactions in edentulous areas as well as to those adjacent to abutment teeth. The periodontal implications of the latter are similar to those for retained roots. These teeth are often neglected until there are serious periodontal implications.

The skeletal structure of the body changes with age. Alterations that affect the jaws frequently result in minute exposures of impacted teeth to the oral cavity via sinus tracts. Resultant infections cause much bone destruction and serious illness for persons who are elderly and not physically able to tolerate the debilitation. Early elective removal of impactions prevents later serious acute and chronic infection with extensive bone loss. Any impacted teeth that can be reached with a periodontal probe must be re-

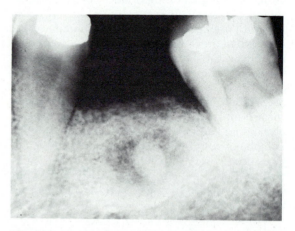

Fig. 12-1. Retained root with associated bone resorption. (From Costich, E.R., and White, R.P., Jr.: Fundamentals of oral surgery, Philadelphia, 1971, W.B. Saunders Co.)

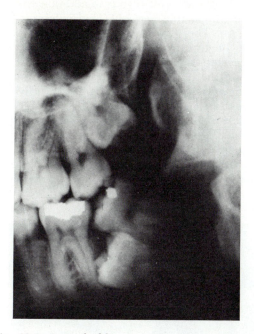

Fig. 12-2. Lateral oblique roentgenogram showing unerupted maxillary third molar and impacted mandibular second and third molars. Maxillary third molar and mandibular second molar could be contacted by periodontal probe. (From Costich, E.R., and White, R.P., Jr.: Fundamentals of oral surgery, Philadelphia, 1971, W.B. Saunders Co.)

moved to treat the periodontal pocket and prevent more extensive damage (Fig. 12-2).

Malposed teeth. The loss of individual teeth or groups of teeth may lead to supraeruption, mesial drifting, or combinations of malpositioning of remaining teeth. In most instances the alveolar bone supporting overly erupted teeth will be carried occlusally as the teeth continue to erupt, providing good support for the teeth that are out of harmony with the dental arches (Fig. 12-3, *A*). Orthodontics may be useful in correcting many occlusal discrepancies. But for some patients, such treatment may not be practical due to lack of teeth for anchorage of the orthodontic appliances or for other reasons. In such situations, individual teeth or groups of teeth and their supporting alveolar bone can be surgically repositioned. This type of surgery can be accomplished in an outpatient setting and should be given serious consideration before condemning additional teeth or compromising the design of removable partial dentures (Fig. 12-3, *B*).

Cysts and odontogenic tumors. Panoramic roentgenograms of the jaws are recommended to survey the jaws for unsuspected pathology. When a suspicious area appears on the survey film, a periapical radiograph should be taken to confirm or deny the presence of a lesion. All radiolucencies or radiopacities observed in the jaws should be investigated by biopsy. Although

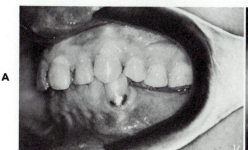 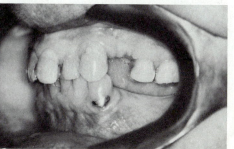

Fig. 12-3. A, Sequelae of unrestored partial edentulism. Maxillary premolars and first molar, unopposed for extended period, have moved inferiorly to such extent that little space remains between occlusal surfaces and mandibular residual ridge at vertical dimension of occlusion. **B,** Results obtained by surgically repositioning supraerupted teeth and supporting bone. Adequate space now exists between residual ridge and opposing teeth to construct removable partial denture without compromising occlusal harmony. Maxillary first premolar will be replaced with fixed partial denture.

the diagnosis may appear obvious from clinical and radiographic examinations, the dentist should confirm that diagnosis through submission of biopsy specimens to the pathologist for microscopic study. The patient should be assured of the diagnosis as well as the successful resolution of the abnormality as confirmed by the pathologist's report.

Exostoses and tori. The existence of abnormal bony enlargements should not be allowed to compromise the design of the removable partial denture. Although modification of denture design can, at times, accommodate for exostoses, more frequently this results in additional stress to the supporting elements and compromised function. The removal of exostoses and tori is not a complex procedure, and the advantages to be realized from such removal are great in contrast to the deleterious effects their continued presence can create (Fig. 12-4). Ordinarily the mucosa covering bony protuberances is extremely thin and friable. Partial denture components in proximity to this type of tissue may cause irritation and chronic ulceration. Also, exostoses approximating gingival margins may complicate the maintenance of periodontal

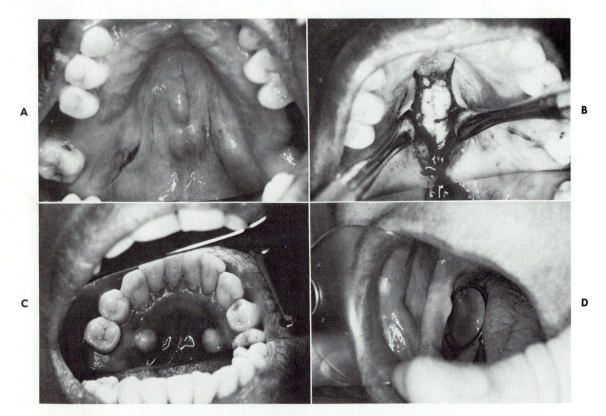

Fig. 12-4. A, Maxillary torus extending to junction of hard and soft palates. If torus is inoperable, its presence would require undersirable U-shaped palatal major connector for removable partial denture. **B,** Torus is exposed and readily visible and accessible for surgical removal. Design of major connector for removable restoration will not be compromised. **C,** Mandibular, lingual tori that should be surgically removed to avoid compromises in design of major connector for Class I removable partial denture. **D,** Sharp, mandibular lingual tuberosity. Removal of this bony projection should be accomplished 3 to 4 weeks before final impression procedures for removable partial denture. Patient comfort during impression procedures and later use of restoration are justifications for surgical removal of sharp bony projection.

health and lead to the eventual loss of strategic abutment teeth.

The air-turbine handpiece is ideal for removing bony irregularities and is much easier to control than a mallet and chisel. The lower speeds (20,000 to 50,000 rpm) provide more torque and thus a better sense of feel for what is being cut. All handpieces used in surgery should be vented outside the mouth to prevent the complication of emphysema. In addition, the assistant should provide copious irrigation to assure against thermal damage to the bone.

Hyperplastic tissue. Hyperplastic tissues are seen in the form of fibrous tuberosities, soft flabby ridges, folds of redundant tissue in the vestibule or floor of the mouth, and palatal papillomatosis (Fig. 12-5). All these forms of excess tissue should be removed to provide a firm base for the denture. This will produce a more stable denture and reduce stress and strain on the supporting teeth and tissues. The appropriate surgical approaches should not reduce vestibular depth. Hyperplastic tissue can be removed with any preferred combination of scalpel, curette, or electrosurgery. Some form of surgical stent should always be considered for these patients so that the period of healing will be more comfortable. An old denture modified properly can serve as a surgical stent. Although hyperplastic tissue has no great malignant propensity, all such excised tissue should be sent to an oral pathologist for microscopic study.

Muscle attachments and freni. As a result of the loss of alveolar bone height, muscle attachments may insert on or near the alveolar crest. The mylohyoid, buccinator, mentalis, and genioglossus muscles are those most likely to introduce problems of this nature. In addition to the problem of the attachments of the muscles themselves, the mentalis and genioglossus muscles occasionally produce bony protuberances at their attachments that may also interfere with denture design. Appropriate ridge extension procedures can reposition attachments and remove bony spines, which will enhance the comfort and function of the removable partial denture.

Repositioning of the mylohyoid muscle is successfully achieved by several methods. The genioglossus muscle is more difficult to reposition, but careful surgery can reduce the prominence of the genial tubercles, as well as provide some sulcus depth in the anterior lingual area.

Surgical procedures using skin or mucosal grafts have largely replaced secondary epithelialization procedures for the facial aspect of the mandible. Mucosal grafts using the palate as a donor site offer the best possibility for success; transplanted skin can be used when large areas must be grafted.

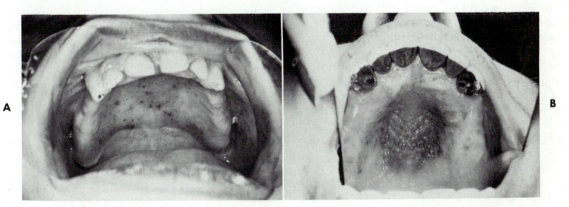

Fig. 12-5. A, Fibrous, unsupported maxillary tuberosities should be vertically reduced to provide supportive basal seat for denture. Stability and longevity of restoration will be enhanced by surgical procedures. **B,** Inflamed palatal papillary hyperplasia. Removal of palatal papillomatosis early in mouth preparation procedures is indicated so that complete healing can take place before final impressions are made in treatment of patient.

The maxillary labial and mandibular lingual freni are probably the most frequent sources of frenum interference with denture design. These can be modified easily with any of several surgical procedures. Under no circumstances should a frenum be allowed to compromise the design or comfort of a removable partial denture.

Bony spines and knife-edge ridges. Sharp bony spicules should be removed and knifelike crests gently rounded. These procedures should be carried out with minimum bone loss. If, however, the correction of a knife-edge alveolar crest results in insufficient ridge support for the denture base, the dentist should resort to vestibular deepening for correction of the deficiency or insertion of rib grafts.

Polyps, papilloma, and traumatic hemangiomas. All abnormal soft tissue lesions should be excised and submitted for pathologic examination before the fabrication of a removable partial denture. Even though the patient may relate a history of the condition's having been present for an indefinite period, its removal is indicated. New or additional stimulation to the area introduced by the prosthesis may produce discomfort or even malignant changes in the tumor.

Hyperkeratoses, erythroplasia, and ulcerations. All abnormal, white, red, or ulcerative lesions should be investigated, regardless of their relationship to the proposed denture base or framework. Incisional biopsy of areas larger than 5 mm should be completed, and if the lesions are large (over 2 cm in diameter), multiple biopsies should be taken. The biopsy report will determine whether the margins of the tissue to be excised can be wide or narrow. The lesions should be removed and healing accomplished before the denture is contructed. On occasion the denture design will have to be radically modified to avoid areas of possible sensitivity, such as after irradiation for malignancy or the excoriations of erosive lichen planus.

Dentofacial deformity. Patients with a dentofacial deformity often have multiple missing teeth as part of their problem. Correction of the jaw deformity can simplify the dental rehabilitation. Before specific problems with the dentition can be corrected, the patient's overall problem must be evaluated thoroughly. Several dentists (prosthodontist, oral surgeon, periodontist, orthodontist, general dentist) may play a role in the patient's treatment. These individuals must be involved in producing the diagnostic data base and in planning treatment for the patient. Information obtained from a general patient evaluation to determine the patient's health status, a clinical evaluation directed toward facial esthetics and the status of the teeth and oral soft tissue, and an analysis of appropriate diagnostic records produce a data base. From this data base the patient's problems can be enumerated, with the most severe problem being placed at the top of the list. Other identified problems would follow in the order of their severity. It is only after this step that input from several dentists can provide a final treatment plan for the patient.

Surgical correction of a jaw deformity can be made in horizontal, sagittal, or frontal planes. Mandibles and maxillae may be positioned anteriorly or posteriorly, and their relationship to the facial planes may be surgically altered to achieve improved appearance (Fig. 12-6). Replacement of missing teeth and development of a harmonious occlusion are almost always major problems in treating these patients.

Osseointegrated devices. A number of new surgical implant devices for the replacement of teeth have been introduced to the dental profession in recent years. One system that demonstrates some very interesting features is the osseointegrated devices of Brånemark and coworkers. The fixtures or endosteal implants are constructed from relatively pure titanium with precisely controlled geometry and surface finish (Fig. 12-7).

The fixtures are placed using very clean and controlled oral surgical procedures and are allowed to heal before surgical exposure and fabrication of a dental prosthesis.

In general, long-term (greater than 15 years) research and clinical programs have demonstrated very good results for the treatment of edentulous dental patients in Sweden. The published reports show highly acceptable success ratios with regard to dental applications.

This titanium implant was designed to provide a direct titanium-to-bone interface (osseointegrated), with the basic laboratory and clinical

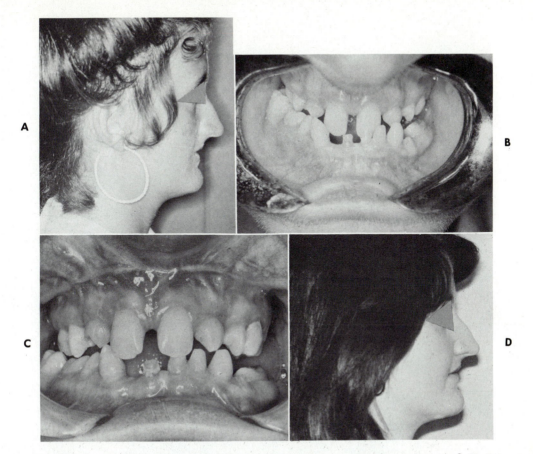

Fig. 12-6. A, Maxillary dental and skeletal deficiency leaves upper lip unsupported. **B,** Pretreatment dental relationships. **C,** Postsurgical relationship of opposing arches after maxillae were repositioned anteriorly and inferiorly. **D,** Profile of patient 3 years after surgery. Prosthodontic treatment consisted of both fixed and removable restorations. (Courtesy Dr. Raymond P. White, University of North Carolina, Chapel Hill, N.C.)

results supporting the value of this situation. This system, although quite demanding technically and quite intricate with respect to prosthetic designs, appears to offer a very promising future for restorative procedures using endosteal implants.

Augmentation of alveolar bone. Considerable laboratory documentation and successful clinical experience have been accomplished in the use of hydroxyapatite as a material for augmentation of deficient alveolar bone (Fig. 12-8). The hydroxyapatite implant materials display a lack of toxicity and demonstrate no inflammatory or foreign body responses.

There is evidence that in addition to providing increase in ridge width and height, the hydroxyapatite material provides a matrix for new bone formation. An additional advantage to the use of this material is its property of being nonresorbable. The hydroxyapatite materials found to be most successful in recent data are those that are nonporous and exhibit a polycrystalline ceramic structure that is fused into a nonporous state in a sintering process.

Clinical evidence suggests that in addition to providing direct bone augmentation, there appears to be the benefit of cessation of further bone resorption at the implant site.

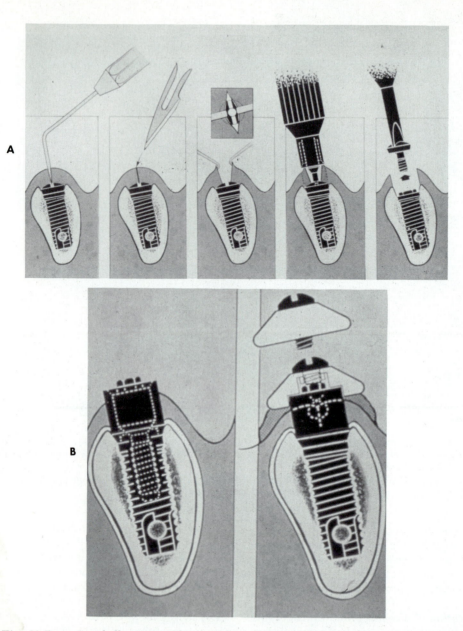

Fig. 12-7. A, Serial illustrations demonstrating location of osseointegrated implant after 6 months of healing and stabilization and removal of temporary obturating screw. **B,** Illustration of integrated post after healing and stabilization of post and placement of transfer stud used in addition of supragingival retainers that may be attached to implant. (Courtesy Dr. Tomas Albrektsson, The Institute for Applied Biotechnology, Gothenburg, Sweden.)

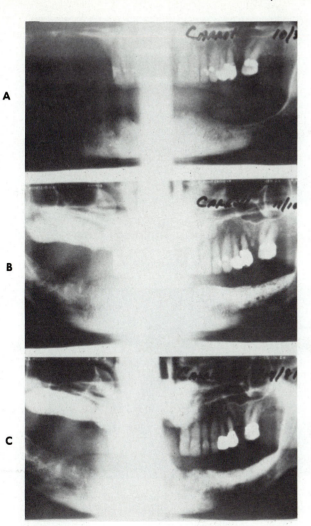

Fig. 12-8. Panoramic series of radiographs of ridge augmentation with hydroxyapatite implant material. **A,** Note excessive loss of alveolar bone in left maxilla and in right mandibular area before augmentation procedures. **B,** Postoperative radiograph of residual ridge augmentation with hydroxyapatite material. **C,** 1 year postaugmentation. Note improved height and volume of residual ridges at augmentation sites.

CONDITIONING OF ABUSED AND IRRITATED TISSUES

Many removable partial denture patients will require some conditioning of supporting tissues in edentulous areas before the final impression phase of treatment. Patients who require con-

ditioning treatment often demonstrate the following symptoms:

1. Inflammation and irritation of the mucosa covering the denture bearing areas
2. Distortion of normal anatomical structures such as incisive papillae, the rugae, and the retromolar pads
3. A burning sensation in residual ridge areas, the tongue, and the cheeks and lips (Fig. 12-9)

These conditions are usually associated with ill-fitting or poorly occluding removable partial dentures. However, nutritional deficiencies, endocrine imbalances, severe health problems (diabetes or blood dyscrasias), and bruxism must be considered in a differential diagnosis.

If a new removable partial denture or the relining of a present denture is attempted without first correcting these conditions, the chances for successful treatment will be compromised because the same old problems will be perpetuated. The patient must be made to realize that fabrication of a denture should be delayed until the oral tissues can be returned to a healthy state. If there are unresolved systemic problems, removable partial denture treatment will usually result in either failure or very limited success.

The first treatment procedure should be an immediate institution of a good home care program. A suggested home care program includes rinsing the mouth three times a day with a prescribed saline solution, massaging the residual ridge areas, palate, and tongue with a soft toothbrush, removing the prosthesis at night, and using a prescribed therapeutic multiple vitamin along with a prescribed high protein, low carbohydrate diet.

Some inflammatory oral conditions caused by ill-fitting dentures can be resolved by removing the dentures for extended periods of time. However, few patients are willing to undergo such inconveniences.

Use of tissue conditioning materials. The tissue conditioning materials are elastopolymers that continue to flow for an extended period, permitting distorted tissues to rebound and assume their normal form. These soft materials apparently have a soothing effect on irritated mucosa, and because they are soft, occlusal forces are probably more evenly distributed.

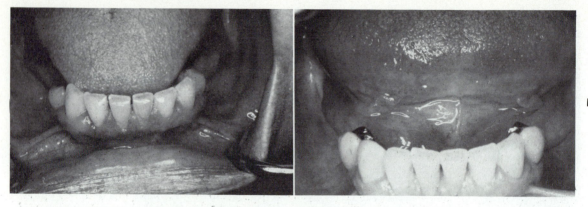

Fig. 12-9. **A,** Distorted and irritated tissue caused by ill-fitting removable partial denture. **B,** Tissues restored to health and retained teeth prepared to receive clasp-retained removable partial denture.

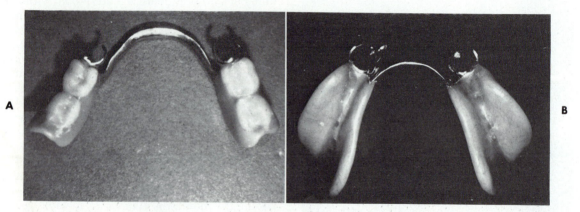

Fig. 12-10. **A,** Mandibular removable partial denture with underextended bases which contributed to tissue irritation. **B,** Denture bases properly extended to enhance support, stability, and retention.

Maximum benefit from using tissue conditioning materials may be obtained by: (1) eliminating deflective or interfering occlusal contacts of old dentures (by remounting on an articulator if necessary), (2) extending denture bases to proper form to enhance support, retention, and stability (Fig. 12-10), (3) relieving the tissue side of denture bases sufficiently (2 mm) to provide space for an even thickness and distribution of conditioning material, (4) applying the material in amounts just sufficient to provide support and a cushioning effect (Fig. 12-11), and (5) following the manufacturer's directions.

The conditioning procedure should be repeated until the supporting tissues display an undistorted and healthy appearance. Many dentists find that intervals of 3 to 4 days between changes of the conditioning material are clinically acceptable. An improvement in irritated and distorted tissues is usually noted within a few visits, and in some patients a dramatic improvement will be seen. Usually three or four changes of the conditioning material are adequate, but in some instances more changes are required.

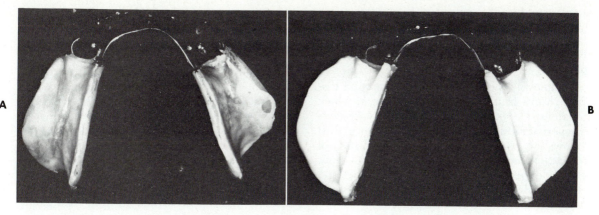

Fig. 12-11. **A,** Unsuccessful attempt to apply tissue conditioning material. Bases **incorrectly** relieved and conditioning material improperly applied. **B,** Tissue conditioning of sufficient thickness and distribution for effective treatment.

PERIODONTAL PREPARATION*

The periodontal preparation of the mouth usually follows, or is performed simultaneously with, the oral surgical procedures employed in the treatment of the conditions described in the previous discussion. Ordinarily tooth extraction and removal of impacted teeth or retained roots or fragments are accomplished before definitive periodontal therapy. The elimination of exostoses, tori, hyperplastic tissue, muscle attachments, and freni, on the other hand, can be incorporated with periodontal surgical techniques. In any situation, periodontal therapy should be completed before restorative dentistry procedures are begun for any dental patient. This is particularly true when a removable partial denture is contemplated because the ultimate success of this restoration depends directly on the health and integrity of the supporting structures of the remaining teeth. The periodontal health of the remaining teeth then, especially those to be used as abutment teeth, must be evaluated carefully by the dentist and corrective measures instituted before partial denture construction.

This discussion will attempt to demonstrate

how periodontal procedures affect diagnosis and treatment planning in a denture service rather than how the procedures are actually accomplished. For technical details the reader is referred to any of several excellent textbooks on periodontics.

Objectives of periodontal therapy

The overall objective of periodontal therapy is the return of health to the supporting and investing structures of the teeth so that the remaining dentition may be maintained in health, function, and comfort. The specific criteria by which the satisfaction of this objective is measured are as follows:

1. Removal of all etiologic factors responsible for periodontal changes
2. Elimination of all pathologic pockets with the establishment of gingival sulci free of inflammation
3. Restoration of a physiologic gingival and osseous architecture
4. Establishment of a harmonious, functional occlusion
5. Maintenance of the result achieved by oral physiotherapy procedures and periodic recall visits to the dentist

At the very least the dentist considering partial denture construction should be certain that these criteria have been satisfied before pro-

---

*Revision by Dr. Samuel B. Low, Department of Periodontics, College of Dentistry, University of Florida, Gainesville, Florida.

ceeding with impression procedures for the master cast.

Periodontal diagnosis and treatment planning

Diagnosis. The diagnosis of periodontal disease results from a **clinical** procedure in which the dentist systematically and carefully inspects the periodontium for deviations from normal. It follows the procurement of the health history of the patient and is performed using direct vision, palpation, periodontal probe, mouth mirror, and other auxiliary aids such as curved explorers, diagnostic casts, and roentgenograms.

In the diagnostic procedure nothing is so important as the careful exploration of the gingival sulcus with a suitably designed instrument—the periodontal probe (Fig. 12-12). Under no circumstances should partial denture construction begin without an accurate appraisal of sulcus

depth and health, as provided by the use of the probe. The probe is inserted gently but firmly between the gingival margin and the tooth surface, and the depth of the sulcus is explored circumferentially around each tooth. A critical assessment of sulcular health, by judging the amount of hemorrhage on probing, is considered more important than the depth itself, for it is the recognition of the inflammatory disease process which mainly concerns the clinician.

Dental roentgenograms are used to supplement the clinical examination but cannot be used as a substitute for it. The extent and pattern of bone loss can be estimated from roentgenograms, and this information serves to substantiate the impression gained from the clinical diagnosis.

Each tooth should be tested carefully for mobility (Fig. 12-13). The degree of mobility present, coupled with a determination of the etio-

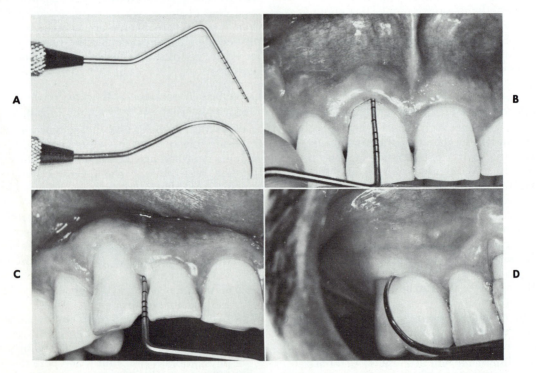

Fig. 12-12. A, Michigan-O periodontal probe graduated in millimeters (top) and Nabers furcation probe (bottom). **B,** Periodontal probe inserted parallel to long axis of tooth on labial surface. **C,** Periodontal probe inserted parallel to long axis of tooth interproximally. **D,** Furcation probe detecting buccal furcation involvement.

logic factor responsible, provides additional information, which is invaluable in planning for the removable partial denture. If the etiologic factor can be removed, many mobile teeth will become stable and can be used successfully to help support and retain the partial denture. Mobility is not in itself an indication for extraction unless the mobile tooth cannot aid in the stability of the partial denture. In general a tooth that is important to the design of the partial denture and has a mobility greater than 2 mm in a buccolingual direction requires immobilization via splinting.

Treatment planning. Depending on the extent and severity of the periodontal changes present, a variety of therapeutic procedures ranging from simple to relatively complex may be indicated. As was the case with the oral surgical procedures discussed, it is the responsibility of the dentist rendering the removable partial denture service to see that the required periodontal care is accomplished for the patient. Periodontal treatment planning can usually be divided into three phases. The first phase is considered disease control or initial therapy, for its objective is to essentially eliminate or reduce all the local etiologic factors and environmental influences before periodontal surgery and restorative dentistry. These procedures include oral hygiene instruction, scaling and planing (curettage), occlusal adjustment, and so forth.

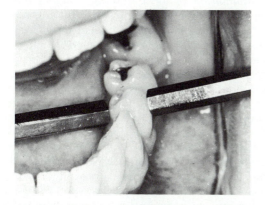

Fig. 12-13. Mobility can be visualized best when pressure is exerted on tooth through instrument handles. If fingers are used for this purpose, movement of soft tissue may mask accurate determination of mobility.

During the second phase, general therapy is administered as periodontal surgery and restorative dentistry. All procedures for maintaining periodontal health are provided in the third phase of therapy considered as the recall or maintenance phase.

Initial disease control therapy (phase 1)

Oral hygiene instruction. Ordinarily dental treatment should be introduced to the patient through instruction in a carefully devised oral hygiene regimen. The cooperation witnessed by the patient's acceptance and compliance with the prescribed procedure, as evidenced by improved oral hygiene, will provide the dentist with a valuable means of evaluating that patient's interest and the long-term prognosis of treatment.

For the oral physiotherapy routine to be successful, the patient must be motivated to follow the prescribed procedure regularly and conscientiously. The most effective motivation is based on the patient's understanding of dental disease and the benefits to be derived from the procedures advocated. Hence an explanation of dental disease, its etiology, initiation, and progression, is an important component of oral physiotherapy instruction. After this discussion the patient should be instructed in the use of disclosing wafers, soft nylon toothbrush, and unwaxed dental floss (Fig. 12-14). At subsequent appointments oral hygiene can be evaluated carefully, and further treatment should be withheld until a satisfactory level has been achieved (Fig. 12-15). This is a particularly critical point for the patient requiring extensive restorative dentistry or a removable partial denture. Without good oral hygiene any dental procedure, regardless of how well it is performed, is ultimately doomed to failure. The wise dentist insists that acceptable oral hygiene be demonstrated and maintained before embarking on an extensive restorative dentistry treatment plan.

Scaling and root planing. One of the most important services rendered to the patient is the removal of calculus and plaque deposits from the coronal and root surfaces of the teeth. Scaling and root planing comprise the definitive treatment for periodontal disease. Without meticulous calculus, plaque, and necrotic cementum

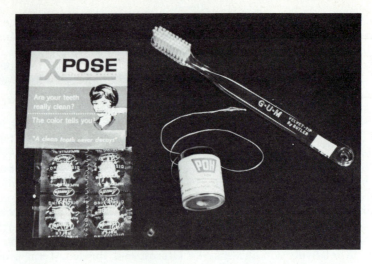

Fig. 12-14. Standard oral hygiene armamentarium prescribed includes disclosing wafers, soft nylon toothbrush, and unwaxed dental floss. Supplementary hygiene aids may be recommended for patients with special needs.

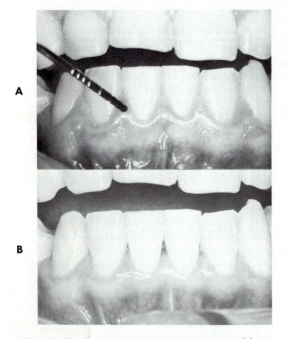

Fig. 12-15. A, Tissue response to poor oral hygiene procedures. Note bulbous papillae in interproximal areas of mandibular anterior teeth. **B,** Same patient shows favorable tissue response after 1 month of effective oral hygiene procedures only. Especially noticeable is reduction of inflamed and edematous interdental papillae.

removal no other form of periodontal therapy can be successful.

Although some of the new ultrasonic instruments may be helpful in calculus removal, hand instrumentation remains the treatment of choice for definitive debridement. The curette is the best designed hand instrument for scaling and root planing (Fig. 12-16). Thorough calculus removal precedes other forms of periodontal therapy that must be completed before impression procedures for the removable partial denture.

Elimination of local irritating factors other than calculus. Overhanging margins (of amalgam alloy and inlay restorations), overhanging crown margins, and open contacts leading to food impaction should be corrected before definitive prosthetic treatment is begun. Although periodontal health predisposes to a much better environment for restorative correction, it is not always possible to delay all restorative procedures until complete periodontal therapy and healing have occurred. This is especially true for patients with deep-seated carious lesions, for whom pulpal exposures are a possibility. Excavation of these areas and placement of adequate restorations must be incorporated early in treatment. Amalgam restorations are far superior to the cements in treating these patients, since the margins can be controlled and the possibility of

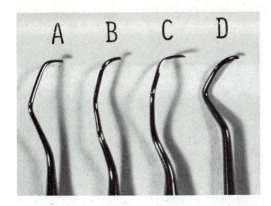

Fig. 12-16. Basic set of curettes for calculus removal and root planning. **A,** 3-4 Gracey for anterior teeth. **B,** 11-12 Gracey for mesial surfaces of posterior teeth. **C,** 13-14 Gracey for distal surfaces of posterior teeth. **D,** Columbia 4R-4L as universal instrument.

washouts is eliminated. The placement of temporary or treatment fillings must not, in itself, become a local etiologic factor.

Elimination of gross occlusal interferences. Oral accretions and poor restorative dentistry cause damage to the periodontium, as also may poor occlusal relationships. Although occlusal interferences may be eliminated by a variety of techniques, at this stage of treatment selective grinding is the procedure generally applied. Particular attention is directed to the occlusal relationships of mobile teeth. Traumatic cuspal interferences are removed by a judicious grinding procedure. An attempt is made to establish a positive centric occlusion that coincides with centric relation. Deflective contacts in the centric path of closure are removed, eliminating mandibular displacement from the closing pattern. After this the relationship of the teeth in the various excursive movements of the mandible is observed, with special attention to cuspal contact, wear, mobility, and radiographic changes in the periodontium. Interferences on both the working and nonworking sides should be observed and, if present, removed.

The mere presence of occlusal abnormalities, in the absence of demonstrable pathologic change associated with the occlusion, does not necessarily constitute an indication for the grinding procedure. The indication for occlusal adjustment is based on the presence of pathology rather than on a preconceived articular pattern. In the natural dentition the attempt to create bilateral balance, in the prosthetic sense, has no place in the occlusal adjustment procedure. Balanced occlusion not only is impossible to obtain on natural dentition but also is apparently unnecessary in view of its absence in most normal healthy mouths. Occlusion on natural teeth needs to be perfected only to a point at which cuspal interference within the patient's functional range of contact is eliminated and normal physiologic function can occur.

Guide to occlusal adjustment. Schuyler has provided the following guide to occlusal adjustment by selective grinding*:

In the study or evaluation of occlusal disharmony of the natural dentition, accurately mounted diagnostic casts are extremely helpful, if not essential, in determining static cusp to fossae contacts of opposing teeth and as a guide in the correction of occlusal anomalies in both centric and eccentric functional relations. Occlusion can be coordinated only by selective spot grinding. Ground tooth surfaces should be subsequently smoothed and polished.

1. A static coordinated occlusal contact of the maximum number of teeth when the mandible is in centric relation to the maxillae should be our first objective.

   a. A prematurely contacting cusp should be reduced only if the cusp point is in premature contact in both centric and eccentric relations. If a cusp point is in premature contact in the centric relation only, the opposing sulcus should be deepened.

   b. When anterior teeth are in premature contact in centric relation, or in both centric and eccentric relations, corrections should be made by grinding the incisal edge of the lower teeth. If premature contact occurs only in the eccentric relation, correction must be made by grinding the lingual incline of the upper teeth.

   c. Usually, premature contacts in the centric relation are relieved by grinding the buccal cusps of the lower teeth, the lingual

*Courtesy Dr. C. H. Schuyler, Montclair, N.J.

cusp of upper teeth, and the incisal edges of the lower anterior teeth. Deepening the sulcus of a posterior tooth or the lingual contact area in centric relation of an upper anterior tooth changes and increases the steepness of the eccentric guiding inclines of the tooth; although this relieves trauma in the centric relation, it may predispose the tooth to trauma in eccentric relations.

2. After establishing a static, even distribution of stress over the maximum number of teeth in the centric relation, we are ready to evaluate opposing tooth contact or lack of contact in eccentric functional relations. Our attention is directed first to balancing side contacts. In extreme cases of pathologic balancing contacts, relief may be needed even before the corrective procedures in the centric relation. Where balancing contacts exist, it is extremely difficult to differentiate the harmless from the destructive because we cannot visualize the influence of these fulcrum contacts on the functional movements of the condyle in the articular fossa. Subluxation, pain, lack of normal functional movement of the joint, or loss of alveolar support of the teeth involved may be evidence of excessive balancing contacts. Balancing side contacts receive less frictional wear than working side contacts, and premature contacts may develop progressively with wear. A reduction in the steepness of the guiding tooth inclines on the working side will increase the proximity of the teeth on the balancing side and may contribute to destructive prematurities. In all corrective grinding to relieve premature or excessive contacts in eccentric relations, care must be exercised to avoid the loss of a static supporting contact in the centric relation. This static support in centric relation may exist between the lower buccal cusp fitting into the central fossae of the upper tooth or between the upper lingual cusp fitting into the central fossae of the lower tooth or may exist in both cases. While both the upper lingual cusp and the lower buccal cusp may sometimes have a static centric contact in the sulcus of the opposing tooth, often only one of these cusps has this static contact. In such instances the contacting cusp must be left untouched to maintain this essential support in centric occlusion, and

all corrective grinding to relieve premature contacts in eccentric positions would be done on the opposing tooth inclines. The lower buccal cusp is in a static central contact in the upper sulcus more often than the upper lingual cusp is in a static contact in its opposing lower sulcus. Therefore corrective grinding to relieve premature balancing contacts is more often done on the upper lingual cusps.

3. To obtain maximum function and the distribution of functional stress in eccentric positions on the working side, necessary grinding must be done on the lingual surfaces of the upper anterior teeth. Corrective grinding on the posterior teeth at this time should always be done on the buccal cusp of the upper premolars and molars and on the lingual cusp of the lower premolars and molars. The grinding of lower buccal cusps or upper lingual cusps at this time would rob these cusps of their static contact in the opposing central sulci in centric relation.

4. Corrective grinding to relieve premature protrusive contacts of one or more anterior teeth should be accomplished by grinding the lingual surface of the upper anterior teeth. Anterior teeth should never be ground to bring the posterior teeth into contact in either protrusive position or on the balancing side. In the elimination of premature protrusive contacts of posterior teeth, neither the upper linqual cusps nor the lower buccal cusps should be ground. Corrective grinding should be done on the surface of the opposing teeth on which these cusps function in the eccentric position, leaving the centric contact undisturbed.

5. Any sharp edges left by grinding should be rounded off.

Temporary splinting. Teeth that are mobile at the time of the initial examination frequently present a diagnostic problem for the dentist. The response of those teeth to temporary immobilization may be helpful in establishing a prognosis for them and may lead to a rational decision as to whether they should be retained or sacrificed. Mobility due to the presence of an inflammatory lesion may be reversible if the disease process has not destroyed too much of the attachment apparatus. Mobility caused by occlusal interference also may disappear after selective grinding. In some cases, however, the teeth

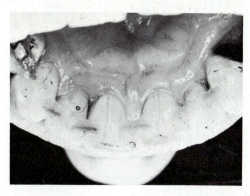

Fig. 12-17. A-splint used to stabilize mobile anterior segment. Markley pins embedded in plastic filling material in dovetail preparations on lingual surfaces. (Courtesy Dr. Daniel R. Trinler, Lexington, Ky.)

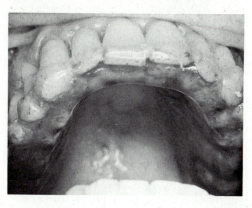

Fig. 12-18. Removable acrylic resin splint with flat occlusal plane can be used effectively as form of temporary stabilization and as means of eliminating excessive lateral forces created by clenching and grinding habits.

must be stabilized because of loss of supporting structure from the periodontal process.

Teeth may be immobilized during periodontal treatment by interdental wiring with acrylic resin splints, with cast removable splints, or with intracoronal attachments (Fig. 12-17). The latter, an example of which is the A-splint, necessitates cutting tooth surfaces and embedding a ridge connector between adjacent teeth.

After periodontal treatment, splinting may be accomplished with cast removable restorations or cast cemented restorations. The preferred form of permanent splinting is with two or more cast restorations soldered or cast together. They may be cemented with either permanent (zinc oxyphosphate or resin) cements or temporary (zinc oxide–eugenol) cements. A properly designed removable partial denture can also stabilize mobile teeth if provision for such immobilization is planned as the denture is designed.

Use of nightguard. The removable acrylic resin splint, originally designed as an aid in eliminating the deleterious effects of nocturnal clenching and grinding, has been used to advantage for the removable partial denture patient. The nightguard may be helpful as a form of temporary splinting if worn at night when the partial denture has been removed. The flat occlusal surface prevents the interdigitation of the teeth, which eliminates lateral occlusal forces (Fig. 12-18).

The nightguard is particularly useful before the fabrication of a partial denture when one of the abutment teeth has been unopposed for an extended period of time. The periodontium of a tooth without an antagonist undergoes deterioration characterized by a loss of orientation of periodontal ligament fibers, loss of supporting bone, and narrowing of the periodontal membrane space. If such a tooth is suddenly returned to full function when it is carrying an increased burden, pain and prolonged sensitivity may result. If, however, a nightguard is used to return some functional stimulation to the tooth, the periodontal changes are reversed and an uneventful course is experienced when the tooth is returned to full function.

Minor tooth movement. The increased use of orthodontic procedures in conjunction with restorative and prosthetic dentistry has contributed to the success of many restorations by altering the periodontal climate in which they are placed. Malposed teeth that were once doomed to extraction should be considered now for repositioning and retention. The additional stability provided for a removable partial denture from uprighting a tilted or drifted tooth may mean much in terms of comfort to the patient. The techniques employed are not difficult to master, and the rewards in terms of a better restorative dentistry service are great (Fig. 12-19).

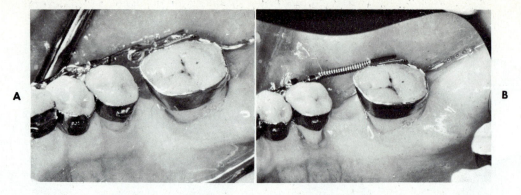

Fig. 12-19. Tooth movement used to upright tilted molar tooth to prepare the segment for receipt of pontic. **A,** Placement of orthodontic appliance. **B,** Space gained after 3 months' active movement.

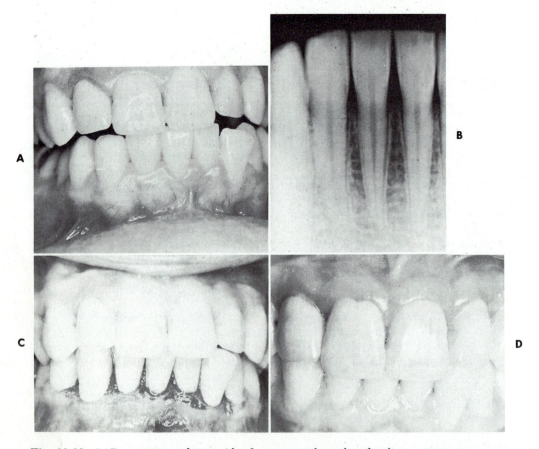

Fig. 12-20. A, Preoperative photograph of patient with pocket depth in anterior segment. Tissue is fibrotic, and pocket depth is confined within band of attached gingiva. **B,** Roentgenograph confirms clinical impression of minimal bone loss and acceptable bony topography. **C,** Immediate gingivectomy view of mandibular anterior segment. Frenectomy is included in operative procedure. **D,** Appearance of maxillary and mandibular anterior segments approximately 3 months after gingivectomy procedures.

General therapy (phase 2)

Periodontal surgery. After initial therapy subsides, the patient is reevaluated for the general treatment phase. If oral hygiene is at an optimum level, yet sulcular depth and inflammation have not resolved, then a variety of periodontal surgical techniques can be employed to advantage in satisfying the objectives of periodontal therapy for the removable partial denture patient. These are largely directed at the elimination of the periodontal pocket, the lesion pathognomonic of periodontal disease, and at a return of physiologic architecture to the area.

Pocket elimination may be achieved by shrinkage, surgical excision, and new attachment procedures. Of these, surgical excision presents the therapist with the most predictable result. Surgical procedures also afford the opportunity for recreating a physiologic architectural pattern, and hence much periodontal therapy is surgical in nature. However, one must keep in mind that elimination of the inflammatory disease process, not just sulcular depth, is the major objective of periodontal surgery.

Gingivectomy. This form of surgical therapy is one of the oldest excision-type procedures and is one that has been used widely for years. When the gingivectomy is indicated, it satisfies the objectives previously stated for periodontal therapy. However, as periodontics has experienced greater refinement in recent years and as the requirements for successful treatment have expanded, situations in which the gingivectomy alone will suffice have been greatly reduced to a minimum.

The gingivectomy is indicated when the following conditions are present (Fig. 12-20).

1. Suprabony pockets of fibrotic tissue
2. Absence of deformities in the underlying bony tissue
3. Pocket depth confined to the band of attached gingiva

If osseous deformities are present or if pocket depth traverses or approximates the mucogingival junction, the gingivectomy is *not* the procedure of choice. The gingivectomy technique is best accomplished with appropriate cutting instruments. However, gingivoplasty or reshaping of the gingiva can also be performed with electrosurgery and assorted diamond stones.

Because most patients with moderate to advanced periodontal disease have experienced various degrees of bone loss, the gingivectomy alone can rarely reestablish the desired physiologic architecture. For that reason more complex forms of treatment, including osseous and mucogingival surgery, have been developed as periodontics has entered an era of plastic and reconstructive surgery.

Periodontal flap. Today the apically repositioned flap is the periodontal surgical procedure of greatest versatility and, consequently, is widely applied in the treatment of periodontal disease (Fig. 12-21). Several healing studies have contributed to a greater understanding of periodontal therapy, and because of these, emphasis is currently placed on closure of the surgical area by various flap techniques.

Indications for the repositioned flap are as follows:

1. Pocket depth traversing the mucogingival junction
2. Presence of osseous deformities that must be corrected to eliminate the pocket and restore physiologic architecture
3. Muscle or frenum attachment at the gingival margin

Adjunctive procedures. In addition to the apically repositioned flap, other adjunctive mucogingival surgical techniques have added to the armamentarium of the therapist in eliminating periodontal disease and in the preparation of the mouth for restorative and prosthetic dentistry. Among these are lateral sliding flaps, pedicle grafts (Fig. 12-22), and free gingival grafts (Fig. 12-23). These procedures have particular application in the reestablishment of an adequate zone of attached gingiva around abutments for the removable partial denture and require at least 2 mm of attached gingiva to preserve gingival health.

Recall maintenance (phase 3)

Several longitudinal studies have now demonstrated the increasing importance of maintenance for all patients who have undergone any periodontal therapy. This not only includes reinforcement of plaque control measures, but also thorough debridement of all root surfaces of supragingival and subgingival calculus and plaque by the dentist or an auxiliary.

The frequency of recall appointments should

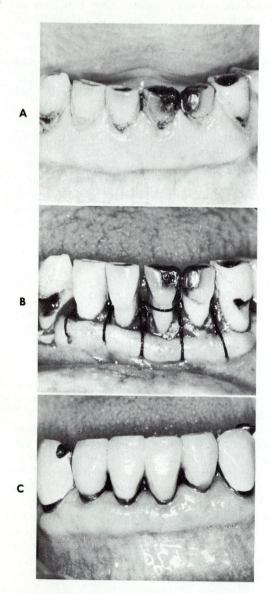

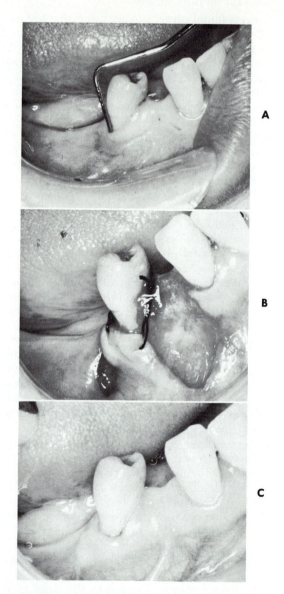

Fig. 12-21. A, Preoperative condition with pocket depth traversing mucogingival junction, osseous deformities and carious lesions extending beneath gingival margin. B, Gingival flap repositioned after osseous correction and crown-lengthening procedure on mandibular right canine tooth. C, Permanent splint with provision for removable partial denture. (Courtesy Dr. Keith Brooks, Lexington, Ky.)

Fig. 12-22. A, Preoperative view of mandibular second premolar with inadequate zone of attached gingiva and pocket depth traversing mucogingival junction. B, Pedicle graft sutured into position. C, Postoperative view showing new zone of attached gingiva with no pocket depth present.

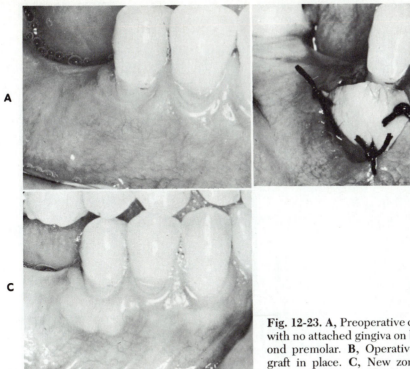

Fig. 12-23. A, Preoperative condition showing patient with no attached gingiva on buccal of mandibular second premolar. **B,** Operative site with free gingival graft in place. **C,** New zone of attached gingiva 9 weeks postoperatively.

be customized for the patient depending on susceptibility and severity of periodontal disease. It is now conceivable that patients with previous moderate to severe periodontitis should be placed on a 3- to 4-month recall system.

Advantages of periodontal therapy

Periodontal therapy before the fabrication of a removable prosthesis has several advantages. First, the elimination of periodontal disease removes a primary etiologic factor in tooth loss. The long-term success of dental treatment is dependent on the maintenance of the remaining oral structures, and periodontal health is mandatory if further loss is to be avoided. Second, a periodontium free of disease presents a much better environment for restorative correction. The elimination of periodontal pockets with the associated return of a physiologic architectural pattern establishes a normal gingival contour at a stable position on the tooth surface. Thus the optimum position for gingival margins of individual restorations can be established with accuracy. The coronal contours of these restorations also can be developed in correct relationships to the gingival margin, assuring the proper degree of protection and functional stimulation to the gingival tissues. Third, the response of strategic but questionable teeth to periodontal therapy provides an important opportunity for reevaluating their prognosis before the final decision is made to include (or exclude) them in the partial denture design. And last, the overall reaction of the patient to periodontal procedures provides the dentist with an excellent indication of the degree of cooperation to be expected in the future.

Even in the absence of periodontal disease, periodontal procedures may be an invaluable aid in partial denture construction. Through periodontal surgical techniques the environment of potential abutment teeth may be altered to the point of making an otherwise unacceptable tooth a most satisfactory retainer for a partial denture.

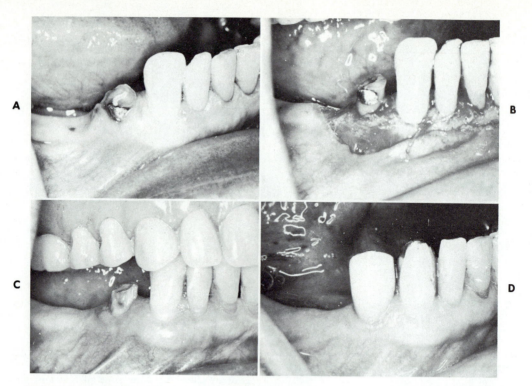

Fig. 12-24. A, Fractured first premolar tooth after endodontic therapy. **B,** Periodontal partial thickness flap retracted for access and apical repositioning of gingival margin. **C,** Appearance of tooth after healing and preparation to receive crown. **D,** Restoration in place, splinted to canine tooth, to act as abutment for removable partial denture.

The lengthening of a clinical crown through the removal of gingival tissue and bone is a common example of the application of periodontal surgical techniques as an aid in partial denture construction (Fig. 12-24).

ABUTMENT TEETH

Abutment restorations. Equipped with the diagnostic casts on which a tentative partial denture design has been drawn, the dentist is able to accomplish preparation of abutment teeth with accuracy. The information at hand should include the proposed path of placement, the areas of teeth to be altered and tooth contours to be changed, and the location of rest seats (Fig. 11-5).

During examination and subsequent treatment planning, in conjunction with a survey of diagnostic casts, each abutment tooth is considered individually as to whether full coverage is indicated. Abutment teeth presenting sound enamel surfaces in a mouth in which good oral hygiene habits are evident may be considered a fair risk for use as partial denture abutments. One should not be misled, however, by a patient's promise to do better as far as oral hygiene habits are concerned. **Good or bad oral hygiene is a habit of long standing and is not likely to be changed appreciably because a partial denture is being worn.** Therefore one must be conservative in evaluating the oral hygiene habits of the patient in the future. It is well to remember that **clasps as such do not cause teeth to decay,** and if the individual will keep the teeth and the partial denture clean, one need not condemn clasps from a cariogenic standpoint. On the other hand, more partial dentures have been condemned as cariogenic because the dentist did not provide for the protection of abutment teeth than because of inadequate care on the part of the patient.

The full cast gold crown is objectionable from an esthetic standpoint, and therefore the veneer type of full crown must be used when a canine or premolar abutment is to be restored or protected. Less frequently does the molar have to be treated in such a manner, and except for maxillary first molars the full gold crown is usually acceptable.

When there is proximal caries on abutment teeth with sound buccal and lingual enamel surfaces, in a mouth exhibiting average oral hygiene and low caries activity, a gold inlay is usually indicated. However, silver amalgam for the restoration of those teeth with proximal caries should not be condemned, although one must admit that an inlay cast of a hard-type gold will provide the best possible support for occlusal rests, at the same time giving an esthetically pleasing restoration. But an amalgam restoration, properly condensed, is capable of supporting an occlusal rest without appreciable flow over a long period of time.

The most vulnerable area on the abutment tooth is the proximal gingival area, which lies beneath the minor connector of the partial denture framework and is therefore subject to the lodgment of debris in an area most susceptible to caries attack. Even when the partial denture is removed for cleaning the teeth, these areas, especially those on the distal surface of an anterior abutment, are often missed by the toothbrush, and bacterial plaque and debris are allowed to remain for long periods of time. Except in a caries-immune mouth or in a mouth in which the teeth are subjected to meticulous brushing, decalcification and caries frequently occur in this region. It is therefore necessary that this area of the tooth be fully protected by whatever restoration is used. When an inlay restoration is used, the preparation should be carried to or beneath the gingival margin and well out onto the buccal and lingual surfaces to afford the best possible protection to the abutment tooth. Even the full crown can be deficient in this most vulnerable area, which lies at and just above the

gingival margin. The full crown, which is cast short of this area, will not afford protection where it is most needed.

All proximal abutment surfaces that are to serve as guiding planes for the partial denture should be prepared so that they will be made as nearly parallel as possible to the path of placement. Preparations may include modifying the contour of existing ceramic restorations, if necessary. This may be accomplished with abrasive stones or diamond finishing stones. A polished surface for the altered ceramic restoration may be restored by using any of several polishing kits supplied by manufacturers.

Contouring wax patterns. Modern indirect techniques using hydrocolloid or rubber base impression materials permit the contouring of wax patterns on the stone abutments with the aid of the surveyor blade. All abutment teeth to be restored with castings can be prepared at one time and an impression made that will provide an accurate stone replica of the prepared arch. Wax patterns may then be refined on separated individual dies or removable dies. All abutment surfaces facing edentulous areas should be made parallel to the path of placement by the use of the surveyor blade. This will provide proximal surfaces that will be parallel without any further alteration in the mouth, will permit the most positive seating of the partial denture along the path of placement, and will provide the least amount of undesirable space beneath minor connectors for the lodgment of debris.

Rest seats. After the proximal surfaces of the wax patterns have been made parallel and buccal and lingual contours have been established, which will satisfy the requirements of retention with the best possible esthetic placement of clasp arms, the occlusal rest seats should be prepared in the wax pattern rather than in the finished gold restoration. The placement of occlusal rests should be considered at the time the teeth are prepared to receive cast restorations so that there will be sufficient clearance beneath the floor of the occlusal rest seat. **Too many times we see a completed gold restoration cemented in the mouth for a partial denture abutment without any provision for the occlusal rest having been made in the wax pattern.** The dentist then proceeds to cut an occlusal rest seat in the gold restoration, being ever conscious of the fact that he may perforate the gold during the process of forming the rest seat. The unfortunate result is usually a **poorly** formed rest seat that is too shallow.

If tooth structure has been removed to provide for the placement of the occlusal rest seat, it may be ideally placed in the wax pattern by using a No. 8 round bur to lower the marginal ridge and to establish the outline form of the rest and then using a No. 6 round bur to deepen slightly the floor of the rest seat inside this lowered marginal ridge. This provides for an occlusal rest that best satisfies the requirements that the rest be placed so that any occlusal force will be directed axially and that there will be the least possible interference to occlusion with the opposing teeth.

Perhaps the most important function of a rest is the division of stress loads to the partial denture to provide for greatest efficiency with the least damaging effect to the abutment teeth. For a distal extension partial denture the rest must be able to transmit occlusal forces to the abutment teeth in a vertical direction only, thereby permitting the least possible lateral stresses to be transmitted to the abutment teeth.

For this reason the floor of the rest seat should incline toward the center of the tooth so that the occlusal forces, insofar as possible, are centered over the root apex. Any other form but that of a spoon shape permits a locking of the occlusal rest and the transmission of tipping forces to the abutment tooth. A ball-and-socket type of relationship between occlusal rest and abutment tooth is the most desirable. At the same time, the marginal ridge must be lowered so that the angle formed by the occlusal rest with the minor connector will stand above the occlusal surface of the abutment tooth as little as possible and avoid interference with the opposing teeth. Simultaneously, sufficient bulk must be provided to prevent a weakness in the occlusal rest at the marginal ridge. The marginal ridge must be lowered and yet not be the deepest part of the rest preparation. To permit occlusal stresses to be directed toward the center of the abutment tooth, the angle formed by the floor of the occlusal rest with the minor connector should be less than 90 degrees. In other words, the floor of the occlusal rest should incline slightly from the lowered marginal ridge toward the center of the tooth.

This proper form can be readily accomplished in the wax pattern if care is taken during crown or inlay preparation to provide for the location of the rest. If an amalgam restoration is used, sufficient bulk must be present in this area to allow proper occlusal rest seat form without weakening the restoration. When the rest seat is placed in sound enamel, it is best accomplished by the use of round diamond points of approximately No. 4, 6, and 8 sizes in the following sequence. First the larger of the diamonds is used to lower the marginal ridge and at the same time create the relative outline form of the rest seat. The result is a rest seat preparation with marginal ridge lowered and gross outline form established but without sufficient deepening of the rest seat preparation toward the center of the tooth. The smaller diamond points or a carbide bur of approximately No. 4 or 6 size may then be used to deepen the floor of the rest seat to a gradual incline toward the center of the tooth. Enamel rods are then smoothed by the planing action of a round bur revolving with little pressure. Abrasive rubber points, followed by the use of wet flour of pumice on a stiff bristle brush, are sufficient to complete the polishing of the rest seat preparation.

Rest seat preparations in existing restorations or on abutment teeth where no restorations are to be placed should always follow, not precede, the recontouring of proximal tooth surfaces. The preparation of proximal tooth surfaces should be done first because if the occlusal portion of the rest seat is placed first and the proximal tooth surface is altered later, the outline form of the rest seat is sometimes irreparably altered.

The success or failure of a removable partial denture may well depend on how well the mouth preparations were accomplished. It is only through intelligent planning and competent execution of mouth preparations that the denture can satisfactorily restore lost dental functions and contribute to the health of the remaining oral tissues.

SELF-ASSESSMENT AIDS

1. A prescribed prosthesis not only must replace what is missing but also, of even greater importance, must _____ what is remaining.

2. Preparation of oral structures most often involves three categories. One of these categories is oral surgical preparation. What are the other two?
3. Which treatment should be accomplished first— oral surgery or preparation of abutment teeth? Why?
4. Generally all retained roots or root fragments should be removed as a mouth preparation procedure. True or false?
5. All impacted teeth should be considered for removal. However, any impacted tooth that can be reached with a periodontal probe must be removed. True or false?
6. Unapposed posterior teeth quite often overly erupt, severely limiting space for a prosthesis and the opportunity to create a harmonious occlusion. Name different methods by which these discrepancies may be corrected, depending of course on the severity of the malpositions.
7. You are viewing a panoramic radiograph of a patient and you see a suspicious radiopaque area. What procedures, listed in chronologic order, would you undertake to resolve the possible problem?
8. Visual examination, carefully conducted, reveals undesirable bony exostoses or tori in some patients. Unless these are removed, the design of the restoration will be compromised. In what areas are these various protuberances likely to be found?
9. Why should hyperplastic tissues seen in the form of fibrous tuberosities, flabby ridges, folds of redundant tissue in vestibular regions, and palatal papillomatosis be surgically removed before the construction of a removable restoration?
10. Discuss the influence of muscle attachments and freni that are inserted on the crest of residual ridges in relation to denture stability.
11. Should all abnormal soft tissue lesions be excised and submitted for pathologic examination before fabrication of a removable restoration?
12. Excessively resorbed residual ridges offer comparatively poor support for removable restorations. Augmentation of alveolar bone to increase ridge height and width is a viable surgical procedure for certain patients. Can you name a material used for such a procedure?
13. What is meant by an "oral osseointegrated device"? What role do you envision for such devices in removable prosthodontics?
14. What are elastopolymers used for in removable prosthodontics?
15. Do you feel that irritated and distorted oral tissues must optimally be returned to a state of health before final impressions are made? Why or why not?
16. Your examination of a patient having removable partial dentures discloses a palatal inflammation. Can you be certain that the inflammation was caused solely by the dentures? What other factors must be considered in a thorough differential diagnosis?
17. Abused and irritated oral tissues most often respond favorably to tissue conditioning procedures. Can you describe an acceptable order of procedures to be undertaken to institute a good tissue conditioning program?
18. Periodontal therapy should be completed before restorative procedures are undertaken. True or false?
19. What is the overall objective of periodontal therapy for the partially edentulous patient?
20. The indication for occlusal adjustment is based on the presence of pathology rather than on a preconceived articular pattern. Can you support and explain this statement?
21. What procedure(s) is most often used to eliminate gross occlusal interferences initially as a phase of periodontal considerations?
22. What is a nightguard and what purpose does it serve?
23. Teeth that demonstrate mobility at the time of the initial examination may be temporarily splinted. How does this help to establish a prognosis?
24. Under what clinical circumstances should minor tooth movement by orthodontic means be considered to enhance treatment?
25. Can you give at least four distinct advantages of performing periodontal therapy (when indicated) before fabricating a removable prosthesis?
26. It is only through intelligent planning and competent execution of mouth preparations that the denture can satisfactorily restore lost dental functions and contribute to health of the remaining oral tissues. True or false?

13 PREPARATION OF ABUTMENT TEETH

Classification of abutment teeth
Sequence of abutment preparations on sound
    enamel or existing restorations
Abutment preparations using conservative cast
    restorations
Abutment preparations using cast crowns
Splinting of abutment teeth

Use of isolated teeth as abutments
Missing anterior teeth
Temporary crowns when a partial denture is
    being worn
The making of crowns and inlays to fit existing
    denture retainers

After surgery, periodontal treatment, and any endodontic treatment of the arch involved, the abutment teeth may be prepared to provide support, stabilization, reciprocation, and retention for the partial denture. **Rarely is the situation encountered where alteration of an abutment is not indicated.**

Endodontic treatment of any teeth elsewhere in the arch, as well as abutment teeth, should precede the making of the partial denture, so that the success of treatment can be reasonably well established before proceeding. Similarly, favorable response to any deep restorations and the results of periodontal treatment should be established before construction of the denture, since if the prognosis of a tooth under treatment becomes unfavorable, its loss can be compensated for by a change in the denture design. The condemned tooth or teeth may then be included in the original denture design, whereas if they are lost subsequently, the partial denture must be added to, remade, or replaced. **Many partial denture designs do not lend themselves well to later additions, although this eventuality should be considered in the design of a denture.**

Particularly when the tooth in question will be used as an abutment, every diagnostic aid should be used to determine the success of previous treatment. It is usually not so difficult to add a tooth or teeth to a partial denture as it is to add a retaining unit when the original abutment is lost and the next adjacent tooth must be used for that purpose.

It is sometimes possible to design a removable partial denture so that a single posterior abutment about which there is some doubt can be retained and used as one end of a tooth-supported base. Then, if that posterior abutment were to be lost, it can be replaced with a distal extension base (Fig. 11-24). Such a design must include provision for future indirect retention, flexible clasping on the future terminal abutment, and provision for establishing tissue support by a secondary impression. Anterior abutments, which are considered to be poor risks, may not be so freely used because of the problems involved in adding a new abutment retainer when the original one is lost. It is rational that such questionable teeth be condemned in favor of a better abutment, even though the original treatment plan must be modified accordingly.

CLASSIFICATION OF ABUTMENT TEETH

The subject of abutment preparations may be grouped as follows: (1) those abutment teeth requiring only minor modifications to their coronal portions, (2) those that are to have cast inlays, and (3) those that are to have cast crowns. The latter group includes abutments for fixed partial dentures, since inlay retainers are not commonly used for such restorations.

Abutment teeth requiring only minor modifications include teeth with sound enamel, those having small restorations not involved in the denture design, those having acceptable restorations that will be involved in the denture design, and those having existing crown restorations. The latter may exist either as an individual crown or as the abutment of a fixed restoration.

The use of unprotected abutments has been discussed previously. Although complete coverage of all abutments may be desirable, it is not always possible or practical to do so. The decision to use unprotected abutments involves certain risks of which the patient must be advised, including his own responsibility for maintaining oral hygiene and caries control. The making of crown restorations to fit existing denture clasps is an art in itself, which will be covered later in this chapter, but the fact that it is possible to do so may influence the decision to use uncrowned but otherwise sound teeth as abutments.

Preferably, silver amalgam alloy should not be used for the support of occlusal rests because of its tendency to flow. Although cast gold will provide the best possible support for occlusal rests, an amalgam alloy restoration, properly condensed, is capable of supporting an occlusal rest without appreciable flow over a long period of time. If the patient's economic status or other factors beyond the control of the dentist prevent the use of cast restorations, any existing silver amalgam alloy fillings about which there is any doubt should be replaced with new amalgam restorations. This should be done before the preparation of guiding planes and occlusal rest seats to permit aging and polishing of the restoration.

SEQUENCE OF ABUTMENT PREPARATIONS ON SOUND ENAMEL OR EXISTING RESTORATIONS

Abutment preparations on either sound enamel or existing restorations should be done in the following order:

1. Proximal surfaces parallel to the path of placement should be prepared to provide guiding planes (Fig. 13-1, *A*).

2. Excessive tooth contours should be reduced (Fig. 13-1, *B* and *C*), thereby lowering the height of contour so that (a) the origin of circumferential clasp arms may be placed well below the occlusal surface, preferably at the junction of the gingival and middle thirds; (b) retentive clasp terminals may be placed in the

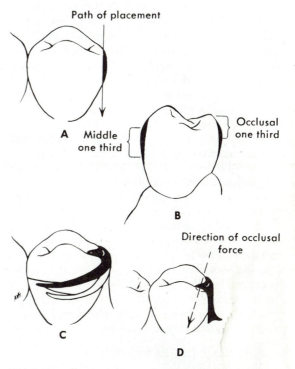

Fig. 13-1. Abutment contours should be altered during mouth preparations in following sequence. **A,** Proximal surface is prepared parallel to path of placement to create guiding plane. **B,** Height of contour on buccal and lingual surfaces is lowered when necessary to permit retentive clasp terminus to be located within gingival third of crown and reciprocal clasp arm on opposite side of tooth to be placed no higher than cervical portion of middle third of crown. **C,** Area of tooth at which retentive clasp arm originates should be altered if necessary to permit more direct approach to gingival third of tooth. **D,** Occlusal rest preparation that will direct occlusal forces along long axis of tooth should be final step in mouth preparations.

gingival third of the crown, for better esthetics and better mechanical advantage; and (c) reciprocal clasp arms may be placed on and above a height of contour that is no higher than the cervical portion of the middle third of the crown of the abutment tooth.

3. **After alterations of axial contours are believed accomplished and before rest seat preparations are instituted, an impression of the arch should be made in irreversible hydrocolloid and a cast poured in a fast-setting stone. This cast can be returned to the surveyor to determine the adequacy of axial alterations before proceeding with rest seat preparations. If axial surfaces require additional axial recontouring, it can be performed during the same appointment and without compromise.**

4. Occlusal rest areas that will direct occlusal forces along the long axis of the abutment tooth should be prepared (Fig. 13-1, *D*).

Mouth preparation should follow a plan that was outlined on the diagnostic cast in red pencil at the time the cast was surveyed and should also follow the design of the partial denture outlined. Better still, proposed changes to abutment teeth actually may be made on the diagnostic cast and **outlined** in red pencil to indicate not only the area but also the **amount** and **angulation** of the modification to be done (Chapter 11). Although occlusal rest seats also may be prepared on the diagnostic cast, indication of their **location** in red pencil is usually sufficient for the experienced dentist, since rest preparations follow a definite pattern (Chapter 5).

ABUTMENT PREPARATIONS USING CONSERVATIVE CAST RESTORATIONS

Each abutment restoration is unique and has to be planned with consideration for the existing circumstances of each patient. Inlay preparations on teeth to be used as removable partial denture abutments differ from conventional inlay preparations in the amount of protection afforded the tooth, the width of the preparation at the occlusal rest, and the depth of the preparation beneath the occlusal rest.

Conventional inlay preparations are permissible on the proximal surface of the tooth not to be contacted by a minor connector of the partial denture. On the other hand, proximal and oc-

clusal surfaces supporting minor connectors and occlusal rests require somewhat different treatment than the conventional inlay preparation. The extent of occlusal coverage (that is, whether or not cusps are capped) will be governed by the usual factors, such as the extent of caries, the presence of unsupported enamel walls, and the extent of occlusal abrasion and attrition.

A primary consideration in the preparation of proximal inlays that will lie beneath minor connectors is the amount of protection afforded vulnerable areas by the inlay. The most vulnerable area on the abutment tooth is the proximal gingival area lying beneath the minor connector of the partial denture because of accumulation of debris and difficulty in keeping the area clean.

Except in a caries-immune mouth or in a mouth in which the teeth are kept meticulously clean, some decalcification and caries attack in this region is inevitable. Even the most conscientious toothbrushing may miss the distal surfaces of abutments because they cannot be seen. It is always important that the patient be instructed, with casts and before a mirror, in the significance of brushing these areas and the correct use of dental floss.

It is necessary that these areas be fully protected by the cast restoration, whether it be an inlay or a partial or full crown. Even the full crown can be deficient in this most vulnerable area, which lies at or just above the gingival margin. A full crown that is short or becomes short because of gingival recession does not afford protection where it is most needed.

When an inlay is the restoration of choice for an abutment tooth, certain modifications of the outline form are necessary. To prevent the buccal and lingual proximal margins from lying at or near the minor connector or the occlusal rest, these margins must be extended well beyond the line angles of the tooth. This additional extension may be accomplished by slicing the conventional box preparation. However, the gold margin produced by such a preparation may be quite thin and may be damaged by the clasp during placement or removal of the partial denture. This hazard may be avoided by extending the outline of the box beyond the line angle, thus producing a strong gold-to-tooth junction (Fig. 13-2).

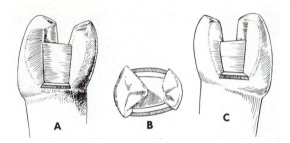

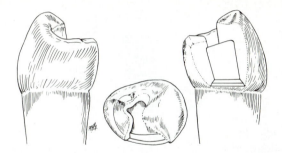

Fig. 13-2. MOD inlay preparation for lower left second premolar to be used as partial denture abutment. **A,** View of distal surface showing broad extension of box, well beyond area that will be covered by minor connector of partial denture. **B,** Occlusal view showing that axial wall is curved to conform with external proximal curvature of tooth. **C,** View of mesial surface where normal tooth contact occurs, being extended into free-cleansing area but not as broadly as distal surface.

Fig. 13-3. MO inlay preparation on lower left first premolar to be used for support of mesially placed occlusal rest. Weak lingual cusp is protected by extension of inlay margin lingually.

In this type of preparation the pulp is particularly vulnerable unless the axial wall is curved to conform with the external proximal curvature of the tooth. When caries is of minimal depth, the gingival seat should have an axial depth at all points about the width of a No. 559 fissure bur. It is of utmost importance that the gingival seat be placed below the free gingival margin. The proximal contour necessary to produce the proper guiding plane surface and the close proximity of the minor connector render this area particularly vulnerable to future caries attack. Every effort should be made to provide the restoration with maximum resistance and retention as well as clinically imperceptible gold margins. The first requisite can be satisfied by preparing opposing cavity walls 5 degrees or less from parallel and producing flat floors and sharp, clean line angles. Through the use of modern impression materials and casting technique the second requisite is not nearly as difficult as it was a few years ago.

The extended box provides the broad occlusoproximal area necessary to accommodate an occlusal rest. Care should be exercised to place the rest area in such a manner that an adequate amount of gold is allowed in both buccal and lingual directions. The proposed depth of the rest must be determined before preparing the tooth to ensure an adequate thickness of gold in the axiopulpal area. Additional depth in this area may be obtained by rounding the axiopulpal line angle of the preparation. In most instances, if the preparation is well into dentin at this point, adequate thickness of gold will be ensured. However, in problem situations a careful study of the roentgenogram will give some indication regarding the depth to which the pulpal floor can be carried with safety.

It is sometimes necessary to use an inlay on a lower first premolar for the support of an indirect retainer. The narrow occlusal width buccolingually and the lingual inclination of the occlusal surface of such a tooth often complicate the two-surface inlay preparation. Even the most exacting occlusal cavity preparation often leaves a thin and weak lingual cusp remaining.

Fig. 13-3 illustrates a modification of the two-surface extended-box inlay preparation, which lends support to a weak lingual cusp. Enough of the tip of the lingual cusp must be removed to allow for sufficient thickness of gold to withstand occlusal forces. Tooth structure should be removed in the direction of the enamel rods, and the cut should be terminated with a bevel just lingual to the proximal embrasure. A short bevel is then placed along the lingual surface of the reduced cusp. A modified inlay preparation such as this permits adequate coverage of a potentially weak cusp and eliminates the necessity of resorting to some type of more extensive restoration such as an MOD inlay or three-quarter crown.

An inlay preparation should be wide enough that the margins will be well beyond the occlusal

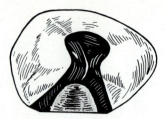

Fig. 13-4. Occlusal view of Class II inlay properly designed to support occlusal rest. Inlay preparation has been made with sufficient width to accommodate occlusal rest without jeopardizing inlay margins.

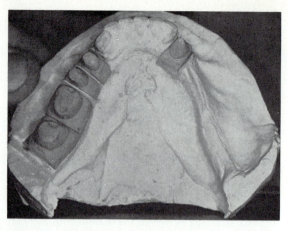

Fig. 13-5. Full arch with removal dies for five abutment crowns. Note depressions in preparations to accommodate occlusal rests.

rest area (Fig. 13-4). Since the rest seat will be carved in the wax pattern, the margins of the inlay should not be jeopardized by their proximity to the rest seat. Generally there should be at least 1 to 1.5 mm of gold between the occlusal rest and the inlay margin. The refinement of the margins, which is the final step in creating an inlay wax pattern, should not infringe on the outline form of the rest seat. The depth of the occlusal rest seat should be provided for in the preparation. If there is any doubt, the axiopulpal line angle should be beveled or made concave to accommodate the occlusal rest.

One of the advantages of making cast restorations for abutment teeth is that mouth preparations that would otherwise have to be done in the mouth may be done on the surveyor with far greater accuracy. It is extremely difficult, and many times impossible, to make several proximal surfaces parallel to one another in preparing them intraorally. The opportunity of paralleling and contouring wax patterns on the surveyor in relation to a path of placement should be used to the fullest advantage whenever cast restorations are being made.

Although it is not always possible, it is best that all wax patterns be made at the same time. A cast of the arch with removable dies may be used if they are sufficiently keyed for accuracy (Fig. 13-5). If preferred, the paralleling and contouring of wax patterns may be done on a solid cast of the arch, using supplementary individual dies to refine margins. Modern impression materials and indirect techniques make either method equally satisfactory.

The same sequence for preparing teeth in the mouth applies to the contouring of wax patterns,

differing only in that it may be done with greater accuracy and precision when indirect methods are used. After the cast has been placed on the surveyor to conform to the selected path of placement, and the wax patterns have been carved for occlusion and contact, proximal surfaces that are to act as guiding planes then may be carved parallel to the path of placement with a surveyor blade. This usually will be extended to the junction of the middle and gingival thirds of the tooth surface involved but not to the gingival margin, since the minor connector must be relieved when it crosses the gingivae. A guiding plane that includes the occlusal two thirds or even one half of the proximal area is usually adequate without endangering gingival tissues.

After the paralleling of guiding planes and any other contouring, occlusal rest seats are carved in the wax pattern. This has been outlined in Chapter 5.

It should be emphasized that critical areas thus prepared in wax should not be destroyed by careless spruing or polishing. The wax pattern should be sprued to preserve paralleled surfaces and rest areas. Polishing should consist of little more than burnishing. Rest areas should need only refining with round finishing burs. If some interference by spruing is unavoidable, the casting must be returned to the surveyor for the refinement of proximal surfaces. However, this can only be done accurately with the aid of a handpiece holder attached to the vertical spindle of the surveyor or some similar machining device. Need for later corrections to the casting can be avoided by carving the wax pattern with care and by spruing and polishing with equal care.

ABUTMENT PREPARATIONS USING CAST CROWNS

Much that has been said in the preceding paragraphs about the preparation of inlays for partial denture abutments applies equally to cast-crown restorations. These may be in the form of three-quarter or full cast gold crowns or porcelain veneer crowns. The latter are, of course, used for esthetic reasons only, but consideration for esthetics must not be allowed to jeopardize the success of the partial denture design. Retentive contours therefore must be provided on veneer crowns the same as on full cast crowns.

The ideal crown restoration for a partial denture abutment is the full cast gold crown, which can be carved to satisfy ideally all requirements for support, stabilization, and retention without compromise for cosmetic reasons. Porcelain veneer crowns can be made equally satisfactory but only by the added step of contouring the veneered surface on the surveyor before the final glaze. If this is not done, retentive contours may be excessive or inadequate. The full cast crown is preferable as an ideal abutment piece whenever esthetics will allow its use.

The three-quarter crown does not permit the creating of retentive areas as does the full crown. However, if buccal or labial surfaces are sound and retentive areas are acceptable or can be made so by slight modification of tooth surfaces, the three-quarter crown is a conservative restoration of merit. The same criteria apply in the decision to leave a portion of an abutment unprotected as in the decision to leave any tooth unprotected that is to serve as a partial denture abutment.

Regardless of the type of crown used, the preparation should be made to accommodate the depth of the occlusal rest seat. This is best accomplished by creating a depression in the prepared tooth at the occlusal rest area (Fig. 13-6). Since the location of any occlusal rests will have

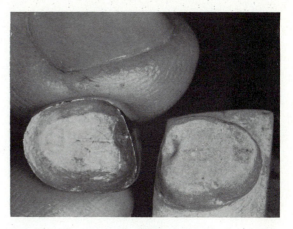

Fig. 13-6. Close-up view of full crown abutment preparation with depression to accommodate depth of occlusal rest.

been established previously during treatment planning, this will be known in advance of any crown preparations. If, for example, double occlusal rests are to be used, this will be known so that the tooth can be prepared to accommodate the depth of both rests. It is almost as bad to find, when waxing a pattern, that a rest seat has to be made more shallow than is desirable because of lack of foresight as it is to have to make a rest seat shallow in an existing crown or inlay because its thickness is not known. Here the opportunity for creating an ideal rest seat depends only on the few seconds it takes to create a space for it.

Ledges on abutment crowns. In addition to providing abutment protection, more nearly ideal retentive contours, definite guiding planes, and optimal occlusal rest support, crown restorations on teeth used as partial denture abutments offer still another advantage not obtainable on natural teeth. This is the crown ledge or shoulder, which provides effective reciprocation and stabilization (Fig. 13-7).

The functions of the reciprocal clasp arm have been stated in Chapter 6. Briefly, these are reciprocation, stabilization, and auxiliary indirect retention. Any rigid reciprocal arm may provide horizontal stabilization if it is located on axial surfaces parallel to the path of placement. To a large extent, since it is placed about the height

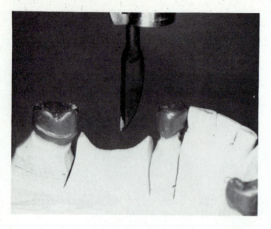

Fig. 13-7. Axial surfaces of abutment crown patterns requiring parallelism are readily contoured with surveyor and carving accessory. Three fourths of lingual surface of molar pattern has been carved with surveyor blade, parallel to path of placement, for crown ledge preparation. Reciprocal element of direct retainer will occupy prepared lingual surface, thus restoring contour of crown when removable partial denture is seated.

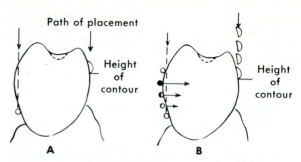

Fig. 13-8. A, Relationship of retentive and reciprocal clasp arm to each other when partial denture framework is fully seated. As retentive clasp arm flexes over height of contour during placement and removal, reciprocal clasp arm cannot be effective because it is not in contact with tooth until denture framework is fully seated. B, Horizontal forces applied to abutment tooth as retentive clasp flexes over height of contour during placement and removal. Open circle at top and bottom illustrates that retentive clasp is only passive at its first contact with tooth during placement and when in its terminal position with denture fully seated. During placement and removal rigid clasp arm placed on opposite side of tooth cannot provide resistance against these horizontal forces.

of convexity, a rigid reciprocal arm may also act as an auxiliary indirect retainer. However, its function as a reciprocating arm against the action of the retentive clasp arm is limited only to stabilization against possible orthodontic movement when the denture framework is in its terminal position. Only when the retentive clasp produces an active orthodontic force, because of accidental distortion or improper design, is such reciprocation needed. Reciprocation is most needed when the restoration is being placed or when a dislodging force is applied, to prevent transient horizontal forces that may be detrimental to abutment stability. Perhaps the term **orthodontic force** is incorrect, since the term signifies a slight but continuous influence that would logically reach equilibrium as soon as the tooth is orthodontically moved. Instead, the transient forces of placement and removal lead to periodontal destruction and eventual instability rather than to orthodontic movement followed by consolidation.

True reciprocation is not possible with a clasp arm that is placed on an occlusally inclined tooth surface because it does not become effective until the prosthesis is fully seated. Immediately, when a dislodging force is applied, the reciprocal clasp arm, along with the occlusal rest, breaks contact with the supporting tooth surfaces, and they are no longer effective. Thus, as the retentive clasp flexes over the height of contour, thereby exerting a horizontal force on the abutment, reciprocation is nonexistent just when it is needed most (Fig. 13-8).

True reciprocation can be obtained only by creating a path of placement for the reciprocal clasp arm that is parallel to other guiding planes. In this manner the inferior border of the reciprocal clasp makes contact with its guiding surface before the retentive clasp on the other side of the tooth begins to flex (Fig. 13-9). Thus reciprocation exists during the entire path of placement and removal. The presence of a ledge on the abutment crown acts as a terminal stop for the reciprocal clasp arm, as well as augmenting the occlusal rest and providing some indirect retention for a distal extension partial denture.

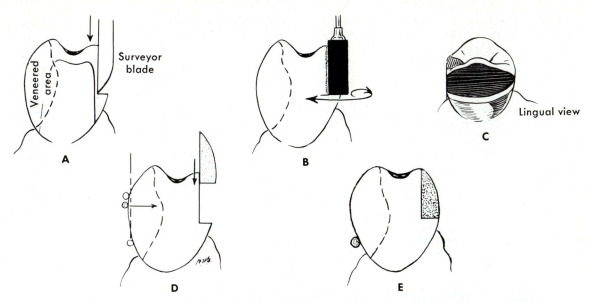

Fig. 13-9. A, Preparation of ledge on wax pattern with surveyor blade parallel to path of placement. **B,** Refinement of ledge on gold casting, using suitable carborundum stone in handpiece attached to dental surveyor or specialized drill press for same purpose. **C,** Approximate width and depth of ledge formed on abutment crown, which will permit reciprocal clasp arm to be inlayed within normal contours of tooth. **D,** True reciprocation throughout full path of placement and removal that is possible when reciprocal clasp arm is inlayed onto ledge on abutment crown. **E,** Direct retainer assembly is fully seated. Reciprocal arm restores lingual contour of abutment.

A ledge on an abutment crown has still another advantage. Although the usual reciprocal clasp arm is half-round, and therefore convex, and is superimposed on an already convex surface, a reciprocal clasp arm built on a crown ledge is actually inlayed into the crown and reproduces more nearly normal crown contours (Fig. 13-9). The patient's tongue then contacts a continuously convex surface rather than the projection of a clasp arm. Unfortunately the enamel cap is neither thick enough nor is the tooth so shaped that an effective ledge can be created on an uncrowned tooth. Narrow enamel shoulders are sometimes used as rest seats on anterior teeth, but these do not provide the parallelism that is essential to reciprocation during placement and removal.

The crown ledge may be used on any full or three-quarter crown restoration that covers the nonretentive side of an abutment tooth. It is used most frequently on premolars and molars but also may be used on canine restorations. It is not ordinarily used on buccal surfaces for reciprocation against lingual retention because of the excessive display of metal, but it may be used just as effectively on posterior abutments when esthetics is not a factor.

The fact that a crown ledge is to be used should be known in advance of crown preparation to assure sufficient removal of tooth structure in this area. Although a shoulder or ledge is not included in the preparation itself, adequate space must be provided so that the ledge may be made sufficiently wide and the surface above it may be made parallel to the path of placement. **The ledge should be placed at the junction of the gingival and middle third of the tooth, curving slightly to follow the curvature of the gingival tissues. On the side of the tooth at which the clasp arm will originate, the ledge** must be kept low enough to allow the origin of the clasp arm to be wide enough for sufficient strength and rigidity.

In forming the crown ledge, which is usually located on the lingual surface, the wax pattern of the crown is completed except for refinement of the margins before the ledge is carved. After the proximal guiding planes and the occlusal rests and retentive contours are formed, the ledge is carved with the surveyor blade so that the surface above is parallel to the path of placement. Thus a continuous guiding plane surface will exist from the proximal surface around the lingual surface, the difference being only that the lingual portion ends in a definite ledge and the proximal portion does not.

The full effectiveness of the crown ledge cannot be obtained with a crown that is not returned to the surveyor for refinement after casting. To afford true reciprocation, the crown casting must have a surface above the ledge that is parallel to the path of placement. This can be accomplished with precision only by machining the casting parallel to the path of placement with a handpiece holder in the surveyor or some other suitable machining device (Fig. 13-10). Similarly, the parallelism of proximal guiding planes needs to be perfected after casting and polishing. Although it is possible to **approximate** parallelism and, at the same time, form the crown ledge on the wax pattern with a surveyor blade, some of its accuracy is lost in casting and pol-

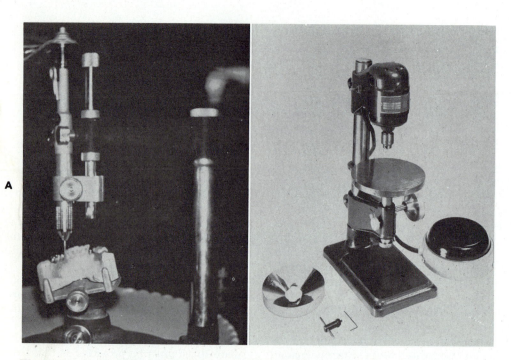

Fig. 13-10. A, Faro laboratory handpiece attached to Ney surveyor by means of handpiece holder. With bur or stone, lingual surface and ledge are machined in relation to previously established path of placement. **B,** Austenal Micro-Drill used to mill internal rest seats and lingual grooves and ledges in cast gold restorations. Such a device permits more precise milling than is possible with dental handpiece attached to dental surveyor. To be effective, cast must be positioned on Micro-Drill in such manner that previously established path of placement is maintained. Movable stage or base therefore should be adjustable until relation of cast to axis of drill has been made same as that obtained when cast was on dental surveyor. (**B** courtesy Austenal, Inc., Chicago, Ill.)

ishing. The use of suitable burs such as No. 557, 558, and 559 fissure burs and true cylindric carborundum stones in the handpiece holder permits the paralleling of all guiding planes on the finished casting with the accuracy necessary for

the effectiveness of those guiding plane surfaces (Figs. 13-11 to 13-13).

The reciprocal clasp arm is ultimately waxed on the investment cast so that it is continuous with the ledge inferiorly and contoured superiorly to restore the crown contour including the tip of the cusp. It is obvious that polishing must not be allowed to destroy the form of the shoulder that was prepared in wax nor to destroy the parallelism of the guiding plane surface. It is equally vital that the denture casting must be polished with great care so that the accuracy of the counterpart is not destroyed. Modern investments, casting alloys, and polishing techniques make this degree of accuracy possible. Only the human element, by carelessness or lack of understanding, may fail to produce a crown and counterpart with the desired accuracy. It is just as necessary for the technician to understand the purpose of the crown ledge as it is for the dentist who designs and plans for its use.

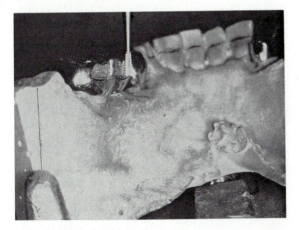

Fig. 13-11. Lingual ledges on cast gold crowns are machined with No. 558 dental bur. Experience has shown that in absence of rigid jig for holding cast, a bur is difficult to use. Therefore it is best that ledge be formed as accurately as possible in wax pattern and that machining of finished casting be done with cylindric carborundum point. Note scratch line on left posterior portion of cast, indicating path of placement.

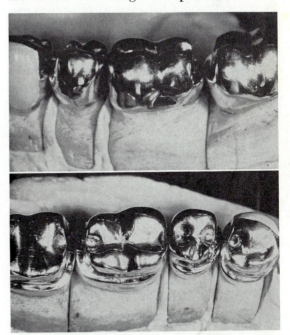

Fig. 13-13. Buccal and lingual views of abutment crowns designed to accept embrasure clasps and lingual reciprocal arms resting on prepared ledges. All surfaces above ledges are made parallel with path of placement. Note size and form of occlusal rests on either side of embrasure ledges.

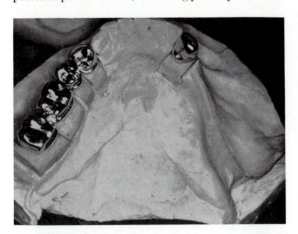

Fig. 13-12. Lingual ledges after machining and polishing. Note that embrasures for clasping are also machined parallel to path of placement and that occlusal rests are used in addition to supporting ledges. These are to prevent tooth separation and to shunt food away from interproximal areas.

Veneer crowns for support of clasp arms. Resin and porcelain veneer crowns are used for cosmetic reasons on abutment teeth that would otherwise display an objectionable amount of metal. They may be in the form of porcelain veneers retained by pins and cemented to the crown, porcelain fused directly to a cast crown, or acrylic resin processed directly to a cast crown.

The retentive clasp terminal should rest on metal when an acrylic resin veneer crown is used as an abutment restoration (Fig. 13-14). In this instance the crown is contoured to be retentive in the desired area, and that area is not included in carving the space for the resin veneer. Whereas the suprabulge portion of the clasp arm crosses the surface of the veneer, the portion that crosses the height of contour and engaged an undercut in which abrasion could occur is supported by the metal of the crown itself. The only disadvantage of a veneer crown so prepared is the display of metal, which more often than not is on the mesial side of the abutment tooth and therefore is cosmetically objectionable. Ceramic-gold crowns do not present this problem. Hopefully, the continued development of abrasion-resistant composites will offer materials suitable for veneering that will withstand clasp contact, thereby eliminating an undesirable display of metal.

If the veneer crown is not contoured to provide retention on metal, suitable retention does not exist until the veneer has been added. This means that the veneer must be slightly overcontoured and then shaped to provide the desired undercut for the location of the retentive clasp arm (Fig. 13-15). If the veneer is of porcelain, this procedure must precede glazing, and if of resin, it must precede final polishing. If this most important step in the making of veneered abutments is neglected or omitted, excessive or inadequate retentive contours may result, to the detriment of effective clasp design.

The flat underside of the cast clasp makes sufficient contact with the surface of the veneer so that abrasion of a resin veneer may result. Although the underside of the clasp may be polished (with some loss in accuracy of fit), abrasion results from the trapping and holding of food debris against the tooth surface as the clasp moves during function. **Therefore unless the retentive clasp terminal rests on metal, glazed porcelain should be used to assure the future retentiveness of the veneered surface.** Present-day acrylic resins, being cross-linked copolymers, are much harder than they have been in the past and will withstand abrasion for considerable time, but not nearly to the same degree as porcelain. Therefore acrylic resin veneers are used best in conjunction with exposed metal supporting the half-round clasp terminal.

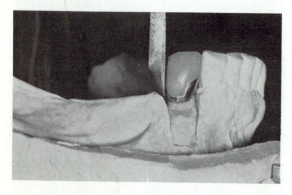

Fig. 13-14. Close-up view of relation of surveyor blade to distal surface of abutment crown. Note that this guiding plane is made parallel to path of placement.

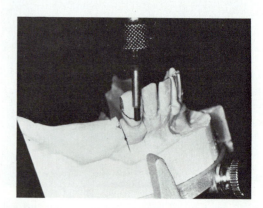

Fig. 13-15. Porcelain veneer crown is resurveyed before glazing. At this stage, veneered portion can be recontoured by grinding to achieve optimal height of contour to place the reciprocal and retentive portion of planned clasp assembly.

SPLINTING OF ABUTMENT TEETH

Frequently a tooth is deemed too weak to use alone as a partial denture abutment because of the short length or excessive taper of a single root or because of bone loss resulting in an unfavorable crown-root ratio. In such instances, splinting of weak abutment teeth to the adjacent tooth or teeth is used as a means of gaining **multiple abutment support.** Thus two single-rooted teeth may be used as a multirooted abutment.

Splinting should not be used to retain a tooth that would otherwise be condemned for periodontal reasons, in the futile hope that by doing so the tooth may be retained. Such a gamble may be justified when, if successful, the need for a prosthetic restoration would be avoided. However, when the length of service of a restoration may depend on the serviceability of an abutment, any periodontally questionable tooth should be condemned in favor of using an adjacent healthy tooth as the abutment, even though the span is increased one tooth by doing so.

The most frequent application of the use of multiple abutments is the splinting of two premolars or a first premolar and a canine (Fig. 13-16). Mandibular premolars generally have round and tapered roots, which are easily loosened by rotation as well as by tipping. They are the weakest of posterior abutments. But maxillary premolars also often have tapered roots, which make them poor risks as abutments, particularly when they will be called on to resist the leverage of a distal extension base. Such teeth are best splinted by casting or soldering two crowns or inlays together. When a first premolar to be used as an abutment has poor root form or support, it is best that it be splinted to the stronger canine in a similar manner.

Anterior teeth on which lingual rests are to be placed frequently need to be splinted together to avoid orthodontic movement of individual teeth. Mandibular anterior teeth are seldom so used, but if they are, splinting of the teeth involved is advisable (Fig. 13-17). When such splinting is impossible for one reason or another, individual lingual rests on cast restorations may be inclined slightly apically to avoid possible tooth displacement, or lingual rests may be used in conjunction with incisal rests, engaging slightly the labial surface of the teeth.

Lingual rests should always be placed as low on the cingulum as possible, and single anterior teeth, other than canines, should not ordinarily be used for occlusal support. Where lingual rests are employed on central and lateral incisors, as many teeth as possible should be included to distribute the load over several teeth, thereby

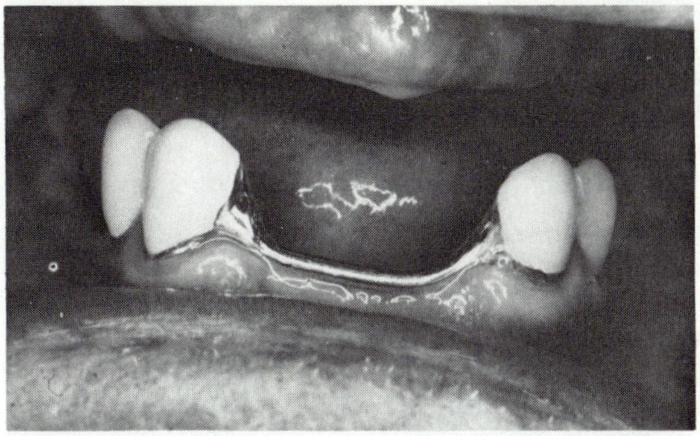

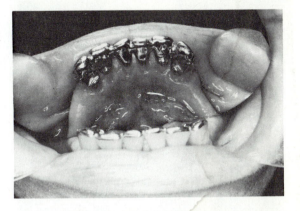

Fig. 13-16. First premolars and canines have been splinted in this Class I, modification 1, partially edentulous arch. Splint bar was added to provide cross-arch stabilization for splinted abutments and to support anterior segment of removable restoration. Prospective longevity of abutments has been enhanced. Fixed partial denture was precluded by unfavorable contours of anterior residual ridge.

Fig. 13-17. Six remaining mandibular anterior teeth are splinted with pin onlays. Lingual rest seats on canines and lateral incisors will support linguoplate major connector. Teeth were prepared for onlays following healing from periodontal surgery. All teeth were slightly mobile.

minimizing the force on any one tooth. Even so, some movement of individual teeth is likely to occur, particularly when they are subjected to the forces of indirect retention. This is best avoided by splinting several teeth with united cast restorations. The condition of the teeth and cosmetic considerations will dictate whether full veneer crowns, three-quarter crowns, or pinledge inlays will be used for this purpose.

Splinting of molar teeth for multiple abutment support is less frequently used, because they are generally multirooted teeth to begin with and a two- or three-rooted tooth that is not strong enough alone is probably a poor abutment risk. However, there may be notable exceptions when, because of fused and conical roots, the abutment would benefit from the effect of splinting.

USE OF ISOLATED TEETH AS ABUTMENTS

Although splinting is advocated for any abutment teeth that are considered too weak to risk using alone, a single abutment standing alone in the dental arch anterior to a distal extension basal seat generally requires the splinting effect of a fixed partial denture (Figs. 13-18 and 13-19). Even though the form and length of the root and the supporting bone seem to be adequate for an ordinary abutment, the fact that the tooth lacks proximal contact endangers the tooth when it is used to support a distal extension base.

The average abutment tooth is subjected to some distal tipping, to rotation, and to horizontal movement, all of which must be held to a minimum by the design of the denture and the quality of tissue support for the distal extension base. The isolated abutment tooth, however, is subjected also to mesial tipping because of lack of proximal contact. Despite indirect retention,

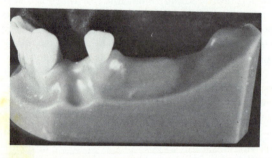

Fig. 13-18. Lone standing premolar should be splinted to canine with fixed partial denture. Not only will design of removable partial denture be simplified, but longevity of abutment service by premolar will be greatly extended.

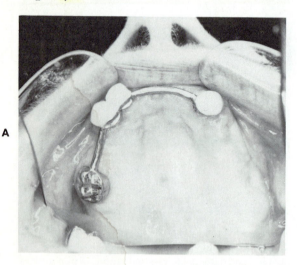
A

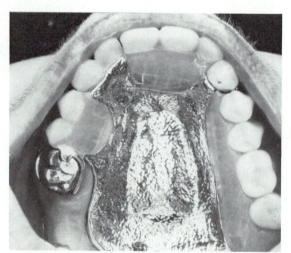
B

Fig. 13-19. A, Isolated abutments have been splinted using splint bars. **B,** Removable partial denture is more adequately supported by splinting mechanism shown in **A** than could be realized with isolated abutments.

some lifting of the distal extension base is inevitable, causing torque to the abutment as the fulcrum of a teeter-totter.

In a tooth-borne prosthesis an isolated tooth may be used as an abutment by using a fifth abutment for additional support. Thus rotational and horizontal forces are resisted by the additional stabilization obtained from the fifth abutment. When two such isolated abutments exist, that is, two second premolars with first premolars missing, the sixth abutments should be used. Thus the two canines, the two isolated premolars, and two posterior teeth are used as abutments.

In contrast, an isolated anterior abutment adjacent to a distal extension base usually should be splinted to the nearest tooth by means of a fixed partial denture. The effect is twofold: (1) the anterior edentulous segment is eliminated, thereby creating an intact dental arch anterior to the space, and (2) the isolated tooth is splinted to the other abutment of the fixed partial denture, thereby providing multiple abutment support. Splinting should be used here only to gain multiple abutment support rather than to support an otherwise weak abutment tooth.

The economic aspect of using fixed restorations as part of the mouth preparations for a partial denture is essentially the same as that for any other splinting procedure: the best design of the partial denture that will assure the longevity of its service makes the additional procedure and expense necessary. Although it must be recognized that **economic considerations, combined with a particularly favorable prognosis of an isolated tooth, may influence the decision to forego the advantages of using a fixed partial denture,** the original treatment plan should include this precautionary measure even though the alternative method is accepted for economic reasons.

A second factor may also influence the decision to use an isolated tooth as an abutment; this is the esthetic consideration for an otherwise sound anterior tooth that would have to be used as an abutment for a fixed restoration. However, neither esthetics nor economics should deter the dentist from recommending to the patient that an isolated tooth to be used as a terminal abutment be given the advantage of splinting by means of a fixed partial denture. Then, if compromises are necessary, the patient must share a measure of the responsibility for using the isolated tooth as an abutment.

MISSING ANTERIOR TEETH

When a partial denture is to replace missing posterior teeth, especially in the absence of distal abutments, any additional missing anterior teeth are best replaced by means of fixed restorations rather than by being added to the denture. In any distal extension situation some teeter-totter action will inevitably result from the adding of an anterior segment to the denture. Here again the ideal treatment plan, which would consider the anterior edentulous space separately, comes in conflict with economic and esthetic considerations. Each situation must be treated according to its own merits. Frequently the best esthetic result can be obtained by replacing missing anterior teeth with the partial denture rather than with a fixed restoration. From a biomechanical standpoint, however, a removable partial denture should replace only the missing posterior teeth **after** the remainder of the arch has been made intact by fixed restorations.

Although the occasional need for compromises is recognized, the decision to include an anterior segment on the denture will depend largely on the support available for that part of the denture. The greater the number of natural anterior teeth remaining, the better the available support for the edentulous segment.

If definite rests are obtainable, the anterior segment may be treated as any other tooth-bounded modification space. Sound principles of rest support apply just as much as elsewhere in the arch. **Inclined tooth surfaces should not be used for occlusal support, nor should rests be placed on unprepared lingual surfaces.** The best possible support for an anterior segment is multiple support extending, if possible, posteriorly across prepared lingual rest seats on the canine teeth to mesial occlusal rest seats on the canine teeth to mesial occlusal rest seats on the first premolars. Such support will permit the missing anterior teeth to be included in the denture, frequently with some cosmetic advantages over fixed restorations.

In some instances the replacement of anterior teeth by means of a partial denture cannot be avoided. However, without adequate tooth support any such prosthesis will lack the stability that would exist from replacing only the posterior teeth with the partial denture and the anterior teeth with fixed restorations. When anterior teeth have been lost through accident or have been missing for some time, resorption of the anterior ridge may have progressed to the point that neither fixed nor removable pontics may be butted to the residual ridge. In such instances, for esthetic reasons, the missing teeth must be replaced with a denture base supporting teeth that are more nearly in their original position, considerably forward from the residual ridge. Although such teeth may be positioned to better cosmetic advantage, the contouring and coloring of a denture base to be esthetically pleasing requires the maximum artistic effort of both the dentist and the technician. Such a partial denture, both from an esthetic and biomechanical standpoint, is one of the most difficult of all prosthetic restorations. **However, a splint bar, connected by abutments on both sides of the edentulous space, will provide much-needed support to the anterior segment of the removable partial denture.** Since the splint bar will act as an occlusal rest, rest seats on abutments adjacent to the edentulous area need not be prepared, thus simplifying an anterior restoration to some extent.

A concept of "dual path of placement" to enhance the esthetic replacement of missing anterior teeth with a removable partial denture is recognized. Sources of information on this concept are made available in the Selected Reading Resources section of this text under Partial Denture Design.

TEMPORARY CROWNS WHEN A PARTIAL DENTURE IS BEING WORN

Occasionally an existing removable partial denture must remain serviceable while the mouth is being prepared for a new denture. In such situations, temporary crowns that will support the old denture and will not interfere with its placement and removal must be made. Only rarely can an aluminum crown be made to serve

this purpose. Instead, an acrylic resin temporary crown that duplicates the original form of the abutment tooth must be made (Fig. 13-20).

The technique for making temporary crowns to fit direct retainers is similar to that for other types of acrylic resin temporary crowns. The principal difference is that an irreversible hydrocolloid impression must be made of the entire arch with the existing partial denture in place. This is wrapped in a wet towel and set aside while the tooth or teeth are being prepared for new crowns.

After the preparations are completed and the impressions and jaw relation records have been made, the prepared teeth are dried and coated with petroleum jelly. The original irreversible hydrocolloid impression is trimmed to eliminate any excess, undercuts, and interproximal projections that would interfere with its replacement in the mouth.

The methyl methacrylate resins exhibit little polymerization shrinkage and serve as excellent materials for temporary crowns in conjunction with removable partial dentures. Tooth-shade resin is sprinkled into the impression in those areas that are to be temporary crowns, and any excess is removed with a pledget of cotton. When the material reaches a soft rubbery state, the impression is seated into the mouth, where it is held by the dentist until sufficient time has elapsed for it to reach a stiff rubbery stage. This again must be based on experience with the particular plastic material being used. At this time the impression is removed, and the crowns remain in the impression. These are then stripped out of the impression; all excess is trimmed away with scissors, and the crowns are reseated on the prepared abutments. The partial denture is then removed from the impression and reseated in the mouth onto the plastic crowns, which are at this time in a stiff rubbery state. The patient may bring the teeth into occlusion to reestablish the former position and occlusal relationship of the existing partial denture.

After the plastic crown or crowns have hardened, the partial denture is removed, and the crowns remain on the teeth. These are then tapped off, trimmed, polished, and temporarily cemented. The result is a temporary crown that

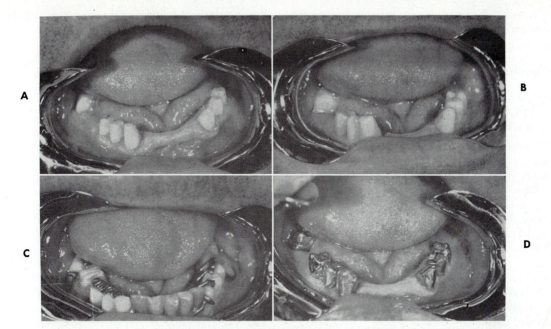

Fig. 13-20. Sequence of mouth preparations with temporary crowns formed to support existing partial denture while new one is being made. **A,** Several abutment teeth have been prepared to receive full coverage crowns. **B,** Acrylic resin temporary crowns duplicating original tooth contour. Impression of teeth before preparation was begun was used to establish shape of temporary crowns. **C,** Existing partial denture, seated onto temporary crowns. These are then removed as often as necessary during succeeding appointments. **D,** Gold castings are tried in before soldering and adding veneers. Temporary crowns and existing partial denture are then returned to mouth until abutment pieces are ready for cementation.

restores the original abutment contours and allows the partial denture to be placed and removed without interference, while providing the same support temporarily to the denture that existed before the teeth were prepared. This service, made possible by modern materials, should be routine for all patients requiring such service.

Cementation of temporary crowns. Cementation of acrylic resin temporary crowns may require slight reaming of the crowns to accommodate the temporary cement and to facilitate removal. The temporary cement should be thin and applied only to the inside rim of the crowns to assure complete seating. As soon as the temporary cement has hardened, the occlusion may be checked and relieved accordingly.

Regardless of the type of temporary cement

used, any excess that might be irritating to the gingivae should be removed. Too frequently the final act before dismissing the patient is the cementation of the temporary crowns. Instead, two considerations are necessary. One is the removal of excess cement after it has hardened. The second is the application of some medication to the slightly abused gingivae to facilitate healing and to prevent discomfort to the patient. Topical application of some antibacterial agent is, at best, a transient treatment that does little to prevent discomfort. Hydrocortisone acetate, 0.5%, in a denture adhesive powder, when applied topically to a freshly lacerated surface, both faciliates healing and prevents afterpain. It should be applied to the lacerated gingivae around each temporary crown and the patient should be dismissed without further rinsing of the mouth. Tissue response to this treatment has been so favorable that it is included here as a specific treatment. Apparently it is effective only on fresh wounds and is of little value as a follow-up treatment.

THE MAKING OF CROWNS AND INLAYS TO FIT EXISTING DENTURE RETAINERS

It is frequently necessary that an abutment tooth be restored with a full crown (and occasionally with an inlay) that will fit the inside of the clasp of an otherwise serviceable partial denture. The technique for doing so is simple enough but requires that an indirect-direct-indirect pattern be made, and therefore justifies a fee for service above that for the usual full crown.

The technique for making a crown to fit the inside of a clasp is as follows: An irreversible hydrocolloid impression of the mouth is made with the partial denture in place. This impression, which is used to make the plastic temporary crown, is wrapped in a wet towel and set aside while the tooth is being prepared. Even though several abutment teeth are to be restored, it is usually necessary that each one be completed before the next one is begun. This is necessary so that the original support and occlusal relationship of the partial denture can be maintained as each new crown is being made.

The abutment tooth is then prepared, during which time the partial denture is replaced frequently enough to ascertain that sufficient tooth structure is being removed to allow for the thickness of the gold casting. When the preparation is completed, a copper band impression of the tooth is obtained, from which a stone die is made.

An acrylic resin temporary crown is then made in the original irreversible hydrocolloid impression as outlined in the preceding paragraphs. It is trimmed, polished, and temporarily cemented, and the denture is returned to the mouth. The patient is dismissed after the excess cement has been removed and the traumatized gingiva treated, as mentioned previously.

On the stone die made from the copper band impression, a thin self-curing resin coping will be formed with a brush technique. The stone die should first be trimmed to the finishing line of the preparation, which is then delineated with a pencil, and the die painted with a tinfoil substitute. A material such as Alcote tinfoil substitute should be used, which will form a thin film on a cold, dry surface. Not all tinfoil substitutes are suitable for this purpose.

With self-curing acrylic resin powder and liquid in separate dappen dishes and a fine sable brush, a coping of acrylic resin of uniform thickness is painted onto the die. This should extend not quite to the pencil line representing the limit of the crown preparation. After hardening, the resin coping may be removed, inspected, and trimmed if necessary. The thin film of foil substitute should be removed before the coping is reseated onto the die.

The wax pattern is usually not begun until the patient returns, at which time it is built up at the chair. First the occlusal portion of the wax pattern is established by having the patient close and carve excursive paths in the wax (Fig. 13-21, A). Additions are made to dull areas until a smooth occlusal registration has been obtained. Except for narrowing the occlusal surface and the carving of grooves and spillways, this will be the occlusal anatomy of the finished restoration.

The second step is the adding of sufficient wax to establish contact relations with the adjoining tooth. At this time the occlusal relation of the marginal ridges also must be established.

Next, wax is added to buccal and lingual surfaces where the clasp arms will contact the crown, and the pattern is again reseated in the mouth. The clasp arms, minor connectors, and occlusal rests involved on the partial denture are warmed with a needle-point flame, carefully avoiding any adjacent resin, and the denture is positioned in the mouth and onto the wax pattern (Fig. 13-21, B). Several attempts may be necessary until the denture is fully seated and the components of the clasp are clearly recorded in the wax pattern. Each time the denture is removed, the pattern will draw with it and must be teased out of the clasp.

When contact with the clasp arms and the occlusal relation of the denture have been established satisfactorily, the temporary crown may be replaced and the patient dismissed. The

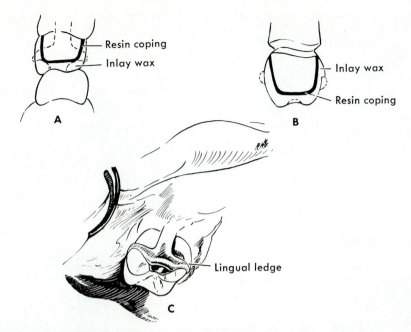

Fig. 13-21. Making of cast crown to fit existing partial denture clasp. **A,** Thin resin coping is first made on individual die of prepared tooth. Inlay wax is then added and coping placed onto prepared tooth when occlusal surfaces and contact relations are established directly in mouth. Clasp assembly is warmed with needle-point flame only enough to soften inlay wax, and partial denture is placed in mouth where it is guided gently to place by opposing occlusion. This step must be repeated several times and excess wax removed or wax added until full supporting contact with underside of clasp assembly has been established, with denture fully seated. Usually wax pattern withdraws with denture and must be gently teased out of clasp each time. **B,** Wax pattern is then placed back onto individual die to complete occlusal anatomy and refine margins. Excess wax remaining below impression of retentive clasp arm must be removed, but wax ledge may be left below reciprocal clasp arm. **C,** Finished casting in mouth. Terminus of retentive clasp is then readapted to engage undercut. It is frequently necessary to remove some interference from casting, as indicated by articulating paper placed between clasp and crown, until clasp is full seated.

crown pattern is completed on the die by narrowing the occlusal surface buccolingually, adding grooves and spillways, and refining the margins.* Any wax ledge remaining below the reciprocal clasp arm may be left to provide some of the advantages of a crown ledge, which were

described earlier in this chapter. Excess wax remaining below the retentive clasp arm, however, must be removed to permit the adding of a retentive undercut later (Fig. 13-21, *C*).

If an acrylic resin veneer is to be added, the veneer space must now be carved in the wax pattern. In such cases the contour of the veneer may be recorded by making a stone matrix of the buccal surface, which can later be replaced onto the completed casting for waxing in the veneer. This stone matrix is then invested with the casting while the acrylic resin veneer is being processed.

---

*Margins on all crown and inlay wax patterns are refined with S. S. White red casting wax, which contrasts with the blue or green wax used for the pattern and permits the carving of delicate margins with accuracy. The preferred wax for the body of crown and inlay patterns is Maves inlay wax. This wax is available in both cone and stick form and has excellent carving properties and color.

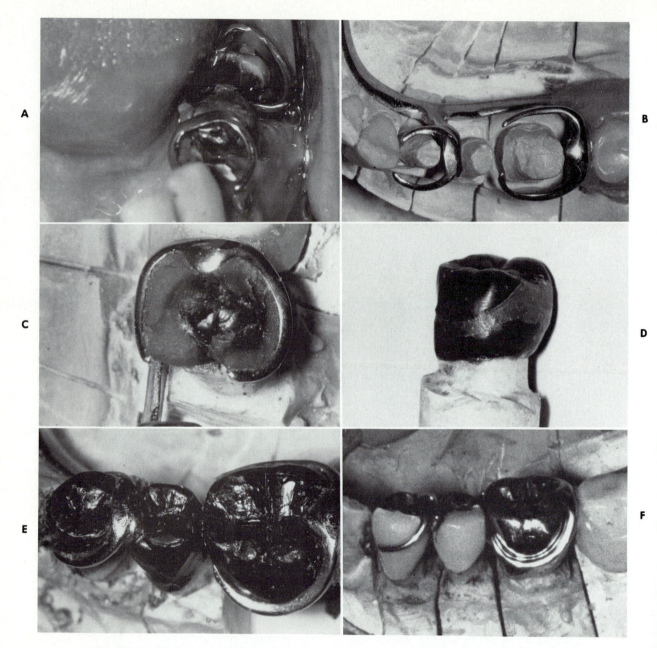

Fig. 13-22. **A**, Coronal portions of premolars and first molar are badly broken down. First premolar and molar are involved in support and retention of removable restoration. **B**, Teeth were prepared for complete coverage crowns. Cast with removable dies and denture in position on cast. **C**, Autopolymerizing acrylic resin coping is first made on molar die. Acrylic resin is built up over coping to fill clasp assembly. Inlay wax is added to develop occlusal surface with opposing mounted maxillary cast. **D**, Pattern is teased out of clasp and finished on die. Note distinctive outline of clasp in acrylic resin. **E**, Patterns for premolars are similarly developed. **F**, Restorations are completed and direct retainers have same relationships to crowns that existed on original abutments.

The wax pattern must be sprued with care so that essential areas on the pattern are not destroyed. After casting, the crown should be subjected to a minimum of polishing, since the exact form of the axial and occlusal surfaces must be maintained.

Since it is impossible to withdraw a clasp arm from a retentive undercut on the wax pattern, the casting must be made without any provision for clasp retention. After the crown has been tried in the mouth with the denture in place, the location of the retentive clasp terminal is identified by scoring the crown with a sharp instrument. Then the crown may be ground and polished slightly in this area to create a retentive undercut. The clasp terminal then may be carefully adapted into this undercut, thereby creating clasp retention on the new crown.

An alternate method for making crowns to fit existing retainers is illustrated in Fig. 13-22. The method mentioned previously involved a functional path technique to develop the occlusal surface for the crown. The method given in Fig. 13-22 uses casts mounted on an articulator to develop the occlusal surfaces for the involved crowns.

The technique for making inlay patterns to fit the inside of denture clasps is essentially the same as for full crowns, except that it may be done entirely in wax. However, patterns for larger inlays that might be distorted during placement of the denture are best supported also by an acrylic resin foundation. In such cases the pattern is started by brushing in the acrylic resin until a supporting frame has been established. The wax pattern is then completed in the mouth as for a full crown.

Ideally all abutment teeth would best be protected with full crowns before the partial denture is constructed. Except for the possibility of recurrent caries because of defective crown margins or gingival recession, abutment teeth so protected may be expected to give many years of satisfactory service in the support and retention of the partial denture. Economically, a policy of insisting on full coverage for all abutment teeth may well be justified from the long-term viewpoint. It must be recognized, however, that in practice full coverage of all abutment teeth is not always possible at the time indicated. Many

factors influence the future health status of an abutment tooth, some of which cannot be forseen. It is necessary therefore that the dentist be able to treat abutment teeth that later become defective in such a manner that their service as abutments may be restored and the serviceability of the partial denture maintained. Although it is not part of the original mouth preparations, this service accomplishes much the same objective by providing the denture with support, stability, and retention, and the dentist must be technically capable to provide this service when it becomes necessary.

SELF-ASSESSMENT AIDS

1. What does the use of a terminal molar abutment contribute to a removable partial denture?
2. Endodontic treatment of any tooth in the arch (when indicated) should be performed before making a final impression for a removable restoration. Why?
3. If you are faced with a single posterior abutment (second molar) about which you have some doubt that it can be retained and used as one end of a tooth-supported base, what options do you have relative to design of the denture?
4. Abutment preparations on sound enamel should be accomplished in a definite order with the altered and designed diagnostic cast used as a blueprint. Give the order of preparation, including a method to check your preparation.
5. What is the danger of preparing an occlusal rest seat before recontouring the adjacent axial surface?
6. Inlay preparations on teeth to be used as removable partial denture abutments differ from conventional inlay preparations in three requirements. What are they?
7. Where is the most vulnerable area on an abutment tooth, with regard to cleanliness?
8. Can you give a sequence of contouring wax patterns for abutment restorations to obtain ideal contours for optimal location of components by using a dental cast surveyor?
9. A rest seat is carved on the occlusal surface of a full gold crown pattern for a posterior abutment. The occlusal morphology has been carved to satisfy occlusal requirements, and axial contours have also been accomplished. The rest seat preparation, however, is inadequate because of its shallowness, created by insufficient room between the preparation and opposing occlusion in the area of the rest seat. What are your options to avoid a compromised result?

10. Crown ledges, parallel to the path of placement, are often carved on the lingual surfaces of abutment crowns. How does this enhance the direct retainer assembly?

11. Contrast the quality of reciprocation afforded by a crown ledge on a molar abutment and that offered by the lingual surface of an unrestored molar abutment.

12. Explain the method of preparing a lingual ledge on the wax pattern for an abutment crown. Include its depth, width, extent, and definitive location.

13. How may the crown ledge be refined after the crown has been cast?

14. Describe the contouring of the component of the direct retainer assembly that occupies the crown ledge preparation.

15. It is rare that the ceramic surface of a ceramometal crown can be fabricated and finished freehand to exhibit the exact planned height of contour for a retentive clasp arm. How may a surveyor be used to assure that the planned location of the height of contour is established? At what stage in the fabrication of the crown should the procedure be undertaken?

16. Splinting of adjacent teeth is sometimes indicated as a means of gaining multiple abutment support. What examination data would indicate that splinting should be performed?

17. Where is the most frequent application of multiple abutments by splinting found in an arch?

18. Quite often the design of a restoration requires lingual rests on lower anterior teeth. How can orthodontic movement of these teeth be minimized?

19. Isolated abutments adjacent and anterior to extension residual ridges usually have a poor prognosis when used in the condition they are found. What is the reason for this?

20. An isolated anterior abutment adjacent to a distal extension base, when splinted to the nearest tooth, provides two beneficial effects. Can you tell what these desirable effects are?

21. An isolated abutment adjacent to an extension base may be splinted to the nearest tooth by either a fixed partial denture or by a _____.

22. Missing anterior teeth should be replaced with fixed partial dentures rather than included in a removable restoration. What are the contraindications for the preceding treatment?

23. On rare occasions an abutment tooth supporting a removable partial denture will have to be restored with an inlay or crown. Can you describe a procedure whereby an abutment crown can be fabricated to an existing direct retainer?

14 IMPRESSION MATERIALS AND PROCEDURES FOR REMOVABLE PARTIAL DENTURES

Rigid materials
Thermoplastic materials
Elastic materials
Impressions of the partially edentulous arch
Individual impression trays

Impression materials used in the various phases of partial denture construction may be classified as being rigid, thermoplastic, or elastic substances. Rigid impression materials are those that set to a rigid consistency. Thermoplastic impression materials are those that become plastic at higher temperatures and resume their original form when the temperature has again been lowered. Elastic impression materials are those that remain in an elastic or flexible state after they have been removed from the mouth.

Most impression materials used in prosthetic dentistry may be included in the following classification:

Rigid materials
    Plaster of Paris
    Metallic oxide pastes
Thermoplastic materials
    Modeling plastic
    Impression waxes and natural resins
Elastic materials
    Reversible hydrocolloids (agar-agar)
    Irreversible hydrocolloids (alginate)
    Mercaptan rubber-base impression materials (Thiokol)
    Silicone impression materials
    Polyethers

Although rigid impression materials may be capable of recording tooth and tissue details ac-

curately, they cannot be removed from the mouth without fracture and reassembly. Thermoplastic materials cannot record minute details accurately because they undergo distortion during withdrawal from tooth and tissue undercuts. Elastic materials are the only ones that can be withdrawn from tooth and tissue undercuts without permanent deformation and are therefore the only ones suitable for impressions of irregular contours of oral tissues. Whereas the rigid and thermoplastic impression materials are most frequently used in various combinations in making impressions for complete dentures, the elastic impression materials are most generally used for the making of impressions for removable partial dentures, immediate dentures, and crowns and fixed partial dentures when tooth and tissue undercuts and surface detail must be recorded with accuracy.

RIGID MATERIALS*

Plaster of Paris. One type of rigid impression material is plaster of Paris, which has been used in dentistry for over 200 years. Although all plaster-of-Paris impression materials are handled in

---

*Much of this discussion has been quoted or paraphrased from McCracken, W.L.: Impression materials in prosthetic dentistry, Dent. Clin. North Am., pp. 671-684, Nov., 1958.

approximately the same manner, the setting and flow characteristics of each manufacturer's product will vary. Some are pure, finely ground plaster of Paris with only an accelerator added to expedite setting within reasonable working limits. Others are modified impression plasters in which binders and plasticizers have been added to permit limited border molding while the material is setting. These do not set as hard or fracture as clean as pure plaster of Paris and therefore cannot be reassembled with as much accuracy if fracture occurs. However, they are preferred by some dentists because of their setting characteristics.

Plaster of Paris was once the only material that could be used for partial denture impressions, but now elastic materials have completely replaced the impression plasters in this phase of prosthetic dentistry. It is still widely used for making accurate transfers of abutment castings or copings in the fabrication of fixed restorations and internal attachment dentures, and for making rigid indexes and matrices for various purposes in prosthetic dentistry. Modified impression plasters are used by many dentists to record maxillomandibular relationships (Fig. 19-2, *M* to *O*).

Metallic oxide pastes. A second type of rigid impression material is classified as metallic oxide pastes, these usually being some form of a zinc-oxide–eugenol combination. A number of these pastes are available today, and they are probably more widely used than any other secondary impression material. They are not used as primary impression materials and are not used in stock impression trays.

Metallic oxide pastes are manufactured with a wide variation of consistencies and setting characteristics. For convenience, most of them are dispensed from two tubes, an arrangement that enables the dentist to mix the correct proportion from each tube onto a glass or paper mixing slab. The previously prepared tray is loaded and positioned in the mouth with or without any attempt at border molding. Generally, border molding of metallic oxide impression pastes is not advisable, as wrinkles will occur if movement is permitted at the time the material reaches its setting state. Therefore, as in most modern impression techniques, the accuracy of the primary impression and of the impression tray has a great influence on the final impression. Some metallic oxide pastes remain fluid for a longer period of time than do others, and some manufacturers claim that border molding is possible. In general, however, all metallic oxide pastes have one thing in common with plaster-of-Paris impression materials: they all have a setting time during which they should not be disturbed and after which no further border molding is effective.

Although metallic oxide pastes, being rigid substances, are widely used as secondary impression materials for complete dentures, they are also used for secondary impressions in removable partial denture techniques. One widely used removable partial denture impression technique uses a paste impression of the edentulous ridge made in a resin or shellac impression tray, which is then finger-loaded through an opening in a stock perforated tray while an overall alginate hydrocolloid impression is made of the entire arch. This technique attempts to relate the zinc oxide impression of the edentulous ridge to the rest of the arch in a relationship similar to that which will be assumed when an occlusal load is applied (Chapter 15).

Metallic oxide pastes are also used as an impression material for relining denture bases and may be used successfully for this purpose if the original denture base has been relieved sufficiently to allow the material to flow without displacement of either the denture or the underlying tissues.

THERMOPLASTIC MATERIALS*

Modeling plastic. Like plaster of Paris, modeling plastic is among the oldest impression materials used in prosthetic dentistry. It is manufactured "in several different colors, each color being an indication of the temperature range at which the material is plastic and workable. A common error in the use of modeling plastic is that it is subjected to higher temperatures than intended by the manufacturer. It then becomes too soft and loses [some of] its favorable working characteristics. If a controlled water bath is not used, a thermometer should be used routinely

---

*Much of this discussion has been quoted or paraphrased from McCracken, W.L.: Impression materials in prosthetic dentistry, Dent. Clin. North Am., pp. 671-684, Nov., 1958.

to maintain a temperature within limits that will not cause a weakening of the material or influence its working characteristics. If modeling plastic is softened at a temperature above that intended by the manufacturer, the material becomes brittle and unpredictable. Also there is the ever-present danger of burning the patient when the temperature used in softening the modeling plastic is too high."

The most commonly used modeling plastic is the red material that, in cake form, softens at about 132° F. It should never be softened at temperatures much above this. Neither it nor any other modeling plastic should be immersed in the water bath for an indefinite period of time. Rather, it should not leave the dentist's fingers during the softening period for more than a few seconds. It should be dipped and kneaded until soft, and it should be subjected to no more heat than necessary before loading the tray and positioning it in the mouth. Then it may be flamed with an alcohol torch for the purpose of border molding, but should always be tempered by being dipped back into the water bath before its return to the mouth to avoid burning the patient. The modeling plastic then may be chilled before removal from the mouth, although this is not necessary if care is used in removing the impression. During sectional flaming and border molding it should be chilled in ice water after each removal from the mouth. Then it may be trimmed with a sharp knife without danger of fracture or distortion.

The red, gray, and green modeling plastics are obtainable in stick form for use in border molding an impression or an impression tray. The green material is the lowest fusing of the modeling plastics. The red and gray sticks have a higher and broader working range than do the cakes of like color so that they may be flamed without harming the material. Because of its contrasting lighter color, the gray material in stick form is preferred by some dentists for border molding. The choice between the use of green and gray sticks is purely optional and entirely up to the dentist.

Although modeling plastic had been used in past years as an impression material for diagnostic casts, it has now been replaced by the elastic materials. Some dentists still prefer to use modeling plastic as a secondary impression material for the recording of edentulous ridges in partial denture construction, but when this is done, the limitations and disadvantages are the same as for making a full modeling plastic impression for complete dentures. Similarly, modeling plastic is sometimes used as a reline impression material for partial denture bases. However, it is generally used only as a means of building up the underside of the denture before recording the tissues with some secondary impression material (Chapter 15).

Impression waxes and natural resins. A second group of thermoplastic impression materials are those impression waxes and resins commonly spoken of as "mouth-temperature waxes." The most familiar of these have been the Iowa wax and the Korecta waxes, both of which were developed for specific techniques. One must be cognizant of the characteristics of mouth-temperature waxes and use them knowingly. Manufacture of Korecta wax has now been discontinued by the Kerr Company.

The Iowa wax was developed for use in recording the functional or supporting form of an edentulous ridge. It may be used either as a secondary impression material or as an impression material for relining the finished partial denture to obtain support from the underlying tissues. "The mouth-temperature waxes lend themselves well to all relining techniques as they will flow sufficiently in the mouth to avoid overdisplacement of tissues. As with any relining technique, it is necessary that sufficient relief be provided. In addition, escapement slots or holes in the original base must be used, to avoid locking the impression material against the tissue without opportunity for escape." Given an opportunity to flow, the fluid waxes record the tissues without overdisplacement and assure uniformity of support for the partial denture base.

The difference between impression wax and modeling plastic is that the impression waxes have the ability to flow as long as they are in the mouth and thereby permit equalization of pressure and prevent overdisplacement; whereas the modeling plastics flow only in proportion to the amount of flaming and tempering that can be done out of the mouth, and this does not continue after the plastic has approached mouth temperature. The principal advantage of mouth-temperature waxes is that given sufficient time they permit a rebound of those tissues that have been overdisplaced.

The impression waxes also may be used to correct the borders of impressions made of more rigid materials, thereby establishing optimal contact at the border of the denture. All mouth-temperature wax impressions have the ability to record border detail accurately and at the same time establish the correct width of the denture border. They have the advantage of being correctable, and if the dentist will take sufficient time in making the correction, not only surface detail may be recorded accurately, but also all border areas that are available for support and retention of the denture.

Some mouth-temperature waxes vary in their working characteristics from those mentioned herein. Among these are the Jelenko Adaptol impression material and the Stalite impression material. Both of these seem to have a more resinous base. They are designed primarily for impression techniques that attempt to record the tissues under an occlusal load. In such techniques the occlusion rim or the arrangement of artificial teeth is completed first. Mouth-temperature wax is then applied to the tissue side of the denture base, and the final impression is made under functional loading, using various movements simulating functional activity. However, these mouth-temperature materials also may be used successfully in open-mouth impression techniques.

The Iowa wax will not distort after removal from the mouth at ordinary room temperatures, but the more resinous waxes must be stored at much lower temperatures to avoid flow when out of the mouth. Resinous waxes are not ordinarily used in partial denture impression techniques except for secondary impressions.

ELASTIC MATERIALS*

Reversible hydrocolloids. Reversible (agar) hydrocolloids, which are fluid at higher temperatures and gel on a reduction in temperature, are used primarily as impression materials for fixed restorations. They are unsurpassed for accuracy when properly used. However, the reversible hydrocolloid impression materials offer few advantages over the irreversible (alginate) hydrocolloids when used as a partial denture impression material. Present-day alginate hydrocolloids are sufficiently accurate for making master casts for partial dentures. However, border control of impressions made with these materials is difficult.

Irreversible hydrocolloids. The irreversible hydrocolloids are used for the making of diagnostic casts, orthodontic treatment casts, and master casts for removable partial denture procedures. Since they are made of colloidal materials, neither reversible nor irreversible hydrocolloid impressions can be stored for any length of time, but must be poured immediately.

Mercaptan rubber-base impression materials. The mercaptan rubber-base (Thiokol) impression materials are used for removable partial denture impressions and especially for secondary or altered cast impressions. To be accurate the impression must have a uniform thickness not exceeding 3 mm (⅛ in). This necessitates the use of a carefully made individual impression tray of acrylic resin or some other material possessing adequate rigidity and stability. It is doubtful that the accuracy of a mercaptan rubber-base impression exceeds that of a properly made alginate hydrocolloid impression, and as with the hydrocolloid impression materials, certain precautions must be taken to avoid distortion of the impression. The mercaptan rubber-base impression materials do have an advantage over the hydrocolloid materials in that the surface of an artificial stone poured against them is of a smoother texture and therefore appears to be smoother and harder than one poured against a hydrocolloid material. This is probably because the rubber material does not have the ability to retard or etch the surface of the setting stone. Despite their accuracy, this has always been a disadvantage of all hydrocolloid impression materials. A cast made from a mercaptan rubber or silicone impression possesses a smoother surface that may possibly lead to a more accurate dental casting. The fact that a smoother surface results does not, however, preclude the possibility of a grossly inaccurate

---

*Much of this discussion has been quoted or paraphrased from McCracken, W.L.: Impression materials in prosthetic dentistry, Dent. Clin. North Am., pp. 671-684, Nov., 1958.

impression and stone cast resulting from other causes. Rubber-base impression materials, possessing a longer setting time than the irreversible hydrocolloid materials, lend themselves better to border molding in adequate supporting trays.

Silicone impression materials. The silicone impression materials are similar in their accuracy and convenience to the rubber-base impression materials. They are used primarily as impression materials for crown and fixed partial denture procedures and require the same precautions as do the rubber-base materials. They are more delicate to handle in the laboratory, and because of their cost and delicate nature they are not widely used as impression materials for removable partial denture master casts. In general, however, they possess many of the same advantages and disadvantages of rubber-base materials and may be similarly used when handled with care.

Polyether impression materials. Polyether impression material is a rubber-type material, as are the polysulfide and silicone materials. A working time of 2 minutes and a setting time of 2.5 minutes for the polyether materials are comparatively short and limit the extensiveness of an impression. The flow characteristics of polyether material are very low—the lowest of any rubber impression material. Its flexibility is also very low (stiffness is high). These characteristics limit its use in removable partial prosthodontics; however, it is widely used in fixed prosthodontics.

IMPRESSIONS OF THE PARTIALLY EDENTULOUS ARCH

An impression of the partially edentulous arch must record accurately the anatomic form of the teeth and surrounding tissues. This is necessary so that the prosthesis may be designed to follow a definite path of placement and removal and so that support and retention on the abutment teeth may be precise and accurate.

Materials that could be permanently deformed by removal from tissue undercuts may not be used. This excludes the use of the thermoplastic impression materials for recording the anatomic form of the dental arch. The rigid materials such as plaster of Paris are capable of recording tissue detail accurately, but they must be sectioned for removal and subsequently reassembled.

Before the advent of the elastic hydrocolloid materials, plaster of Paris and modeling plastic were the only impression materials available for impressions of the partially edentulous arch. Modeling plastic was used for making preliminary impressions for diagnostic casts, despite its distortion on removal from undercuts. Such diagnostic casts were grossly inaccurate and permitted only approximate evaluation of tooth contours. Impressions for master casts were made of plaster of Paris, which was scored and sectioned for removal and then reassembled. This was time consuming and discomforting to the patient.

Plaster of Paris is accurate, dimensionally stable, and inexpensive and requires no special equipment for its use. Its main disadvantages are its inflexibility and the fact that some separating medium must be used before pouring the cast to prevent the cast material, which is usually also a gypsum product, from adhering to it. Damage to the resulting cast can easily occur during removal of the impression from the cast. Since it must be removed from the mouth sectionally, small pieces from essential areas may be lost, and reassembly of the pieces may take considerable time.

The introduction of hydrocolloids as impression materials was a long step forward in dentistry. For the first time impressions could be made of undercut areas with a material that was elastic enough to be withdrawn from those undercuts without permanent distortion. It permits the making of a one-piece impression, which does not require the use of a separating medium, and it is an extremely accurate material when handled properly.

Phillips has reduced the complicated chemistry of the hydrocolloid impression materials to its simplest form in the following paragraphs:

Hydrocolloids can be classified into two general types: reversible and irreversible. These materials are suspensions of aggregates of molecules in a dispersing medium of water, the water being held by capillary action. Gelation of the reversible hydrocolloids is primarily a physical change in which a latticework of fibrils forms as the temperature is lowered. This gel can be readily dispersed by merely heating the material—thus the term reversible. An example of a reversible hydrocolloid is ordinary gelatin. When gelatin is dissolved in boiling water, it forms a colloidal sol which gels upon cooling. This gel can be returned to the liquid sol by heating, formed again by cooling, etc.

The base for dental reversible hydrocolloids is agar-agar, a material that can be liquefied at temperatures compatible to oral tissues and then solidified to a firm, yet elastic, gel at temperatures slightly above 100° F. This gelation is acocmplished by means of water-cooled impression trays. Such factors as ability to secure routinely accurate reproductions of cavity preparation with one impression, reproductions of minor undercuts without rupture or distortion, and actual saving in chair time have been instrumental in the successful adaptation of this material for use in the indirect inlay technique. It is unexcelled when used in this procedure.

The irreversible hydrocolloids, or alginates, are not thermally reversible and their gelation is induced by an actual chemical reaction rather than by physical means. The powder is essentially sodium alginate and calcium sulphate which when mixed with water react to form a latticework of fibrils of insoluble calcium alginate. These materials have been used extensively in prosthetics and orthodontia. . . .

In general it can be said that the alginates approach the accuracy of reversible hydrocolloid but, due to the greater number of variables both in their manufacture and use, they are not routinely quite as accurate.*

The principal differences between agar and alginate hydrocolloids are as follows:

1. Agar converts from the gel form to a sol by the application of heat. It may be reverted to gel form by a reduction in temperature. This physical change is reversible.

2. Alginate hydrocolloid becomes a gel via a chemical reaction as a result of mixing alginate powder with water. This physical change is irreversible.

Agar hydrocolloid does have some disadvantages. It must be introduced into the mouth while warm enough to be a sol, converting to an elastic gel on cooling. Therefore there is an ever-present danger of burning the tissues of the mouth, a burn that is painful and slow to heal. It requires warming and tempering equipment that is thermostatically controlled and necessitates the use of water-jacketed impression trays for cooling.

All hydrocolloids are dimensionally stable only during a brief period after removal from the mouth. If exposed to the air, they rapidly lose water content, with a resulting shrinkage and other dimensional changes. If immersed in water, they imbibe water, with an accompanying swelling and dimensional changes. All hydrocolloid impressions should be poured immediately, but if they must be stored for a brief period of time, it should be in a saturated atmosphere rather than in water. This is accomplished simply by wrapping the impression in a damp towel.

All hydrocolloids also exhibit a phenomenon known as syneresis, which is associated with the giving off of a mucinous exudate. This mucinous exudate has a retarding effect on any gypsum material, which results in a soft or chalky cast surface. Sometimes this is only detected by a close examination of the impression after removal from the cast. Nevertheless, such a cast surface is inaccurate, and an inaccurate denture casting ultimately results in proportion to the inaccuracy of the master cast. This can only be prevented by pouring the cast immediately and using some chemical accelerator such as potassium sulfate to counteract the retarding effect of the hydrocolloid.

Agar hydrocolloid impressions should be immersed in a 2% solution of potassium sulfate for 5 to 10 minutes before the cast is poured, even though some accelerator may have been incorporated by the manufacturer. Almost all modern alginate hydrocolloid impression materials have an accelerator incorporated into the powder and no longer need to be treated with a "fixing solution" unless one is supplied by the manufacturer. However, an alginate hydrocolloid impression material that is compounded to require a "fixing solution" consistently gives a smoother cast surface than those that do not require immersion in such a solution. It is probably because of the popular demand for alginate impression materials that do not require fixing that the suppliers have all but abandoned the manufacture of those requiring a fixing solution.

---

*From Phillips, R.W.: The physical properties of hydrocolloids and alginates and factors influencing their work qualities and accuracy, Fortn. Rev. Chic. Dent. Soc. **26**:9-12, 1953.

Since no heat is employed in the preparation of alginate hydrocolloid, there is no danger of burning the patient. For this reason the patient will be more relaxed and cooperative during the positioning of the tray. However, some disadvantages are associated with the use of alginate hydrocolloid. This material gels by means of a chemical reaction that is accelerated by the warmth of the tissues, whereas agar hydrocolloid gels from the tray in toward the tissues, because of the cooling action of the water circulating through the tray. In the former, gelation takes place first next to the tissues, and any movement of the tray during gelation of the remote portions results in internal stresses that are released on removal of the impression from the mouth. A distorted and therefore inaccurate impression results from an alginate hydrocolloid impression that is not held immobile during gelation.

Another disadvantage of alginate hydrocolloid is that it must be introduced into the mouth at approximately 70° F, which causes an immediate increase in the viscosity and surface tension of the saliva. Air bubbles are therefore harder to dispel, and it is inevitable that more air will be trapped in an alginate impression than in an agar impression. Every precaution must be taken to avoid the entrapment of air in critical areas.

Important precautions to be observed in the handling of hydrocolloid. Some important precautions to be observed in the handling of hydrocolloid are as follows:

1. Impression should not be exposed to air because some dehydration will inevitably occur, resulting in shrinkage.

2. Impression should not be immersed in water because some imbibition will inevitably result, with an accompanying expansion.

3. Impression should be protected from dehydration by placing it in a humid atmosphere or wrapping it in a damp towel until a cast can be poured. To avoid volume change, this should be within 15 minutes after removal from the mouth.

4. Exudate from hydrocolloid has a retarding effect on the chemical reaction of gypsum products and results in a chalky cast surface. This can be prevented by pouring the cast immediately and by first immersing the impression in a solution of accelerator.

Step-by-step procedure for making a hydrocolloid impression. The step-by-step procedure and important points to observe in the making of a hydrocolloid impression are as follows:

1. Select a suitable, sanitary, perforated impression tray that is large enough to provide a 4 to 5 mm border thickness of the impression material.

2. Build up the palatal portion of the maxillary impression tray with wax or modeling plastic to ensure even distribution of the impression material and to prevent the material from slumping away from the palatal surface (Fig. 14-1, *A*).

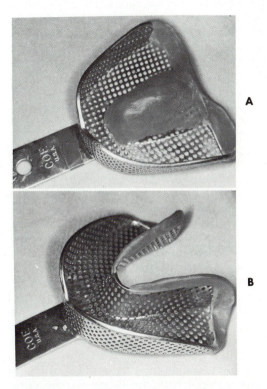

Fig. 14-1. **A,** Maxillary impression tray with palatal portion built up with beeswax to prevent impression material from sagging away from palatal surface. Beeswax is also added across posterior border of tray to cover maxillary tuberosities and to prevent impression material from being expelled posteriorly when impression is made. **B,** Mandibular impression tray with beeswax added to lingual flanges to prevent tissues of floor of mouth from rising inside tray. Posterior end of tray is extended with beeswax to cover retromolar pad regions.

If gelation occurs next to the tissues while the deeper portion is still fluid, a distorted impression of the palate may result, which cannot be detected in the finished impression. This may result in the major connector of the finished casting not being in contact with the underlying tissues. The maxillary tray frequently has to be extended posteriorly to include the tuberosities and vibrating line region of the palate. Such an extension also aids in correctly orienting the tray in the patient's mouth when the impression is being made.

3. The lingual flange of the mandibular tray may need to be lengthened with beeswax in the retromylohyoid area or to be extended posteriorly, but it rarely ever needs to be lengthened elsewhere. Beeswax may need to be added **inside** the distolingual flange to prevent the tissues of the floor of the mouth from rising inside the tray (Fig. 14-1, *B*).

4. Place the patient in an upright position, with the involved arch nearly parallel to the floor.

5. When using alginate hydrocolloid, place the measured amount of water (at 70° F) in a clean, dry, rubber mixing bowl (600 ml capacity). Add the correct measure of powder. Spatulate rapidly against the side of the bowl with a short, **stiff** spatula. This should be accomplished in less than 1 minute. The patient should rinse his mouth with cool water to eliminate excess saliva while the impression material is being mixed and the tray is being loaded.

6. In placing the material in the tray, try to avoid entrapping air. Have the first layer of material lock through the perforations of the tray to prevent any possible dislodgment after gelation.

7. After loading the tray, quickly place (rub) some material with the finger on any critical areas such as rest preparations and abutment teeth. If a maxillary impression is being made, place material in the highest aspect of the palate and over the rugae.

8. Use a mouth mirror or index finger to retract the cheek on the side away from you as the tray is being rotated into the mouth from the near side.

9. Seat the tray first on the side away from you, next on the anterior area while reflecting the lip, and then on the near side, using the mouth mirror or finger for cheek retraction. Finally make sure that the lip is draping naturally over the tray.

10. Be careful not to seat the tray too deeply, leaving room for a thickness of material over the occlusal and incisal surfaces.

11. Hold the tray immobile for 3 minutes with light finger pressure over left and right premolar areas. Do not allow the tray to move during gelation to avoid internal stresses in the finished impression. Do not allow the patient or the assistant to hold the tray in position. Some movement of the tray is inevitable during the transfer, and at a critical time of gelation, movement will produce an inaccurate impression. Do not remove the impression from the mouth until the impression material has completely set.

12. After releasing the surface tension, remove the impression quickly in line with the long axis of the teeth to avoid tearing or other distortion.

13. Rinse the impression free of saliva with slurry water, or dust with plaster and rinse gently, then examine critically. Cover the impression immediately with a damp towel.

A cast should be poured immediately into a hydrocolloid impression to avoid dimensional changes and syneresis. Circumstances often necessitate some delay, but this time lapse should be kept to a minimum. A delay not exceeding 15 minutes may not be deleterious if the impression is kept in a humid atmosphere.

Step-by-step procedure for making a stone cast from a hydrocolloid impression. The step-by-step procedure for making the stone cast from the impression is as follows:

1. Have the measured dental stone at hand, along with a measured quantity of water, as recommended by the manufacturer. For most laboratory stones, 28 ml of water for each 100 g is recommended; for improved stones the proportion is 24 ml of water for each 100 g. A clean 600 ml mixing bowl, a stiff spatula, and a vibrator complete the preparations. A No. 7 spatula also should be within reach.

2. First pour the measure of water into the mixing bowl and then add the measure of stone. Spatulate thoroughly for 1 minute, remembering that a weak and porous stone cast may result

from insufficient spatulation. **Mechanical spatulation or vacuum spatulation if such facilities are available may be used to advantage.** After any spatulation other than in a vacuum, place the mixing bowl on the vibrator and knead the material to permit the escape of any trapped air.

3. The hydrocolloid impression material used may require a fixing solution. If so, follow the manufacturer's instructions. Any fixing is done just before pouring the cast and is not meant to be used as a storing medium. After removing the impression from the damp towel or fixing solution, gently shake out surplus moisture and hold the impression over the vibrator, impression side up, with only the handle of the tray contacting the vibrator. The impression material must not be placed in contact with the vibrator because of possible distortion of the impression.

4. With a small spatula add the first cast material to the distal area away from you. Allow this first material to be vibrated around the arch from tooth to tooth toward the anterior part of the impression (Fig. 14-2). Continue to add small increments of material at this same distal area, each portion of added stone pushing the mass ahead of it. This avoids the entrapment of air. The weight of the material causes any excess water to be pushed around the arch and to be expelled ultimately at the opposite end of the impression. Discard this fluid material. When the impressions of all teeth have been filled, continue to add artificial stone in larger portions until the impression is completely filled.

5. The filled impression should be placed on a supporting jig and the base of the cast completed with the same mix of stone (Fig. 14-3). The base of the cast should be 16 to 18 mm (⅔ to ¾ in) at its thinnest portion and should be extended beyond the borders of the impression so that buccal, labial, and lingual borders will be recorded correctly in the finished cast. **A distorted cast may result from an inverted impression.**

6. As soon as the cast material has developed sufficient body, trim the gross excess from the sides of the cast. Wrap the impression and cast in a wet paper towel or place it in a humidor until the initial set of the stone has taken place. The impression is thus prevented from losing water by evaporation, which might in turn de-

prive the cast material of sufficient water for crystallization. Chalky cast surfaces around the teeth are often the result of the hydrocolloid's acting as a sponge and robbing the cast material of its necessary water for crystallization.

7. After the cast and impression have been in the humid atmosphere for 30 minutes, separate the impression from the cast. Thirty minutes is sufficient for initial setting. Any stone interfering with separation must be trimmed away with a knife.

8. Clean the impression tray immediately while the used impression material is still elastic.

9. The trimming of the cast should be deferred until final setting has occurred. The sides

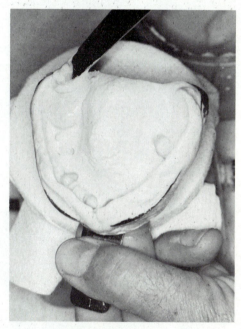

Fig. 14-2. Small portions of mechanically spatulated stone are applied at posterior section of impression and vibrated around arch, pushing moisture and diluted stone ahead of mass. Stone is applied at this point only until impressions of teeth are filled and diluted stone is discarded at opposite end. Only then is remainder of impression filled with larger portions, using larger spatula. Only handle of impression tray should be allowed to touch vibrator so that distortion of impression material will be avoided. (Note that vibrator is protected with paper towel as impression is being filled.)

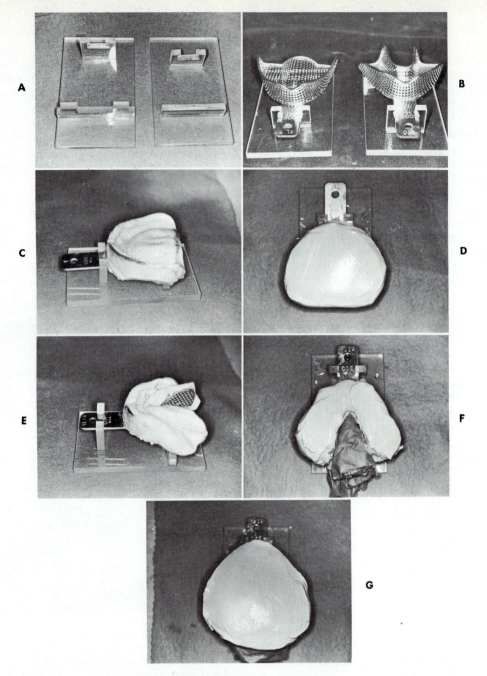

Fig. 14-3. A, Homemade plastic jigs are used to support impressions. Handle of tray is placed in slotted portion, and posterior end of tray is supported by elevated cross-members. Jig used to support mandibular impression is on left. **B,** Note that impression trays are elevated and contact jigs at only three points. **C,** An impression could be easily distorted when cast is being poured if tray was placed on laboratory bench. Since impression is elevated by jig, distortion of impression is minimized. **D,** After impression is filled with stone, as previously demonstrated, it is placed in jig and additional stone is added to form base of cast. **E,** Mandibular impression placed in jig to demonstrate support by jig. Note that impression is supported by contact of tray only at handle and on either side posteriorly. **F,** Impression is returned to supporting jig after being filled with stone. Wet paper is placed in tongue space to support stone base in this region and to avoid locking impression tray to cast. **G,** Additional stone is added to impression to form base for cast.

of the cast then may be trimmed to be parallel, and any blebs or defects resulting from air bubbles in the impression may be removed. If this is a cast for a permanent record, it may be trimmed to orthodontic specification to present a neat appearance for demonstration purposes. Master casts and other working casts are ordinarily trimmed only to remove excess stone.

Possible causes of an inaccurate cast of a dental arch. The possible causes of an inaccurate cast are as follows:

1. Distortion of the hydrocolloid impression (a) by partial dislodgment from tray, (b) by shrinkage caused by dehydration, (c) by expansion caused by imbibition (this will be toward the teeth and will result in an undersize rather than oversize cast), (d) by attempting to pour the cast with stone that is too resistant.

2. A ratio of water to powder that is too high. While this may not cause volumetric changes in the size of the cast, it will result in a weak cast.

3. Improper mixing. This also results in a weak cast or one with a chalky surface.

4. Trapping of air, either in the mix or in pouring, because of insufficient vibration.

5. Soft or chalky cast surface resulting from the retarding action of the hydrocolloid or the absorption of necessary water for crystallization by the dehydrating hydrocolloid.

6. Premature separation of the cast from the impression.

7. Failure to separate the cast from the impression for an extended period of time.

INDIVIDUAL IMPRESSION TRAYS

This chapter has dealt previously with making an impression in a stock tray of the anatomic form of a dental arch for making a diagnostic cast, a working cast for restorations, or a master cast. There are times, however, when a stock tray is not suitable for making the final anatomic impression of the dental arch. Most tooth-borne partial dentures may be made on a master cast from such an impression. Some maxillary distal extension partial dentures with broad palatal coverage, particularly those for a Kennedy Class I arch, may also be made on an anatomic cast, but usually these necessitate the use of an individually made tray.

Unless a stock tray can be found that will fit the mouth with about 6 mm clearance for the impression material, yet without interference with bordering tissues, an individual tray made of some resin tray material should be used for the final anatomic impression.

Most partial denture trays are either of the rim-lock or perforated varieties. Both are made in a limited selection of sizes and shapes. One manufacturer in particular has gone to considerable length to provide a wide selection of perforated trays, including trays for both bilateral and unilateral edentulous areas, trays with built-in occlusal stops, and trays for particular techniques* (Fig. 14-4).

All these trays have reinforced borders. Although a complete denture impression tray is, or should be, made of material that permits trimming and shaping to fit the mouth, the existence of a beaded border and the rigidity of a stock partial denture tray allow no trimming and little shaping. **The resulting impression is often a record of border tissues distorted by an ill-fitting tray rather than an impression of tissues draping naturally over a slightly underextended impression tray.**

An individual acrylic resin tray, on the other hand, can be made with sufficient clearance for the impression material and can be trimmed just short of the vestibular reflections to allow the tissues to drape naturally without distortion. The partial denture borders may then be made as accurate as complete denture borders with equal advantages.

Although techniques have been proposed for making individual impression trays that incorporate plastic tubing for water-cooling agar hydrocolloid impressions, the final anatomic impression usually will be made with alginate hydrocolloid, mercaptan rubber, or silicone impression materials.

Technique for making individual acrylic resin impression trays. The diagnostic cast is often adequate for the preparation of the individual tray. However, if extensive surgery or extractions were performed after making the diagnostic cast, a new impression in a stock tray and a new cast must be made. The procedures for making the new cast are identical to those described previously.

*Nevin, J.J.: Tray selection for partial denture impressions, Cal **26:**10-16, July, 1963.

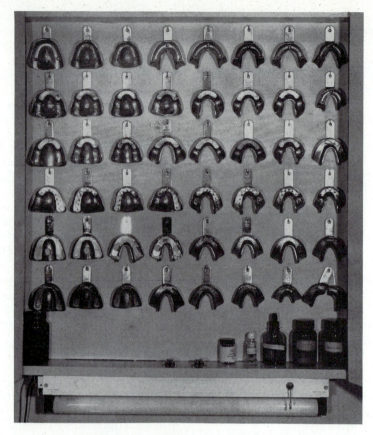

Fig. 14-4. Impression tray cabinet with doors open, exposing wide selection of perforated impression trays for alginate hydrocolloid impressions. Beginning at top are impression trays for completely edentulous mouths, depressed anterior trays, trays with unilateral occlusal stops, Hindels trays for use with double impression technique, and more commonly and regularly used perforated trays.

A duplicate of the diagnostic cast, on which the individual tray can be fabricated, should be made. The cast on which an individual tray is made is often damaged or must be mutilated to separate the tray from the cast. Obviously the original diagnostic cast must be retained as a permanent record in the patient's file.

The technique for making an individual maxillary acrylic resin tray is as follows:

1. Outline the extent of the tray on the cast with a pencil. The tray must include all teeth and tissues that will be involved in the removable partial denture. Adequate space must be provided for frenal attachments. Mark the area of the posterior palatal seal on the maxillary cast

and cut a 1 mm × 1 mm groove following the line designating the posterior extent of the tray (Fig. 14-5, *A*).

2. Adapt one layer of baseplate wax over the tissue surfaces and teeth of the cast to serve as a spacer for impression material. The wax spacer should be trimmed to the outline drawn on the diagnostic cast. Wax covering the posterior palatal seal area should be removed so that intimate contact of the tray and tissue in this region may serve as an aid in correctly orienting the tray when making the impression (Fig. 14-5, *B*).

3. Adapt an additional layer of baseplate wax over the teeth if the impression is to be made in irreversible hydrocolloid (alginate). This step

is not necessary if the choice of impression material is a rubber-base or silicone type of material.

4. Expose portions of the incisal edges of the central incisors to serve as anterior stops when placing the tray in the mouth. Bevel the wax so that the completed tray will have a guiding incline that will help position the tray on the anterior stop.

5. Paint the exposed surfaces of the cast that may be contacted by the acrylic resin tray material with a tinfoil substitute (Alcote) to facilitate separation of the cured tray from the cast.

6. Mix the correct proportions of auto polymerizing acrylic resin (8 ml of monomer to 24 ml of polymer) in a mixing jar or paper cup. When the resin mix is no longer stringy and can be handled without adhering to the fingers, form it into a wafer the size and thickness of a cake of modeling plastic or use special stone templates to form the wafer (Fig. 14-5, *C* to *E*). A wooden roller and wafer-forming block are also available from dental supply houses in kit form.

7. Carefully transfer the resin wafer to position on the cast and adapt the resin with the fingers, covering the wax spacer and palatal seal area and maintaining a uniform thickness. Remove the gross excess with a sharp knife while the resin is still soft.

8. Form a handle with the excess resin. The handle should be about 12 mm (½ in) in width, about 6 mm (¼ in) in thickness, and about 5 cm (2 in) long.

9. Attach the handle to the tray over the region of the central incisors and shape it to extend 12 mm (½ in) downward and 2.5 cm (1 in) outward (Fig. 14-5, *F*). It is usually necessary to place additional monomer on the handle and tray to provide a satisfactory union.

10. Allow the resin to cure, and remove the tray from the cast. The wax spacer can be removed from the tray with any suitable instrument.

11. Perfect the borders of the tray with rotary instruments (vulcanite burs, acrylic resin trimmers) and roughly polish the external surface of the tray (Fig. 14-5, *G*).

12. Place perforations (No. 8 bur size) in the resin tray at 4.5 mm (³⁄₁₆ in) intervals, with the exception of the alveolar groove areas, if an irreversible hydrocolloid impression material is to be used (Fig. 14-6).

13. The tray must be **sanitized** and tried in the mouth so that any necessary corrections to the tray can be accomplished before the impression is made.

The technique for making an individual mandibular acrylic resin tray follows the same procedures. The buccal shelf regions on the lower cast are left uncovered by the wax spacer to serve as posterior stops in orienting the tray in the patient's mouth and at the same time will permit selective placement of tissues in the mandibular stress-bearing areas (Fig. 14-7).

Perforations in a resin tray are not easily made with a round bur because after a few revolutions the bur becomes clogged. Instead a bi-beveled surgical drill is used, which will make the holes rapidly without clogging (Fig. 14-8). These are available in various sizes No. 100 through 106, the higher number being the smaller size. The size of the perforations should be slightly larger than those in a stock tray, and only about one third as many are used. This will be sufficient to lock the impression material in the tray and thereby avoid distortion of the impression on removal from the mouth.

If mercaptan rubber or silicone is to be used, perforations are not usually necessary to lock the material in the tray, as the adhesive provided by the manufacturer provides reliable retention, and some confinement of these materials is desirable. However, a series of perforations are placed in the median palatal raphe and incisive papilla areas of the maxillary tray so that excess impression material will escape through them, thus providing relief of the tissues in this area. For the same reasons, perforations are placed in the alveolar groove of the mandibular tray. With the use of adhesives the impression material is not easily removed from the tray should a faulty impression have to be remade, but this is an inconvenience common to all newer elastic materials and does not prevent reuse of the impression tray.

The pouring of a cast in an irreversible hydrocolloid impression made in an individual tray presents a minor problem, since the tray is usually covered with the elastic material and is delicate to handle. Some of the excess material in

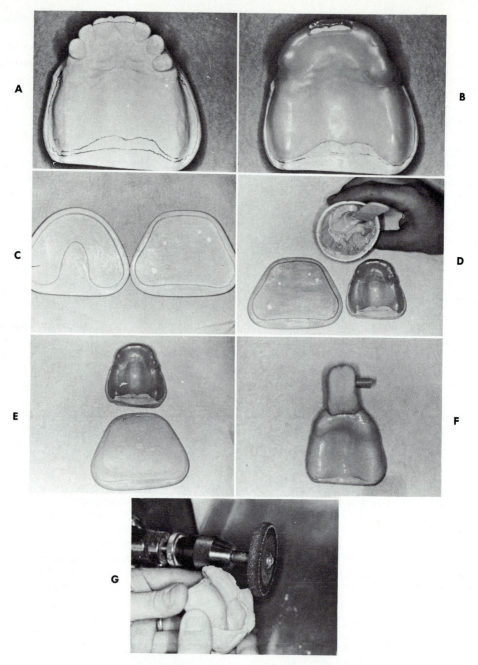

Fig. 14-5. For legend, see opposite page.

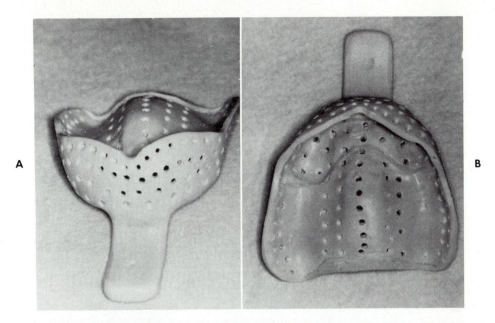

A　　　　　　　　　　　　　　　　　　　　　　　B

Fig. 14-6. **A,** Holes are drilled through tray, being spaced approximately 4.5 mm (³⁄₁₆ in) apart. These holes will serve to lock impression material in tray. In addition, excess impression material is forced out of holes when impression is made, thereby minimally displacing soft oral tissues. **B,** Note elevated posterior palatal seal region of tray and incisal stop. These two features will assist in correctly orienting individualized impression tray in mouth.

Fig. 14-5. **A,** Desired outline of tray is drawn on duplicate diagnostic cast. Posterior palatal seal region and portion of incisal edges of central incisors are outlined. **B,** One thickness of baseplate wax is adapted to cast and is trimmed to penciled outline. Posterior palatal seal region is not covered by wax but will be included in finished tray. Two thicknesses of baseplate wax cover teeth. Window is created in wax spacer over incisal edges. Tinfoil substitute is painted on stone surfaces of cast that will be contacted by autopolymerizing acrylic resin. **C,** Stone templates are used to form uniform wafers of acrylic resin dough about 3 mm thick. Left template is used in making mandibular impression trays. These templates may be made by embedding double thick shellac baseplate form in 12 mm (½ in) thick patty of stone. They are lightly lubricated with petroleum jelly so that soft tray material will not adhere to stone when acrylic resin wafer is being made. **D,** Tray resin is mixed in paper cup with wooden tongue depressor. Tray material is spatulated onto stone template when it reaches "nontacky" stage. **E,** Uniform acrylic resin wafer is made on stone template by using tongue depressor as trowel to fill mold and to remove excess tray material. **F,** Resin wafer is carefully removed from template and adapted over cast with fingers. Excess tray material is removed from borders of cast with sharp knife while resin is still doughy. Excess material is used to shape handle, which is attached over incisal edges of anterior teeth. It is supported by piece of baseplate wax until resin has become hard. **G,** As soon as tray material has hardened, tray is removed from cast, and wax spacer is removed from rough tray. Acrylic resin trimmer in lathe is used to rough finish the tray.

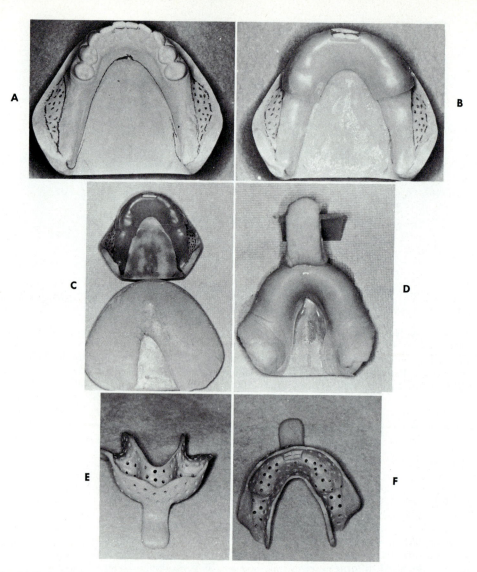

Fig. 14-7. A, Outline of tray is penciled on duplicate mandibular diagnostic cast. Buccal shelf region is outlined on each side of cast (dotted portion). **B,** Single sheet of baseplate wax is adapted to outline of tray, and another sheet of baseplate wax is adapted over teeth. Buccal shelves are uncovered, and window is cut in spacer to expose incisal edges of lower central incisors. **C,** Acrylic resin wafer is formed in stone template as described in Fig. 14-5. **D,** Tray material wafer is adapted over cast and spacer, and handle is formed with excess tray material as previously described. **E** and **F,** Multiple holes are placed throughout tray with the exception of buccal shelf regions of tray and also the elevated incisal stop in tray. Buccal shelf region of tray on either side and incisal stop will assist in correctly orienting tray in patient's mouth.

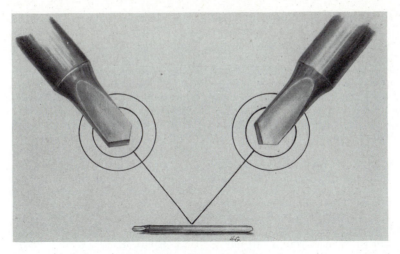

Fig. 14-8. Bi-beveled drill used for making holes in resin impression trays. Such a drill will not clog and facilitates making a perforated impression tray for use with alginate hydrocolloid, mercaptan rubber, or silicone impression materials. They can be readily made with shank portion of straight handpiece bur.

the handle area may have to be cut away to expose enough of the rigid tray to make contact with the vibrator. The impression may then be vibrated while being filled, as with any other hydrocolloid impression.

Master casts made from impressions in individual resin trays are generally more accurate than are those made in stock trays. The use of individual trays should be considered a necessary step in making the majority of removable partial dentures when a secondary impression technique is not to be used. Reasons and methods for making a secondary impression will be considered in Chapter 15.

Final impressions for maxillary tooth-borne removable partial dentures often may be made in carefully selected and recontoured stock impression trays. However, an individual acrylic resin tray is preferred in those situations in the mandibular arch in which the floor of the mouth closely approximates the lingual gingiva of remaining anterior teeth. Recording the floor of the mouth at the elevation it assumes when the lips are licked is important in selecting the type of major connector to be used (Chapter 4). Modification of the borders of an individual tray to fulfill the requirements of an adequate tray is much easier than is the modification of a metal stock tray.

SELF-ASSESSMENT AIDS

1. Impression materials used in various phases of partial denture construction may be classified as rigid, thermoplastic, or elastic. Give two examples for each of the three categories.
2. Which type of impression material has been used the longest in prosthodontics?
3. Why should the metallic oxide paste types of impression material not be used for primary impressions of partially edentulous arches?
4. Modeling plastic (compound) may be used effectively in making secondary impressions of Class I and II partially edentulous arches. Why is it not used for primary impression for the partial denture patient?
5. What is an impression wax? Do its characteristics make it appropriate for use as a primary impression or for a secondary impression?
6. There are two types of hydrocolloid impression materials used in dentistry. What are the two types?
7. Are the hydrocolloid impression materials elastic or thermoplastic?
8. What is the advantage in using an elastic material versus a rigid material in making impressions of partially edentulous arches?
9. Briefly compare reversible and irreversible hydrocolloid impression materials from the standpoints of composition, gelation mechanism, trays, and relative accuracy.
10. Mercaptan rubber-base impression material may be used for primary or secondary impressions.

Its characteristics make it best suited, however, for the _____ impression.

11. Does the use of mercaptan rubber-base material and silicone impression material require the use of a stock tray or an individualized tray? Why?

12. There are many different artificial stones used in dentistry and equally as many impression materials. Are these varied materials necessarily compatible with each other when used to make casts? What precautions should be taken to ensure compatibility?

13. What is syneresis? What effect will this phenomenon have on a cast poured in a hydrocolloid impression?

14. What is meant by the word *imbibition* in relation to hydrocolloid impressions? What effect does it have on a hydrocolloid impression?

15. How long should you wait to pour a cast into a hydrocolloid impression after it is removed from the mouth? Why?

16. What would be the quality of a cast poured in a hydrocolloid impression that had been exposed to air for thirty minutes?

17. The thickness of impression material when rubber-base type material is used should be about 3 mm (⅛ in) for accuracy and stability. Does this equally apply to a hydrocolloid impression material? If not, can you give a rule of thumb for the desirable thickness of the hydrocolloid material in the impression?

18. What are the advantages of using perforated stock trays vs. nonperforated stock trays when making impressions of partially edentulous arches with an irreversible hydrocolloid?

19. Inaccuracies of a cast made from a hydrocolloid impression may result from many causes. Can you think of at least six causes of such inaccuracy?

20. Why should impressions into which stone casts have been poured not be inverted until the initial set of the stone has taken place?

21. An individual acrylic resin impression tray has two distinct advantages over any type of stock tray. Can you think of these two advantages?

22. Describe the procedures for making individual maxillary and mandibular impression trays, paying special attention to relief of the casts with wax spacers.

23. Holes about 3 mm (⅛) in diameter should be placed at strategic locations in both maxillary and mandibular individualized trays. Give the location of the holes and what is accomplished by their presence.

24. What is the advantage of drilling holes in acrylic resin trays with a bi-bevel drill rather than with fissure or round burs?

25. Under what circumstances would you use a stock tray in preference to an individual acrylic resin tray?

15 SUPPORT FOR THE DISTAL EXTENSION DENTURE BASE

Distal extension removable partial denture
Factors influencing the support of a distal extension base
Methods for obtaining functional support for the distal extension base

In a tooth-supported removable partial denture, a metal base or the framework supporting a resin base is connected to and is part of a rigid framework that permits the direct transfer of occlusal forces to the abutment teeth through the occlusal rests. Even though the base of a tooth-supported (Kennedy Class III) partial denture supports the supplied teeth, the residual ridge beneath the base is not called on to aid in the support of the denture. Therefore the resiliency of the ridge tissues and the conformation and type of bone supporting these tissues are not factors in denture support. Regardless of the length of the span, if the framework is rigid, the abutment teeth are sound enough to carry the additional load, and the occlusal rests are properly formed, support comes entirely from the abutment teeth at either end of that span. Support may be augmented by splinting and by the use of additional abutments, but in any event the abutments are the sole support of the removable restoration.

An impression (and resulting reproduction in stone) that records faithfully the anatomic form of the teeth and their surrounding structures and the residual ridges of a dental arch is the only impression needed in making a tooth-borne removable partial denture. The impression also should record the moving tissues that will border the denture in an unstrained position so that the relationship of the denture base to those tissues may be as accurate as possible, being neither overextended nor underextended. Although underextension of the denture base in a tooth-supported prosthesis is the lesser of two evils, an underextended base may lead to food impaction and inadequate contours, particularly on the buccal and labial sides. For this reason, and also to record faithfully the moving tissues of the floor of the mouth in the mandibular arch, an individual impression tray should be used rather than an ill-fitting or overextended stock tray. This has been discussed at length in Chapter 14.

DISTAL EXTENSION REMOVABLE PARTIAL DENTURE

The distal extension denture does not have the advantage of total tooth support, since one or more bases are extensions onto the residual ridge from the last available abutment. It therefore is dependent on the residual ridge for a portion of its support.

The distal extension partial denture not only must depend on the residual ridge for some **support** but also should obtain **retention** from its base, aided by indirect **retention** to prevent the denture's lifting away from the residual ridge. Whereas the tooth-supported base is secured at either end by the action of a direct retainer and supported at either end by a rest, this degree of support and direct retention are lacking in the distal extension restoration. **For this reason a distal abutment should be preserved whenever possible.** In the event of the loss or absence of a distal abutment tooth, the patient must be made aware of the movements to be expected with a distal extension partial denture and the limitations imposed on the dentist when the residual ridge must be used for both support and retention for that part of the prosthesis.

FACTORS INFLUENCING THE SUPPORT OF A DISTAL EXTENSION BASE

Support from the residual ridge becomes greater as the distance from the last abutment increases and will depend on several factors:

1. Quality of the residual ridge
2. Extent of residual ridge coverage by the denture base
3. Type and accuracy of the impression registration
4. Accuracy of the denture base
5. Design of the partial framework
6. Total occlusal load applied

Quality of the residual ridge. The ideal residual ridge to support a denture base would consist of cortical bone covering relatively dense cancellous bone, a broad flat crest, and high vertical slopes and would be covered by firm, dense, fibrous connective tissue. Such a residual ridge would optimally support vertical and horizontal stresses placed on it by denture bases. Unfortunately this ideal is seldom encountered.

Easily displaceable tissue will not adequately support a denture base, and tissues that are interposed between a sharp, bony residual ridge and a denture base will not remain in a healthy state. Not only must the nature of the bone of the residual ridge be considred in developing optimal support for the denture base, but also its positional relationship to the direction of forces that will be placed on it.

The crest of the bony mandibular residual ridge is most often cancellous in nature. Pressures placed on tissues overlying the crest of the mandibular residual ridge usually result in inflammation of these tissues, accompanied by the sequelae of chronic inflammation. Therefore the crest of the mandibular residual ridge cannot

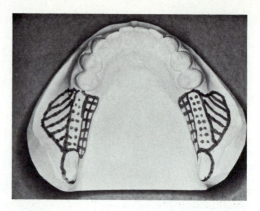

Fig. 15-1. Dotted portion outlines crest of residual ridge, which should be recorded in its anatomic form in impression procedures. Similarly, retromolar pads should not be displaced by impression. Buccal shelf regions are outlined by herringbone pattern, and selected additional pressures may be placed on these regions for vertical support of denture base. Lingual slopes of residual ridge (cross-hatched) may furnish some vertical support to restoration; however, these regions principally resist horizontal rotational tendencies of denture base and should be recorded by impression in undisplaced form.

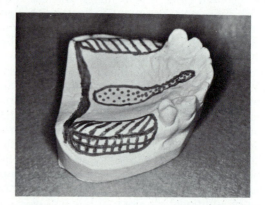

Fig. 15-2. Crest of maxillary residual ridge (herringbone pattern) is primary supporting region for maxillary distal extension denture base. Buccal and lingual slopes may furnish limited vertical support to denture base. It seems logical that their primary role is to counteract horizontal rotational tendencies of denture base. Dotted portion outlines incisive papilla and median palatal raphe. Relief must be provided these regions, especially if tissues covering palatal raphe are less displaceable than those covering crest of residual ridge.

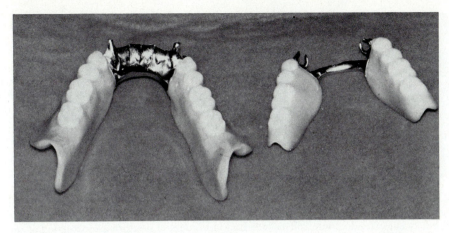

Fig. 15-3. Comparison of two removable partial dentures for same patient. Denture on right has grossly underextended bases. Its replacement, with properly extended bases, is on left. Occlusal forces are more readily distributed to denture bearing areas by replacement denture.

become a primary stress-bearing region. The buccal shelf region (bounded by the external oblique line and crest of alveolar ridge) seems to be more ideally suited for a primary stress-bearing role because it is covered by relatively firm, dense, fibrous connective tissue supported by cortical bone. In most instances this region bears more of a horizontal relationship to vertical forces than do other regions of the residual ridge (Fig. 15-1). The slopes of the residual ridge then would become the primary stress-bearing region to resist off-vertical forces.

The immediate crest of the bone of the maxillary residual ridge may consist primarily of cancellous bone. Oral tissues overlying the maxillary residual alveolar bone are usually of a firm, dense nature or can be surgically prepared to support a denture base. The topography of a partially edentulous maxillary arch imposes a restriction on selection of a primary stress-bearing area. In spite of impression procedures the crestal area of the residual ridge will become the primary stress-bearing area to vertically directed forces. Some resistance to these forces may be obtained by the immediate buccal and lingual slopes of the ridge. Palatal tissues lying between the medial palatal raphe and the lingual slope of the edentulous ridge posteriorly are readily displaceable and cannot be considered as primary stress-bearing sites (Fig. 15-2). The tissues covering the crest of the maxillary residual ridge

must be less displaceable than are the tissues covering palatal areas, or relief of palatal tissues must be provided either in the denture bases or for palatal major connectors.

Extent of residual ridge coverage by the denture base. The broader the coverage, the greater the distribution of the load, thereby resulting in less load per unit area (Fig. 15-3). Most prosthodontists agree that a denture base should cover as much of the residual ridge as possible and be extended the maximum amount within the physiologic tolerance of the limiting border structures or tissues (Fig. 15-4). A knowledge of these border tissues and the structures that influence their movement is paramount to developing broad coverage denture bases. In a series of experiments, Kaires has shown that "maximum coverage of denture-bearing areas with large, wide denture bases is of the utmost importance in withstanding both vertical and horizontal stresses."

It is not within the scope of this text to review the anatomic considerations related to denture bases. The student is referred to several articles concerning this subject that are listed in Selected Reading Resources.

Type of the impression registration. The residual ridge may be said to have two forms, the **anatomic** and the **functional** form (Figs. 15-5 and 15-6, *A*). The **anatomic form,** is the surface contour of the ridge when it is not supporting

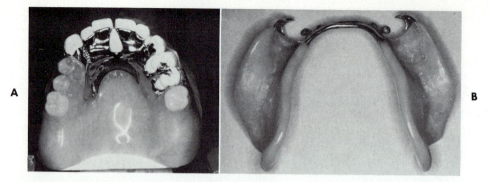

Fig. 15-4. A, Denture base is extended posteriorly to cover maxillary tuberosities, ending in pterygomaxillary notches. Posterior border of denture is located at junction of hard and soft palate but is not extended onto soft palate. Buccal borders of denture are extended as much as possible but within physiologic tolerance of bordering structures. B, Fully extended mandibular bases. Lingual flange extended into retromylohyoid space. S curve of lingual flange permits unrestricted contraction of mylohyoid muscle. Buccal portions of bases are supported by buccal shelves.

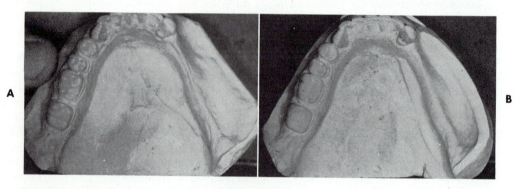

Fig. 15-5. Comparison of anatomic and functional ridge forms. A, Original master cast with edentulous area recorded in its anatomic form, using elastic impression material. B, Same cast after edentulous area has been repoured to its functional form as recorded by secondary impression.

an occlusal load. It is this resting form that is recorded by a soft impression material such as plaster of Paris or a metallic oxide impression paste **if the entire impression tray is uniformly relieved.** Depending on the viscosity of the particular impression material used and the impression tray, it is also the form recorded by mercaptan rubber, silicone, and hydrocolloid impression materials. Distortion and tissue displacement by pressure may result from confinement of the impression material within the tray and from insufficient thickness of impression material between the tray and the tissues, as well

as from the viscosity of the impression material, but none of these factors is selective or physiologic in its action. These are accidental distortions of the tissues occurring through faulty technique.

Some dentists use the anatomic form of the residual ridge in constructing complete dentures, believing this is the most physiologic form for support of the dentures. Such dentures are said to be made from anatomic impressions. However, many other dentists believe that certain regions of the residual ridge are more capable of supporting dentures than are other re-

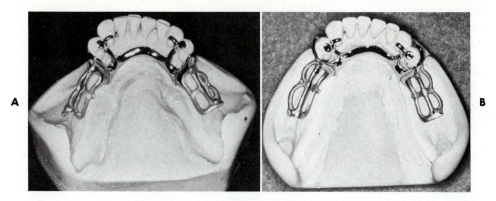

Fig. 15-6. Comparison of functional and anatomic forms of same edentulous ridge. **A,** Master cast with edentulous area reproduced in its anatomic form from hydrocolloid impression. **B,** Same master cast after edentulous areas have been repoured in their functional or supporting form, as recorded with secondary impression. Note not only difference in surface anatomy but also that functional impression has recorded width available for support of denture base. New acrylic resin base may now be made by sprinkling method to establish occlusal relationship on base almost identical with that of finished denture.

gions. Their impression methods are directed to placing more stress on primary stress-bearing regions with specially constructed individual trays and at the same time recording the anatomic form of other basal seat tissues, which cannot assume a stress-bearing role. Of the two rationalizations, the latter seems to be more logical

Since there is no tooth support with which the denture base must be made compatible, and since the basal seat tissues are recorded with a predominantly anatomic impression, the complete denture fits the resting form of those tissues. When it may be presumed that occlusion is harmonious throughout the dental arch, the complete denture may move tissueward under function until the tissues beneath assume a supporting form or a compactness that will support an occlusal load. The same principle would apply to a removable partial denture made without abutment support, differing only in that the area of tissue support is less and the tissues adjacent to the remaining teeth would be impinged by tissueward movement of the denture. Without occlusal support from the natural teeth, occlusion on the tissue-supported partial denture would be negative, leaving only the remaining natural teeth to carry the masticatory load.

Several years ago, McLean and others recognized the need for recording the tissues supporting a distal extension partial denture base in their **functional form,** or supporting state, and then relating them to the remainder of the arch by means of a secondary impression. This was called a **functional impression** because it recorded the ridge relation under simulated function (Fig. 15-6, *B*).

The technique consisted of making an impression of the edentulous areas in a vulcanite or denture base tray, which was provided with modeling plastic occlusion rims. Impression paste was used to record the ridge areas while they were under biting stress. This impression was then related to the remainder of the arch by making a hydrocolloid impression with the original impression seated in the mouth. On removal of the impression from the mouth, a master cast was poured in the composite impression, with the edentulous areas recorded under functional loading. Although the tray used for the overall impression was in contact with the occlusion rims, finger pressure was necessary to hold the original impression in its functional position while the hydrocolloid material gelled. Finger pressure thus applied could at best be only an approximation of the occlusal loading under which the original impression was recorded. This variable tended to nullify the advantage of making the original impression under occlusal loading.

A variation of this technique eliminated the occlusion rims as such but provided stops of modeling plastic against the underside of the hydrocolloid impression tray for finger loading the original impression. In this method, also, the impression of the edentulous areas was made with impression paste but with the tissues in their resting form. A finger load was then applied to the hydrocolloid tray for relating the edentulous areas under some loading to the remainder of the arch as the hydrocolloid gelled. The resulting master cast recorded the anatomic or resting form of the ridge in a pseudofunctional relationship to the rest of the arch.

Hindels and others have used with apparent success a method of finger loading the anatomic impression through a hole in the hydrocolloid impression tray. These trays are available for use with the technique and eliminate the possibility of error arising from ineffective or incorrectly placed modeling plastic stops. It does not eliminate the variable of the dentist's individual interpretation of what constitutes functional loading. The occlusal loading of McLean was unquestionably a more accurate and less variable method of recording the residual ridge beneath a distal extension base, but it became a variable finger-loading relationship in the final impression. That such methods are better than making a partial denture from a one-piece anatomic impression cannot be denied, because they recognize the need for adequate support of the distal extension base.

Any method, whether it records the **functional relationship** of the ridge to the remainder of the arch, or the **functional form** of the ridge itself, may provide acceptable support for the partial denture. On the other hand, those who use the static ridge form or ridge relationship for the partial denture should seriously consider the need for some mechanical stressbreaker to avoid the possible cantilever action of the distal extension base against the abutment teeth.

The one-piece colloidal or plaster impression will produce a cast that represents not a functional relationship between the various supporting structures of the mouth but only the hard and soft tissues at rest. With the partial denture in position in the dental arch, the occlusal rest will fit the rest seat of the abutment tooth, while the denture base will fit the surface of the mucosa at rest. When a masticatory load is applied to the extension base, the rest will act as a definite stop, which will prevent the part of the base near the abutment tooth from transmitting the load to the underlying anatomic structures. The distal end of the base, however, being able to move freely, will transmit the full masticatory load.

It is obvious that the soft tissues covering the ridge cannot by themselves carry any load applied to them. They act as a protective padding for the bone, which in the final analysis is the structure that receives and carries the masticatory load. Distribution of this load over a maximum area of bone is a prime requisite in preventing trauma.

A denture constructed from a one-piece impression, only recording the anatomic form of basal seat tissues, places the masticatory load only on the abutment teeth and that part of the bone that underlies the distal end of the extension base. The balance of the bony ridge will not function in carrying the load. The result will be a traumatic load to the bone underlying the distal end of the base and to the abutment tooth, which in turn will result in bone loss and loosening of the abutment tooth. Yet the use of a properly prepared individualized impression tray can be a means to record the primary stress-bearing areas in a functional form and the non-stress-bearing areas in an anatomic form, just as is often accomplished by many dentists in making impressions for complete dentures.

Some believe that every partial denture should be relined before its final placement in the mouth. Some believe that tissue can be evenly displaced and use impression materials of heavy consistency. This process introduces traumatic stresses to the underlying tissues. Some use easy-flowing pastes that produce an impression of the soft tissues at rest. During the functioning of a partial denture so relined, the sequence of events will be similar to that of a partial denture constructed from a one-piece impression. The occlusal rest will act as a stop, preventing an even distribution of the masticatory load by the base to the edentulous ridge.

An impression technique as given by Hindels is as follows:

An acrylic resin tray is processed on a cast made from an impression that should include all areas of future tissue support of the partial denture. The tray is selectively relieved and, when checked in the mouth, should cover the edentulous areas up to the border tissue attachments and should include the retromolar pads. The bases of the tray should be connected with each other by means of an acrylic resin lingual bar. The bar should cover the area between the muscle attachments of the floor of the mouth and the lingual gingivae of the anterior teeth. The tray should clear the free gingivae around the abutment teeth to prevent future impingement and stripping.

This tray is loaded with an easy-flowing zinc-oxide–eugenol paste and is brought into position in the mouth, care being taken that the soft tissues are left in their passive state. After the material has hardened, the tray is removed and the impression examined. In a successful impression, the tissue side of the tray is fully covered with impression material, and no part of the tray itself is visible. The material that has flowed from the tray onto the abutment teeth should now be cut away and the tray reinserted in the mouth and tested for stability.

The next step is to make an impression of the teeth and to establish a relationship between the teeth and the mucosa in a displaced state. For this purpose a perforated tray that has been provided with two circular openings of approximately 18 mm diameter in the region of the first molars is used. The impression of the soft tissue areas is placed in the mouth. Then, while the tray is being loaded with an irreversible hydrocolloid impression material, some of this material is used to fill the space between the soft tissue impression and the remaining teeth. The loaded metal tray is then inserted over both the teeth and the acrylic resin tray. The index fingers are passed through the openings in the perforated tray until they contact the underlying tray; then pressure is exerted on it. This pressure should be maintained until the alginate impression material has hardened. The completed impression is then removed as one unit. The cast made in this impression will be a reproduction of both the surface of the teeth and the undistorted surface of the mucosa, but the two will be related to each other with the mucosa in a functional state as it would be found under the partial denture base during mastication. While the base is related to the occlusal rest with the mucosa in a functional state, the tissue surface of the base is actually a reproduction of the passive and undistorted mucosa as obtained with zinc oxide–eugenol paste in the individual impression tray.*

The form of the residual ridge recorded under some loading, whether by occlusal loading, finger loading, specially designed individual trays, or the consistency of the recording medium, is called the **functional form.** This is the surface contour of the ridge when it is supporting a functional load. How much it will differ from the anatomic form will depend on the thickness and structural characteristics of the soft tissues overlying the residual bone. It will also differ from the anatomic form in proportion to the total load applied to the denture base.

The objective of any functional impression technique is to provide maximum support for the removable partial denture base, thereby maintaining occlusal contact to distribute the occlusal load over both natural and artificial dentition and at the same time minimize movement of the base, which would create leverage on the abutment teeth. While some tissueward movement of the distal extension base is unavoidable and dependent on the six factors listed previously, it can be minimized by providing the best possible support for the denture base.

Steffel has classified advocates of the various methods for treating the distal extension partial denture as follows:

1. Those who believe that ridge and tooth supports can best be equalized by the use of stressbreakers or resilient equalizers
2. Those who insist on bringing about the equalization of ridge and tooth support by physiologic basing, which is accomplished

---

*Paraphrased from Hindels, G.W.: Load distribution in extension saddle partial dentures, J. Prosthet. Dent. **2:**92-100, 1952.

by a pressure impression or by relining the denture under functional stresses

3. Those who uphold the idea of extensive stress distribution for stress reduction at any one point

It would seem that there is little difference in the philosophy behind methods 2 and 3 as given by Steffel, for both the equalization of tooth and tissue support and stress distribution over the greatest area are objectives of the functional type of impression. **Many of the requirements and advantages that may be given for the distributed stress denture apply equally well to the functionally or physiologically based denture.** Some of these requirements are (1) positive occlusal rests; (2) an all-rigid, nonflexible framework; (3) indirect retainers, wherever practical, to add stability; and (4) well-adapted, broad-coverage bases.

Those who do not accept the theory of physiologic basing, for one reason or another, should use some form of stressbreaker between the abutment and the distal extension base. The advantages and disadvantages of doing so have been given in Chapter 8.

Accuracy of the denture base. Support of the distal extension base is enhanced by intimacy of contact of the tissue surface of the base and the tissues covering the residual ridge. The tissue surface of the denture base must optimally represent a true negative of the basal seat regions of the master cast. Denture bases have been discussed in Chapter 8.

In addition, the denture base must be related to the partial denture framework the same as the basal seat tissues were related to the abutment teeth when the impression was made. Every precaution must be taken to ensure this relationship when the altered-cast technique of making a master cast is used.

Design of the partial denture framework. Some rotation movement of a distal extension base around posteriorly placed direct retainers is inevitable under functional loading. It must be remembered that the extent to which abutment teeth are subjected to rotational forces resulting from masticatory function is directly related to the position and resistance of the food bolus. The greatest movement takes place at the most posterior extent of the denture base. The

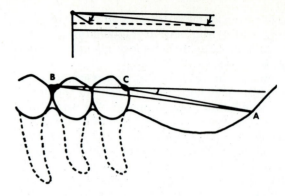

Fig. 15-7. Acute dip of short denture base is compared with that of long one in upper figure. In lower figure, when point of rotation is changed from *C* to *B*, it can be seen that proportionally greater area of residual ridge is used to support denture base than occurs when fulcrum line passes through *C*. Line *AC* represents length of denture base.

retromolar pad region of the mandibular residual ridge and the tuberosity region of the maxillary residual ridge therefore are subjected to the greatest movement of the denture base (Fig. 15-7). **As the rotational axis (fulcrum line) of the denture is moved anteriorly, more of the residual ridge is used to support the denture base, thereby distributing stresses over a proportionally greater area.** Steffel and Kratochvil have excellently demonstrated this concept in dental periodical literature (Fig. 15-8). In many instances, occlusal rests may be moved anteriorly to better use the residual ridge for support without jeopardizing either vertical or horizontal support of the denture by occlusal rests and guiding planes (Fig. 15-9).

Total occlusal load applied. The total occlusal load applied is influenced by the number of supplied teeth, the width of their occlusal surfaces, and their occlusal efficiency. Kaires conducted an investigation under laboratory conditions and concluded that "the reduction of the size of the occlusal table reduces the vertical and horizontal forces acting on the partial dentures and lessens the stress on the abutment teeth and supporting tissues."*

*From Kaires, A.K.: Effect of partial denture design on bilateral force distribution, J. Prosthet. Dent. **6:**373-389, 1956.

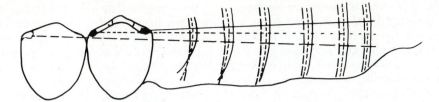

Fig. 15-8. Assuming that rotation of distal extension base occurs around nearest rest, as rest is moved anteriorly, more of residual ridge will be used to resist rotation. Compare more nearly vertical arcs of "long-dash" broken line with arcs of solid line.

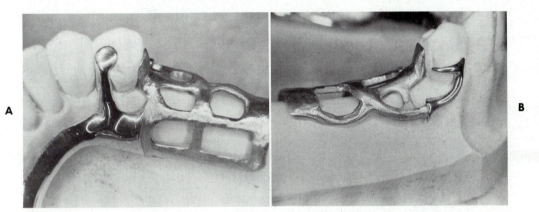

Fig. 15-9. A, Occlusal rest is placed on mesio-occlusal surface of lower first premolar to move point of rotation anterior to conventionally placed disto-occlusal rest. Occlusal rest is connected to lingual bar by minor connector, which contacts small mesiolingual prepared guiding plane. Note vertical extension of denture base minor connector contacting guiding plane surface also. Lingual guiding plane is prepared to extend from occlusal surface inferiorly to approximately one fifth the height of lingual surface and is as broad as contacting minor connector. Distal guiding plane extends from distal marginal ridge gingivally to about two thirds the height of distal surface. Such preparations will not lock tooth in viselike grip when denture base rotates toward residual ridge. **B,** Buccal view of **A.** Direct retainer assembly is completed by bar-type clasp with only retentive tip engaging undercut. It is possible that rotation toward basal seat will occur around anterior portion of direct retainer retentive arm located occlusally to height of contour. In any event, rotation will occur around some portion of direct retainer assembly.

METHODS FOR OBTAINING FUNCTIONAL SUPPORT FOR THE DISTAL EXTENSION BASE

A thorough understanding of the characteristics of each of the impression materials leads to the obvious conclusion that no single material can record both the anatomic form of the teeth and tissues in the dental arch and, at the same time, the functional form of the residual ridge.

Therefore some secondary impression method must be used.

This may be accomplished by several methods. Each seems to satisfy the two requirements for providing adequate support to the distal extension partial denture base, which are (1) that it records and relates the tissues under some loading and (2) that it distributes the load over as large an area as possible.

Selective tissue placement impression method. Soft tissues covering basal seat areas may be **placed, displaced,** or recorded in their **resting** or **anatomic form.** Placed and displaced tissues differ in degree of alteration from their resting form and in their physiologic reaction to the amount of displacement. For example, the palatal tissues in the vicinity of the vibrating line can be slightly displaced to develop a posterior palatal seal for the maxillary complete denture and will remain in a healthy state for extended periods of time. On the other hand, these tissues develop an immediate inflammatory response when they have been overly displaced in developing the posterior palatal seal.

Oral tissues that have been overly displaced attempt to regain their anatomic form. When not permitted to do this by the denture bases, the tissues become inflamed and their physiologic functions become impaired, accompanied by bone resorption. Tissues that are minimally displaced (placed) by impression procedures respond favorably to the additional pressures placed on them by resultant denture bases if these pressures are intermittent rather than continuous.

The selective tissue placement impression method is based on the previously stated clinical observations, the histologic nature of tissues covering the residual alveolar bone, the nature of

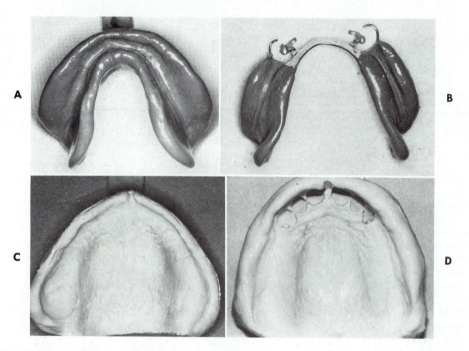

Fig. 15-10. **A,** Impression of mandibular edentulous arch using individualized tray and rubber-base impression material. Tray was so constructed and impression so made that buccal shelves of mandible could assume primary stress-bearing role. **B,** Rubber-base secondary impression of Class I partially edentulous arch made in individualized trays attached to framework. Just as in **A,** buccal shelves will assume primary stress-bearing role. Note similarity of two impressions. In each instance, individualized acrylic resin impression trays permitted dentist to carry out his philosophy of impression making for support of denture bases. **C,** Impression of edentulous maxillary arch made with impression plaster in individualized tray. **D,** Impression of Class I partially edentulous arch made with irreversible hydrocolloid material in individualized tray. Again, without individualized tray, properly constructed, a philosophy of impression making is most difficult to carry out.

the residual ridge bone, and its positional relationship to the direction of stresses that will be placed on it. It is further believed that by use of specially designed individual trays for impressions, denture bases can be developed that will use those portions of the residual ridge that can withstand additional stress and at the same time relieve the tissues of the residual ridge that cannot withstand functional loading and remain healthy.

There should be no difference philosophically in the requirement of support and coverage by bases of distal extension removable partial dentures and complete dentures, either maxillary or mandibular (Fig. 15-10). The tray is unquestionably the most important part of an impression. A tray must, however, be so formed and modified that the impression philosophy of the dentist can be carried out. The making of individualized acrylic resin impression trays was illustrated in the preceding chapter.

An impression for a mandibular distal extension partially edentulous arch may adequately be made in an individualized, full-arch tray. To do so, not only must the tray be formed to provide proper space for the particular impression material, but provision must also be made so that the functional form of primary stress-bearing areas may be recorded. Such an impression procedure, properly executed, can be used when metal bases are to be incorporated in the design of the restoration. There is little difference, if any, between recording the basal seats in the partially edentulous arch and recording like areas for complete dentures on an edentulous arch. A secondary impression made in trays attached to the framework only makes definitive border control and tissue placement a bit easier, compared with the individualized full arch tray.

A method of attaching custom trays to a removable partial denture framework is illustrated in Fig. 15-11. Before the trays are attached, the framework must be fitted in the mouth as illustrated in Fig. 15-12. After the framework has been fitted and the custom trays attached, the selective tissue placement impression and cast formation can be accomplished as described in Fig. 15-13.

Fluid wax functional impression method. One must differentiate between the wax "wash,"

or correction impression, as originally developed by Earl S. Smith of the University of Iowa, and the fluid-wax impression, as developed by O. C. Applegate of the University of Michigan and S. G. Applegate of the University of Detroit. The latter method used an impression wax (Korecta wax No. 4) that is slightly more fluid than the Iowa wax. Border extension was established by the impression wax and then reinforced by backing it up with a special hard wax (Korecta wax No. 1).*

The Applegate method may be used for making a reline impression or for the correction of the original master cast. In either application the thickness of wax permits a greater flow of material and therefore less tissue displacement than does the wax "wash." However, if adequate space (1 to 2 mm) exists in the tray, the Iowa wax is most acceptable. The fluid-wax impression is used with an open-mouth procedure; therefore there is less danger of overdisplacement of tissues by the application of vertical forces. If adequate space for the flow of the material is provided and sufficient time is allowed for the escape of excess material, the fluid-wax impression will not overdisplace tissues. Only those soft tissues that can readily be displaced or made more compact by the consistency of the wax itself will be recorded in a different form from that recorded by the anatomic impression.

In addition to less displacement of tissues, the fluid-wax technique records the moving border tissues physiologically, resulting in an accurate denture border. Both the length and the width of the border are thus established in wax and reproduced in the denture base. The harder wax (Kerr Ivory Inlay wax) is used only to back up the impression and should not be allowed to influence the impression record.

O. C. Applegate has named this method the **fluid-wax functional impression.** Although it may be used for relining purposes, it is designed primarily for making a secondary impression to correct a master cast. The anatomic ridge form, as recorded in hydrocolloid, is thus replaced with the functional form, as recorded in fluid

---

*Korecta waxes are no longer available. Iowa wax is a suitable substitute for Korecta No. 4 wax, and Kerr Ivory Inlay wax may be used in lieu of Korecta No. 1 wax.

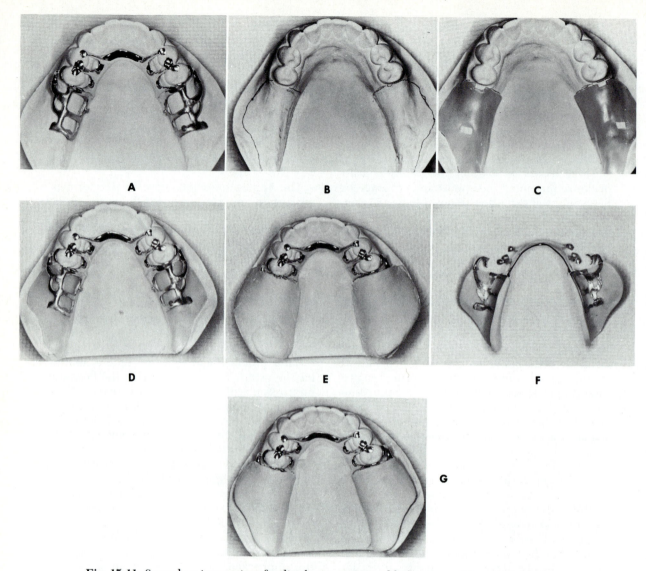

Fig. 15-11. Secondary impressions for distal extension mandibular removable partial dentures are made in individual tray attached to denture framework. **A,** Framework has been tried in mouth and fits mouth and master cast as planned. **B,** Outline of resin tray is penciled on cast. **C,** One thickness of baseplate wax is adapted to outline to act as spacer so that room for impression material exists in finished tray. Windows are cut in wax spacer corresponding to regions on cast contacted by minor connectors for denture bases. **D,** Framework is warmed and pressed to position on relieved master cast. All regions of cast that will be contacted by autopolymerizing acrylic resin dough are painted with tinfoil substitute (Alcote). **E,** Autopolymerizing acrylic resin is mixed, and wafers of material are made as described in Chapter 14. Resin material is adapted to cast and over framework with finger pressure. Excess material over borders of cast is removed with sharp knife while material is still soft. **F,** Cured resin trays and framework are removed from cast, and trays are trimmed to outline of wax spacer. **G,** Borders of trays will be adjusted to extend within 2 mm of tissue reflections. Holes will then be placed in trays corresponding to crest of residual ridge and retromolar pads to allow escape of excess impression material when impression is made.

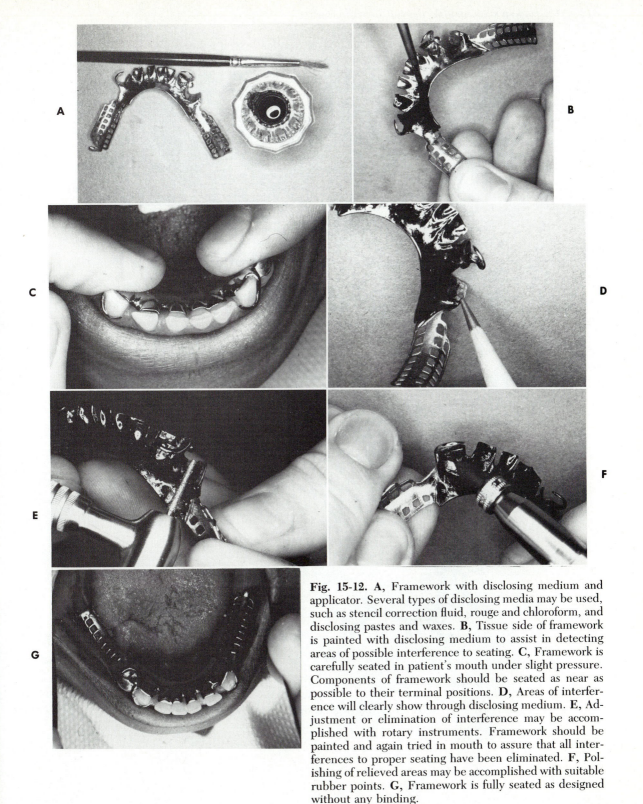

Fig. 15-12. A, Framework with disclosing medium and applicator. Several types of disclosing media may be used, such as stencil correction fluid, rouge and chloroform, and disclosing pastes and waxes. B, Tissue side of framework is painted with disclosing medium to assist in detecting areas of possible interference to seating. C, Framework is carefully seated in patient's mouth under slight pressure. Components of framework should be seated as near as possible to their terminal positions. D, Areas of interference will clearly show through disclosing medium. E, Adjustment or elimination of interference may be accomplished with rotary instruments. Framework should be painted and again tried in mouth to assure that all interferences to proper seating have been eliminated. F, Polishing of relieved areas may be accomplished with suitable rubber points. G, Framework is fully seated as designed without any binding.

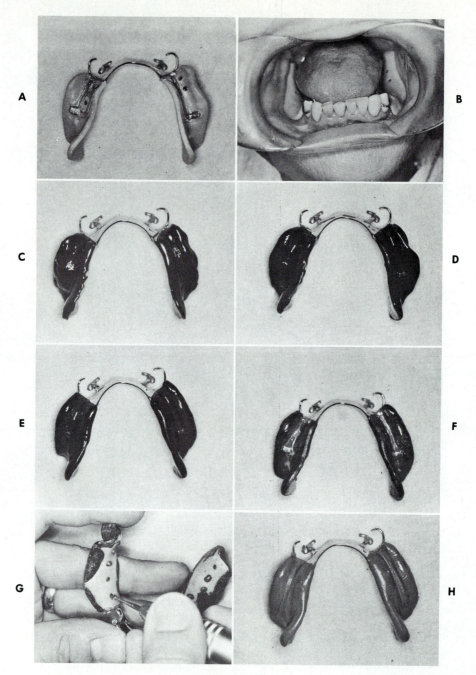

Fig. 15-13. For legend see opposite page.

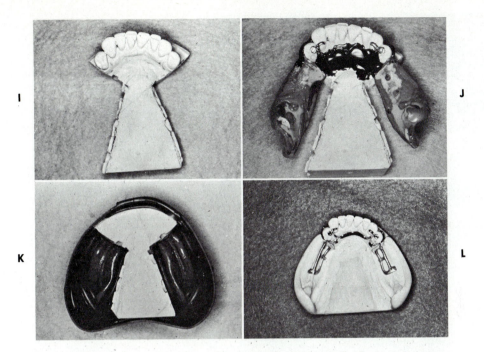

Fig. 15-13. Selective tissue placement impression method. **A,** Individual acrylic resin impression trays are attached to framework. Holes are placed in tray along alveolar groove to allow escape of excess impression material. **B,** Framework and attached trays are tried in patient's mouth. Borders of tray are adjusted so that they are 2 to 3 mm short of all reflections but cover retromolar pads. **C,** Thin layer of red stick modeling plastic is painted on tissue sides of impression trays by first softening modeling plastic with flame. **D,** Modeling plastic has been softened by flame, tempered in 135° F water, and placed in patient's mouth. This procedure is repeated (usually three times) until basal seat tissues are not displaced and framework is correctly positioned. Impression trays will be stable at this time and border-molding procedures can begin. **E,** Borders are perfected by heating individual areas, placing tempered tray in mouth, manipulating cheeks, and having patient form lingual borders by tongue movements. Note that lingual flanges have assumed an **S** shape. This S shape has been formed by action of mylohyoid muscle. Note also that lingual flange has been extended into retromylohyoid fossa. There would be **no difference** in form of impression of edentulous regions at this stage from complete denture impression of same regions if patient was edentulous. **F,** Borders of compound impression are shortened 1 to 1.5 mm, and whole inside of impression, **with exception of buccal shelf region,** is relieved approximately 1 mm. **G,** Modeling plastic is removed from holes in tray. **H,** Final impression is completed with rubber-base impression material wash. Framework must be perfectly seated and maintained in position while impression material is setting. **I,** Edentulous regions of cast are eliminated. Cut surfaces are grooved for additional retention of stone poured to make altered cast. **J,** Framework and impression are returned to cast and are luted with sticky wax to avoid displacement during boxing and pouring procedures. **K,** Utility wax is used to box impression. **L,** Altered master cast with framework in position. Buccal shelf regions have been recorded in functional form. Other regions of basal seats have been recorded in anatomic form.

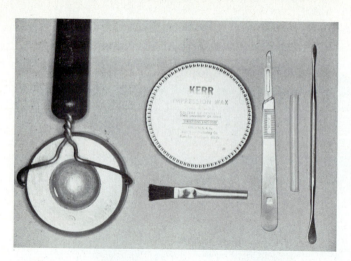

Fig. 15-14. Armamentarium for making secondary, functional impression of mandibular residual ridges with mouth temperature wax: heavy metal crucible for melting wax, impression wax of Iowa formula, brush for applying wax, scalpel used for bisecting impression wax at borders before adding Kerr Ivory inlay wax for reinforcement, stick of Ivory inlay wax, and No. 7 wax spatula for applying reinforcing wax.

Fig. 15-15. Nine steps in making fluid-wax functional impression. **A,** Fluid Iowa wax is painted evenly over impression base. **B,** Denture framework is placed in mouth and held by the dentist in its terminal position with three fingers, one on each principal occlusal rest and a third in between, holding framework forward in its terminal position with any indirect retainers fully seated. Chin is supported with other hand. **C,** While dentist is holding framework down, cheek on each side is pulled vertically against border of impression. This limits buccal extension to extreme positions of limiting structures. **D,** While dentist is keeping framework fully seated, patient is asked to place tongue forcibly into each cheek. This records extreme movement of sublingual tissues on opposite side. **E,** While dentist is still holding framework down, patient is asked to press tongue forward against lingual surface of anterior teeth. This limits distolingual extension of impression on both sides. After this movement, patient is asked to open wide, to make pterygomandibular raphe taut and to limit extreme distal portion of impression. **F,** Impression is removed and examined for glossy surface, which is evidence of tissue contact. Once this has been checked, border is reinforced by bisecting the impression wax at border with No. 11 Bard-Parker blade, leaving impression wax extending beyond impression base unsupported. **G,** Hard Kerr Ivory Inlay wax is applied with hot No. 7 spatula to reinforce impression wax at border. This must be applied hot enough to effect good attachment to impression base. Sufficient hard wax is used to act as reinforcing extension of impression base and to prevent any undesirable shifting of impression wax at border. **H,** More Iowa wax is brushed on, just inside border, to provide excess that will then be turned at border by repetition of previous movements. Wax must be fluid enough that it can be brushed on with broad sweeping strokes free of brush marks. **I,** Completed functional impression. Note border extension buccally and lingually and thickness of border permissible with this particular patient. This varies widely with each patient, but border recorded by this method should always be reproduced in finished denture.

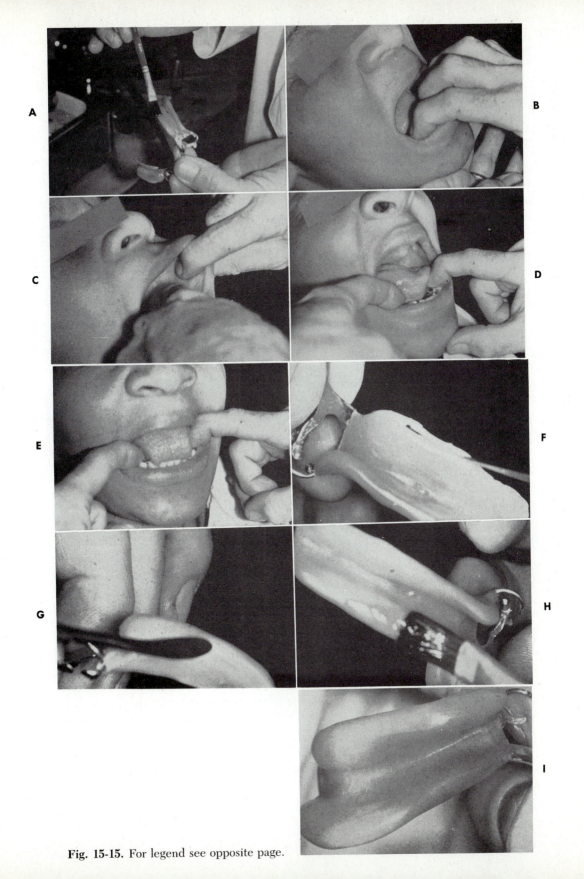

Fig. 15-15. For legend see opposite page.

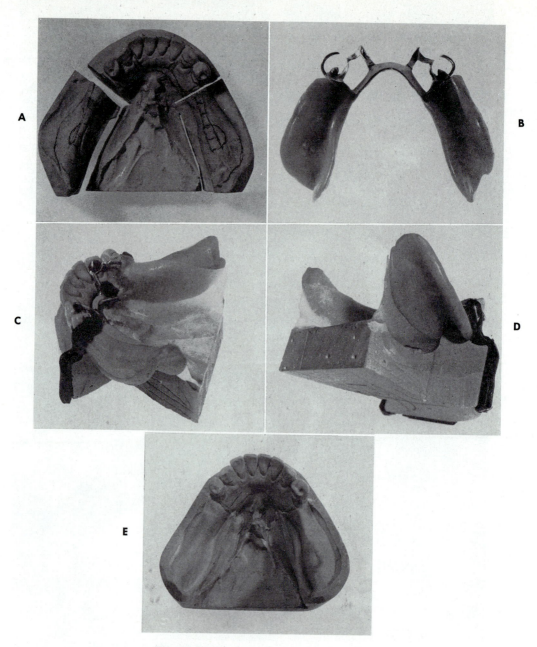

Fig. 15-16. For legend see opposite page.

Fig. 15-16. A, After making acrylic resin impression trays attached to partial denture framework, ridge areas recorded in their static or anatomic form are removed from master cast by sawing with spiral saw blade in two planes. One cut is made at right angles to longitudinal axis of ridge, 1 mm distal to abutment tooth. Second cut is made just lingual and parallel to lingual sulcus as recorded in original impression. The two are joined anteriorly, and anatomic reproduction of ridge is removed. At this time, if saw cuts are not rough enough, cut surfaces of cast should be scored with knife to provide mechanical retention for attachment of new stone to old. **B,** Completed fluid-wax functional impression. **C,** Completed wax functional impression is seated on remainder of cast after anatomic ridges have been removed. Note scored surface for added retention. Cast metal framework is secured to dry cast with sticky wax after first making sure that no debris interferes with seating and that all occlusal rests and indirect retainers are seated. Utility wax is placed on original cast just anterior to saw cut and sealed anteriorly with hot spatula. Sheet wax of adhesive type is placed lingually and sealed to cast and along side of impression base. It must be sealed anteriorly, but hot spatula must not come in contact with impression. Surface of cast anteriorly is then painted with sodium silicate or some other separator, such as Microfilm. Just before pouring new ridge areas, base of cast is immersed in 12 mm (½ in) of water for 5 minutes to provide saturation of dry stone. **D,** Wax functional impression attached to master cast. Anatomic ridge form has been removed, and cut portion of cast has been undercut to assure attachment of new stone to old. Cast has been saturated by placing it base downward in 12 mm (½ in) of water for 5 minutes before pouring. In adding new mix of stone, vibrating is only necessary to prevent trapping air at junction of wax impression with cut surfaces of stone cast. **E,** Ridge areas are poured with stone of different color, using no more vibration than necessary, and then are inverted into additional stone on glass or ceramic slab immediaely after new stone has lost its surface sheen. Stone must be brought up well around distal ends of impression. After stone has hardened, excess is trimmed away until margins of impression wax are exposed. Sticky wax is chilled with ice or cast is chilled and sticky wax flaked off. Cast is then immersed in water at 110° F, just sufficient to soften mouth-temperature wax, and framework with attached impression base is lifted. Usually, impression wax remains on impression base, leaving clean cast as shown.

wax, and the denture base is processed to the latter form. The fluid-wax functional impression is a rather time-consuming procedure but will produce desired results when properly executed.

Objectives in making a fluid-wax impression. Three objectives must be considered in making a fluid-wax impression, as in other impression procedures. These objectives are recording primary stress-bearing areas in their functional form, recording other basal seat or nonbearing areas in their anatomic form, and maximum extension of borders within the physiologic tolerance of bordering structures.

Armamentarium and procedures in making a fluid-wax impression and pouring a cast are illustrated in Figs. 15-14 to 15-16.

SELF-ASSESSMENT AIDS

1. Support for a tooth-borne removable partial denture is provided by what oral structures?

2. Support for a distal extension denture is provided by what oral structures?
3. Residual ridges may be recorded by an impression in their anatomic form or functional form. A Class III arch may be recorded in its _____ form; however, the residual ridges in Class I or II arches should be recorded in their _____ form.
4. There are at least six important factors that influence the support of a distal extension denture base by the residual ridges. You should be able to state them without omission.
5. Describe what you would consider to be an ideal residual ridge to support a distal extension denture base.
6. What areas of the residual ridge are considered to be the primary stress-bearing areas for a mandibular distal extension base? A maxillary distal extension base?
7. Why can the crest of the mandibular residual ridge not assume a stress-bearing role?
8. Which type of tissue interposed between a denture base and the underlying bone would prob-

ably afford a more favorable reaction to stress—firm, dense, fibrous connective tissue or easily displaceable connective tissue?

9. The space that is available for a distal extension denture base is controlled by the moving structures that surround the space. True or false?

10. A denture base should cover as much of the residual ridge as possible and be extended the maximum amount within the physiologic tolerance of the limiting border structures. True or false?

11. The objective of any functional impression technique is to provide maximum support for the removable partial denture base. When this objective is attained, what advantages accrue to the denture environment?

12. How does accuracy or inaccuracy of the denture base influence the quality of support by the residual ridge?

13. Since some rotational movement of the extension denture is bound to occur, and since use of as much of the primary stress-bearing areas as possible is desirable, in what manner may the design of the framework (location of rests) influence the greatest use of the primary stress-bearing areas? Can you illustrate your answer by a simple diagram?

14. Total occlusal load applied to a denture base certainly influences the quality of support for the base. What can be done to lessen the total occlusal load applied in relation to the prosthetically supplied teeth?

15. There are many approaches to recording the functional form of residual ridges in Class I and II arches and relating this form accurately to the rest of the dental arch. The various methods are only means to an end. A basic understanding of anatomy, histology, physiology, materials, and principles will permit each dentist to develop his own philosophy and a technique of impression-making to carry out his philosophy. Therefore you should be able to rationalize the functional relining method and the selective tissue placement method, whether with fluid waxes or other materials, or to relate the anatomic form under functional loading to the rest of the arch (Hindels' approach).

16. What are the risks involved in using a closed-mouth method when performing a functional impression procedure?

17. You will note in some of the various methods of making functional impressions of residual ridges that a series of holes are placed in the alveolar groove of the trays. What is accomplished by such a procedure?

18. What is the most important part of an impression? If you said the **tray,** you are correct. Can you rationalize why this must be true in relation to what you are trying to accomplish in an impression procedure?

19. In your opinion, should there be any difference in the support characteristic, extension, and form of a removable partial denture extension base and a complete denture base occupying the same area?

20. One method discussed in the text is the selective tissue placement of impression making. What is meant by tissue placement?

21. Can you fully describe a selective tissue placement procedure for making impressions of mandibular extension residual ridges?

22. What is meant by a secondary impression?

23. What is meant by an "altered cast" in relation to impression making?

24. Some dentists prefer to use mouth temperature waxes in trays attached to the framework to record the functional form of mandibular residual ridges. Two dental pioneers stand out in the development of wax as an impression material. Can you recall their names?

25. Try describing a fluid-wax functional impression method.

26. Would you anticipate any gross differences in the form of a residual ridge on a cast made from a selective tissue placement impression method and the same ridge recorded by a fluid-wax functional impression method?

16 OCCLUSAL RELATIONSHIPS FOR REMOVABLE PARTIAL DENTURES

**Desirable occlusal contact relationships for
    removable partial dentures**
Methods for establishing occlusal relationships
Materials for artificial posterior teeth
**Establishing jaw relations for a mandibular
    removable partial denture opposing a
    maxillary complete denture**

The fourth phase* in the treatment of patients with removable partial dentures is the establishment of a functional and harmonious occlusion. Therefore occlusal harmony between a partial denture and the remaining natural teeth is a major factor in the preservation of the health of their surrounding structures.

In the treatment of patients with complete dentures, the inclination of the condyle path is the only factor not within the control of the dentist. All other factors may be altered to obtain occlusal balance and harmony in eccentric positions to conform to a particular concept and philosophy of occlusion.

Balanced occlusion is desirable on complete dentures because occlusal stresses may cause instability of the dentures or trauma to the supporting structures. These stresses can reach a point beyond which movement of the denture takes place. The stresses therefore are overcome at the expense of denture stability and retention. In partial dentures, however, because of the fixation to abutments, occlusal stresses are transmitted directly to the abutment teeth and other supporting structures, resulting in sustained

stresses, which may be more damaging than those transient stresses found in complete dentures. Failure to provide and maintain adequate occlusion on the partial denture is primarily a result of (1) lack of support for the denture base, (2) the fallacy of establishing occlusion to a single static jaw relation record, and (3) an unacceptable occlusal plane.

In establishing occlusion on a partial denture the influence of the remaining natural teeth is usually such that the occlusal forms of the teeth on the denture must conform to an already established occlusal pattern. This pattern may have been altered by occlusal adjustment or reconstruction, but the pattern present at the time the partial denture is made dictates the occlusion on the partial denture. The only exceptions are those in which an opposing complete denture can be made to harmonize with the partial denture or in which only anterior teeth remain in both arches and the incisal relationship can be made noninterfering. In these situations the recording of jaw relations and the arrangement of the teeth may proceed in the same manner as with complete dentures, and the **same general principles apply.**

With all other types of partial dentures the remaining teeth must dictate the occlusion. The

---

* See Chapter 2, under discussion on the six phases of partial denture service.

319

dentist should strive for planned contacts in centric occlusion and no interferences in lateral excursions. Some claim that a functional relationship of the partial denture to the natural dentition may be adjusted satisfactorily in the mouth. It is doubtful that this is or ever can be done adequately. Partial denture occlusion thus established **can at best only perpetuate malocclusions** that existed previously and help to maintain the existing vertical relationship, however inadequate it may be.

The establishment of a satisfactory occlusion for the partial denture patient should include the following: (1) an analysis of the existing occlusion, (2) the correction of existing occlusal disharmony, (3) the recording of centric relation or an adjusted centric occlusion, (4) the recording of eccentric jaw relations or functional eccentric occlusion, and (5) the correction of occlusal discrepancies created in processing the denture.

DESIRABLE OCCLUSAL CONTACT RELATIONSHIPS FOR REMOVABLE PARTIAL DENTURES

The following occlusal arrangements are recommended to develop a harmonious occlusal relationship of partial dentures and to enhance stability of the dentures:

1. Simultaneous bilateral contacts of opposing posterior teeth must occur in centric occlusion.

2. Occlusion for tooth-borne dentures may be arranged similar to the occlusion seen in a har-

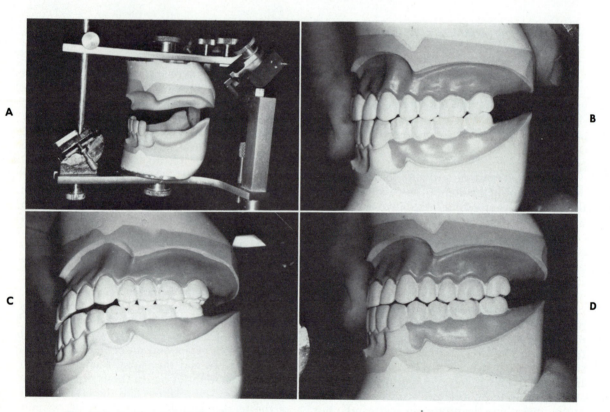

Fig. 16-1. A, Class I partially edentulous arch opposed by edentulous maxillary arch. Stability of maxillary complete denture can be promoted by developing balanced occlusion. **B,** Linear working contacts. **C,** Balancing contacts are arranged, thus minimizing tipping stresses to complete denture. **D,** Protrusive contact of posterior teeth will better distribute forces to entire basal seat of complete denture in contrast to contacts only by opposing anterior teeth.

monious natural dentition. Stability of the dentures is assured by direct retainers at both ends of the denture base.

3. Balanced occlusion in eccentric positions should be formulated when the partial denture is opposed by a maxillary complete denture (Fig. 16-1). This is accomplished primarily to promote the stability of the complete denture. However, simultaneous contacts in a protrusive relationship do not receive priority over appearance, phonetics, and a favorable occlusal plane.

4. Working side contacts should be obtained for the mandibular distal extension denture (Fig. 16-2). These contacts should occur simultaneously with working side contacts of the natural teeth to distribute the stress over the great-

est possible areas. Masticatory function of the denture is improved by such an arrangement, especially if the patient chews in a teardrop or elliptical pattern.

5. Simultaneous balancing and working contacts should be formulated for the maxillary bilateral distal extension partial denture whenever possible (Fig. 16-3). Such an arrangement will compensate in part for the unfavorable position the maxillary artificial teeth must occupy in relation to the residual ridge, which is usually lateral to the crest of the ridge. This desirable relationship often must be compromised, however, when the patient's anterior teeth have an excessively steep vertical overlap with little or no horizontal overlap. Even in this situation, working side contacts can be obtained without

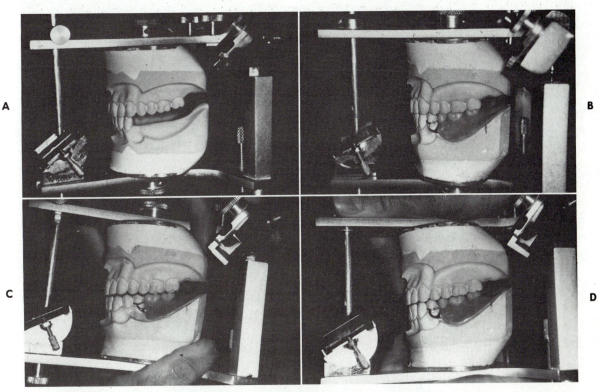

Fig. 16-2. A, Bilateral distal extension mandibular arch opposed by natural dentition in maxillary arch. Master casts have been oriented to articulator in centric relation. **B,** Acrylic resin record bases attached to framework are used to support artificial teeth that have been arranged in maximum intercuspation. **C,** Working contacts have been developed after articulator was programmed with eccentric records. **D,** Balancing and protrusive contacts are purposefully avoided, since they would not enhance stability of restoration.

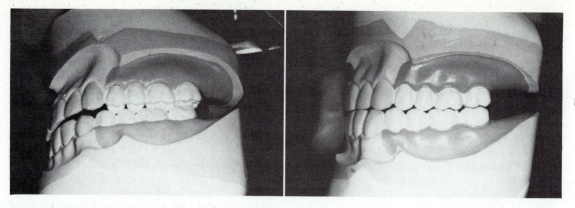

Fig. 16-3. Casts of opposing Class I edentulous arches correctly oriented on programmed articulator. **A,** Resultant restoration has linear working side contacts of opposing posterior teeth occurring simultaneously with contact of opposing canines on working side. **B,** Balancing contact should be arranged to minimize tipping of maxillary removable partial denture and to broadly distribute forces accruing to its supporting structures (abutments and residual ridges).

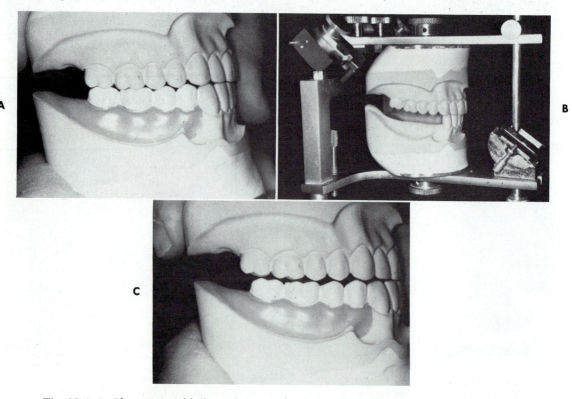

Fig. 16-4. A, Class III mandibular arch opposed by natural dentition. **B,** Artificial teeth were arranged for simultaneous contact in centric occlusion and linear working contacts. **C,** Protrusive and balancing contacts have been avoided, since such arrangement would not enhance stability of the unilateral restoration.

resorting to excessively steep cuspal inclinations.

6. Only working contacts need to be formulated for either the maxillary or mandibular unilateral distal extension denture (Fig. 16-4). Balancing side contacts would not enhance the stability of the denture, since it is entirely tooth supported by the framework on the balancing side.

7. In the Class IV removable partial denture situation, contact of opposing anterior teeth in centric occlusion is desirable to prevent a continuous eruption of the opposing natural incisors (Fig. 16-5). Contact of the opposing anterior teeth in eccentric positions should not be developed. Such contact would be detrimental to the residual ridge and in no way enhances the stability of the denture.

8. Contact of opposing posterior teeth in a straightforward protrusive relationship is not desirable in any situation except when an opposing complete denture is placed (Fig. 16-6).

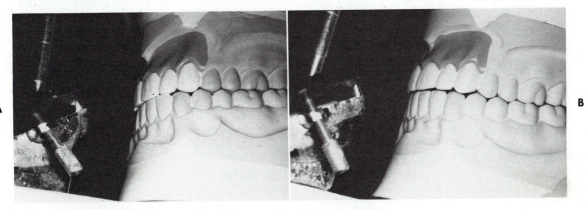

Fig. 16-5. Class IV maxillary arch opposed by mandibular dentulous arch. **A,** Contact of prosthetically supplied teeth and opposing mandibular teeth has been developed in centric occlusion to prevent continued eruption of mandibular teeth. **B,** Contact of anterior teeth in eccentric positions is avoided to eliminate unfavorable forces to maxillary anterior residual ridge.

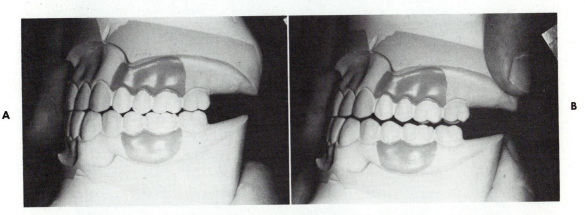

Fig. 16-6. Opposing partially edentulous arches having prospective abutments bounding all edentulous spaces. **A,** Linear working contacts may be developed if canine guidance does not take molars out of contact in working position. **B,** Balancing and protrusive contacts would not add to stability of either restoration and should be avoided.

9. Artificial posterior teeth should not be arranged farther distally than the beginning of a sharp upward incline of the mandibular residual ridge or over the retromolar pad (Fig. 16-7). To do so would have the effect of shunting the denture anteriorly.

A harmonious relationship of opposing occlusal and incisal surfaces alone is not adequate to assure stability of distal extension removable partial dentures. In addition, the relationship of the teeth to the residual ridges must be considered. Bilateral eccentric contact of the mandibular distal extension denture need not be formulated to stabilize the denture. The buccal cusps may be favorably placed over the buccal turning point of the crest of the residual ridge, and in such positions the denture is not subjected to excessive tilting forces (Fig. 16-8). On the other hand, the artificial teeth of the bilateral, distal extension, maxillary denture often must be placed laterally to the crest of the residual ridge (Fig. 16-9). Such an unfavorable position is conducive to tipping the denture, restrained only by direct retainer action on the balancing side. To enhance the stability of the denture, it seems logical to provide simultaneous balancing and working contacts in these situations if possible.

METHODS FOR ESTABLISHING OCCLUSAL RELATIONSHIPS

Five methods of establishing interocclusal relations for removable partial dentures will be briefly described. Before describing any of these, it is necessary that the use of a face-bow mounting of the maxillary cast and the pertinent factors in partial denture occlusion be considered. The technique for applying the face-bow has been described briefly in Chapter 11.

Whereas a hinge axis mounting may be desirable for complete oral rehabilitation procedures, any of the common arbitrary type of face-bow will facilitate mounting of the maxillary cast in relation to the condylar axis of the articulating instrument with reasonable accuracy. As suggested in Chapter 11, it is still better that the plane of occlusion be related to the axis-orbital plane. Since the dominant factor in partial denture occlusion is the remaining natural teeth and their proprioceptor influence on occlusion, a

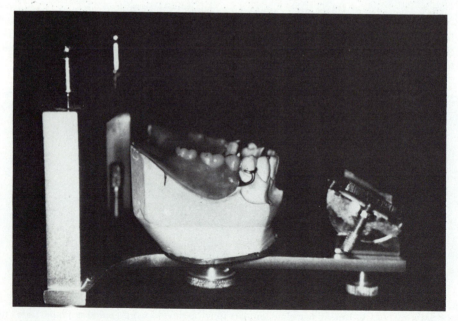

Fig. 16-7. Posterior teeth should not be arranged distal to upward incline of residual ridge. Note that this beginning incline has been marked on land of cast as reference point.

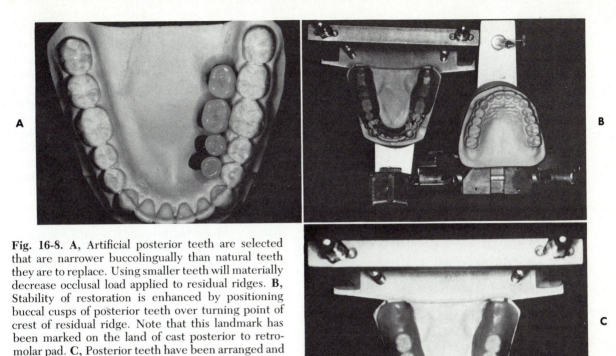

Fig. 16-8. A, Artificial posterior teeth are selected that are narrower buccolingually than natural teeth they are to replace. Using smaller teeth will materially decrease occlusal load applied to residual ridges. B, Stability of restoration is enhanced by positioning buccal cusps of posterior teeth over turning point of crest of residual ridge. Note that this landmark has been marked on the land of cast posterior to retromolar pad. C, Posterior teeth have been arranged and occlusal surfaces have been adjusted for harmonious occlusion.

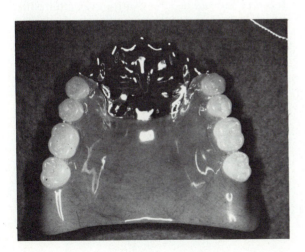

Fig. 16-9. It is often necessary to arrange posterior teeth for maxillary distal extension removable restoration lateral to crests of residual ridges to accommodate positions of posterior teeth in opposing arch. This position is unfavorable; however, stability can be improved by arranging simultaneous working and balancing contacts.

comparable radius at the oriented plane of occlusion on an acceptable instrument will allow reasonably valid mandibular movements to be reproduced. Such instruments are the Hanau models (158 and 96-H2), the Dentatus model ARH, the Whip-Mix, and similar instruments.

Articulators can simulate but not duplicate jaw movement. A realization of the limitations of a specific instrument and a knowledge of the procedures that can overcome these limitations are necessary if an adequate occlusion is to be created.

The recording of occlusal relationships for the partially edentulous arch may vary from the simple apposition of opposing casts by occluding sufficient remaining natural teeth to the recording of jaw relations in the same manner as for a completely edentulous patient. As long as there are natural teeth remaining in contact, however, the cuspal influence that those teeth will have on functional jaw movements must be considered.

The horizontal jaw relation (centric occlusion or centric relation) in which the restoration is to be constructed should have been determined during diagnosis and treatment planning. Mouth preparations also should have been accomplished based on this determination, including occlusal adjustment of the natural dentition, if such was indicated. Therefore one of the following conditions should exist: (1) centric relation and centric occlusion coincide; (2) centric relation and centric occlusion do not coincide but the decision has been made to construct the restoration in centric occlusion; (3) posterior teeth do not contact and the restoration is to be constructed in centric relation; and (4) posterior teeth are not present in one or both arches and the denture will be constructed in centric relation.

Then occlusal relationships may be established by using the most appropriate of the following methods to fit a particular partially edentulous situation.

Direct apposition of casts. The *first method* is used when there are sufficient opposing teeth remaining in contact to make the existing jaw relationship obvious and when only a few teeth are to be replaced on short denture bases. In

this method, opposing casts may be occluded by hand. The occluded casts should be held in apposition with wire nails attached with sticky wax to the bases of the casts until they are securely mounted on the articulator.

At best, this method can only perpetuate the existing vertical dimension and any existing occlusal disharmony present between the natural dentition. **Occlusal analysis and the correction of any existing occlusal disharmony should precede the accepting of such a jaw relation record.** The limitations of such a method are obvious. Yet, such a jaw relation record is better than an inaccurate interocclusal record between the remaining natural teeth. Unless a record is made that does not influence the closing path by reason of its bulk and the consistency of the recording medium, direct apposition of opposing casts at least eliminates the possibility of the patient's giving a faulty jaw relationship.

Interocclusal records with posterior teeth remaining. A *second method*, which is a modification of the first, is used when sufficient teeth remain to support the partial denture (Kennedy Class III), but the relation of opposing teeth does not permit the occluding of casts by hand. In such situations, jaw relations must be established as for fixed restorations using some kind of interocclusal record.

The least accurate of these is the interocclusal wax record. The successful recording of centric relation with an interocclusal wax record will be influenced by the bulk and the consistency of the wax and the accuracy of the wax after chilling. Excess wax contacting mucosal surfaces may distort soft tissues, thereby preventing accurate seating of the wax record onto the stone casts. Distortion of wax during or after removal from the mouth may also interfere with accurate seating. Therefore a definite procedure for making interocclusal wax records is given as follows:

A uniformly softened, reinforced wafer of impression wax is placed between the teeth, and the patient is guided to close in centric relation (Fig. 16-10). Correct closure should have been rehearsed before placement of the wax so that there will be no hesitancy or deviation on the part of the patient. The wax is then removed and immediately chilled thoroughly in room-

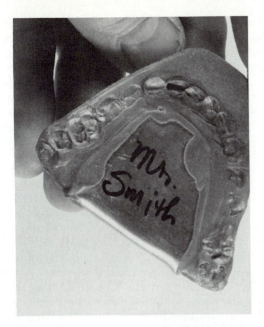

Fig. 16-10. Impression wax (Aluwax) wafer is reinforced with ash No. 7 metal. Reinforcement is folded over wafer and should be shaped to just clear lingual surfaces of teeth in lower arch. Water bath is used to uniformly soften impression wax.

temperature water. It should be replaced a second time to correct the distortion resulting from chilling and again chilled after removal.

All excess wax should now be removed with a sharp knife. It is most important at this time that all wax contacting mucosal surfaces be trimmed free of contact. The chilled wax record again should be replaced to make sure that no contact with soft tissue exists.

A wax record should be further corrected with an impression paste, which is used as the final recording medium. Some impression pastes are more suitable than others for this purpose. Generally a material that sets quite hard is preferred.

In making such a corrected wax record, the opposing teeth (and also the patient's lips and the dentist's fingers) should first be lightly coated with petroleum jelly or a silicone preparation. The impression paste is then mixed and applied to both sides of the metal-reinforced wax record. It is quickly placed, and the patient is assisted

with closing in the rehearsed path, which will this time be guided by the previous wax record. After the paste has set, the corrected wax record is removed and inspected for accuracy. Any excess projecting beyond the wax matrix should then be removed with a sharp knife.

Such a record should seat on accurate casts without discrepancy or interference and will provide an accurate interocclusal record. When an intact opposing arch is present, use of an opposing cast is not necessary. Instead, a hard stone may be poured directly into the impression paste record to serve as an opposing cast. However, although this may be an acceptable procedure in the construction of a unilateral fixed partial denture, the advantages of having casts properly oriented on a suitable articulator contraindicates the practice. The only exception to this is if the maxillary cast on which the partial denture is to be fabricated has been mounted previously with the aid of a face-bow. In such an instance an intact lower arch may be reproduced in stone by pouring a cast directly into the interocclusal record.

An interocclusal record also may be made with an adjustable frame. Reference to this method was made in Chapter 11 (Fig. 11-15). The adjustable frame was devised for use with materials that offer no resistance to closure, such as zinc oxide and eugenol impression pastes.

Some of the advantages of using a metallic oxide paste over wax as a recording medium for occlusal records follow: (1) uniformity of consistency, (2) ease of displacement on closure, (3) accuracy of occlusal surface reproduction, and (4) dimensional stability; also (5) some modification in occlusal relationship is possible after closure, if made before the material sets, and (6) distortion is less likely during mounting procedures.

Three important details to be observed when you are using such a material are as follows:

1. Make sure that the occlusion is satisfactory before making the interocclusal record.
2. Be sure that the casts are accurate reproductions of the teeth being recorded.
3. Trim the record with a sharp knife whenever it engaged undercuts, soft tissues, or deep grooves.

Occlusal relations using occlusion rims on record bases. A *third method* is used when one or more distal extension areas are present, when a tooth-bounded edentulous space is large, or when opposing teeth do not meet. In these instances, occlusion rims on accurate jaw relation record bases must be used. **It should not be necessary to add that simple wax records of edentulous areas are never acceptable, despite the unfortunate continuation of this practice. Any wax, however soft, will displace soft tissues. It is totally impossible to seat such a wax record on a stone cast of the arch with any degree of accuracy.**

In this method the recording proceeds much the same as in the second method, except that occlusion rims are substituted for remaining teeth (Fig. 16-11). It is essential that accurate bases be used to help support the occlusal relationship. Shellac bases may be adapted to the casts and then corrected with some kind of impression paste. This is best done by first burnishing tinfoil onto the lubricated cast, mixing a suitable zinc oxide and eugenol impression paste and applying it to the shellac base, and then seating the shellac base onto the cast until the paste has set. The tinfoil adheres to the impression paste, giving a tinfoil-lined correction of the original base. Such a corrected base is entirely acceptable for jaw relation records. Shellac bases also may be lined with some autopolymerizing resin to accomplish the same purpose. In either case, undercuts on the cast must first be blocked out, and tinfoil is required. When resin is employed, a tinfoil substitute is required.

Record bases also may be made entirely of autopolymerizing resin. Those **materials used in dough form lack sufficient accuracy for this purpose unless they are corrected by relining.** A resin base may be formed by sprinkling monomer and polymer into a shallow matrix of wax or clay after blocking out any undercuts. If the matrix and blockout have been formed with care, interference to removal will not occur, and little trimming will be necessary. When the sprinkling method is used and sufficient time is allowed for progressive polymerization to occur, such bases are the most stable and accurate obtainable short of using cast metal, vulcanite, or

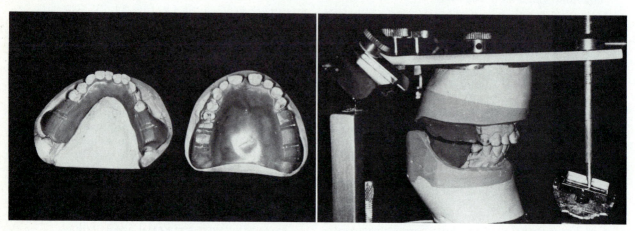

A   **B**

Fig. 16-11. Relationship and distribution of remaining teeth for this patient require that record bases and occlusion rims be used for accurate mounting of casts. **A,** Acrylic resin record bases and hard baseplate wax occlusion rims. These record bases are very stable and were formed by sprinkling autopolymerizing acrylic resin. Note that occlusion rims have been indexed. Occlusion rims substitute for missing posterior teeth and provide an opportunity for posterior support when making interocclusal records. **B,** Casts have been oriented to articulator in centric relation. Recording was made as near vertical dimension of occlusion as possible, yet permitting no contact of occlusion rims or teeth when recording was made.

compression molded and processed resin bases for jaw relation records (Fig. 17-42).

Jaw relation records made by this method accomplish essentially the same purpose as the two previous methods. The fact that record bases are used to support edentulous areas does not alter the effect. Therefore in any of these three methods the skill and care used by the dentist in making occlusal adjustments on the finished prosthesis will govern the accuracy of the resulting occlusion.

Methods for recording centric relation on record bases. There are many ways by which centric relation may be recorded when record bases are used. The least accurate is the use of softened wax occlusion rims. Modeling plastic occlusion rims, on the other hand, may be uniformly softened by flaming and tempering, resulting in a generally acceptable occlusal record. This method is time proved, and when competently done, it is equal in accuracy to any other method.

When wax occlusion rims are used, they should be reduced in height until just out of occlusal contact. A single stop is then added to maintain its terminal position while a jaw relation record is made in some uniformly soft material, which sets to a hard state. Quick-setting impression plaster, impression paste, or autopolymerizing resin may be used. With any of these materials, opposing teeth must be lubricated to facilitate easy separation. Whatever the recording medium, it must permit normal closure into centric relation without resistance and must be transferable with accuracy to the casts for mounting purposes.

Relative to the third method, some mention must be made of the ridge on which the record bases are formed. If the prosthesis is to be tooth supported or a distal extension base is to be made on the anatomic ridge form, the bases will be made to fit that form of the residual ridge. But **if a distal extension base is to be supported by the functional form of the residual ridge, it is necessary that the recording of jaw relations be deferred until the master cast has been corrected to that functional form.** Record bases must be as nearly identical as possible to those of the finished prosthesis. Jaw relation record bases are useless unless they are made on the same cast to which the denture will be processed, or a duplicate thereof, or are themselves the final denture bases. The latter may be either of cast alloy or a processed resin base.

Jaw relation records made entirely on occlusion rims. The *fourth method* is used when no occlusal contact exists between the remaining natural teeth, such as when an opposing maxillary complete denture is to be made concurrently with a mandibular partial denture. It may also be used in those rare situations in which the few remaining teeth do not occlude and will not influence eccentric jaw movements. Jaw relation records are made entirely on occlusion rims when either arch has only anterior teeth present (Fig. 16-12).

In any of these situations, jaw relation records are made entirely on occlusion rims. The occlusion rims must be supported by accurate jaw relation record bases. Here the choice of method for recording jaw relations is much the same as that for complete dentures. Either some direct interocclusal method or a stylus tracing may be used. As with complete denture construction the use of a face-bow, the choice of articulator used, the choice of method for recording jaw relations, and the use of eccentric positional records are optional according to the training, ability, and desires of the individual dentist.

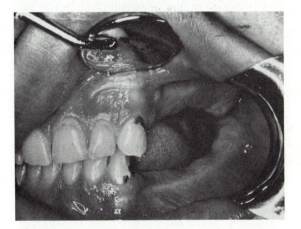

Fig. 16-12. Opposing Class I dental arches with remaining anterior teeth only. Recording of maxillomandibular relations can be accomplished accurately only by using stable record bases and occlusion rims.

Establishing occlusion by the recording of occlusal pathways. The *fifth method* of establishing occlusion on the partial denture is the registration of occlusal pathways and the use of an occluding template rather than a cast of the opposing arch. **When a static jaw relation record is used, with or without eccentric articulatory movements, the prosthetically supplied teeth are arranged to occlude according to a specific concept of occlusion.** On the other hand, **when a functional occlusal record is used, the teeth are modified to accept every possible eccentric jaw movement.**

These movements are made more complicated by the influence of the remaining natural teeth. Occlusal harmony on complete dentures and in complete mouth rehabilitation may be obtained by the use of several different instruments and techniques. Schuyler has emphasized the importance of establishing first the anterior tooth relation and incisal guidance before proceeding with any complete oral rehabilitation. Others have shown the advantages of establishing canine guidance as a key to functional occlusion before proceeding with any functional registration against an opposing prosthetically restored arch. This is done on the theory that the canine teeth serve to guide the mandible during eccentric movements when the opposing teeth come into functional contact. It also has been pointed out that the canine teeth transmit periodontal proprioceptor impulses to the muscles of mastication and thus have an influence on mandibular movement even without actual contact guidance. However, as long as the occlusal surfaces of unrestored natural teeth remain in contact, as in many a partially dentulous mouth, these will always be the primary influence on mandibular movement. The degree of occlusal harmony obtainable on a fixed or removable restoration will depend on the occlusal harmony existing between these teeth.

Regarding occlusion, Thompson has said: "Observing the occlusion with the teeth in static relations and then moving the mandible into various eccentric positions is not sufficient. A dynamic concept is necessary in order to produce an occlusion that is in functional harmony with the facial skeleton, the musculature, and the temporomandibular joints."[*] By adding "and with the remaining natural teeth," the requirements for partial denture occlusion will be more completely defined.

Whereas some of the methods described previously may be applied to the construction of partial dentures in both arches simultaneously, the registration of occlusal pathways requires that an opposing arch be intact or restored to the extent of planned treatment. If partial dentures are planned for both arches, a choice is necessary as to which denture is to be made first and which is to bear a functional occlusal relation to the opposing arch. Generally the maxillary arch is restored first and the mandibular partial denture occluded to that restored arch. Similarly, if the maxillary arch is to be restored with a complete denture or a fixed partial denture or crowns, this is done before establishing the occlusion on the opposing partial denture.

Regardless of the method used for recording jaw relations, when one arch is completely restored first, that arch is treated as an intact arch even though it is wholly or partially restored by prosthetic means. The dentist should consider at the time of treatment planning the possible advantages of establishing the final occlusion to an intact arch.

Step-by-step procedure for registering occlusal pathways. After the framework has been adjusted to fit the mouth, the technique for the registration of occlusal pathways is as follows:

1. Support the wax occlusion rim by a denture base having the same degree of accuracy and stability as the finished denture base. Ideally, this would be the final denture base, which is one of the advantages of making the denture with a metal base. Otherwise, make a temporary base of sprinkled autopolymerizing acrylic resin, which is essentially identical to the final resin base. In any distal extension partial denture, make this base on a cast that has been corrected to the functional or supporting form of the edentulous ridge (Fig. 16-13).

---

[*]From Thompson, J.R.: In Sarnat, B.S., editor: Temporomandibular disorders: diagnosis and dental treatment in the temporomandibular joint, Springfield, Ill., 1951, Charles C Thomas, Publisher.

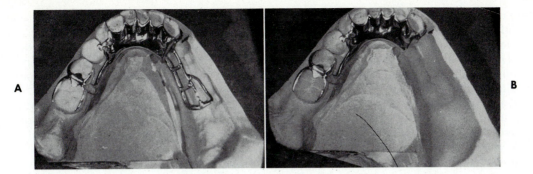

Fig. 16-13. A, After correction of edentulous area to functional form, framework is reseated accurately on corrected master cast, any undercuts are blocked out with clay, and tinfoil substitute is applied to surface of cast. **B,** New resin base is made with autopolymerizing acrylic resin by sprinkling to form record base that is as nearly as possible identical to form of finished denture base. After curing, framework is lifted and any flash or excess is trimmed away. This base is then used to establish occlusal relations by whatever method is indicated, depending on opposing dentition and dentist's preference.

Place a film of sticky wax on the base before the wax occlusion rim is secured to it. The wax used for the occlusion rim should be hard enough to support biting stress and should be tough enough to resist fracture. Peck's purple hard inlay wax has proved to be suitable for the majority of patients. However, some individuals with weak musculature or tender mouths may have difficulty in reducing this wax. In such situations use a slightly less hard wax. Make the occlusion rim wide enough to record all extremes of mandibular movement.

2. Inform the patient that the occlusion rim must be worn for a period of 24 hours or longer. It should be worn constantly, including nighttime, except for removal during meals. By wearing and biting into a wax occlusion rim, a record is made of all extremes of jaw movement (Fig. 16-14). The wax occlusion rim must maintain positive contact with the opposing dentition in all excursions and must be left high enough to assure that a record of the functional path of each cusp will be carved in wax. This record should include not only voluntary excursive movements but also involuntary movements and changes in jaw movement caused by changes in posture. Extreme jaw positions and habitual movements during sleep should also be recorded.

The occlusal paths, thus recorded, will represent each tooth in its three-dimensional aspect. Although the cast poured against this will resemble the opposing teeth, it will be wider than the teeth that carved it because it represents those teeth in all extremes of movement. The recording of occlusal paths in this manner eliminates entirely the need to reproduce mandibular movement on an instrument.

Instruct the patient in the removal and placement of the partial denture supporting the occlusion rim and explain that by chewing and gliding, the wax will be carved by the opposing teeth. Therefore the opposing teeth must be cleaned occasionally of accumulated wax particles. It is necessary that the patient comprehend what is being accomplished and understand that both voluntary and involuntary movements must be recorded.

Before dismissing the patient, add or remove wax where indicated to provide continuous contact throughout the chewing range. To accomplish this, repeatedly warm the wax with a hot spatula and have the patient carve the warmed wax rim with the opposing dentition, each time adding to any areas that are deficient. Support with additional wax any wax left unsupported by its flow under occlusal forces. It is important that the wax rim be absolutely dry and free of saliva before additional wax is applied. Each addition of wax must be made homogeneous with the larger mass to avoid separation or fracture of the occlusion rim during the time it is being worn. Leave the wax occlusion rim from 1 to 3 mm high, depending on whether vertical dimension is to be increased.

3. After 24 hours, the occlusal surface of the wax rim should show a continuous gloss, indicating functional contact with the opposing teeth in all extremes of movement (Fig. 16-14). Any areas deficient in contact should be added to at this time. **The reasons for maintaining positive occlusal contact** throughout the time the occlusion rim is being worn are that (a) all opposing teeth may be placed in function; (b) an opposing denture, if present, will become fully seated; and (c) vertical dimension in the molar region will be increased, thus repositioning the head of the mandibular condyle and allowing temporomandibular tissues to return to a normal relationship.

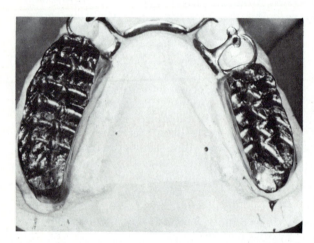

Fig. 16-14. Example of completed occlusal registration in hard inlay wax supported by accurate record bases. Note that width of each cusp in all extremes of mandibular movement is recorded as continuous glossy surface. Yet, anatomy of each opposing tooth is well defined. Completed registration must be placed back onto master cast without intervening debris or discrepancy and secured there with sticky wax so that accuracy of occlusal registration will be maintained.

If during this period the wax occlusion rim has not been reduced to natural tooth contact, warm it by directing air from the air syringe through a flame onto the surface of the wax. By holding the wax rim with the fingers while warming it, a gradual softening process will result, rather than a melting of the surfaces already established. Repeatedly warm the occlusion rim and replace it in the mouth until the occlusal height has been reduced and lateral excursions have been recorded. At this time, support with additional wax those areas left unsupported by the flow of the wax to the buccal or lingual surfaces. At the same time, trim the areas obviously not involved, thus narrowing the occlusion rim as much as possible. Remove also those areas projecting above the occlusal surface, which by their presence might limit functional movement.

Having accomplished seating of the denture and changes in mandibular position by the previous period of wear, it is possible to complete the occlusal registration at the chair. However, if all involuntary movements and those caused by changes in posture are to be recorded, the patient should again wear the occlusion rim for a period of time.

4. After a second 24 to 48 hour period of wear the registration should be complete and acceptable. The remaining teeth serving as vertical stops should be in contact, and the occlusion rim should show an intact glossy surface representing each cusp in all extremes of movement.

Not all natural teeth formerly in contact will necessarily be in contact on completion of the occlusal registration. Those teeth that have been depressed over a period of years and those that have been moved to accommodate overclosure or mandibular rotation may not be in contact when mandibular equilibrium has been reestablished. Such teeth may possibly return to occlusal contact in the future or may have to be restored to occlusal contact after initial placement of the denture. Since the mandibular position may have been changed during the process of occlusal registration, the cuspal relation of some of the natural teeth may be different than before. This fact must be recognized in determining the correct restored vertical dimension.

Occlusion thus established on the partial denture will have more complete harmony with the opposing natural or artificial teeth than can be obtained by adjustments in the mouth alone, because occlusal adjustment to accommodate voluntary movement does not necessarily prevent occlusal disharmony in all postural positions or during periods of stress. Furthermore, occlusal adjustment in the mouth without occlusal analysis is limited by the dentist's ability to interpret correctly occlusal markings made intraorally, whether by articulating ribbon or by other means.

The registration of occlusal pathways has still further advantages. It makes possible the obtaining of jaw relations under actual working conditions, with the denture framework in its terminal position, the opposing teeth in function, and an opposing denture, if present, fully seated. In some instances it also makes possible the recovery of lost vertical dimension, either unilaterally or bilaterally, when overclosure or mandibular rotation has occurred, rather than perpetuating an abnormal mandibular relationship.

The completed registration is now ready for conversion to an occluding template. This is usually done by boxing the occlusal registration with modeling clay after it has been reseated and secured onto the master or processing cast (Figs. 16-15 to 16-18). Only the wax registration and areas for vertical stops are left exposed. It is then filled with a hard stone to form an occluding template (Chapter 17).

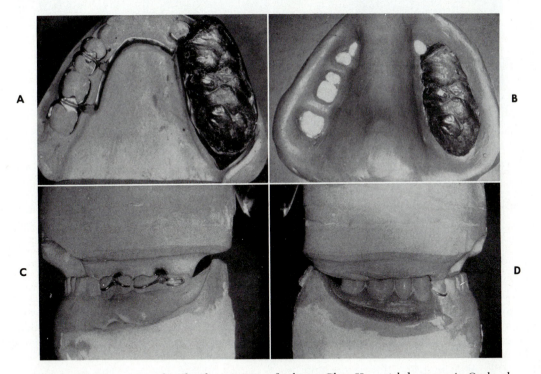

Fig. 16-15. Four views of occlusal registration for lower Class II partial denture. **A,** Occlusal registration in wax returned to master cast. Note extreme horizontal movement recorded. **B,** Same cast boxed with clay, leaving multiple occlusal surfaces exposed as vertical stops. **C,** Effect of occlusal stops, eliminating any possible changes in vertical dimension on articulator. **D,** Processed denture remounted for occlusal readjustment. Note modification in occlusal anatomy of stock artificial teeth and slight increase in height of occlusal plane. This is in harmony with natural tooth contact elsewhere in arch.

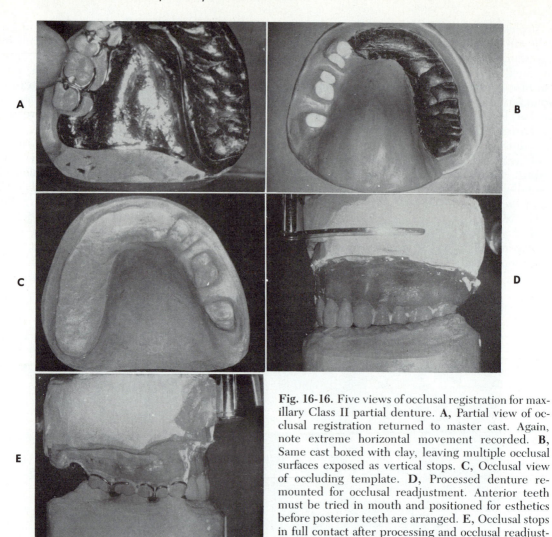

Fig. 16-16. Five views of occlusal registration for maxillary Class II partial denture. **A,** Partial view of occlusal registration returned to master cast. Again, note extreme horizontal movement recorded. **B,** Same cast boxed with clay, leaving multiple occlusal surfaces exposed as vertical stops. **C,** Occlusal view of occluding template. **D,** Processed denture remounted for occlusal readjustment. Anterior teeth must be tried in mouth and positioned for esthetics before posterior teeth are arranged. **E,** Occlusal stops in full contact after processing and occlusal readjustment following remounting.

It is necessary that stone stops be used to maintain the vertical relation rather than relying on some adjustable part of the articulating instrument, which might be changed accidentally (Fig. 16-19). Also, by using stone stops and by mounting both the denture cast and the template before separating them, a simple hinge instrument may be used.

Because of its simplicity and the accessibility it affords in arranging teeth, the Hagman Junior Balancer is preferred as an articulating instrument for use with an occluding template (Fig.

16-20). In this application the instrument is used as a hinge only, with all other moving elements securely locked in a fixed position. However, any hinged articulator may be similarly used.

MATERIALS FOR ARTIFICIAL POSTERIOR TEETH

Modern resin teeth are preferred by some over porcelain teeth because they are more readily modified and thought to more nearly resemble enamel in their action against opposing teeth. Resin teeth with gold occlusal surfaces

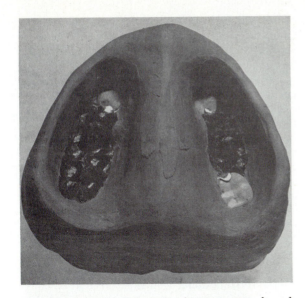

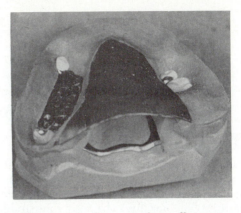

Fig. 16-17. Completed occlusal registration boxed with clay before pouring template in hard die stone. Occlusal surfaces of adjacent abutment teeth are left exposed to serve as stone-to-stone vertical stops. Clay is trimmed just to margins of registration and raised in center to provide arch for lingual access while arranging teeth to occlude with template.

Fig. 16-18. Rather than use clay sufficient to arch across from one side to another, same may be done with wax using less time and material. It is better that the wax form a more acute angle with occlusal wax registration and exposed occlusal surfaces than illustrated here.

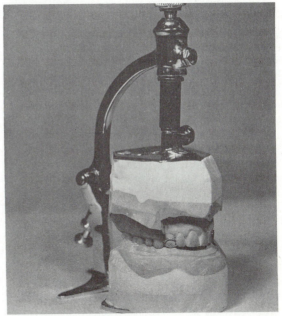

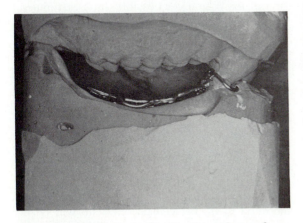

Fig. 16-19. Profile view of occlusal template and one of its vertical stops. Despite fact that this is a record of all extremes of mandibular movement for this patient, anatomy of occluding teeth can easily be identified.

Fig. 16-20. Completed maxillary partial denture with artificial teeth arranged and modified to occlude with template made from wax occlusal registration. Hagman Junior Balancer is used as hinge alone, with all adjustable elements securely locked before the cast and template are mounted. Stone stops are used to preserve vertical relation. Note notch in upper cast for keying cast to articulator to facilitate accurate remounting after processing.

are preferably used in opposition to natural teeth, restored natural teeth, and gold occlusal surfaces, whereas porcelain teeth are generally used in opposition to other porcelain teeth.

Some changes in this concept have occurred in recent years. Sears and, later, Myerson have introduced the feasibility of using porcelain and resin teeth in opposition and the advantage of reduced frictional resistance by doing so. Myerson has compared the effect of porcelain teeth against resin teeth to that of a diamond stylus against a vinyl phonograph record, which results in less wear by friction than does the less hard sapphire stylus. For this to be truly comparable, the porcelain tooth should possess a glazed surface, but experience has shown that even a polished vacuum-fired porcelain surface causes limited wear and reduced frictional resistance when in opposition to a modern resin artificial tooth.

A second fact also has been recognized, which is that resin tooth surfaces may in time become impregnated with abrasive particles, thereby becoming an abrasive substance themselves. This may explain why resin teeth are sometimes capable of wearing opposing gold surfaces. **An evaluation of occlusal contact or lack of contact, however, should be meticulously accomplished at each 6-month recall appointment regardless of the choice of material for posterior tooth forms.**

Although some controversy still may exist in regard to the use of porcelain or resin artificial teeth, there is broad agreement that narrow occlusal surfaces are desirable. Posterior teeth that will satisfy this requirement should be selected, and the use of tooth forms having excessive buccolingual dimension should be avoided.

It has been observed that artificial posterior resin teeth become excessively abraded in comparatively short periods of time regardless of the material by which they are opposed. The attendant ills of excessive abrasion of occlusal surfaces may often be avoided by using porcelain teeth to oppose porcelain teeth, gold occlusals to oppose other gold occlusal surfaces or natural teeth, and removal of the denture on retiring.

Acrylic resin teeth are easily modified and readily lend themselves to construction of cast gold surfaces on their occlusal portions. A simple procedure for fabricating gold occlusal surfaces and attaching them to acrylic resin teeth is described in Chapter 17 under posterior tooth forms.

Arranging teeth to an occluding template. The occlusal surface of the artificial teeth, porcelain or resin, must be modified to occlude with the template. In this method they are actually only raw materials from which an occlusal surface that is in harmony with an existing occlusal pattern is developed. Therefore the teeth must be occluded too high and then modified to fit the template at the established vertical dimension.

Teeth arranged to an occluding template ordinarily should be placed in the center of the functional range. Whenever possible, the teeth should be arranged buccolingually in the center of the template. When natural teeth have registered the functional occlusion, this may be considered the normal physiologic position of the artificial dentition regardless of its relation to the residual ridge. On the other hand, if some artificial occlusion in the opposing arch has been recorded, such as that of an opposing denture, the teeth should be arranged in a favorable relation to their foundation, even if this means arranging them slightly bucally or lingually from the center of the template.

The teeth are usually arranged to intercuspate with the opposing teeth in a normal cuspal relationship. Whenever possible, as is customary, the mesiobuccal cusp of the maxillary first molar is located in relation to the buccal groove of the mandibular first molar and all other teeth arranged accordingly. With functional occlusion, however, it is not absolutely necessary that a normal anterior-posterior relation be reestablished (Fig. 16-21). In the first place the opposing teeth in a broken dental arch may not be in normal alignment, and intercuspation may be difficult to accomplish. In the second place the occlusal surfaces will be modified so that they will function favorably regardless of their anterior-posterior position (Fig. 16-22). Since cusps modified to fit an occlusal template will be in harmony with the opposing dentition, it is not necessary that the teeth themselves be arranged to conform to the usual concept of what constitutes a normal anterior-posterior relationship.

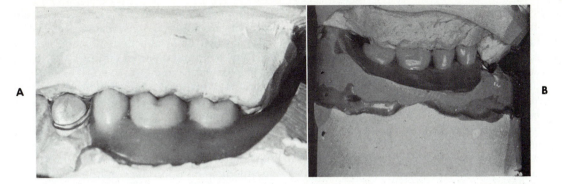

Fig. 16-21. **A,** View of intercuspation sometimes possible when teeth are arranged to occlusal template. This is possible only when gross migration of opposing teeth has not occurred. **B,** View of modification to occlusal surfaces necessary when customary intercuspation would create objectionable spaces. Note that original cusp-to-cusp relation of artificial teeth has been altered until marginal ridges have actually become cusps. Such occlusal relationship is entirely permissible and effective.

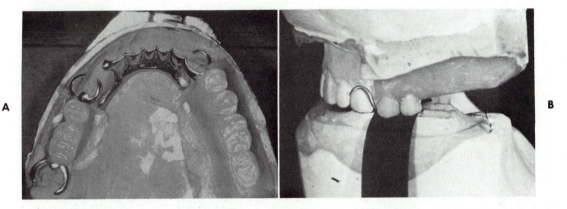

Fig. 16-22. **A,** Occlusal surfaces after remounting and final occlusal readjustment to template. Note functional occlusal anatomy resulting. This is entirely different occlusal surface from that which was present on stock artificial teeth as manufactured. **B,** When dentist is arranging teeth to occluding template, marking tape should be used in positioning and modifying each tooth to fit template. Note that at this early stage articulator has been opened approximately 0.5 mm, as evidenced by slight space at vertical stop.

ESTABLISHING JAW RELATIONS FOR A MANDIBULAR REMOVABLE PARTIAL DENTURE OPPOSING A MAXILLARY COMPLETE DENTURE

It is not uncommon for a mandibular removable partial denture to be made to occlude with an opposing maxillary complete denture. The maxillary denture may already be present or it may be made concurrently with the opposing partial denture. In any event, the establishment of jaw relations in this situation may be accomplished by one of several methods previously outlined.

If an existing maxillary complete denture is satisfactory and the occlusal plane is oriented to an acceptable anatomic, functional, and esthetic position, then the complete denture need not be replaced and the opposing arch is treated as an intact arch as though natural teeth were present. A face-bow transfer is made of that arch and the cast mounted on the articulator in the usual manner. Maxillomandibular relations may be recorded on accurate record bases attached to the mandibular partial denture framework, using one of the recording mediums previously outlined, such as wax, modeling plastic, quick-setting plaster, impression paste, or autopolymerizing acrylic resin. Centric relation is thus recorded and transferred to the articulator. Eccentric records can then be made to program the articulator.

In rare instances, when the mandibular partial denture replaces all posterior teeth and the anterior teeth are noninterfering, a central bearing point tracer may be mounted in the palate of the maxillary denture and centric relation recorded by means of an intraoral stylus tracing against a stable mandibular base.

If the relationship of the posterior teeth on the maxillary denture to the mandibular ridge is favorable and the complete denture is **stable,** jaw relations may be established by recording occlusal pathways in the mandibular arch the same as for any opposing intact arch. The success of this method depends on the stability of the denture bases, the quality of tissue support, the relation of the opposing teeth to the mandibular ridge, and the interrelation of existing artificial and natural teeth.

More often than not, the existing maxillary complete denture will have been made to occlude with malpositioned mandibular teeth, which have since been lost, or the teeth will have been arranged without consideration for the future occlusal relation with a mandibular partial denture. Too frequently one sees a maxillary denture with posterior teeth arranged close to the residual ridge without regard for interarch relationship and with an occlusal plane that is too low. In such instances the least that can be done is to reposition the posterior teeth on the maxillary denture before establishing maxillomandibular relations. This can only be justified when the maxillary denture is otherwise satisfactory as to fit, appearance, and occlusion elsewhere in the arch. **Usually, however, a new**

maxillary denture must be made concurrently with the mandibular partial denture, and jaw relations may be established in one of two ways.

If the mandibular partial denture will be tooth supported (a Kennedy Class III arch accommodating a bilateral removable prosthesis), that arch is restored first. The same applies to a mandibular arch being restored with fixed partial dentures. In either situation the mandibular arch is completely restored first, and jaw relations are established as they would be to a full complement of opposing teeth. Thus the maxillary complete denture is made to occlude with an intact arch, and the procedure for doing so need not be included here.

On the other hand, as is more frequently the situation, the mandibular partial denture may have one or more distal extension bases. The situation then requires that either the occlusion be established on both dentures simultaneously or the maxillary denture be completed first.

After making final impressions, which include the correction of the mandibular cast to establish optimal support for the bases of the partial denture (the denture framework must be made previously), the maxillary occlusion rim is contoured, vertical relation with the remaining lower teeth is established, and a face-bow transfer of the maxillary arch is made. The maxillomandibular relations may be recorded by any one of the several methods previously outlined and the articulator mounting completed. Occlusion may be established as for complete dentures, taking care to establish a favorable tooth-to-ridge relationship in both arches, an optimal occlusal plane, and cuspal harmony between all occluding teeth.

After try-in, either of two methods may be used. Both dentures may be processed concurrently and remounted for occlusal correction, or the maxillary denture may be processed first, and after it is remounted, the teeth, still in wax on the partial denture, are adjusted to any discrepancies occurring.

Up to the point of establishing the final occlusion on the partial denture, jaw relations, articulator mounting, and try-in are accomplished as though both dentures were to be completed at the same time. The teeth on the mandibular partial denture are arranged in wax so that a favorable ridge relationship and occlusal plane will have been established. The maxillary denture alone is then remounted to adjust the occlusion to the remaining natural teeth and is placed in the mouth as a completed restoration.

The teeth in wax are removed from the partial denture base and replaced with hard inlay wax occlusion rims secured to acrylic resin bases, which are attached to the denture framework. A functional occlusal record is then accomplished by registering occlusal pathways, treating the opposing complete denture as an intact arch. The occlusal registration thus obtained is placed back on the master cast, boxed with clay, and an occluding template is formed complete with stone-to-stone vertical stops. The same articulator may be used, replacing the original upper cast with the template, or the mandibular cast and the template may be mounted on a simple hinge-type articulator.

It is necessary that the acrylic resin record base be removed by softening it over a flame before the teeth are rearranged to occlude with the template. The teeth that were formerly arranged to occlude with the maxillary denture are then modified to fit the template, and the denture bases are waxed and processed. Investing must be done in such a manner that the cast may be recovered intact and remounted for occlusal refinement to the template.

Occlusion thus established on a mandibular partial denture opposing a maxillary complete denture provides occlusal harmony. Not only does stability of both dentures result, but trauma conducive to tissue changes beneath both dentures is held to a minimum. The harmony of occlusion thus established justifies the added steps necessary to accomplish such results.

Correction of occlusal discrepancies created during processing must be accomplished before the patient is permitted to use the denture(s). Methods by which these discrepancies may be corrected are discussed in Chapter 17.

SELF-ASSESSMENT AIDS

1. See if you believe this statement: Occlusal harmony exists when the masticating mechanism can carry out its physiologic functions while the factors of occlusion remain in a healthy state; the factors of occlusion being the temporomandibular joints, the neuromuscular mechanism, and the teeth and their supporting structures.
2. Occlusal harmony between a removable partial denture and the remaining natural teeth is a major factor in preserving the health of the supporting structures of the natural teeth. True or false?
3. The establishment of a satisfactory occlusion for a partial denture patient should include five considerations or procedures by the dentist. Can you recall these five "musts"?
4. Define **centric relation** in your own words.
5. What is **centric occlusion**?
6. What is meant by **eccentric occlusion?**
7. Describe a **balanced occlusion.**
8. Two methods are commonly used to develop an acceptable occlusion for a removable partial denture patient. Can you give a brief description of these two methods?
9. What records are necessary to correctly orient casts to an arcon type articulator and to program the articulator?
10. A harmonious relationship of opposing occlusal and incisal surfaces, in itself, is not adequate to assure stability of distal extension removable partial dentures. What other factor must be recognized and dealt with to minimize unwanted leverages?
11. There are differences among dentists in devloping contacts of opposing teeth in centric and eccentric positions for partially edentulous patients. When you answer the following queries correctly, honestly try to rationalize the recommendations contained in this text:
    a. Simultaneous contacts of opposing posterior teeth must occur in centric occlusion. True or false?
    b. Occlusion for tooth-borne removable partial dentures may be arranged to duplicate the occlusion seen in a harmonious natural dentition. True or false?
    c. Under what circumstances is a balanced occlusion desirable for the partially edentulous patient?
    d. Should working side contacts be developed when a mandibular distal extension denture is opposed by natural teeth (assuming all mandibular posterior teeth are missing)?
    e. You are treating a patient with a Class I maxillary arch. Is it beneficial to develop balancing and working contacts? Explain your answer. What about protrusive contacts?
    f. Are balancing side contacts for a Class II maxillary arch desirable?
    g. What are the desirable contact relationships

of artifical-natural teeth when one arch is a Class IV arch?

h. What is the most distal extent that an artificial tooth should be arranged in a Class I or II mandibular arch?

12. A patient requires a tooth-borne mandibular removable partial denture. The remaining teeth are maximally intercusping; however, this position does not coincide with centric relation. There is no TMJ pathology, no neuromuscular disorders, and no periodontal conditions aggravated by occlusion. Would you insist that the patient be restored to have maximum intercuspation coincide with centric relation? Why or why not?

13. Under what circumstances would you develop an occlusion for a partially edentulous patient so that maximum intercuspation coincided with centric relation?

14. When must the dentist determine the horizontal jaw relation in which he will develop the occlusion for the partially edentulous patient? Why?

15. After the horizontal relationship of the jaws to which the occlusion will be developed has been determined, occlusal relationships may be established by five methods. The choice of method will be determined by the existing partially edentulous situation of the patient, location of remaining teeth in each arch, and the prior correction of any existing occlusal discrepancies. These five methods are (a) direct opposition of casts, (b) interocclusal records with posterior teeth remaining, (c) occlusal relations using occlusal rims, (d) jaw relation records made entirely on occlusion rims, and (e) recording functionally generated paths. You should be able to rationalize and briefly discuss each of the five methods.

16. What are the disadvantages of using wax alone for making interocclusal records?

17. When developing an occlusion for a partially edentulous patient using the functionally generated path technique, why may occluding frames be used rather than an articulator?

18. What are the disadvantages in developing an occlusion to a stone template or stone teeth on a cast?

19. Materials of which the occlusal surfaces of artificial posterior teeth are made deserve serious consideration by the dentist. These considerations should be based on minimizing attrition of occlusal surfaces, maintaining the established vertical dimension of occlusion, and maintaining positive contact of posterior teeth as planned. To best accomplish the preceding, please give the material of choice for opposing occlusal surfaces for (a) porcelain, (b) enamel, (c) restored natural teeth, and (d) fixed partial denture pontics with gold occlusal surfaces.

20. Acrylic resin posterior teeth lend themselves to easier modification than do porcelain teeth when the interresidual ridge distance is small or when an edentulous space to be restored with the denture is grossly restricted. However, acrylic resin teeth have one big drawback when occluded against any other occlusal surface, including acrylic resin. Do you know what this drawback is?

21. The occlusal surfaces of acrylic resin teeth attached to a denture may be duplicated in gold and attached to the same teeth. Did you consult Chapter 17 to see how this is accomplished?

22. Occlusal discrepancies created during processing procedures *must* be corrected before the patient is given possession of the dentures. True or false?

17 LABORATORY PROCEDURES

This chapter will cover only those phases of dental laboratory procedures that are directly related to partial denture construction. Familiarity with laboratory procedures relative to the making of fixed restorations and complete dentures is presumed. Such information is already available in the numerous excellent textbooks on those subjects and will not be duplicated here. For example, the principles and techniques involved in the waxing, casting, and finishing of single inlays, crowns, and fixed partial dentures are adequately covered in lecture material and textbooks and in manuals available to the dental student, the dental laboratory technician, and the practicing dentist. Similarly, knowledge of the principles and techniques for mounting casts, articulating teeth, and waxing, processing, and polishing complete dentures is presumed as a necessary background for the laboratory phases of partial denture construction. Therefore this chapter will be directed specifically toward the laboratory procedures involved in making a removable partial denture.

DUPLICATING A STONE CAST

A stone cast may be duplicated for one of three purposes. One is the duplication in stone of the original or corrected master cast to preserve the original. On this duplicate cast the denture

framework may be fitted without danger of abrading or fracturing the surface of the original master cast. Most of the better commercial dental laboratories have adopted a policy of doing all work on a duplicate cast, including the fitting procedures. The finished casting is then returned to the dentist after all fitting has been completed on the duplicate cast.

Students or dentists doing their own laboratory work should likewise follow the policy of making a duplicate cast for fitting the denture framework. Although some dental laboratories also may use the duplicate cast for blockout, it is preferable to do the blockout on the master cast just before a second duplication rather than to use the duplicate cast for this purpose. After blockout of the master cast a second duplication is done for making an investment cast. On this investment cast the wax or plastic pattern is formed, and the metal framework is ultimately cast against its surface.

A blocked out master cast should be duplicated in stone if wrought-wire retainers are planned as components of the framework for the removable partial denture. The contouring of wrought-wire retainers may be accomplished on this cast and transferred to the duplicate investment cast in the exact same relationship to which it was contoured on the duplicate stone

341

cast. This use of a duplicate stone cast of the blocked out master cast avoids marring the master cast or investment cast. (See Fig. 17-10.)

Although both the fitting cast and the investment cast must be an accurate reproduction of the original, the fitting cast is made of a hard stone and is not directly involved in making the metal framework. The investment cast, on the other hand, must possess the properties of a casting investment, such as the ability to withstand burnout temperatures while providing the necessary mold expansion. Gold alloys and also Ticonium are cast to plaster-bound silica investments, whereas the higher melting Stellite alloys are cast to investments containing quartz held together by a suitable binder so that they will withstand the higher casting temperatures necessary with these alloys. Although the latter are generally harder than are gypsum investments, any investment cast may be easily abraded and must be handled carefully to preserve the accuracy of its surface. The practice of treating the dried investment cast by lightly spraying it with a model spray reduces considerably the danger of its becoming abraded during subsequent handling.

The use of preformed plastic patterns eliminates some of the danger of altering the surface of the investment cast in the process of forming the pattern (Fig. 17-6). With freehand waxing, considerable care must be taken not to score or abrade the investment cast. The student, however, needs the experience of freehand waxing to obtain a better comprehension of the bulk and contours necessary to produce an acceptable denture framework. A continuation of this practice is recommended. For the same reasons it is also recommended that the laboratory technician be experienced in the use of wax shapes and freehand waxing before being allowed to use preformed patterns.

Duplicating materials and flasks. Duplicating materials are colloidal materials, which are made fluid by heating and return to a gel on being cooled.

The cast to be duplicated must be placed in the bottom of a suitable flask, called a duplicating flask. It is necessary that a duplicating flask

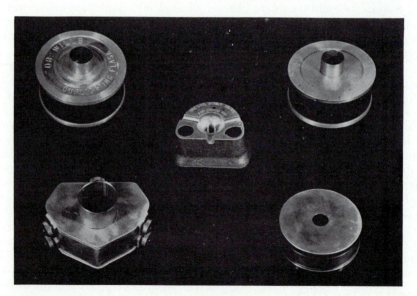

Fig. 17-1. Five types of duplicating flasks. Upper left, Wills flask, type E; upper right, Wills flask, type F. Both these flasks have Formica ring, 4-inch inside diameter and are 2 inches in height. Formica is used for its non-heat–conducting property and is machined with 5-inch inside taper. In center is bell-shaped flask; lower left, Kerr duplicating flask; lower right, lightweight brass flask in common usage.

contain the fluid material to facilitate cooling, to facilitate removal of the cast from the mold without permanent deformation or damage to the mold, and to support the mold while it is being filled with the cast material. Numerous duplicating flasks are on the market (Fig. 17-1). One type is a metal bell with holes in the top for pouring. Another is a simple metal ring with removable bottom and top, the latter having a center hole for pouring. Still another has the top and bottom secured with thumb screws.

Noble G. Wills is due much credit for his untiring efforts in furthering the development of accurate cast duplication equipment. Two of these duplicating flasks are illustrated in Fig. 17-1. They consist of a machined metal top and bottom fitting onto a Formica ring 2 or 2¼ inches high. Formica rather than metal is used for the ring because Formica acts as an insulator to prevent too rapid cooling through the sides of the flask. The center hole in the top of each type is provided with a filling reservoir, or "feeder ring." Although not all duplicating flasks provide a filling reservoir, it is most desirable that a ring superstructure be provided to serve as a reservoir for feeding the warm material into the mold. Thus as cooling and subsequent shrinkage occur, additional fluid material is fed into the mold from the reservoir above. This is similar to the cooling of dental gold after casting. Gold requires an additional bulk of metal so that on cooling, the piece being cast can draw on additional metal from the reservoir, which is called the **button.** Without the additional bulk of metal the casting would likely show porosity. In duplication, cooling from the bottom of the flask causes the duplicating material to shrink, which has a tendency to draw the chilling solution into closer adaptation to the cast.

The technique for duplicating is the same for any cast, whether or not blockout is present. However, if wax or clay blockout is present, the temperature of the duplicating material must not be any higher than recommended by the manufacturer to avoid melting and distorting the blockout material.

Any clay used for blockout before duplication must be of the insoluble type (Chapter 10). Therefore only an oily base clay may be safely used for this purpose.

Although ordinary baseplate wax may be used for paralleled blockout and ledges, care must be taken that the temperature of the duplicating material is not high enough to melt the wax. The use of prepared blockout material may be preferred, such as Ney blockout wax or Wills undercut material. A formula has been given in Chapter 10 for those preferring to prepare their own blockout material.

Duplicating procedure. The equipment needed for duplication is as follows (Fig. 17-2).

Bunsen burner and tripod
Enamel or stainless steel double boiler (aluminum utensils should not be used, as aluminum seems to have a deleterious effect on the composition of the duplicating colloid)*
Duplicating flask
Plaster bowl (600 ml)
Stiff spatula (Kerr laboratory spatula or Buffalo dental No. 4 R)
Vibrator
Rubber suction cup
No. 7 spatula

Step-by-step procedure (Fig. 17-4). Although the procedure given describes the use of the Wills flask, it applies as well to the use of any duplicating flask.

1. New hydrocolloid duplicating material is usually packaged in a semidried state. It may be in the form of a crumbled meal. In such a case, further chopping is unnecessary. If in bulk form, it must be chopped into fine particles. This is greatly facilitated by running it through a kitchen food chopper. Any duplicating material being reused should similarly be reduced to small pieces before heating.

Heat the duplicating material in the top of the double boiler, stirring to dissipate lumps. New material must be diluted with water in the proportions recommended by the manufacturer; material being reused may be diluted if needed to replace water lost by evaporation. Remember that duplicating material may be further thinned with warm water during preparation as it becomes necessary, but the incorporation of dry material into a mix that is too thin is much more difficult to accomplish. Therefore it is best that

---

*Ready Duplicator may be used in lieu of an enamel or stainless steel double boiler (Fig. 17-3).

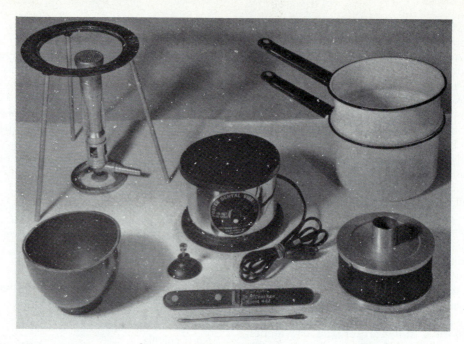

Fig. 17-2. Armamentarium for preparing material for duplicating: double boiler, ring stand, Bunsen burner, stiff laboratory spatula for stirring duplicating material and for mixing cast material in plaster bowl, No. 7 wax spatula for directing stream of fluid duplicating material over critical areas of cast, vibrator, duplicating flask with feeder ring, and rubber suction cup for extracting cast from chilled mold.

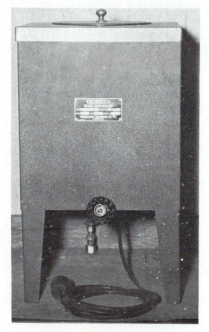

Fig. 17-3. Ready Duplicator maintains duplicating material at controlled temperature and ready for immediate use. Duplicating hydrocolloid flows through rubber hose at base of duplicator, and rate of flow is controlled by manually operated shut-off valve. Its use is particularly suited when several duplications are accomplished daily. (Courtesy Ticonium Division, CMP Industries, Inc., Albany, N.Y.)

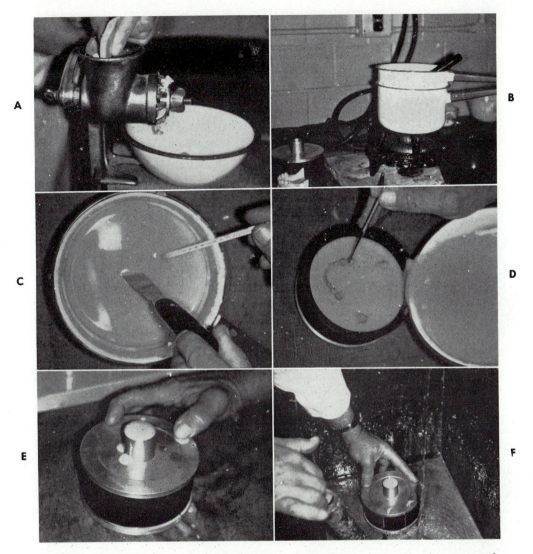

Fig. 17-4. Ten steps in process of duplication. **A,** If duplicating material is being reused, it should be ground into small pieces before being heated, to avoid lumps and uneven consistency. **B,** Material is then placed in top of double boiler and stirred well with spatula until it reaches smooth, creamy consistency. Warm water may be added sparingly to dilute it if necessary, but avoid overdilution. **C,** Remove pan from double boiler and continue stirring until temperature has dropped to about 120° F. At this temperature finger may be immersed without burning, but it is more accurately checked with thermometer. **D,** Cast to be duplicated, which has been immersed in water just before duplication, is placed in bottom of duplicating flask, over small pellet of clay. Small continuous stream of duplicating material is poured in at posterior end of cast while material is guided over critical areas with No. 7 spatula held in other hand. **E,** After filling flask, top and feeder ring are positioned, and duplicating material is added to completely fill feeder ring. **F,** Flask is placed in running tap water about 2.5 cm deep until material in feeder ring has completely gelled, with depression in its center to show that shrinkage has occurred. Then flask may be completely immersed in running tap water for additional 30 minutes.

Continued.

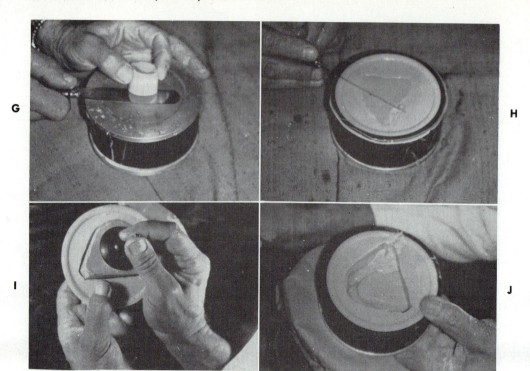

Fig. 17-4, cont'd. G, Feeder ring is removed and projecting material cut off flush with top of flask. **H,** Flask is inverted and bottom of flask removed, exposing base of cast. In this position, open end now becomes top of mold and original top of flask becomes bottom. Excess duplicating material is then removed around base of cast. **I,** Rubber suction cup is applied to base of cast **under water.** Mold is then removed from flask and flexed gently around sides as cast is removed with suction cup acting as handle. **J, Mold** is inspected for defects. It is then returned to flask precisely in its original position, original lid placed on bottom for support, and stone or investment, properly proportioned and spatulated, is slowly vibrated around arch, tooth by tooth, to avoid trapping air or diluting material with moisture. Mold is then completely filled and covered with wet towel or bell jar to prevent dehydration of mold at expense of water of crystallization of cast material. Although duplicating mold will not be poured a second time, its dimensional accuracy must be preserved until cast material has completely set.

any thinning be done by adding water slowly until the right consistency has been obtained.

When a smooth, creamy mix has been obtained, remove the upper pan of the double boiler from the burner and **continue stirring** until the temperature has dropped to 120° F. At this temperature, which is just low enough not to burn a finger immersed in it, the duplicating material is ready to pour.

2. For 4 minutes just before duplication, immerse the cast in water at about 85° F, preferably in water (slurry) that has lost its ability to etch the surface of the stone. Do this while the duplicating material is being cooled to a usable temperature. Immerse the cast upside down to allow the escape of any air trapped beneath sheets of wax placed on the master cast for relief. Another effective method is to immerse the blocked-out cast in clear slurry water in a rubber mixing bowl and place the bowl in an activated vacuum bell jar for 2 minutes just before duplication (Fig. 17-5).

Water that has been allowed to stand for some time with pieces of dental stone or plaster in it

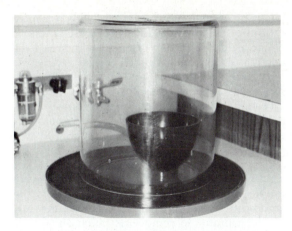

Fig. 17-5. Entrapped air in blocked-out master stone cast may be eliminated before duplication by placing cast in rubber mixing bowl, three-fourths filled with clear slurry water, and placing bowl under bell jar and activating vacuum for 2 minutes.

will have lost its ability to etch the surface of a stone cast. **Therefore any soaking of a stone cast should be done in water prepared for that purpose rather than in tap water.**

When pieces of plaster or stone have been previously placed in tap water, solution will occur until the water becomes saturated with calcium sulfate. Once the water has become saturated, an equilibrium occurs with no further dissolution taking place. A stone cast placed in such water will not become etched because the water already contains all the calcium sulfate it can hold. A container of such water should be available in the laboratory for use any time a cast needs to be soaked, such as before duplication or before repouring a portion of the original cast.

The broken pieces of plaster or stone should be small to medium in size but not fine enough to remain suspended in the water when it is agitated. These pieces should remain in the water at all times to maintain the equilibrium of the calcium sulfate. When used, the water should be clear.

Gently blow surface moisture off of the cast with compressed air, and center the cast in the bottom of the duplicating flask over a small pellet of clay. Press the base of the cast firmly against the bottom of the flask.

3. With one hand, slowly pour the duplicating material into the flask just behind one posterior end of the cast. A stream of duplicating material about 3 mm in diameter should be poured continuously at this point until the base of the cast has been completely covered. At this time, with the No. 7 spatula in the other hand, guide the material around the teeth, into interproximal spaces, and on critical tooth surfaces. This prevents trapping air bubbles in critical areas.

After the teeth have been completely covered, fill the flask within 3 mm of the top. Then interrupt the pouring while positioning the metal top and feeder ring, after which completely fill the mold to the top of the feeder ring.

4. Now place the flask in about 2.5 cm of cold (preferably running) water. The water should cover no more than the metal base and the lower 12 mm of the Formica ring so that initial cooling will occur only through the metal bottom.

Although cooling **must** be done slowly and from the bottom to control shrinkage and avoid distortion, it is not absolutely necessary that cooling be hastened by using cold water. Time permitting, a hydrocolloid mold may be bench cooled without affecting its accuracy, whereas too rapid cooling may cause distortion. With this in mind, allow the mold to set completely in a shallow water bath. However, to facilitate early separation of the mold, when the feeder ring has gelled, immerse the flask in cold running water, where it should be left for at least 15 minutes to assure chilling throughout.

5. After thorough chilling, remove the flask from the water bath and remove the feeder ring. Cut off the hydrocolloid projecting above the lid flush with the top of the lid. Then invert the flask and remove the bottom, exposing the base of the cast. Remove any hydrocolloid covering the base of the cast and the flattened piece of clay, leaving the smooth base of the cast exposed.

The inside of the Formica ring is tapered; therefore it may be removed by sliding it away from the top, leaving the mold attached only to the top. In the inverted position the top now has become the bottom and will remain so during the subsequent procedures. The original bottom, now removed, will not be replaced on the mold, as this becomes the open end into which the cast material is poured.

If the top of the flask is undercut, the mold is not removed from it, and it becomes the base for supporting the mold. If the flask has a top that is keyed but not undercut, the mold is removed from it also to facilitate flexing as the cast is being removed from the mold. In either case, removal is best accomplished by applying a rubber suction cup to the base of the cast under running tap water and lightly flexing the mold while extracting the cast.

The suction cup is used as a convenient handle. Without it, the mold would have to be cut away to expose enough of the sides of the cast for a finger grip. After pouring and removing the duplicate cast, an excess would result where the mold has been cut away. Although this may be trimmed on the cast trimmer, it must be remembered that the base of the cast has been scored in three places to facilitate repositioning on the surveyor. If the scored areas are inadvertently trimmed away, there will be no record of the path of placement on the duplicate cast to aid in positioning it on the surveyor for locating contour lines. This necessity does not exist when clasp ledges (indices) were formed on the master cast. However, when waxing is to be done in relation to a survey line only, it is necessary that the original cast position be recorded on the duplicate cast. On the other hand, such a record always must be preserved on a duplicate stone cast to be used for fitting. This is particularly true when wrought-wire clasp arms must be accurately adapted in relation to the height of contour of the abutment teeth.

6. After removing the cast, replace the mold in the flask in exactly the same position as before. This is made possible by the keyed relationship of the parts of the flask. Reposition the hydrocolloid in the tapered Formica ring so that the longer of the three grooves in the hydrocolloid mold points to the centering screw on the outside of the ring. Replace the keyed top, which is to become the bottom, and invert the ring so that the open end of the mold is up. If the reassembly is properly done, the mold is in exactly the same relation to the flask as before; otherwise distortion of the mold may result.

Remove any free moisture from the mold by inverting it and blowing it out with a gentle stream of compressed air. Care must be taken not to hold the stream of air on any area long enough to cause dehydration of that area.

With the correct amount of water in the plaster bowl, add a measured amount of stone or investment, following the manufacturer's recommendations. The correct water-powder ratio is given by the manufacturer for each 100 g of powder.

Mix thoroughly with a stiff spatula or a mechanical mixer. **Vacuum mixing is always preferable for eliminating entrapped air.** If this equipment is not available, knead the mixture on the vibrator to remove as much air as will come to the surface. Many of the small air voids in a cast are the result of air bubbles being carried into the mold in the mix rather than to air trapped in the mold during pouring.

Fill the hydrocolloid mold in much the same manner as an impression of a dental arch. With the No. 7 spatula, add small amounts of material only at one posterior end while using the vibrator. The material is thus made to flow around the arch by the weight of the material behind it. Add material only at the original site until all critical areas of the mold have been filled. In this manner, excess moisture is pushed ahead of the material until it reaches the opposite end of the mold, where it should be expelled and discarded. This avoids any dilution of the mix by the moisture remaining in the mold, minimizes the chances of trapping air, and results in a uniformly dense cast.

7. Immediately on filling the mold, partially immerse it in still water and allow it to set for about 30 minutes. Partial immersion supplies the cast material with needed water of crystallization, some of which may otherwise be taken up by the hydrocolloid, resulting in a chalky cast surface. On the other hand, partial immersion should not be for longer than approximately 45 minutes, and never overnight, or etching of the surface of the cast will result. The filled mold may also be covered with a damp towel to supply the cast material with needed water of crystallization while hardening.

After the cast material has hardened, remove the flask from the mold and **break the mold away from the cast** rather than attempt to remove the cast from the intact mold. The mold should not be poured a second time anyway, and fresh surfaces of the cast may be rubbed off in withdrawing it from the mold. **Therefore the mold should always be broken away from the cast.**

Duplicating material may be washed and placed in water in a covered jar for reuse, especially when it will likely be reused in the near future. However, if any doubt exists as to its texture, it should be discarded. One should not attempt to revitalize old duplicating material by replenishing with new. Instead, any questionable material should be discarded and a new batch of material mixed as needed.

A freshly duplicated cast should not be handled unnecessarily, particularly one made of investment material, until it has been allowed to dry in air or in an oven. **An investment cast should not be trimmed on a cast trimmer, as this causes a slurry of investment to splash over the cast, which may not then be entirely removed by rinsing.** For that matter an investment cast should not be rinsed at all. Instead it should be hand-trimmed with a sharp knife, and any powdered residue should be carefully blown off.

After initial drying and trimming, an investment cast should be dried in an oven at 180° to 200° F for 60 to 90 minutes depending on the size of the cast. Then it should be removed and immediately lightly sprayed with a plastic model spray. A buildup of the plastic spray on the investment cast must be avoided.

Some of the advantages of spraying an investment cast are (1) it provides a smooth dense surface on the investment cast, (2) it facilitates the development of wax and plastic patterns in that these substances will adhere better to the sprayed cast than they will to an untreated refractory cast, and (3) it helps prevent marring of the cast during handling.

The use of microwave ovens as a means of rapid drying investment casts is being investigated and may eventually prove to be an acceptable time-saving procedure.

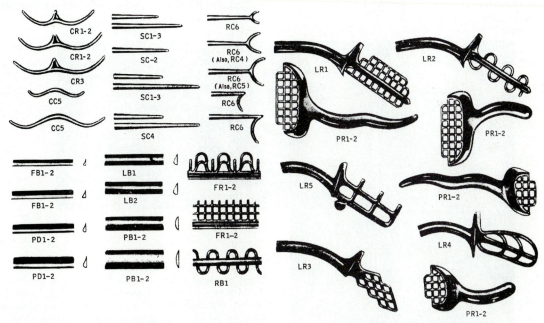

Fig. 17-6. Preformed plastic patterns are available in many shapes and sizes. Being made of soft plastic material, they tend to stretch on removal from their backing. Therefore care must be exercised when removing patterns. Their use generally requires that "tacky" liquid be first applied to investment cast at their area of placement. (Courtesy, J.F. Jelenko and Company, Armonk, N.Y.)

WAXING THE PARTIAL DENTURE FRAMEWORK

Experience with freehand waxing and the use of ready-made wax shapes is recommended as a prerequisite to the use of preformed plastic patterns (Fig. 17-6). Unless plastic patterns are selected and used with care, they are better not used at all. The fact that they facilitate rapid production of partial denture castings has led to their widespread use in commercial laboratories, but this alone does not justify their use. Even when plastic patterns are used, parts of the denture framework must be waxed freehand to avoid excessive bulk and to create the desired contours. (See Fig. 17-7.)

The use of ready-made wax shapes facilitates freehand waxing to the point that an experienced dentist or dental laboratory technician can complete a wax pattern in little more time than is necessary when plastic patterns are used. Much of the speed with which a wax pattern may be produced depends on how well the step-by-step procedure is organized to take fullest advantage of the wax shapes.

The students in the preclinical laboratory should begin a waxing experience on a stone cast rather than on the softer investment cast, so that they may be free to modify and correct their errors as they are pointed out. Only after having a clear understanding of the location, bulk, and contours of the various parts of the wax pattern being done should they be allowed to wax on the investment cast. Since corrections on the investment cast may result in a rough casting, it is imperative that the waxing on the investment cast be done in a positive manner with a minimum of changes and corrections.

The same applies to making a removable partial denture framework in the undergraduate dental clinic. Although typical dental students probably will not fabricate their own partial denture castings after graduation, it is essential that they have a background and experience in dental laboratory procedures that will enable them to design the denture framework and prescribe how it is to be fabricated (Fig. 17-8). Not only this, but they must also be capable of evaluating the finished product to the end that the

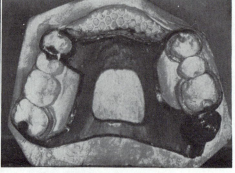

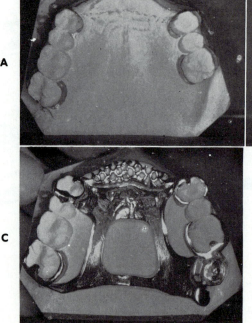

Fig. 17-7. Three steps in making denture framework using blockout ledges and ready-made pattern forms. **A,** Master cast with shaped blockout ledges for location of retentive and nonretentive clasp arms. **B,** Completed pattern using anatomic replica pattern, plastic clasp forms resting on investment ledges, and open retention mesh anteriorly. Pattern is then waxed to completion. **C,** Finished casting returned to master cast. Blockout ledges may be seen below three lingual clasp arms.

quality of dental laboratory services is maintained (Fig. 17-9).

With this in mind, it is desirable that two or more partial denture frameworks be waxed to completion, if not cast and finished, by the clinical student. To avoid discrepancies occurring as a result of inept waxing and subsequent corrections on the investment cast, it is most desirable that the student first do a practice wax pattern on a duplicate stone cast. After all corrections

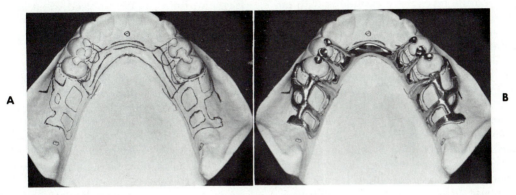

Fig. 17-8. A, Technician should receive from dentist master cast that has been surveyed and had reference lines scratched on two sides and dorsal aspect of base of cast or has been marked for tripoding. On this cast, outline of denture framework should be drawn precisely, without marring cast, where components parts of framework are to be placed and their dimensions indicated. In addition, written instructions, including waxing specifications, which ideally should accompany the outlined master cast, must be included (Fig. 18-2). From such work authorization, the technician may be expected to return polished casting that accurately conforms to penciled design, as in B.

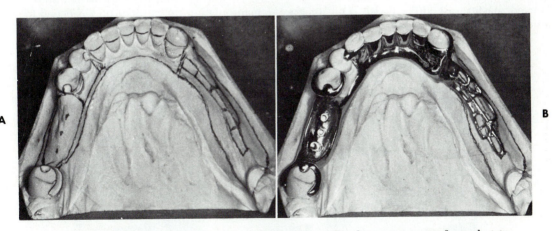

Fig. 17-9. A, Design of partial denture framework is outlined on master cast for technician to follow in waxing and casting framework. B, Cast framework as returned from laboratory, superimposed on penciled design. Note contouring of thin lingual apron continues with half-pear–shaped lingual bar major connector. In the modification space metal base is used with undercut finishing lines and nailhead retention for attachment of artificial posterior teeth later with resin base material. Also note use of lingual ledges on abutment teeth of modification space. (From McCracken, W.L.: J. Prosthet. Dent. 8:71-84, 1958.)

have been approved by the instructor, waxing on the investment cast may be done with confidence and dispatch, resulting in a casting of high quality. Although this policy may be criticized as time-consuming, the total time spent should be little more than that required when it is done on the investment cast alone with numerous corrections. A higher percentage of satisfactory castings and fewer remakes will result when this policy is followed in the undergraduate clinic. The quality of the finished product and the knowledge and experience gained by the student more than justify the additional time spent.

Forming the wax pattern for a mandibular Class II removable partial denture framework. One waxing exercise will be given that embodies many of the essentials of waxing a partial denture framework. This exercise includes the waxing of three types of direct retainers—circumferential, combination, and bar type. A lingual bar major connector is used and also a cast denture base for the tooth-bounded edentulous space. The adaptation of a round, 18-gauge wrought wire is required for the formation of the retentive arm of a combination-type direct retainer.

The student should be furnished two stone casts that are duplicates of the blocked-out and relieved master cast (Fig. 17-10). One of the stone casts will be used to adapt a wrought-wire,

retentive direct retainer arm, and the other stone cast will be used to simulate a refractory cast on which the wax pattern will be completed.

1. On one of the stone casts, outline lightly the pattern for the framework, being guided by the transfer indices (Fig. 17-11). A color pencil (Eagle Verithin) should be used when outlining the pattern on a refractory cast or on the stone cast for this exercise. In either instance, extreme caution must be used in this procedure to avoid the slightest abrasion of the cast.

2. Forming the wrought-wire retentive arm is the next step in the procedure. The design for the mandibular partial denture framework calls for the use of a tapered, round, 18-gauge wrought-wire retentive direct retainer arm on the lower left second premolar. The wrought wire to be used may be selected according to the guidelines discussed in Chapter 11.

Any wrought wire may be fatigued by repeated bending and straightening, and prolonged manipulation with pliers causes nicks in the wire. Either may result in early failure of the clasp arm through no fault of the material itself. To avoid having to correct mistakes by rebending, the student should practice first with paper-clip wire of similar gauge. After having learned to contour the wire with a minimum of manipulation the student may proceed to adapt the tougher 18-gauge wrought wire.

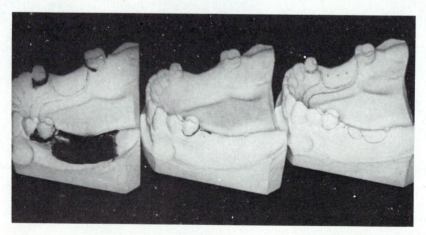

Fig. 17-10. Blocked out master cast is on left. Wrought-wire direct retainer arm is adapted to one of duplicate stone casts (center figure). Right figure is duplicate stone cast simulating refractory cast on which outline of framework has been lightly drawn.

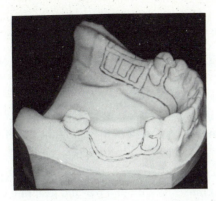

Fig. 17-11. Penciled outline of framework. Outline of major connector and borders of cast denture base were scratched lightly on master cast and duplicated in refractory cast. Ledge indices of direct retainers and outlined major connector and denture base permit exact duplication of penciled outline on master cast to refractory cast.

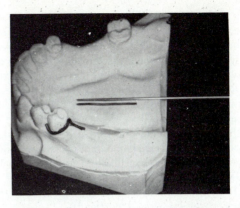

Fig. 17-12. Outline for retentive wrought-wire arm is outlined on cast following ledge index. An 18-gauge round wax strip is adapted to penciled outline. Wax strip straightened out determines length of 18-gauge wrought wire required to form direct retainer arm.

We have found that round wrought wire may be contoured to almost any usable configuration by using only one type of pliers—Dixon No. 139 or similar pliers of other manufacturers. The wire should be contoured around the round beak of the pliers to avoid acute angles to the greatest extent possible.

The procedure for forming wrought-wire direct retainer arms is as follows:

a. On the second stone cast, being guided by the ledge index, outline in pencil the design of the wrought-wire retentive arm (Fig. 17-12). Extend the outline just lingual to the center of the guiding plane area on the abutment and then continue the outline downward to the gingival area. Extend the line posteriorly on the cast for approximately 8 to 9 mm. This is the outline for the right-angle "foot," which will be embedded in the casting just lingual to the crest of the residual ridge. Since it should be assumed that only a mechanical attachment with the casting alloy may result, the "foot" is necessary to secure the wrought wire to the casting.

b. Determine the length of the wire needed by adapting a piece of 18-gauge round wax to the penciled outline of the wrought-wire retainer. Straighten this wax form and cut a piece of the selected 18-gauge wire about 2 mm longer than the wax form (Fig. 17-12).

c. Round one end of the wire with an abrasive rubber wheel. Measure the length of the penciled outline of the wrought-wire direct retainer arm on the cast from its proposed terminal tip to its junction with the envisioned minor connector on the distal of the second premolar. Taper the rounded end portion of the wire uniformly the measured length of the retainer arm using a 2-inch cut-off carborundum disk in a bench lathe and an abrasive rubber polishing wheel. The wire should be so tapered that the terminal portion of the wire engaging the undercut is approximately one half the diameter of the 18-gauge wire. (See Chapter 11.)

d. With contouring pliers, contour the tapered portion of the wire to contact the buccal surface of the premolar starting the contour near the tapered terminal end of the wire. The wire must accurately follow the ledge index on the cast. Continue contouring the wire to contact the tooth slightly lingual to one-half the width of the distal surface of the tooth.

e. With the contoured portion of the wire held in position against the abutment tooth, mark the wire with a pencil at the exact spot where the wire must turn inferiorly toward the residual ridge. Also, carefully estimate the length of this upright portion of the wire according to the outline on the cast. Make a bend in the wire at the previously marked spot so that the vertical portion of the wire will contact the guiding plane area of the abutment tooth. The wire cannot be placed back on the cast at this time. Having estimated the length of the vertical portion of the wire, make a bend so that the remaining portion of the wire contacts the residual ridge region of the cast and is directed posteriorly. Two millimeters from the untapered end of the wire, make a bend so that the end of the wire projects almost vertically.

f. The formed wire should accurately and passively conform to the outline on the stone cast (Figs. 17-13 and 17-14). Wrought wire can be accurately and rather quickly adapted without nicks or having become strain-hardened. Practice first with paper clips. Place the formed wire and cast aside until the wax pattern has been developed on the other stone cast.

3. Adapt one thickness of 24-gauge casting sheet wax (green or pink) or adhesive wax on the lingual aspect of the alveolar ridge to cover the outline of the lingual bar major connector. Be careful not to stretch the wax, thereby altering its thickness.

4. Adapt a piece of 6-gauge half-pear–shaped wax over the sheet wax to conform to the pencil lines denoting the lingual bar and showing through the sheet wax. The greater bulk of the half-pear shape must be at the lower border, with the tapered edge near or along the top pencil line. The thickness of the wax shape and the sheet wax previously adapted, plus a small amount of wax added to maintain a half-pear shape, will be the thickness of the major connector before polishing.

5. Cut away the sheet wax extending above the outline of the lingual bar and also below the half-pear–shaped wax, which has now become the lingual bar, and cut off both the bar and sheet wax even with the distal aspects of the premolar abutments or according to the outline of these areas (Fig. 17-15). Use a fairly dull instrument (Roach carver) for this purpose to avoid scoring the cast.

6. Seal the inferior and superior borders of the bar to the cast. It is important that the wax be sealed to the cast throughout its course, yet that the original half-pear shape be preserved. Should any part of the wax pattern not be sealed to the cast, the pattern may become dislodged during the application of the outer investment, resulting in the investment's seeping under the

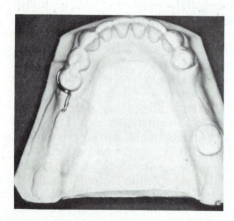

Fig. 17-13. Wrought-wire arm is closely and passively adapted to abutment tooth. Note taper of arm from distobuccal aspect of abutment to retentive end. "Foot" is just lingual to crest of residual ridge to provide space for cervical end of artificial molar.

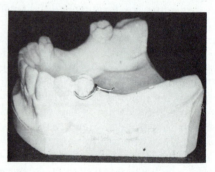

Fig. 17-14. Portion of wrought wire contacting distal of abutment is placed as far inferiorly as possible, since master cast was blocked out in this area. Such position will have less tendency to "top-load" the tooth in resisting horizontal rotation of denture. Small angled piece of wire at distal of conformed arm facilitates handling of warm clasp arm with cotton forceps in later waxing procedures and provides mechanical attachment of retainer arm, which will be embedded in cast framework.

pattern. This would result in a false undersurface on the casting.

7. Adapt a piece of 8-gauge half-round wax to the full extent of the guiding plane on the distal surface of the left premolar (flat side to the guiding plane surface). Cut the wax off slightly inferior to the marginal ridge and seal the wax to the cast. Taper the wax superiorly to a feather edge (Fig. 17-16).

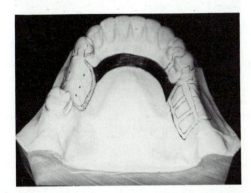

Fig. 17-15. Lingual bar pattern is made of half-pear–shaped, 6-gauge wax form, reinforced on tissue surface with 24-gauge sheet wax for rigidity. Bar is trimmed to conform to outline of denture base on one side and minor connector outlined on distal extension side.

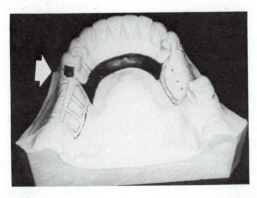

Fig. 17-16. This minor connector (arrow) forms part of direct retainer assembly for abutment tooth. Its contact with guiding plane, in conjunction with guiding plane surfaces on opposite side of arch, will assure only one path of placement and removal of completed restoration.

8. Adapt a piece of 10-gauge round wax strip from the superior border of the lingual bar up the embrasure between the first and second premolars, then over the marginal ridges, and into the rest seats prepared in the premolars. This minor connector should pass perpendicularly from the lingual bar up the interdental embrasure. A rule previously stated is that any crossing of gingival tissues by components of the framework should be abrupt and definite. A second rule to be followed is that minor connectors should conform to interdental embrasures whenever possible and should be so shaped to present as little bulk to the tongue as possible. Seal the wax shape to the cast, converting it to an embrasure form, and wax the occlusal rests to conform to the outline of the rest seat preparations (Fig. 17-17). Strengthen the wax at the marginal ridges if necessary. The final form of the pattern for the occlusal rests should be representative of the occlusal anatomy before the rest seats were prepared.

9. Cut two pieces of 24-gauge casting sheet wax (green or pink), which, when joined at the crest of the tooth-bounded edentulous ridge, will cover the penciled outline of the cast base (Fig. 17-18). Adapt the lingual portion first,

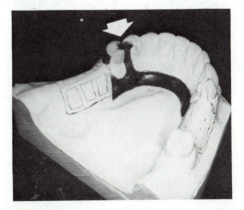

Fig. 17-17. Gingival margins were relieved and interproximal undercuts were blocked out on master cast parallel to path of placement. Therefore this minor connector does not engage undercut. In fact, the only components of framework engaging undercuts are terminal ends of retentive direct retainer arms. See Fig. 4-43 for interproximal conformation of this component on finished framework.

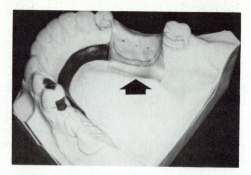

Fig. 17-18. Twenty-four–gauge sheet wax is adapted over outline of lingual portion of cast denture base area. Outline will show through pink sheet wax, thus permitting accurate trimming of wax. Use of 24-gauge sheet wax permits some adjustment of denture base to alleviate sore spots if such occur after patient uses restoration.

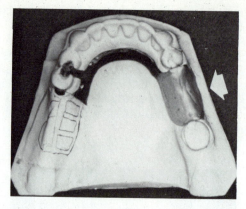

Fig. 17-19. Buccal portion of cast base pattern is added, and wax is trimmed to conform to outline of framework. Forming this portion of cast base pattern is best done in two steps as described to avoid thinning 24-gauge sheet wax. Two halves are then carefully joined and sealed at crest of residual ridge.

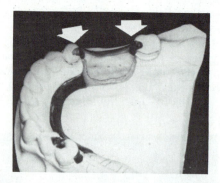

Fig. 17-20. Occlusal rests may be carved to form before other components of direct retainer assemblies are formed in wax. Rests should conform to occlusal morphology present before rest seats were prepared.

being careful not to stretch the wax. Trim this wax just 0.5 mm inferior to the penciled outline of the lingual portion of the cast base area. Seal the wax along its edges and to the adjacent end of the major connector.

10. In a like manner, adapt and seal the other piece of 24-gauge sheet wax over the buccal portion of the cast base, joining both pieces over the crest of the ridge in a smooth junction (Fig. 17-19).

11. Adapt a length of 8-gauge half-round wax on the guiding plane, proximal surfaces of the right side abutments (flat side against the guiding plane), attaching one end to the cast base pattern gingivally and carrying the other end over the marginal ridge and into the rest seat preparations (Fig. 17-20). Seal the wax along its edges and to the cast base pattern after the wax has been trimmed to conform to the outline of the rests and guiding plane areas.

12. Being guided by the index ledge, adapt a piece of 12-gauge half-round wax on the lingual surface of the right premolar abutment, and connect the distal end of the strip of wax to the previously formed minor connector on the same tooth. On this particular abutment and also on the molar abutment, the retentive clasp arms will be on the buccal surfaces and the reciprocal arms on the lingual surfaces. Reciprocal arms are nonretentive and therefore should not be tapered except to avoid abruptness and irritation to the tongue by the terminal end of the clasp arm. Reinforce the junction of the reciprocal arm pattern with the minor connector to which it is attached (Fig. 17-21).

13. Adapt a piece of 8-gauge half-round wax to the lingual surface of the molar abutment, being guided by the lingual ledge of the abutment crown. Connect the strip of wax to the previously formed minor connector. Add suffi-

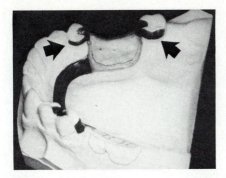

Fig. 17-21. Reciprocal components must be rigid and, since they do not engage undercuts, need not be tapered for sake of flexibility. Reciprocal arm on molar restores lingual anatomy of abutment crown.

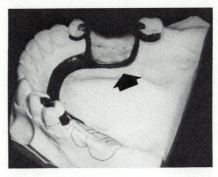

Fig. 17-22. Fourteen-gauge round wax added as described forms trough to support and retain acrylic resin supporting artificial teeth. Therefore smooth junction between framework and acrylic resin is made without danger of cracks in resin appearing after denture has been in use. Since border of cast base pattern is thickened by addition of 14-gauge round wax, resultant casting can be gently rounded at borders, making it more comfortable for patient than having borders finished as sharp edges.

cient wax to have the lower portion of this reciprocal arm as thick as the lingual extent of the ledge on the crown. Superiorly, wax must be added to restore the normal contour of the lingual surface of the crown and feathered to the lingual height of the crown (Fig. 17-21). The terminal end of the reciprocal arm should have a taper corresponding to the taper of the lingual ledge in this area as viewed from above.

14. Beginning at the inferior border of the reciprocal arm of the right premolar at its junction with the minor connector, adapt a piece of 14-gauge round wax over the outline of the lingual portion of the border of the cast base. Carry the wax form up to the inferior border of the reciprocal arm on the molar abutment. Seal this piece of wax on the outside border without appreciably altering its form. This piece of wax will provide an adequate thickness for the border of the cast base and at the same time will form an undercut finishing line on the cast base (Fig. 17-22).

15. Up to this point the forming of the wax pattern has been done primarily on the lingual surfaces of the cast. The rationale of this procedure is to avoid distortion of any buccal components of the pattern by handling of the cast while accomplishing the heavier lingual waxing.

16. Perfect the waxing done thus far by smoothing and adding to the weak points. Smoothing does not mean polishing or flaming the wax pattern, either of which affects only the highest part of the convex surfaces and serves only to flatten and alter the shape of the wax. Rather, smoothing should be done by gentle carving, which preserves the original form of the wax pattern. Therefore, as weak areas become evident, reinforce them by flowing on additional wax and blending it into the original waxing with a hot spatula and by carving. In the process of smoothing, gently trim away all excess wax around the borders of the pattern with a Roach carver. Exercise caution to avoid any alteration of the surface of the cast.

17. Retention for the attachment of resin base on the distal extension side is added next. This consists of two parallel pieces of 12-gauge half-round wax connected with cross rungs to form a ladderlike framework. Beginning at the base of the vertical minor connector on the left second premolar, adapt a piece of 12-gauge half-round wax along the lingual surface of the residual ridge at the ridge crest (convex side up). Extend this piece of wax approximately two thirds the length of the edentulous area. Seal and blend the proximal end of the wax into the minor connector at its point of origin and just tack the distal end to the cast. The retentive frame need

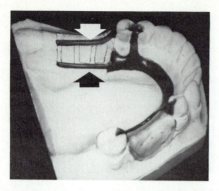

Fig. 17-23. Twelve-gauge half-round wax form is attached to minor connector on guiding plane and runs posteriorly just lingual to crest of residual ridge. Placed in this position, interference to arranging artificial posterior teeth will be minimized. Lower portion of ladderlike structure should be superior to inferior portion of major connector. Otherwise, butt-type junction of major and minor connector would be difficult to construct.

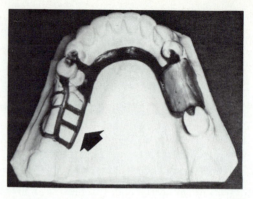

Fig. 17-24. Longitudinal pieces forming portion of minor connector are joined with 12-gauge half-round wax forms (arrow). Two buccal loops of 18-gauge round wax form are attached to longitudinal piece of wax near crest of residual ridge. Minor connector extending on both buccal and lingual slopes of residual ridge will, in all probability, strengthen acrylic resin denture base and minimize warping.

not be sealed to the cast throughout its course (Fig. 17-23).

About 5 to 7 mm inferior to the longitudinal piece of wax, adapt another piece of 12-gauge half-round wax parallel to the first piece and of the same length. The anterior end of the lower wax strip will be attached to the distal end of the major connector. At its point of origin, add wax to reinforce and blend it into the major connector (Fig. 17-23).

At equally spaced intervals of about 4 to 5 mm join the two longitudinal pieces with connecting bars of 12-gauge half-round wax strips. This forms the rungs of the ladderlike construction (Fig. 17-24). Each end of the rung must be attached securely to the longitudinal pieces with additional wax so that reinforcement rather than weakness will exist at each junction point. None of these crossbars need be sealed to the cast except at their ends.

From one rung of the ladder, usually the third from the end, curve a piece of 18-gauge round wax over the buccal side of the ridge to join the most distal rung at the end of the framework. This will provide additional support to the buccal flange of the resin denture base. To facilitate casting from lingually placed sprues, this buccal

loop should be continuous with any two cross rungs. Attach the buccal loop securely with additional wax but do not seal it to the cast in its entire length. In a long span, such as a distal extension situation from a canine or first premolar abutment, two such buccal loops should be used; otherwise one will usually suffice (Fig. 17-24).

A butt-type joint finishing line of the major connector and the resin base retention ladder (minor connector) is made. The purpose of this type joint and finishing line is twofold. First, a smooth, flat, continuous surface between the major connector and the acrylic resin denture base will result, which is less noticeable to the tongue than is a "hump" surface. Second, a butt-type joint is stronger and more resistant to "working" the resin and producing strain fissures than other type joints. Place a strip of 14-gauge round wax about halfway up the lingual surface of the guiding plane minor connector and continue the wax strip inferiorly and on top of the previously formed joint between the ladder and the major connector. Seal this wax to the cast and to the superior border of the major connector. In the process of sealing the 14-gauge round wax, a half-round shape should result. Then ad-

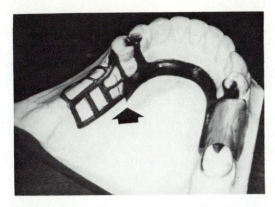

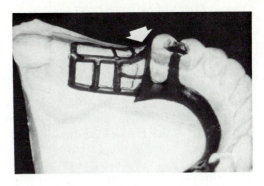

Fig. 17-25. Round 14-gauge wax is used to form direct connection of major connector to minor connector contacting guiding plane surface (arrow). Round form is modified to present flat surface facing posteriorly and angled surface anteriorly, thus forming desired butt joint between major and minor connector.

Fig. 17-26. Eighteen-gauge round wax form is used to strengthen connection between major and minor connector (arrow). This could be accomplished with half-round 12-gauge wax form also. It is absolutely necessary that strong, rigid union exist between major connector and minor connector to which acrylic resin denture base will be attached.

ditional wax may be added to provide the greatest bulk toward the lingual surface. The minor connector contacting the guiding plane surface is thickest at its gingival portion and tapers to a very thin form as it approaches the marginal ridge of the abutment. A minor connector thus established (a rectangular, wedge shape) provides the least interference with the placement of the adjacent artificial tooth. Blend the anterior side into the major connector with a hot wax spatula. Flatten the posterior portion with a warm spatula and carve it to form (Fig. 17-25).

All junctions with the major connector should be reinforced and blended smoothly into its contour (Fig. 17-26). After the butt-type joint is formed, in most instances and especially in those instances where the longitudinal sections of the ladder are separated by more than 4 to 5 mm, an 18-gauge round wax reinforcing element should be provided between the butt joint and the most anterior rung of the ladder (Fig. 17-26).

18. Accomplish the procedure described in 14 on the buccal portion of the cast base pattern.

19. Small "nailheads," as additional acrylic resin retentive elements, are now placed on both the cast base and the minor connector (ladder) for attachment of the resin base on the distal extension side (Fig. 17-27). For the latter the

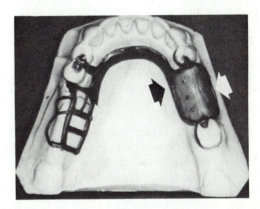

Fig. 17-27. Small mushroom "nailhead" configurations are attached to cast base portion of wax pattern (arrows). These nailheads serve as additional retentive elements for acrylic resin supporting artificial teeth. They should be so positioned that no interference to arranging artificial teeth will be encountered. Six to eight nailheads are quite sufficient on short-span bases (not more than two missing posterior teeth).

nailheads serve to attach a resin tray for making a secondary impression and are removed before the denture base is processed.

A nailhead is quickly and easily made by holding one end of a 5 to 7.5 cm piece of 18-gauge round wax to the area the nailhead is to occupy, sealing the end to the pattern with a hot waxing instrument, holding the strip until the junction has hardened, and then cutting the 18-gauge wax strip about 2 mm above the junction. With a warm wax spatula the protruding end of the wax can be "mushroomed" by simply applying a little pressure.

Nailheads on the cast denture base are confined within the undercut finishing lines and must be placed so that they will neither interfere with the arrangement of the artificial teeth nor protrude through the resin supporting the artificial teeth. Two rows of three or four nailheads are ample. One row should be placed lingually and about halfway between the border of the cast base pattern and the crest of the residual ridge. The other row is similarly located but placed on the buccal side of the cast base pattern.

20. Form the cast retentive direct retainer arms. The creation of the wax pattern has now progressed up to the point of adding the planned retentive clasp arms. These have been classified in Chapter 6. When a cast retentive clasp of any type (other than an l-bar type) is to be used, it must be waxed in relation to the height of contour with the terminal one fourth of the tapered clasp arm progressively engaging a retentive undercut.

The location and extent of the undercut to be used as well as the remaining portion of the retentive arm are established first on the master cast, and the clasp arm is outlined from its origin to its terminus. A wax ledge is carved to establish the location of the inferior border of the clasp arm. In fact, this ledge should be carved the width of a pencil line cervically to the planned inferior border and terminus of the arm to allow for smoothing and polishing the completed casting. Otherwise the inferior border of the cast arm would occupy a position occlusal to its planned position. This ledge is duplicated on the refractory cast, and the clasp arm is waxed or the plastic pattern is placed with its inferior border along the ledge.

Cast retentive clasp arms are most satisfactorily made using preformed plastic patterns that are uniform in dimensions and taper (Fig. 17-6). Students and technicians alike, however, should have had experience in freehand waxing and in the use of wax shapes. Twelve-gauge half-

round wax is used to form the outline of the clasp, which is then sealed to the cast. Some reinforcement at the point of origin and addition of wax along the length of the arm is necessary to create a tapered arm by carving. Of course, some trimming along the sealed edges will also be necessary. The finished pattern should have a uniform taper throughout its course, terminating in a predetermined infrabulge area. With a circumferential clasp the height of contour is crossed at about three-fourths of the length of the retentive arm (never less) as the diameter of the clasp arm decreases and the terminal one fourth progressively engages the tooth undercut.

With a bar-type clasp arm the height of contour is not always crossed by the clasp arm, but the clasp must have a uniform taper from its point of origin to its termination in the undercut area. The point of origin of a bar clasp arm is at the cast denture base or where it emerges from an acrylic resin denture base. Its taper therefore should begin at this point rather than at its attachment to minor connectors of the denture framework. Any portion thereof that will be embedded in a resin base must be considered a rigid connector and not part of the retentive clasp; therefore only the exposed part is tapered to form the bar-type clasp arm.

A cast clasp arm should not be indiscriminately polished and then pliered to place. Rather, waxing should be done in such a manner that a minimum of finishing is necessary and its intended relationship to the abutment tooth is maintained.

With the preceding information and suggestions the patterns for the cast retentive arms may be accomplished. Being guided by the index ledge on the buccal surface of the molar abutment tooth, adapt a piece of 12-gauge half-round wax (flat side to abutment) and attach it to the minor connector (body of the direct retainer). Add a small amount of wax to the clasp arm so that it can be carved to a taper that conforms to the relative dimensions of a cast retentive arm as illustrated in Fig. 6-10. Reinforce the junction of the clasp arm with the body of the clasp by adding sufficient wax to provide a uniform taper from the body to the terminal end of the arm (Fig. 17-28). The student is reminded that in

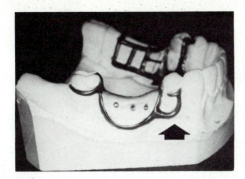

Fig. 17-28. Wax pattern for cast circumferential retainer arm on buccal surface of molar abutment. Since this is retentive arm, it is tapered from its attachment area to its terminus. Bar-type direct retainer arm (arrow) joins cast base pattern. From its retentive tip to its junction with cast base pattern, clasp is carved to tapering, half-round form. Note that inferior portion of assembly is 6 to 7 mm inferior to gingival sulcus to avoid impingement of tissue and possible strangulation. The only portion of bar-type retainer arm occupying undercut is terminal one third to one fourth of horizontal portion in contact with tooth.

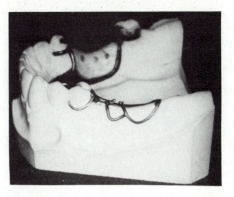

Fig. 17-29. Previously formed wrought-wire retainer arm is attached to wax pattern and is in passive relation to both abutment tooth and pattern.

the formation of **all** wax pattern junctions, the end result must be a solid, homogeneous pattern without pits, voids, cracks, or fissures.

The bar-type retainer is formed next by first adapting a piece of 12-gauge half-round wax (flat side to abutment) on the buccal aspect of the right premolar abutment, being guided by the ledge index on the simulated refractory cast. Carefully cut (vertically) this piece of wax at the designated anterior portion of the retainer. Join another piece of 12-gauge half-round wax (flat side to cast) to the anterior end of the crosspiece on its underneath side. Adapt the wax to follow the inferior border of the outline of the retainer assembly and seal the end of the cast base pattern. Add sufficient wax with a hot spatula to provide a continuous taper from the retentive tip of the bar-type arm to its junction with the pattern for the denture base. The bar retainer is sealed to the cast in its entire length. Carve the wax to the outline form on the cast (Fig. 17-28). The thickest and broaded portion of the bar retainer will be at its junction with the denture base.

21. Perfect the waxing done thus far by carving, smoothing, and adding to weak points. The use of binocular loops (or any magnifying systems) to carefully inspect the pattern at this stage will probably disclose discrepancies heretofore unobserved.

22. Attach the wrought-wire retentive arm. Hold the previously formed wrought-wire retainer in a pair of cotton forceps by the small upright portion of the "foot" and warm it **over** a flame. Place the wire on the cast in its intended position in the wax pattern. It is usually necessary to hold a hot instrument against the retentive arm to dissipate enough heat so that the foot and upright portions of the retainer will be passively and completely embedded in the wax pattern (Fig. 17-29). However, the wrought wire need not be hot enough to excessively pool the wax pattern and change its desired form. Carefully inspect the area where the retentive arm emerges from its embedded position in the minor connector to ascertain that the wire arm is positively surrounded by wax without evidence of wax fissures or cracks.

The wax pattern is now completed and ready for sprung and investing (Figs. 17-30 and 17-31). Spruing is discussed later in this chapter.

An alternate method for forming the wrought-wire retentive clasp arm is illustrated in Fig. 17-32. The method illustrated is particularly applicable to short abutment teeth and will avoid two right-angle bends in the wrought wire.

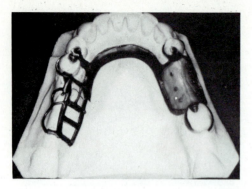

Fig. 17-30. Completed wax pattern for mandibular Class II partial denture framework.

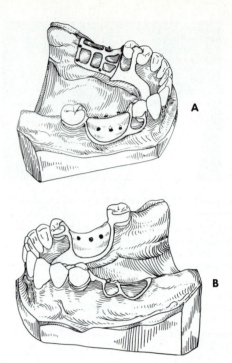

Fig. 17-31. Meticulous attention to detail and neatness in forming wax patterns not only assures quality of framework but also saves time in finishing resultant casting. **A,** Right side view. Note retentive "nailheads" on both cast base pattern and minor connector for denture base. Three nailheads on minor connector serve to retain impression tray for making secondary impression and are of no further use after this procedure has been accomplished. **B,** Left side view. Buccal loops have been so placed that they will not interfere with arranging artificial posterior teeth. In some instances, because of lack of interresidual ridge space, acrylic resin teeth must be used but almost always having their occlusal surfaces duplicated in gold.

Attaching wrought-wire retainer arms by soldering. Wrought-wire retainers may be attached to a partial denture framework after it has been cast and finished (Fig. 17-33). The soldering procedure may be accomplished by electric soldering or by a direct heat method with an oxygen-gas flame. In either method, care must be taken to use an appropriate solder and flux in conjunction with the careful application of controlled heat.

The student is encouraged to review the Chapter 11 discussion of the selection of metal alloys to enhance an understanding of the properties of solder, flux, the effect of heat on metal alloys, and the necessity for quality control in soldering procedures.

Waxing metal bases. A technique for forming the retentive framework for the attachment of resin bases has been given. Two basic types of metal bases may be used instead of the resin base. The advantages of using cast metal bases in preference to resin bases have been discussed in Chapter 8.

The type of base to be used must be determined before blockout and duplication so that the relief over each edentulous ridge may be provided or eliminated as required. For a resin base, relief for the retentive frame must be provided. For a complete metal base, no relief over the ridge is used. For a partial metal base, the junction between metal and resin must be clearly defined by trimming the relief along a definite, previously determined line (Fig. 8-9).

One type of metal base is the complete base with a metal border to which tube teeth, cast copings, or a resin superstructure may be attached. If porcelain or plastic tube or grooved teeth are used, they must be positioned first and the pattern waxed around them to form a coping (Fig. 8-11). The teeth are then attached to the metal base by cementation or, with the use of resin teeth, attached with additional acrylic resin under pressure, a so-called "pressed-on" meth-

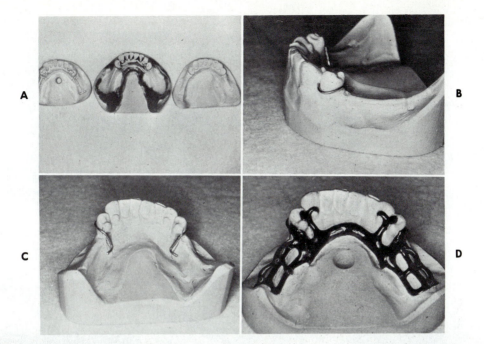

Fig. 17-32. A, Blocked-out master cast is duplicated in refractory investment and also in dental stone. **B,** Eighteen-gauge, round wrought-wire clasp is carefully adapted to duplicate stone cast being guided by ledge index created in wax on master cast for its placement. Required length of wire for making clasp is easily determined by laying 18-gauge, round wax strip to planned outline and then measuring wax strip. **C,** Lingually, wrought wire is contoured to conform to thickest portion of finishing line at junction of lingual bar and minor connector used to retain denture base. **D,** Contoured clasp is transferred to duplicate refractory cast and will occupy exact position that it occupied on duplicate stone cast. Waxing pattern for framework is completed in usual manner.

od of attaching resin teeth to a metal base. Another method of attaching teeth is to wax the base to form a coping for each tooth, either by carving recesses in the wax or by waxing around dummy teeth. Rather than attaching a stock tooth, the full tooth may be waxed into occlusion, the base invested, and the wax patterns replaced with a processed acrylic resin tooth. This method permits some variation in the dimension and form of the supplied teeth not possible with stock teeth. It is particularly applicable to abnormally long or short spaces or when a stock tooth of desired width is not available. With modern cross'linked acrylic resins, such processed teeth are fairly durable; however, the addition of gold occlusal surfaces is indicated.

Wax patterns of the teeth to be supplied may be waxed directly onto a metal base and then cast in gold and attached to the base by soldering. In this method the prosthetically supplied teeth are carved as for resin veneer fixed partial denture pontics. After attachment to the metal base, resin veneers are then processed to match any adjacent veneered abutment crowns. Visible teeth are generally abutted to the ridge, and cast flanges are used only in the posterior part of the mouth. This method is generally used only in conjunction with full mouth reconstruction. Both the denture framework and the cast pontics are usually made of gold to facilitate assembly by soldering.

When artificial teeth are to be arranged to occlude with an opposing cast or an opposing template, the metal base must be formed with

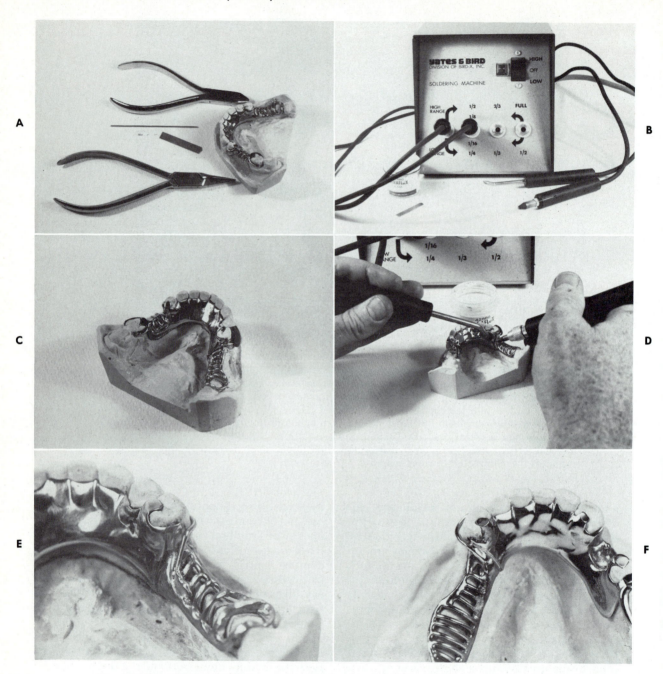

Fig. 17-33. A, Electric soldering machine with selection of heat ranges for various soldering requirements. **B,** Armamentarium for adapting (contouring) wrought wire direct retainer arm. Note tapered wire and section of electric solder. **C,** Contoured retainer arm is in position and is held in place with modeling clay. **D,** Area to be soldered is coated with small amount of appropriate flux. Solder is positioned and electrodes are applied until solder flows. **E,** Clasp arm has been soldered to framework. **F,** Alternative attachment of retainer arm by soldering at minor connector contacting guiding plane. **Student is referred to Chapter 21 for detailed information on electric soldering.**

a boxing for the attachment of the tissue-colored denture resin supporting the teeth. This is the most common method of attaching teeth to a metal base. The wax pattern for the base is formed from one thickness of 24-gauge casting wax, which is then reinforced at the border, and a boxing is formed for the retention of the resin superstructure. Since metal borders are more difficult to adjust than resin, they are usually made somewhat short of the area normally covered with a resin base. Also, since border thickness adds objectionable weight to the denture, it is made with only a slight border roll. This is one disadvantage of the complete metal base, in that the border accuracy of the impression registration cannot be used to fullest advantage, and the contouring of facial and lingual surfaces cannot be as effective as with a resin base in which added bulk can sometimes be used to advantage.

The border is first penciled lightly on the investment cast, and then the 24-gauge sheet casting wax is smoothly adapted. Considerable care must be taken not to stretch and thin the sheet wax in adapting it to the cast. To avoid wrinkling, the wax should be adapted in at least two longitudinal pieces and joined and sealed together at the ridge crest. The wax is then trimmed along the penciled outline with a dull instrument to avoid scoring the investment cast.

A single piece of **14-gauge round** wax is now adapted around the border **over** the sheet wax. With a hot spatula this must be sealed to the cast along its outer border. The inner half of the round wax form remains untouched. Then, sufficient wax is flowed onto the round wax to blend it smoothly into the sheet wax, thus completing a border roll. Wax is added when needed to facilitate carving without trimming the original 24-gauge thickness. The result should be a rounded border blending smoothly into the sheet wax.

The boxing for the resin, which will in turn support the artificial teeth, is now added, again using **14-gauge round** wax. The proposed outline for the boxing is identified by lightly scoring the sheet wax. On this scored line the 14-gauge round wax is adapted, thus forming the outline of the boxing.

With additional wax the ditch between the sheet wax and the outer border of the round wax is filled in and blended smoothly onto the sheet wax. This is done in the same manner as the border, adding sufficient wax to allow for smoothing and carving. As mentioned previously, the pattern should not be flamed or polished with a cloth. Instead the pattern must be smoothed by carving.

The result thus far should be a pattern reinforced at the border and at the boxing and slightly concave in between, with some of the original sheet wax exposed. The inside of the boxing is not sealed to the sheet wax, thus leaving a slight undercut for the attachment of the resin. With a sharp blade the margins of the boxing are then carved to a knife-edge finishing line. With the back side of the large end of the No. 7 wax spatula this margin may be lifted slightly, further deepening the undercut beneath the finishing line.

In addition to the undercut finishing line, retention spurs, loops, or nailheads are added for retention of the resin to be added later. Spurs are usually made of 18-gauge or smaller round wax attached at one end only at random acute angles to the sheet wax. Loops are small-gauge round (wax, resin, or metal) circles attached either vertically or horizontally with space beneath for the resin attachment. Nailheads are made of short pieces of 18-gauge round wax attached vertically to the sheet wax, with the head flattened with a slightly warmed spatula. Any method of providing retention is acceptable if it permits positive attachment of the resin and will not interfere with the placement of artificial teeth.

A metal base waxed as described will provide optimal contours with a minimum of bulk and weight and with adequate provision for the attachment of artificial teeth to the metal base. Properly designed, the more visible portions of the metal base will be covered with the acrylic resin supporting the supplied teeth.

ANATOMIC REPLICA PATTERNS

A technique for obtaining a duplication of the palatal portion of a maxillary cast was developed originally by William Thompson as an aid to phonetics. This was called the **Thompson Tru-Rugae technique.** It was soon discovered that many other advantages also resulted from anatomic replica patterns (Fig. 4-35). It was found that patients became accustomed to an anatomic replica palate much more readily than to a smooth highly polished surface or to the concentrated bulk of palatal bars. It has been claimed that an irregular palatal surface seems to improve mastication by giving the tongue a "washboard" surface against which to press out the softer food particles and thereby separate them for mastication by the teeth.

The appearance of the denture to the patient is seemingly improved by its anatomic form and by the fact that the surface is never highly polished. This fact is readily recognized and makes the patient aware that it is a personalized reproduction of his own palate rather than a foreign body to be tolerated.

The irregular contour of the anatomic replica palate adds rigidity to the casting by its corrugated shape, thus permitting the use of thinner castings than would be permissible with a smooth, uncorrugated surface. This adds to patient acceptance and comfort by decreasing both weight and bulk.

To the laboratory the anatomic replica palate means a saving in polishing time and in finishing and polishing materials.

The original Thompson technique was cumbersome but worthy of note because it led to later developments in anatomic replica techniques. Walker and Orsinger are credited with originating the present technique for palate reproduction, a description of which appeared in 1954. It is now almost a universally accepted technique for making complete and partial palate reproductions.

The material is available as a Tru-Rugae kit and contains all the materials needed to make anatomic replica palates for complete and partial dentures.* Whether used as a pattern to be burned out and cast or, in slightly thicker form, as an anatomic pattern of the palate to be discarded when boiling out a flasked denture, the technique is essentially the same. Walker and Orsinger listed the equipment and material required as follows:

Cardboard box approximately 6 by 6 by 2 inches deep [to permit reuse of the polymer]
Camel's-hair brush, large water coloring size, or larger
Small nasal atomizer (DeVilbiss Economy Atomizer No. 182 is satisfactory)*
Wax spatula
Iris or cuticle scissors
Powder: Ethyl methacrylate powder, Dupont Lucite HG-24 or equal
Liquid: Methyl methacrylate monomer, or any denture base liquid acrylic resin
Coloring material for liquid: Prussian blue, artist's color ground in oil
Pattern cement: Pre-formed plastic pattern scraps dissolved in acetone
Plasticizers: Methyl salicylate, camphor, rosin, or suitable commercial plasticizers such as Dow Resin 276. . . . [The plasticizer is added to the liquid in the atomizer or spray gun only, about six drops to the small atomizer, correspondingly more to the larger spray gun.]†

The following formula for a liquid is used at Lackland Air Force Base and contains a plasticizer:

Camphor	75 ml
Oil of wintergreen	75 ml
Acrylic resin monomer	350 ml
Sudan red	Pinch

Procedure for making an anatomic replica pattern. The procedure for making the anatomic replica pattern (or wafer) is as follows:

1. Make an alginate impression of the master cast. The buccal and labial borders of the impression extending beyond the impression tray should be shortened to provide better access to the palatal area. Rinse the impression to remove any loose particles, and remove excess moisture with compressed air. Leave the surface damp but free of surface moisture.

2. Fill the impression with powder from the cardboard box. (It is suggested that only enough

---

* Ticonium Company, 413 N. Pearl St., Albany, N.Y.

---

*Compressed air–operated spray guns give a much finer and more uniform spray than the hand-operated atomizer and are not subject to clogging. Two of these are the Thayer-Chandler air brush and the Dupli-Color touch-up spray gun, model A, both of which require compressed air for operation.
†From Walker, T.J., and Orsinger, W.O.: Palate reproduction by the hydrocolloid-resin method; J. Prosthet. Dent. 4:54-66, 1954.

powder be kept in the box to completely fill a hydrocolloid impression rather than to reuse larger quantities. Since this material becomes contaminated, it can be screened to remove foreign particles and replenished with fresh powder from the original container.)

3. Invert the impression over the cardboard box and dump out the surplus powder. Give the back of the hand holding the impression three or four slaps to remove more excess powder. This leaves powder layer No. 1 in the impression, which now has a fine sugar-coated appearance.

4. Using the atomizer, or preferably an air gun giving a fine misty spray, spray the face of the impression, as it is held in the other hand, with monomer. In this manner the liquid is prevented from building up in deeper areas of the impression. The monomer should contain several drops of plasticizer, depending on the size of the container.

5. Immediately fill the impression again, and dump and tap out the excess powder. This is powder layer No. 2, which is then sprayed with monomer as before. Use sufficient liquid to saturate the powder particles.

Ordinarily three layers of powder are sufficient to make a pattern thick enough for casting. (For palate reproductions on complete dentures, five or six layers may be necessary.) The thickness will be determined by how hard the operator shakes or taps out the excess powder from the impression and also by the length of time the second and third applications of powder are left on the impression before they are tapped off. The longer they remain on the impression, the thicker the wafer will be, because the powder picks up more liquid as it stands.

6. Set the impression under an inverted container or in a bell jar to prevent evaporation of the monomer and to allow the liquid to penetrate more thoroughly the grains of powder. This results in a finer surface and a more uniform thickness after cementation on the refractory cast. (This precaution applies equally well to any procedure in which denture bases are made by a sprinkling method.) An inverted bowl or glass refrigerator jar prevents evaporation and allows more thorough penetration of the monomer during polymerization.

7. When the plastic wafer has reached a flexible polymerized state (in about 30 minutes), strip it out of the impression completely. With fine iris scissors, trim the wafer to correspond to the outline of the palatal coverage previously penciled lightly on the refractory cast. Discard the cuttings, leaving only the wafer to be cemented to the refractory cast. If a definite ledge for a finishing line was established on the master cast with relief wax, the plastic wafer should extend about 2 mm beyond the platform that has been reproduced on the investment cast. This establishes the finishing line on the tissue side of the casting. (The undercut finishing line on the exposed side will be waxed on the plastic wafer about 2 mm in front of its trimmed edge.)

8. With a fine camel's-hair brush, paint a uniform layer of pattern cement on the investment cast inside the penciled outline. If preferred, this cement can be made up by dissolving plastic pattern forms in acetone. If it becomes too thick, it may be thinned with monomer. Excess cement should be avoided because it will cause irregular borders to be reproduced in the casting. Press the plastic wafer to place on the cast, making sure it conforms to the penciled outline. The remainder of the pattern then may be completed in the usual manner. If it is necessary to store the wafer overnight before completing the pattern, it should be covered with an inverted glass container or placed under a bell jar to maintain its plasticity. Refrigeration will also maintain the plasticity of anatomic replica patterns for extended periods.

In making cast palate reproductions for a complete maxillary denture the method is essentially the same as that used for a partial denture. For resin palate reproductions an alignate hydrocolloid impression of the master cast is also used. The wafer is sprayed into the impression somewhat thicker than for a metal casting, then it is removed after polymerizing and trimmed as above. The wafer is not cemented to the master cast but merely waxed to place to form the palate of the denture. This is done before the denture is invested for processing. The palate of the original base is then cut out and replaced with the anatomic palate wafer. This is discarded during boilout, leaving a mold that results in an anatomic replica palate on the completed denture.

SPRUING, INVESTING, BURNOUT, CASTING, AND FINISHING OF THE PARTIAL DENTURE FRAMEWORK

Brumfield has listed some of the factors that influence the excellence of a dental casting:

1. Care and accuracy with which the model [cast] is reproduced.
2. Intelligence with which the case [framework] is designed and proportioned.
3. Care and cleanliness in waxing up the model [cast].
4. Consideration of the expansion of the wax due to temperature.
5. The size of the sprues.
6. The length of the sprues.
7. The configuration of the sprues.
8. Points of attachment and manner of attachment of the sprues to the cast.
9. Choice of investment.
10. The location of the pattern in the mold.
11. The mixing water: amount, temperature, and impurities.
12. The spatulation of the investment during mixing.
13. The restraint offered to the expansion of the investment, due to the investment ring.
14. Setting time.
15. Burn-out temperature.
16. Burn-out time.
17. Method of casting.
18. Gases: adhered, entrapped, and absorbed.
19. Force used in throwing the metal into the mold.
20. Shrinkage on cooling.
21. Removal from the investment after casting.
22. Scrubbing, pickling, etc.
23. Polishing and finishing.
24. Heat handling.*

Spruing. Brumfield describes the function of the sprues as follows:

The sprue channel is the opening leading from the crucible to the cavity in which the appliance [framework] is to be cast. Sprues have the purpose of leading the molten gold from the crucible into the mold cavity. For this purpose, they should be large enough to accommodate the entering stream, and of the proper shape to lead it into the mold cavity as quickly as possible, but with the least amount of turbulence. The sprues have the further purpose of providing a reservoir of molten metal from which the casting may draw during solidification, thus avoiding porosity due to shrinkage. The spruing of the cast may be roughly summarized in three general rules.

1. The sprues should be large enough that the molten metal in them will not solidify until after the metal in the casting proper has frozen. (8- to 12-gauge round wax is usually used for multiple spruing of partial denture castings.)
2. The sprues should lead into the mold cavity as directly as possible and still permit a configuration which will induce a minimum amount of turbulence in the stream of molten metal.
3. Sprues should leave the crucible from a common point and be attached to the case [pattern] at its bulkier sections. That is, no thin sections of casting should intervene between two bulky, unsprued portions.

The configuration of the sprues, from their point of attachment at the crucible, until they reach the mold cavity may be influential in reducing turbulence. One of the more important sources of difficulty in casting is the entrapment of gases in the mold cavity, before they have a chance to escape. If the sprue channels contain sharp right angle turns, great turbulence is induced which is calculated to entrap such gases and so lead to faulty castings. Sprue channels should make long radii, easy turns and also enter the mold cavity from a direction designed to avoid splashing at this point.

As pointed out, the sprues should be attached to the bulky points of the mold [pattern]. If two bulky points exist with a thin section between them, each of the bulky spots should be sprued. The points of attachment should be flared out and local constrictions avoided. If this practice is followed, the sprue, being bulky enough to freeze after the case [framework] has frozen, will continue to feed molten metal to the case [framework] until it has entirely solidified, thus providing sound metal in the casting proper with all shrinkage porosity forced into the sprue rod, which is later discarded.*

There are two basic types of sprues: multiple and single (Figs. 17-34 and 17-35). The majority of partial denture castings require multiple spruing, using 8- to 12-gauge round wax shapes for the main sprues and 12- to 18-gauge round wax shapes for auxiliary sprues. Occasionally, however, a single sprue is preferred for cast palates and cast metal bases for the mandibular arch

---

*From Brumfield, R.C.: Dental gold structures, analysis and practicalities, New York, 1949, J.F. Jelenko & Co., Inc.

*From Brumfield, R.C.: Dental gold structures, analysis and practicalities, New York, 1949, J.F. Jelenko & Co., Inc.

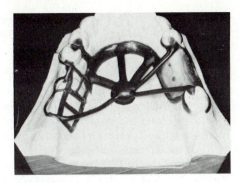

Fig. 17-34. View of sprued wax pattern. Three 8-gauge sprues attached to lingual bar and three 12-gauge sprues attached to denture base minor connector and direct retainer assemblies are joined at central sprue hole in investment cast.

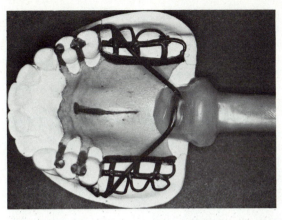

Fig. 17-35. Broad palatal coverage patterns are best sprued with single main sprue located posteriorly. Where cast denture base for completely edentulous arch is being sprued, single sprue may be located anteriorly.

when these are used as complete denture bases. With partial dentures the use of a single sprue is limited to those maxillary frameworks in which, because of the presence of a palatal plate, it is impossible to locate multiple sprues centrally. In such situations the single sprue may be used advantageously. A single sprue must be attached to the wax pattern so that the direction of flow of the molten metal will be parallel to the long axis of the single sprue. In some instances the investment cast may have to be cut away anteriorly to make room for the attachment of the sprue; in others the sprue may be attached posteriorly. One disadvantage of using a single sprue for large castings is that an extra long investment ring must be used.

Some important points to remember in multiple spruing are as follows:
1. Use a few sprues of large diameter rather than several smaller sprues.
2. Keep all sprues as short and direct as possible.
3. Avoid abrupt changes in direction; avoid T-shaped junctions as much as possible.
4. Reinforce all junctions with additional wax to avoid constrictions in the sprue channel and to avoid V-shaped sections of investment that might break away and be carried into the casting.

Step-by-step procedure. The laboratory procedure for multiple spruing is essentially the same for all mandibular castings and maxillary castings except those with a palatal plate. The following technique is given for a typical mandibular Class II partial denture casting:

1. Reduce the base of the cast to about 12 mm thickness. Trim all edges of the cast until it is slightly larger than the wax pattern and tapers from the occlusal aspect toward the base.

2. Cut a 9 mm hole through the cast centered on a line joining the distal ends of the major connector on each side. The hole must be large enough to accommodate the main sprue from which other sprues will lead to the framework. (Stainless steel sprue cones may be purchased for forming the main sprue hole. These are available in several sizes and shapes and are used to form the hole in the investment cast at the time the cast is poured into the duplication mold.)

3. Roll one-half sheet of softened pink baseplate wax into a rod of such diameter that it will just pass through the hole cut in the base of the cast when it is inserted from the bottom. Allow the wax rod to protrude slightly on the wax pattern side of the cast. Seal this portion to the cast all around its border. The long portion protruding from the underside of the cast will serve as a handle during investment. The slight projection on the wax pattern side serves as an extrusion, with the sprue leads attached approxi-

mately 4.5 mm below the tip of the main sprue. By using this overjet principle of spruing, the initial thrust of molten metal is directed against the tip of the main sprue reservoir, and the turbulence that is created is confined to this area rather than at the entrance to the pattern mold cavity.

4. From this main sprue, attach three pieces of 8-gauge round wax extending radially to the lower border of the lingual bar major connector. Direct one piece to the central portion of the connector and the other two to just anterior to the finishing lines where the major connector joins the base retention on one side and the cast base on the other side. Thus the molten metal is fed to portions of the clasp assembly as well as to the bar itself. Attach these sprues to the bulkiest part of the major connector, being careful not to involve any critical margins. In spruing a tooth-borne partial denture framework consisting of four clasp assemblies, four such sprues should be used, each attached to the major connector just below the clasp assembly.

5. In a similar manner, using pieces of 12-gauge round wax, connect the main sprue to the retentive framework or to any metal bases. In attaching to a retentive framework, make sure this is at the junction of a crossbar, thus assuring a free flow of metal with a minimum of changes in direction. A 12-gauge, round wax sprue is attached to the body of each direct retainer assembly on the cast denture base side. These sprues so placed will ensure the casting of the bar-type retainer, the circumferential retainer, and the buccal portion of the cast base pattern.

6. Reinforce all points of junction between the sprues and the denture framework with additional wax. The spruing is now completed (Fig. 17-36).

Investing the sprued pattern (Fig. 17-37). The investment for a partial denture casting consists of two parts: the investment cast on which the pattern is formed and the outer investment surrounding the cast and pattern. The latter is confined within a metal ring, which may or may not be removed after the outer investment has set. If the metal ring is not removed, it must be lined with a layer of asbestos to allow for both setting and thermal expansion of the mold in all directions.

The investment must conform accurately to the shape of the pattern and must preserve the configuration of the pattern as a cavity after the pattern itself has been eliminated through vaporization and oxidation. Brumfield has listed the purposes of the investment as follows:

1. Investment provides the strength necessary to hold the forces exerted by [the] entering stream of molten metal until this metal has solidified into the form of the pattern.
2. It provides a smooth surface for the mold cavity so that the final casting will require as little finishing as possible and in some cases a deoxidizing agent to keep surfaces bright.

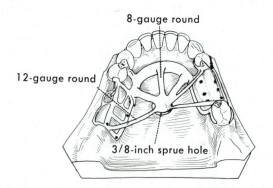

Fig. 17-36. Wax pattern is sprued.

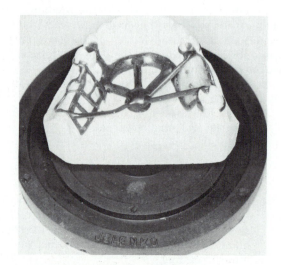

Fig. 17-37. Trimmed investment cast and sprued pattern are secured to sprue former.

3. It provides an avenue of escape for most of the gases entrapped in the mold cavity by entering stream of molten metal.

4. It, together with other factors, provides necessary compensation for the dimensional changes of the gold [alloy]* from the molten to the solid, cold state.†

The investment for casting gold alloys is a plaster-bound silica material, so compounded that the total mold expansion will offset the casting shrinkage of the gold, which varies from 1% to 1.74% (the highest figure being the shrinkage of pure gold). Generally, the higher the percentage of gold in the alloy, the greater the contraction of the casting on solidifying.

Only one chromium-cobalt alloy has a sufficiently low melting temperature to be cast into a plaster-silica investment mold. According to Peyton, for the others having a higher melting temperature, an investment containing quartz powder held together by an ethyl silicate or sodium silicate binder is generally used. Expansion to offset casting shrinkage for the chromium-cobalt alloys is accomplished primarily through thermal expansion of the mold and must be sufficient to offset their greater casting shrinkage, which is in the order of 2.3%. For this reason the metal ring is usually removed after the mold has hardened, to allow for the greater mold expansion necessary with these alloys. Since the investments for chromium-cobalt alloys are generally less porous, there is greater danger of entrapping gases in the mold cavity by the molten metal. Spruing must be done with greater care, and in some instances, provision for venting the mold is necessary to avoid defective castings.

Step-by-step procedure. The technique for applying the outer investment is usually referred to as "investing the pattern." Actually, the cast on which the pattern is formed is part of the investment also. The following technique is given as being representative of, and applicable to, all partial denture castings:

1. Just before mixing the investment, line the ring with one layer of sheet casting ring liner. The liner should be 6 mm shorter than the ring at the crucible end. The liner permits hot gases to escape; yet some investment in contact with the ring at the crucible end prevents the investment from falling out during handling of the ring after heating. Wet the liner after it is in place, but do not pack it tightly against the walls of the ring. (Step 1 is omitted if a split-type forming flask is used that will be opened and removed as soon as the investment has set.)

2. The investment cast must be soaked in room-temperature water before painting. Immerse the cast with the sprued pattern in a pan of water at about 85° F no longer than 4 minutes. Water saturation of an investment cast assures a good bond between the old investment and the new, but cold water must not be used for fear the pattern will shrink and be loosened from the cast.

3. Mix 100 g of investment, using 2 ml more water than was used to make the investment cast. (If the investment for the cast required 28 ml of water per 100 g of powder, the painting mix should be 30 ml of water per 100 g.) Spatulation must be thorough and should continue for about 60 seconds to distribute water throughout the mix when mixed by hand. Remember that a well-spatulated mix gives greater expansion and that mechanical spatulation, under vacuum conditions, usually results in the best mix possible.

Paint the pattern with a wetting agent (debubblizer) just before applying the investment to reduce the surface tension of the wax so that the outer investment readily covers and adheres to the pattern. With a brush carrying the mixed investment, start at one end of the cast and work the investment under the sprues. Use only indirect vibration, the hand supporting the cast being between it and the vibrator. Keep working the investment under the wax sprues, working from one side of the cast around to the other. Proceed to invest the remainder of the pattern in the same manner. Wrought-wire retentive clasp arms also must be covered with investment. The entire pattern should be covered with

---

*Note the substitution of the word **alloy**, as the same principles apply whether the metal be a precious metal alloy or a chromium-cobalt alloy. In some of the latter alloys the cobalt is partially replaced by nickel; such alloys are sometimes described as "Stellite" alloys.

†From Brumfield, R.C.: Dental gold structures, analysis and practicalities, New York, 1949, J.F. Jelenko & Co., Inc.

about 6 mm of investment. An even layer of investment is necessary to assure uniform expansion of the mold. Set the invested pattern aside until the outer investment has set (unless the vibrator will remain off, do not place the pattern on the same bench or vibration transferred through the bench will cause the investment to pull away from the pattern).

4. After the painting investment has reached its initial set (in about 10 minutes), it may be invested in the casting ring or flask former. Just before investing the assembly in the casting ring, dip the assembly in water to again wet the outer investment, shaking off any excess water. Four hundred grams of powder will be ample, mixed with the same proportion of water as before. **Only hand spatulation for about 60 seconds should be used, since some air in the outer investment is necessary to aid in venting the mold.**

One type of casting ring (Ney partial denture casting ring) has no crucible former and consists of a large heavy metal ring with an opening at one end about the diameter of an inlay casting ring. The other end is open to accommodate the

invested pattern. To use this ring the invested pattern is inserted with its main sprue protruding through the center of the smaller opening. The invested cast in this position should have sufficient space above for an adequate bulk of investment to cover it. In this position, connect the main wax sprue with the sides of the ring at its mouth, thus closing the opening. The main sprue protruding through the wax seal may be held between two fingers while the ring is held inverted in the palm of the hand. The invested cast is now completely covered with investment, filling the ring to the top. A glass slab may be slid over the top of the filled ring to permit inverting the ring on the bench while the investment sets. The crucible is then cut into the hardened investment at the main sprue.

A second type of ring has a crucible former. Representative of this type are the Kerr and Jelenko partial denture casting rings. This type is perhaps the most frequently used. The invested cast is attached to the crucible former by placing the main sprue into the hole and sealing it to the crucible former. Care must be taken that the invested cast is centered in the ring, with sufficient space all around and at the top for adequate thickness of outer investment. The

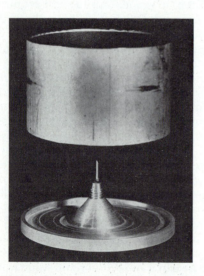

Fig. 17-38. Wills threaded sprue former and matching casting ring. Base and ring may be either Kerr or Jelenko size, but both must match. Projection on ⅜-inch rod threaded with No. 16 thread is for positioning lubricated sprue into duplication mold before pouring investment cast.

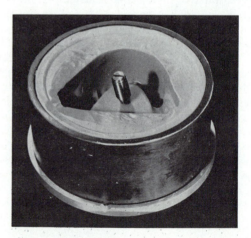

Fig. 17-39. Threaded sprue being held in duplication mold by pointed projection. Sprue is first lubricated with petrolatum or silicone jelly. Note slotted end to facilitate withdrawal from cast and, later, to adjust with small screwdriver height of wax pattern in casting ring.

casting ring is seated onto the crucible former and filled with investment, thus embedding the cast in investment as previously outlined.

Wills developed an innovation to the spruing and investing of a partial denture, which is a valuable aid in securing the investment cast to the sprue former and in regulating the height of the cast in the ring.

For a long time a tapered sprue cone of metal has been used to form the sprue hole in the investment cast, thus eliminating the need for cutting a 9 mm sprue hole in the base of the cast later. The sprue is then reinserted into the cast just before investment, where it is retained by friction.

The Wills sprue pin is a machined brass, untapered screw, ⅜ inch in diameter and threaded with a No. 16 thread. This fits into a threaded hole in a metal sprue former made to accommodate the Kerr or the Jelenko partial denture casting ring (Fig. 17-38). Projecting from the screw is a pin that is used to retain the threaded sprue in the hydrocolloid mold as the investment cast is being poured into it (Fig. 17-39). The threaded sprue must be lubricated with petrolatum or silicone jelly so that it may be removed from the cast with ease. A screwdriver is then used to remove the sprue from the cast, leaving a threaded sprue hole comparable to that in the sprue former.

After the wax pattern is completed and ready to invest, the brass sprue pin is screwed halfway into the base of the cast, and the other half is screwed into the sprue former. Thus the investment cast is held securely to the sprue former, and by inserting a screwdriver through the hole in the sprue former and engaging the slot in the threaded sprue, its height in relation to the ring can be adjusted.

Since there is some probability that the sharp edges of investment making up the threaded sprue channel may become broken off by the force of the molten metal and thus be carried into the mold proper, the threaded sprue hole should be reamed slightly and the particles eliminated just before placing the investment in the furnace.

A third type of casting ring is the split-type forming flask, which is opened and removed as soon as the investment has set. This flask is available in various diameters and heights, but the medium size will accommodate about 90% of all wax patterns. This type of casting ring does not use a crucible former. Instead the flask is placed on a glass slab and nearly filled. Then the invested cast (sprue up) is embedded into it, using the sprue as a handle until the investment reaches a consistency sufficient to support the weight of the cast. Sometimes a copper screen is used inside the split-type flask to support the investment during heating and casting. This is not necessary if care is taken to avoid too rapid burnout or careless handling of the heated mold.

5. Allow the investment to set for at least an hour. At the end of this time, if the first type of ring was used, cut away the wax and protruding main sprue in such a manner as to form a concavity in the investment with the deepest part at the sprue. If the second type was used, merely remove the crucible former, which will leave the investment concaved or funnel shaped. The concavity may be deepened if desired by trimming the walls uniformly smooth, maintaining the funnel shape. If a split-type flask is used, a crucible may be formed by carving a funnel in the mold at the main sprue. Finally, trim the two faces of the mold to be parallel, using the edges of the ring as a guide. This is done by rubbing the mold over piece of wire mesh screening (Fig. 17-40).

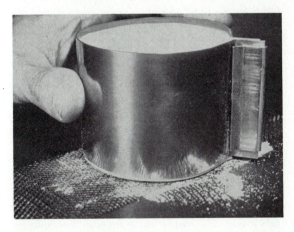

Fig. 17-40. Excess investment may be trimmed flush with rim of casting ring or flask by rubbing it over piece of wire mesh or screening material. (Courtesy Ticonium Division, CMP Industries, Inc., Albany, N.Y.)

If the split-type ring was used, it is now removed by sliding off the retaining clip, which allows the ring to be opened.

Burnout. The burnout operation serves three purposes: it drives off moisture in the mold, it vaporizes and thus eliminates the pattern, leaving a cavity in the mold, and it expands the mold to compensate for contraction of the metal on cooling.

Brumfield has this to say about burnout:

The time required to drive off the water is mainly a function of the amount of heat available and of the closeness of the heating element to the investment when placed in the furnace. If the furnace is large and a number of molds are burned out at the same time, the burn-out will require more time than would be the case with a single mold in the same furnace. . . .

The temperature of the mold is held down during early stages of burn-out by the vaporization of the water. Water will not rise appreciably above its boiling point until it is all vaporized. At the end of 60 minutes, the water is practically all driven off and the temperature at the inside of the mold will rise fairly rapidly to near the temperature of the furnace. Complete equalization, however, requires another 70 minutes, giving a total burn-out time of about two and one-quarter hours for eliminating the water and raising the temperature of the mold approximately 1300° F. The so-called soaking period often recommended to be given the mold, after furnace pyrometer shows the full burn-out temperature, is designed to allow time for the water to be eliminated from the mold and the mold temperature to rise to that of the furnace.

During the time the water is being eliminated, the wax is being eliminated through vaporization and oxidation of carbon. Vaporization of wax ordinarily does not require as much time as that for vaporization of the water and will often have been completed when the temperature on the inside of the furnace has risen to about 1000° F. The carbon residue may require more time for elimination. The more oxidizing the atmosphere of the eliminating furnace the better from the standpoint of eliminating wax. . . .

It is essential that the time of burn-out be sufficient to entirely eliminate the moisture. If the moisture is not eliminated, its presence has two bad effects on the casting. The casting made from an incompletely eliminated ring is apt to be porous due to the continued emission of steam by the investment. Second, the venting of the mold cavity is largely accomplished through the interstices of the investment itself. Although the investment is finely ground and these interstices are invisible to the eye, they nevertheless exist in very considerable amounts. Most investments contain voids (that is, spaces not occupied by investment particles), which amount to as much as 50 per cent of the total volume occupied. It is through these void spaces that the gases entrapped in the mold cavity by the entering stream of molten metal are able to depart with sufficient rapidity to avoid porosity in the casting. If these spaces are already occupied by steam from the incompletely eliminated mold or by finely divided particles of carbon residue from the wax, the entrapped gases cannot escape and porosity results from their inclusion in the casting. It is better to err on the side of too long a burn-out than in the opposite direction.*

For the investment to heat uniformly it should be moist at the start of the burnout cycle. Steam will then carry the heat into the investment during the early stages of the burnout. Therefore if the investment is not burned out on the same day it is poured, it should be soaked in water for a few minutes before being placed in the burnout furnace.

Just before being placed in the furnace, the mold should be placed in the casting machine to balance the weight against the weight of the mold. At this time the mold should be properly oriented to the machine and its crucible and a scratch line made at the top for later repositioning of the hot mold.

The mold should be placed in the oven with the sprue hole down and the orientation mark forward. Burnout should be started with a cold oven, or nearly so. Then the temperature of the oven should be increased slowly to a temperature of 1250° F over a period of 2 hours. This temperature than should be maintained for at least a 30-minute "heat-soaking" period to ensure uniform heat penetration. More time must be allowed for plastic patterns, particularly palatal anatomic replica patterns.

It is important that this temperature not be exceeded during the burnout period. (When a high heat investment is used, the manufacturer's instructions as to burnout temperature should be followed.) For all plaster-bound investments, contraction of the mold occurs beyond **1350° F,**

*From Brumfield, R.C.: Dental gold structures, analysis and practicalities, New York, 1949, J.F. Jelenko & Co., Inc.

and breakdown of the binder begins at about **1450° F.** To avoid loss of expansion and possible cracking, the soaking temperature should not exceed **1250° F.**

Casting. The method of casting will vary widely with the alloy and equipment being used. All methods use force to inject quickly the molten metal into the mold cavity. This force may be either centrifugal or air pressure; the former is more commonly used. In any case, either too much or too little force is undesirable. If too little force is used, the mold is not completely filled before the metal begins to freeze. If too much force is used, excessive turbulence may result in the entrapment of gases in the casting. With centrifugal casting machines this is regulated by the number of turns put on the actuating spring. For the Thermotrol casting machine, for example, this is two to three turns.

The metal may be melted with a gas-oxygen blowtorch or by an electric muffle surrounding the metal. In some commercial casting procedures and in some dental laboratories the induction method may be used, which provides a rapid and accurate method of melting the metal. The cost of induction equipment prohibits its wide-spread use.

The blowtorch method may produce consistently excellent results, but the lack of temperature control leaves much responsibility on the skill and judgment of the dentist or technician. Since the temperature at which the metal is thrown into the mold has an important bearing on the excellence of the casting, the use of controlled melting with an electric muffle, such as the Thermotrol, eliminates many of the variables common to the blowtorch method. Properly adjusted, this machine indicates the temperature of the molten metal at the instant it is thrown into the mold.

Removing the casting from the investment. Chromium-cobalt alloys are usually allowed to cool in the mold and are not cleaned by pickling. Finishing and polishing, which are done with special high-speed equipment, require a technical skill in the use of bench lathes not ordinarily acquired by the dental student. The average dentist is more adept in the use of the dental handpiece, whereas the average technician is, by reason of his training, more proficient in the use of bench lathes for finishing and polishing larger castings. Just before being polished (high-shine), chromium-cobalt castings are electropolished, which is a controlled deplating process. The following therefore applies specifically to gold alloy castings being completed by the dental student or dentist.

After the casting is completed, allow the mold to cool until the sprue button has changed in color from red to black when viewed in shaded light. This will be about eight to twelve minutes after completion of a large casting. At this time, quench the hot ring in water. With most gold castings this will produce a fairly soft and ductile condition in the metal. However, the larger the flask and the greater the amount of investment surrounding the casting, the longer the period required for bench cooling before quenching. It has been pointed out that when the Ney partial denture flask is used, a cooling period of 8 to 12 minutes is sufficient, but that if a flask with straight sides is used, it will hold approximately 60% more investment and therefore will require considerably more time for cooling. For the latter type of flask (such as the Kerr or Jelenko flask) it is suggested that 20 minutes be allowed for bench cooling to avoid the possibility that the casting will be too soft.

The practice of allowing the casting to completely cool in the investment is not recommended for gold alloys. Although it is true that all gold alloys capable of being hardened by slow cooling will harden if allowed to cool slowly in the investment, the difference between the outside and the center at any given instant may vary 200° F or more. Not only is heat hardening by this method uneven but shrinkage also is non-uniform, resulting in an inaccurate casting.

After removal of the investment from the casting by brushing under water with a stiff-bristle brush, the casting should be further cleaned by **pickling**. Before pickling, detergent powder may be used to aid in removing investment particles.

When the casting is clean, it should be pickled in an acid pickling solution. Prevox, Jel-Pac, dilute sulfuric acid, or 30% to 50% hydrochloric acid may be used for pickling. The latter is objectionable because of the fumes and the fact that these fumes corrode laboratory instruments. It is essential that the pickling acid be clean and relatively colorless rather than have the typical greenish blue color of contaminated acid. Contamination results not only from repeated use of the solution but also from handling the casting with metal tongs during pickling. A contaminated acid contains excessive copper and other salts that will contaminate the surface of the casting, leading to tarnish and discoloration in the mouth.

When surface pits and irregularities on the casting become contaminated with foreign salts, later finishing and polishing may fail to remove them completely. When such a restoration comes in contact with sulfur-bearing foods, metallic sulfides are formed that exude from the pits and irregularities. Dark rings of stain and discoloration subsequently spread over a larger area, giving a tarnished appearance to the polished metal. This is the result of using an unclean pickling bath.

Under no conditions should the casting be heated and plunged into the pickling solution. Pickling is properly done by placing the casting in a clean porcelain dish and pouring the clean pickling solution over it to a depth sufficient to cover it. The dish then should be heated over a flame until the surface of the casting brightens. The pickling solution is poured off (flushing generously with water or base solution) and the casting washed with an abundance of water. If the acid solution is fresh and clean, no base metal deposits will occur to cause later discoloration of the polished casting in the mouth.

Finishing and polishing. Some authorities hold that the sprues should not be removed from the casting until most of the polishing is completed. Although it is true that this policy may prevent accidental distortion, it is difficult to adhere to and is therefore somewhat impractical. Instead, reasonable care should be exercised to avoid any distortion resulting from careless handling.

Actual polishing procedures may vary widely according to personal preference for certain abrasive shapes and sizes. However, several rules in finishing the casting are important. These are as follows:

1. High speeds are preferable to low speeds. Not only are they effective but in experienced hands there also is less danger of the casting's being caught and thrown out of the hands by the rotating instrument.

2. The wheels or points and the speed of their rotation should do the cutting. Excessive pressure heats the work, crushes the abrasive particles, causes the wheels to clog and glaze, and slows up the cutting.

3. A definite sequence for finishing should be adopted and followed in every case. Such a sequence for finishing a gold casting is given by Berger:

(a) Remove sprues with a jeweler's saw rather than separating discs. This saves gold and prevents accidentally cutting into essential parts of the case [framework].

(b) Grind off sprue stubs with ¾" or ⅞" heatless stones, ¹⁄₁₆" thick. Rough grind entire case [framework] and shape bars, clasps, and saddles [metal denture bases]. Always grind bars and clasps lengthwise. Cross-grinding can weaken a bar or clasp by grinding it too thin in spots. [If the location of clasps has been properly surveyed, it should not be necessary to grind the insides of the clasps. Smoothing the inner surface and polishing should be all that is needed.]

(c) Finish grinding with barrel-shaped mounted stones of medium grit. Use above precaution in grinding bars and clasps.

(d) Sandpaper the entire appliance [framework] using fine arbor bands, following the above precautions as to bars and clasps.

(e) . . . rubber wheel the entire case [framework] carefully to remove all scratches. The better the case [framework] is rubber-wheeled, the easier the subsequent polishing steps become.

(f) The insides of the clasps and other inaccessible points may be polished readily and rapidly with a pointed rubber cylinder. Retentive clasps should be shaped with a uniform taper in both width and thickness throughout their entire length.

(g) The case [framework] is now ready for final polish. Use a B-20, 2-row brush wheel, with pumice or tripoli, or both, to remove all traces of rubber wheel marks.

(h) Finish this step with a tripoli-charged cloth buff or felt wheel and cones to get a velvety smooth finish.

(i) High gloss is imparted with a rouge-charged cloth or chamois buff.

(j) Boil case [framework] in a solution of [detergent] for several minutes and then with a hard brush remove all traces of polishing media. [This may also be accomplished by brushing with a solution of soap and household ammonia, or with commercial cleaning solutions.]*

4. Clean polishing wheels should be used. If contaminated wheels are used, foreign particles may become embedded in the surface, which will lead to later discoloration.

5. Be sure each finishing operation completely removes all scratches left by the preceding one. Remember that each successive finishing step uses a finer abrasive and therefore cuts more slowly and requires more time to accomplish.

Heat hardening. If the gold casting has been quenched in the investment, it is removed from the investment in its softest and most ductile condition. All grinding and finishing operations are performed while it is in this condition. **After finishing, and just before final polishing, precious metal alloys should be heat hardened.** Although chromium-cobalt alloys cannot be heat hardened, they have satisfactory physical properties in their original state as cast, plus whatever work-hardening occurs from manipulation and use.

Hardening gold castings by heat soaking.† Dental gold castings, which are subject to heat hardening, may be effectively hardened as follows when the casting is finished and ready for the final high polish:

1. Stabilize the furnace at the desired temperature by proper adjustment of the dial. See manufacturer's instructions for correct temperature for each alloy. (Yellow casting golds heat harden at temperatures between 600° and 700° F. White gold alloys heat harden more effectively at temperatures as high as 800° F, except Jelenko Palloro and alloys of its type, which require somewhat different treatment. These should be quenched in the investment as soon as the casting machine stops, while the button is still red, and heat hardened by soaking for 5 minutes in a furnace stabilized at 600° F.)

2. Place the casting on a metal tray in the furnace, close the door, and allow to heat soak for 15 minutes.

3. Remove the tray at the end of this period with the casting on it (do not touch the casting with cold tongs) and allow it to bench cool.

This treatment will produce from 85% to 100% of the strength given by the variable cooling–heat hardening process and will avoid any possibility of warpage because of heat treatment.

MAKING OF RECORD BASES

Bases for jaw relation records should either be made of materials possessing accuracy or be relined to provide such accuracy. Relining may be accomplished by seating the previously adapted base onto the tinfoiled or lubricated cast with an intervening mix of some zinc oxide–eugenol paste or with autopolymerizing resin. Some use has been made of the mercaptan and silicone impression materials for this purpose, but the wisdom of using an elastic lining for jaw relation record bases is questionable. However, when rigid setting materials are used for this purpose, any undercuts on the cast must be blocked out with wax or clay to facilitate their removal without damage to the cast.

The ideal jaw relation record base is one that is processed (or cast) to the form of the master cast, becoming the permanent base of the completed prosthesis. Cast metal bases for either complete or partial dentures offer this advantage over resin-based dentures. Resin bases may be processed directly to the master cast, thus becoming the permanent denture base. When undercuts are present, the master cast must be destroyed during removal of the base. Then existing undercuts must be blocked out inside the denture base before a cast is poured into it to make an articulator mounting. A second cast, which includes the undercuts, must be poured against the entire base to support it during the processing of the resin superstructure. When both the base and the superstructure are of resin, some care must be taken to avoid visible junction lines between the original resin base and the resin that supports the teeth and establishes facial contours.

Some autopolymerizing acrylic resin materials are sufficiently accurate for use as jaw relation bases. These are used with a sprinkling tech-

*From Berger, H.R.: Finishing and polishing requires a careful technic, Jelenko Thermotrol Technician 1:7, Oct. 1947.
†From information taken from the physical properties chart of J.F. Jelenko & Co., Inc., New York, N.Y.

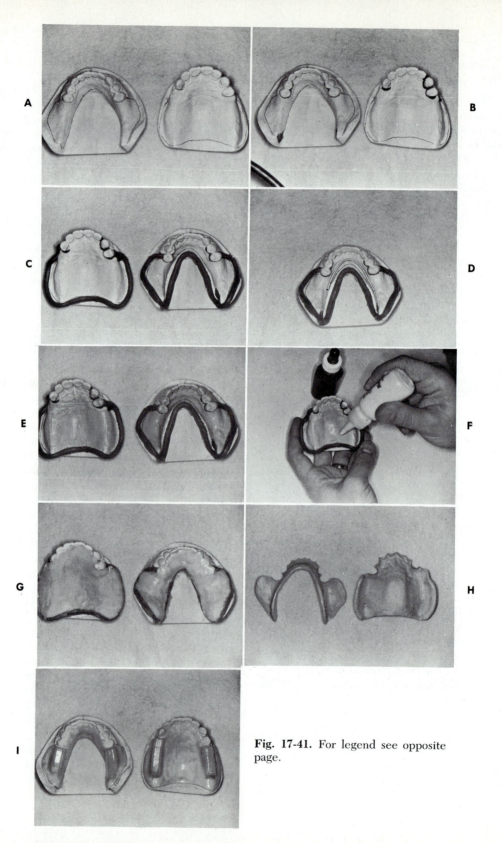

Fig. 17-41. For legend see opposite page.

nique, which when properly done permits a base to be made that compares favorably with a processed base. A material must be selected that will polymerize in a reasonable time (usually a 12-minute monomer) and will retain its form during the sprinkling process. Since polymerization with typical shrinkage toward the cast begins immediately, alternate addition of monomer and polymer in small increments results in reduced overall shrinkage and greater accuracy.

Technique for making a sprinkled acrylic resin record base. The technique for sprinkling a record base will be given here. Some blockout of the cast is necessary. Relief of undercut areas on the cast is best accomplished with a water-soluble modeling clay or baseplate wax. Modeling clay is easily formed and shaped on the cast and is easily removed from either the cast or the base with a natural-bristle toothbrush under warm running water. Wax, on the other hand, must be flushed off the cast with hot water. It must be removed from the inside of the base by scraping and with a wax solvent, followed by flushing with water only hot enough to eliminate any residual wax.

Bases for jaw relation records must have maximum contact with the supporting tissues. The accuracy of the base will be in proportion to the total area of intimate tissue contact provided. Those areas most frequently undercut and requiring blockout are the distolingual and retromylohyoid areas of the mandibular cast, the distobuccal and labial aspects of the maxillary cast, and, frequently, small multiple undercuts in the palatal rugae. These areas and any others are blocked out with a minimum of clay, to obliterate as little of the surface of the cast as possible. A close-fitting base may then be made that will have the necessary accuracy and stability and yet may be lifted from and returned to the master cast without abrading it (Fig. 17-41).

The cast and the blockout or relief is then painted with a tinfoil substitute of a type that may be painted onto a cold surface without leaving a heavy or uneven film, such as Alcote. This is essential to the accuracy of a denture base, but not all tinfoil substitutes are suitable for this purpose.

As soon as the tinfoil substitute has dried, the cast is wet with the monomer from a dropper bottle. The ordinary medicine dropper is not suitable for this purpose because the lumen is too large, resulting in an uncontrollable excess of monomer. The glass may be drawn to a fine tip over a flame but it easily broken. Instead the

Fig. 17-41. Stable record bases are required to correctly orient diagnostic casts representative of distal extension removable partial denture situations. Such bases are made with an autopolymerizing acrylic resin. **A,** Extent of record bases is outlined in pencil. Note that outline includes cingula of anterior teeth and distal surface of prospective terminal abutments. **B,** Interproximal undercuts are blocked out with wax. Other undercut areas involved in denture base design are also eliminated by blockout. Prominent or undercut rugae must be blocked out. **C,** Utility wax is adapted to outline of cast in edentulous regions to confine acrylic resin when it is being applied. Wax should be adapted approximately 2 mm from penciled outline to provide adequate thickness of record base borders. **D,** Stiff 16-gauge wire is bent to conform to lingual alveolar ridge of lower cast and becomes part of record base. This wire will strengthen final record base and will eliminate some flexibility of base. **E,** Tinfoil substitute Alcote is painted on cast to act as separator. Two thin coats are applied, allowing first coat to dry before application of second coat. **F,** Acrylic resin is sprinkled on cast, alternating application of monomer and polymer. **G,** Uniform thickness (2 mm) of acrylic resin is sprinkled within record base outline. **H,** Record bases have been removed (after curing) and trimmed to establish outlines. Note tissue detail and border thickness. **I,** Occlusion rims have been added to polished record bases. Occlusal surfaces of occlusion rims should be only as wide as occlusal surfaces of natural teeth they are representing. Attention must be given fabrication of occlusion rims so that natural arch form is maintained. In fact, occlusion rims should be thought of as replacements for lost natural teeth and their supporting structures for record-making purposes.

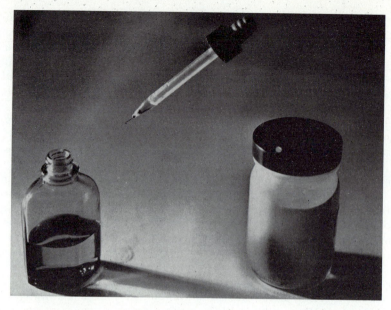

Fig. 17-42. Autopolymerizing acrylic resin in bottles used for sprinkling resin bases. Twenty-three–gauge hypodermic needle has been sealed into tip of dropper barrel to limit size of drop and facilitate wetting monomer without flooding. Large-mouthed bottle is of size that can easily be held in hand, and it has hole in rim the size of No. 8 or 10 round bur to allow powder to be applied selectively to area involved.

simple addition of a hypodermic needle of about 23 gauge to the glass lumen by flaming the glass tip around the needle provides a suitable syringe tip for the application of monomer in small quantities as needed (Fig. 17-42).

After the surface is wetted with the monomer, the polymer is sprinkled or dusted onto the wet surface until all the monomer has been absorbed. Sprinkling is best accomplished with a large-mouthed bottle with a single hole in the lid near the rim (Fig. 17-42). This facilitates the placement of the polymer without excess in any one area. A flexible bottle with suitable applicator tip also may be used. The objective should be the uniform application of polymer over the entire ridge rather than allowing excess to accumulate at the border to be trimmed later. An autopolymerizing acrylic resin material must be used that will retain its form during the sprinkling procedure without objectionable flow into low areas.

Once the polymer has been sprinkled in slight excess, the monomer is again added. Flooding must be avoided; therefore the monomer must be directed over the entire surface gradually until the polymer has just absorbed the monomer. **A few seconds' delay before the addition of excess monomer will allow the mass to reach a tacky consistency and prevent it from flowing when more monomer is added.** Then the monomer may be added in excess, which is immediately absorbed by the application of more polymer as before. This process is repeated selectively until a uniform layer has been built up just thick enough so that none of the underlying cast or relief may be seen. Some areas will require further addition, particularly ridge crests and other prominent areas.

The final step in sprinkling is the addition of monomer sufficient to leave a wet surface. **Immediately,** the cast should be placed in a covered glass dish or covered with an inverted bowl. This permits final polymerization in a saturated atmosphere of monomer and prevents evaporation of surface monomer. The cast should not be placed in water nor any attempt made to accelerate polymerization. Slow polymerization is necessary so that shrinkage **toward** the cast will occur, earlier layers polymerizing first. Only thus will overall shrinkage be negligible and accuracy of fit be assured. Whereas this is of little consequence in making an impression tray, it is most essential in making a sprinkled resin base.

Although polymerization will be about 90% complete within an hour, and an impression tray may even be lifted within a half hour, a sprinkled denture base should be left **overnight** before being separated from the cast. It should then be lifted either dry or under lukewarm tap water. It should not be immersed in hot water, or some warpage may occur.

A sprinkled acrylic resin base made with the precautions outlined above will retain its accuracy for days, or even for an indefinite period, comparable to that of a heat-cured resin base (Figs. 17-41 and 17-43). Failure to do so can be attributed to faulty technique rather than to any inherent inaccuracy in the material itself, provided the proper material has been used.

OCCLUSION RIMS

It has been explained that jaw relation records for partial dentures always should be made on accurate bases that are either part of the denture casting itself or attached to it in exactly the same relation as the final denture base will be. Further, it has been stated that although the use of the final denture base is best for jaw relation records, a sprinkled or corrected acrylic resin base may be used satisfactorily. In any case, accuracy of the base supporting a maxillomandibular record must be assured before the function of occlusion rims can be considered.

Occlusion rims may be made of several materials. The material that is most commonly used to establish static occlusal relationships is the hard baseplate wax rim. However, use of a wax occlusion rim is likely to be inaccurate when the occlusal portion of the rim is pooled with a hot instrument or flamed, because of the fact that uniform softening cannot be assured. Also, some errors in repositioning opposing casts against wax occlusion rims for mounting on the articulator are likely to occur. When some soft material that sets to a rigid state, such as impression plaster or impression paste, is used in conjunction with wax rims to record static occlusal relations, many of the errors common to wax rims are eliminated provided some space exists between the occlusion rims or the opposing teeth or both at the desired vertical dimension to be recorded. Occlusion rims for static jaw relation records should be so shaped that they represent the lost teeth and their supporting structures (Figs. 17-41, *I* and 17-43, *H*). An occlusion rim that is too broad and extended beyond where prosthetically supplied teeth will be located is inexcusable. Such rims will substantially alter the shape of the palatal vault and arch form of the mandibular arch, crowd the patient's tongue, have a nonwelcomed effect on the patient, and will offer more resistance to jaw relation recording media than will a correctly shaped occlusion rim.

Modeling plastic may be used rather than wax for occlusion rims, with several advantages. It may be softened uniformly by flaming, yet becomes rigid and sufficiently accurate when chilled. It may be trimmed with a sharp knife to expose the tips of the opposing cusps to recheck or position an opposing cast into the record rim. Opposing occlusion rims of modeling plastic may be keyed with greater accuracy than opposing wax rims. Preferably, however, even those should be trimmed short of contact at the vertical dimension of occlusion, and plaster or impression paste should be interposed for the final record. As with wax rims, an adjustable frame to support the final record also may be used.

Occlusion rims of either extra hard baseplate wax or modeling plastic may be used to support intraoral central bearing devices or intraoral tracing devices or both. However, because of its greater stability, modeling plastic is preferable for this purpose also when the edentulous situation permits the use of flat plane tracings. An example of such a situation is when an opposing denture is being made concurrently with the partial denture. In such a case, modeling plastic occlusion rims provide greater stability than wax rims, with corresponding improvement in the predictable accuracy of such a jaw relation record. Although sealing opposing occlusion rims or using clips for complete denture jaw relation records, particularly for an initial articulator mounting, may be acceptable, the existence of

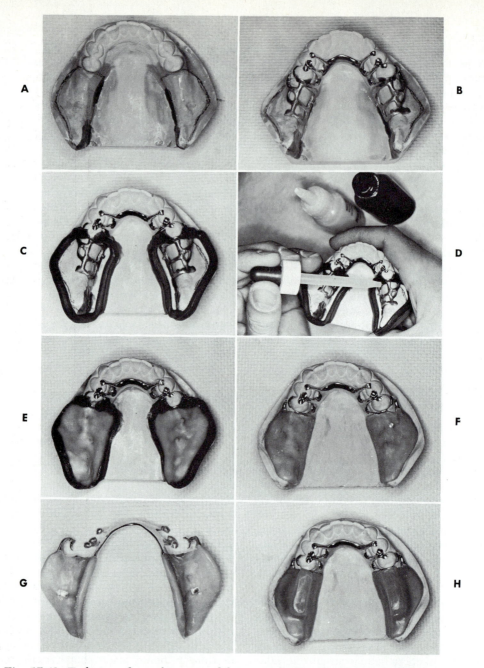

Fig. 17-43. Technique for making record base attached to framework for distal extension removable partial denture. **A,** Tissue undercuts are blocked out only enough to eliminate undercuts, and edentulous ridges are painted with tinfoil substitute (Alcote). **B,** Framework is positioned on cast after tinfoil substitute has dried. Small amount of wax is added on either side of minor connector extension touching distal surface of premolars to avoid having acrylic resin "run under" connector at gingival of abutment tooth. **C,** Utility wax strips are used to confine "sprinkled-on" acrylic resin, and they outline extent of record base. Wax strips do not cover finishing lines of direct retainers and lingual bar. **D,** Cast is wet with monomer in small area, and just enough polymer is added to take up monomer. This procedure is repeated until overall thickness of 2 mm is obtained. **E,** All areas within wax boxing have been covered by acrylic resin. **F,** Record base has been removed from cast and trimmed. Only borders of record base are polished. **G,** View of tissue surfaces. **H,** Occlusion rims are added to record base.

a partial denture framework makes this practice hazardous. Since it is necessary that the dentist be able to see that the partial denture framework is in its original relation to the supporting teeth before the casts are articulated, the framework and attached base should be seated accurately on its cast before the opposing cast is repositioned in occlusion to it.

Occlusion rims for recording functional, or dynamic, occlusion must be made of a hard wax that can be carved by the opposing dentition. This method, outlined in Chapter 16, presumes that the opposing arch is intact or has been restored. Functional occlusion records by this method cannot be made when both arches are being restored simultaneously.

Rather, an opposing arch must be as intact as the treatment plan calls for or must be restored by whatever prosthetic means the situation dictates. Opposing partial dentures or an opposing complete denture may be carried concurrently up to the final occlusal record. One denture is then completed and placed and the functional record made in opposition to it. Frequently this requires that all opposing teeth be articulated first in wax to establish optimal ridge relations and the correct occlusal plane. One denture is then carried to completion, and the teeth remaining in wax on the opposing denture are removed while the functional occlusal record is being made.

No single wax has been manufactured specifically for establishing functional occlusal records. Some inlay waxes are used for this purpose because they can be carved by the opposing dentition and because most of them are hard enough to support occlusion over a period of hours or days. A wax for recording functional crown and bridge occlusion, since it is established entirely in the dental office, is selected on the basis of how well it may be carved by the opposing dentition in a relatively short period of time. Therefore a softer wax may be used than is required for the recording of occlusal paths over a period of 24 hours or more. For this latter purpose, Peck's purple hard inlay wax seems to satisfy best the requirements for a wax that is durable yet capable of recording a functional occlusal pattern. This wax is packaged in the form of sticks. A layer of sticky wax is first flowed onto the surface of the denture base. Two sticks of the inlay wax are then laid parallel along the longitudinal center of the denture base and secured to it with a hot spatula. This is the only preparation before the dental appointment. Since neither the height nor the width of the occlusion rim can be known in advance and since deep warming of a chilled wax rim is difficult, the rim is not completed before the appointment.

With the patient in the chair a hot spatula is inserted into the crevice between the two sticks of wax, making the center portion fluid between two supporting walls. Some transfer of heat to the supporting walls occurs, resulting in the occlusion rim's becoming uniformly softened. The patient is asked to close into this wax rim until the natural teeth are in contact, which establishes both the height and the width of the occlusion rim. Wax is then added or carved away as indicated and the patient asked to go into lateral excursions. Any excess wax is then removed, and any unsupported wax is supported by addition. Finally, wax is added to increase the vertical dimension sufficient to allow for (1) denture settling, (2) changes in jaw relation brought about by the reestablishment of posterior support, and (3) carving in all mandibular excursions. When sufficient height has been established, as well as sufficient width to accommodate all excursive movements, the patient is instructed and dismissed.

Although this discussion has been included in this chapter on laboratory procedures, the entire procedure of establishing occlusion rims for recording functional occlusion should be considered a chariside procedure rather than a laboratory procedure. It is necessary, however, that the purpose of a functional occlusal record be clearly understood so that subsequent laboratory steps may be accomplished in a manner that the effect of such an occlusal record may be reproduced on the finished denture.

MAKING A STONE OCCLUSAL TEMPLATE FROM A FUNCTIONAL OCCLUSAL RECORD

After final acceptance of the occlusal record as registered by the patient, the effectiveness of this method for establishing functional occlusion on the partial denture will depend on how accurately the following procedures are carried out. For this reason it will be given as a step-by-step procedure (Figs. 16-14 to 16-19).

1. If the base of the master cast (or processing cast) has not been keyed previously, do this before proceeding. Reduce the thickness of the base if it is so thick that difficulty will be encountered in flasking. The base may not be reduced on this account after removal from the articulator, since the mounting record would be lost.

Keying may be done in several ways, but a method whereby the keyed portions are visible on the articulator mounting eliminates some possibility of remounting error. According to the preferred method, form a 45-degree bevel on the base of the cast by hand or with the model trimmer and then add three V-shaped grooves on the anterior and the posterior aspects of the base of the cast at the bevel (Fig. 17-44). The bevel serves to facilitate reseating the cast on the articulator mounting, and the mounting surfaces are made still more definite by the triangular grooves. Being placed at the beveled margin, the triangular grooves are visible at all times, and any discrepancy may be clearly seen.

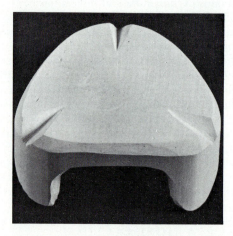

Fig. 17-44. Base of any cast should be beveled and keyed as shown before mounting on articulator. Petroleum jelly is used as separating medium to facilitate removal and remounting subsequent to processing. Keying should always be done before boxing and pouring occlusal registration because cast and template must be mounted on articulator before they are separated.

2. Inspect the underside of the cast framework and denture bases, removing any particles of wax or other debris. Similarly, inspect and clean the master cast of any particles of stone, wax, blockout material, or any other debris that might prevent the casting from being seated accurately on it.

Now seat the denture framework on the cast in its original terminal position. This is the position that was maintained by securing it with sticky wax while the trial denture base was being made, with all the occlusal rests seated. It is also the position that the casting assumed in the mouth while the occlusal record was being made and that must be duplicated on returning the denture framework to the master cast. Holding the framework in this terminal position, secure it again with sticky wax. (If a processing cast is being used in place of the master cast, the denture base will have been made on that cast and the same precautions in returning the framework to its original position apply.)

3. With the denture framework and the occlusal record in position, form a matrix of clay around the occlusal record to confine the hard stone, which will form the stone occlusal template. (The clay matrix is the same for a metallized surface as for the wax record.)

The clay matrix should rise at a 45-degree angle from the buccal and lingual imits of the occlusal registration. Then arch either clay or a sheet of wax across from one side to the other, forming a vault that will permit lingual access when articulating the teeth.

Leave the occlusal surfaces of a processing cast exposed so that they may act as vertical stops. This will serve to maintain the vertical relation on the articulator. Unless such stone-to-stone stops are used, the vertical relation on the articulator may be altered by the technician, either accidentally or otherwise. Any change in vertical relations is incompatible with a concept of dynamic conclusion, since the occlusal pattern is directly related to the degree of jaw separation. Although it may be true that vertical dimension may be changed when casts are mounted in relation to the opening axis of the mandible, **as long as natural cusps remain to influence mandibular movement, the vertical relation established with a functional occlusal record must not be changed on the articulator.**

Treat the surfaces of the adjacent abutment teeth left exposed with sodium silicate, Microfilm, or some other separating medium to ensure separation of the stone vertical stops.

4. If the wax record has not been metallized, use a hard dental stone to form the opposing template. This may be an improved stone such as Duroc, but the use of a stone die material such as Vel-Mix is preferred. Only the occluding surface need be poured in the harder stone, a less costly laboratory stone being used to back it up. If this is done, add the second layer to the first before the former takes its initial set, to avoid any possibility of accidental separation between the two materials.

Vibrate the stone only into the wax registration and against the stone stops. Pile on the rest of the stone and leave it uneven to facilitate firm attachment to the mounting stone. Attach the occlusal template to the articulator without provision for remounting, since only the working cast need by keyed for remounting.

5. After the stone template has set, attach the occluded casts to both arms of the articulator before separating the casts. The type of articulating instrument used is of little importance, since all eccentric positions are recorded on the template, and whatever instrument is used acts purely as a simple hinge or a tripod. Therefore any laboratory articulator or tripod may be used. Because of the easy access afforded in arranging artificial teeth and adjusting occlusion, the Hagman Junior Balancer is preferred over most other instruments for this purpose.

Casts should be attached to the articulating instrument selected with stone rather than with plaster. Mounting stones are available that have been especially formulated and prepared to minimize the setting expansion inherent in most gypsum products. The least amount of setting expansion of the mounting medium is most desirable to maintain the intended relationship of the opposing casts.

It must be remembered which arch is represented by the working cast, and the articulator mounting should be made accordingly. For example, for a mandibular denture the template is attached to the upper arm of the articulator, whereas for a maxillary denture the template is mounted upside down on the lower arm. The keyed base of the working cast attached to the opposing arm must be coated with a light coat of mineral oil or petroleum jelly to facilitate its separation from the mounting stone.

6. After the mounting has been completed, separate the casts and remove the clay. The template with its mounting may be removed from the articulator if a mounting ring or mounting stud permits; otherwise trimming must be done on the articulator. With pencil, outline the limits of the occlusal registration and carefully knife-trim any excess stone around its borders. Trim the vertical stops to a sharp edge on the buccal surface where they contact the working cast. Also remove any overhanging stone, leaving the occluding template and vertical stops clearly visible and accessible.

Remove the wax registration preparatory to arranging artificial teeth to the occluding template.

ARRANGING POSTERIOR TEETH TO AN OPPOSING CAST OR TEMPLATE

Whether posterior teeth are to be arranged to occlude with an opposing cast or an occlusal template, unless metal bases are part of the denture framework, the denture base on which the jaw relation record has been made must first be removed and discarded. This statement is based on the assumption that where an adjustable articulator has been used to develop the occlusion, the trial dentures have been evaluated, the articulator mounting has been proved, and the articulator has been programmed for eccentric positions. Since record bases that are entirely tissue supported have no place in recording occlusal relations for partial dentures, the bases must be attached to the denture framework. Metal bases being part of the prosthesis present no problem. The teeth may be arranged in wax or replaced on the metal base, depending on the type of posterior tooth being used, and these occluded directly to the opposing cast or template.

Unless occlusal relations are recorded on final resin bases, autopolymerizing acrylic resin bases by the sprinkling method are the most accurate and stable of bases that may be used for this purpose. (An alternate method is the relining of the original impression bases, thus accomplishing the same purpose.) Although static relations may be recorded successfully on corrected bases, functional registrations are best accomplished on new resin bases made for that purpose. In either case the denture cannot be completed on these bases, nor can the bases be removed conveniently from the retentive framework during the boilout after flasking. Therefore the metal framework must be lifted from the cast, and the original record base removed by flaming its underside: **Care must be taken not to allow the resin to catch on fire, or the cast framework will become discolored with carbon.** The framework is repolished and is then returned to its original position on the master cast and secured there with sticky wax before arrangement of the artificial teeth is begun.

Posterior tooth forms. Posterior tooth forms for partial dentures should not be selected arbitrarily. One should bear in mind at all times that the objective in partial denture occlusion is harmony between natural and artificial dentition. Whether the teeth are arranged to occlude with an opposing cast or to an occlusal template, they should be modified to harmonize with the existing dentition. In this respect, partial denture occlusion may differ from complete denture occlusion. In the latter, posterior teeth may be selected and articulated according to the dentist's own concept of what constitutes the most favorable complete denture occlusion, whereas partial denture occlusion must be made to harmonize with an existing occlusal pattern. Thus the occlusal surfaces on the finished partial denture may bear little resemblance to the original occlusal surfaces of the teeth as manufactured.

Artificial tooth forms should be selected to restore the space and fulfill the esthetic demands of the missing dentition. Manufactured tooth forms usually require modification to satisfactorily articulate with an opposing dentition. The original occlusal form therefore is of little importance in forming the posterior occlusion for the partial denture.

Whereas the posterior teeth may be made of porcelain or resin, resin teeth are more easily modified and subsequently reshaped for masticating efficiency by adding grooves and spillways. Resin teeth are also more easily narrowed buccolingually to reduce the size of the occlusal table without sacrificing strength or esthetics. They also may be more easily ground to fit minor connectors and irregular spaces and to avoid retentive elements of the denture framework. **However, it is reemphasized that when acrylic resin teeth are used without gold occlusal surfaces, the occlusion must be evaluated quite frequently to make sure that the occlusal sur-**

Fig. 17-45. Gold occlusal surfaces, duplicating occlusal morphology of adjusted acrylic resin posterior teeth, are readily fabricated. **A,** Denture has been used by patient and all necessary occlusal adjustments have been accomplished on resin teeth in first 2 weeks of use. **B,** Stone matrix is poured over occlusal surfaces and extended over top one fourth of buccal surfaces. **C,** Stone matrix is extended to cover depth of lingual flange so that it can be positively relocated in same position after artificial teeth have been prepared for reception of gold occlusal surfaces. Buccal portion of matrix is trimmed so that wax patterns for gold surfaces will be about 1.5 mm thick. **D,** Stone matrices are painted with separating medium, and wax patterns of occlusal surfaces are formed by flowing inlay wax into occlusal portions of matrix. Small retention loops are placed—one in each individual occlusal pattern. Patterns are sprued and cast in Type III gold. **E,** Wax patterns have been cast and polished. **F,** Acrylic resin artificial teeth are prepared for reception of gold occlusal surfaces by reducing their occlusal portion about 2 mm and making undercut groove through central fossa of resin teeth. Groove should only be deep enough to accommodate retention loops on gold occlusal surfaces. **G,** Gold occlusals, stone matrix, and denture are assembled. Matrix is held in position with sticky wax. Tooth shade acrylic resin (autopolymerizing) is used to attach gold occlusal surfaces to denture by using the "sprinkling" method of application. **H,** Procedure is completed by finishing and polishing tooth shade resin. Although original occlusal surfaces have been duplicated in gold and now occupy same position as original resin surfaces, remounting cast should be made so that any possible resulting occlusal discrepancies can be corrected on articulator, using new interocclusal records to mount lower cast and denture. (From Morris, A.L., and Bohannon, H.M., editors: Dental specialties in general practice, Philadelphia, 1969, W.B. Saunders Co.)

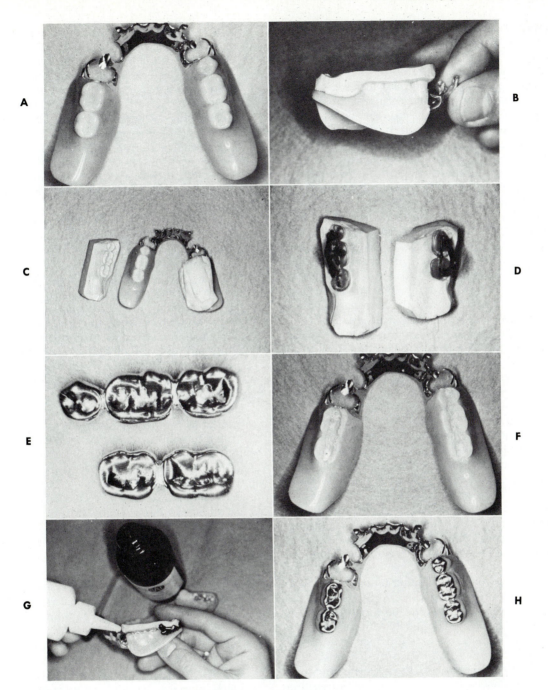

Fig. 17-45. For legend see opposite page.

faces of the resin teeth have not worn out of contact in centric occlusion. Aside from economics, the occlusal surfaces of acrylic resin teeth should be duplicated in gold to prevent excessive wear of the occlusal surfaces, thereby maintaining the planned occlusion for artificial posterior teeth (Fig. 17-45). It seems that the best combinations of opposing occlusal surfaces to maintain the established occlusion and avoid deleterious abrasion are porcelain to porcelain surfaces, gold surfaces to natural or restored natural teeth, and gold surfaces to gold surfaces.

Arranging teeth to an occluding surface. The procedure for arranging teeth to a static relationship with an opposing cast is essentially the same as for arranging teeth to an occluding template. On the other hand, articulation of artificial teeth on an adjustable instrument, which reproduces to some extent mandibular movement, will follow more closely the customary pattern for complete denture occlusion.

Step-by-step procedure. The procedure for arranging posterior teeth to an occluding template is as follows:

1. Raise the vertical adjustment of the articulator approximately 1 mm. If vertical stops are used, this will separate the stone stops by that amount.

2. With the aid of marking tape or articulating ribbon, mark the mesial and the ridge lap surfaces of the tooth to be placed against the most anterior minor connector on either side. Continue to mark and relieve this tooth until it conforms to and fits around the minor connector, occluding with the opposing surface at the existing vertical dimension. Modify the cusps of this tooth as required to occlude with the opposing surface.

3. Arrange the remaining teeth on that side in order, progressing posteriorly. Relieve the ridge lap and modify the occlusal surfaces as required to occlude optimally with the opposing surfaces. One or more teeth may have to be narrowed mesiodistally to establish a satisfactory mesiodistal relation with the opposing teeth. In other instances it may be necessary to leave a space between the first two teeth to accomplish this effect. Although intercuspation is desirable in most instances, it is not absolutely necessary when arranging to an occlusal template, since modified occlusal surfaces will function satisfactorily in any mesiodistal relation.

4. If a posterior abutment is present, the last tooth may have to be narrowed mesiodistally to fit the remaining space. This tooth also should be ground to conform to the contour of the minor connector, thereby effecting a more natural marginal contact relation with the abutment tooth.

5. Proceed to the opposite side of the arch and arrange the tooth or teeth in the same sequence, with each tooth lying adjacent to a minor connector being ground to fit that minor connector.

6. When all teeth have been arranged to the opposing surfaces, having been modified to occlude optimally at the existing vertical dimension, release the vertical element (pin or screw), leaving the occlusion uniformly high. When vertical stops of stone are used, the vertical element on the articulator may be removed entirely, since the absolute vertical dimension will be ultimately maintained by the stone stops. Otherwise the pin or screw should be returned to its original position. (This is difficult to reestablish without a calibrated pin; hence the value of having definite stone stops.)

Using marking tape or articulating ribbon as an indicator, the occlusal surfaces are now further modified until an optimal occlusal relationship at the selected vertical dimension of occlusion has been established. At least three factors must be considered:

a. The template surface may be easily abraded or otherwise damaged by repeated closure against the teeth being arranged. This does not apply when opposing artificial teeth are being arranged and modified concurrently. When arranging teeth on a single denture, however, an opposing surface made of hard metal is the only way of eliminating this possibility; otherwise, violent tapping must be avoided.

b. Unreliable markings usually result when articulating paper is used. Areas of heavy contact become perforated, leaving only a small mark, whereas areas of lesser contact may make a heavier mark. This may be avoided by using a marking tape or an inked ribbon, which better conforms to irregular occluding surfaces, does not tear or become perforated, and remains constant with repeated use. Markings are thus more reliably interpreted. A ribbon holder has been described in Chapter 16 under the discussion on arranging teeth to an occluding template.

c. Wax from articulating paper eventually is deposited on opposing surfaces, having the effect of increasing the vertical dimension of occlusion and leading to false interpretation of occlusal interference. This too is avoided by using a marking tape or an inked ribbon, since the ink or dye does not create a false surface.

Regardless of the type of indicator used, stone stops are best left unmarked for better interpretation of absolute contact. Wax from articulating paper may create a false surface here also, changing the vertical relation. Although marking ink does not do this, it does make visualization of the vertical relation at the stops more difficult to interpret.

7. Except for the addition of spillways, perfect the occlusion while the teeth are still in wax. Only those errors occurring as a result of processing will then need to be corrected by remounting. Final waxing may be done off of the articulator, but the cast should be returned to it to correct any tooth displacement resulting from waxing and carving.

TYPES OF ANTERIOR TEETH

Anterior teeth on partial dentures are concerned primarily with esthetics and the function of incising. These are best arranged in the mouth, since an added appointment for try-in would be necessary anyway. They may be arranged arbitrarily on the cast and then tried in, but a stone index of their labial surfaces should be made on the master cast after the final arrangement has been established.

From a purely mechanical standpoint, all missing anterior teeth are best replaced with fixed restorations rather than with the partial denture. However, for economic or cosmetic reasons or in situations in which several missing anterior teeth are involved, such as in a Class IV partially edentulous arch, their replacement with the partial denture may be unavoidable.

Some types of anterior teeth used on partial dentures are as follows:

1. Porcelain or resin teeth, attached to the framework with acrylic resin.

2. Ready-made resin teeth processed directly to retentive elements on the metal framework with a matching resin. This is called a **pressed-on** method and has the advantage of permitting prior selection and trying of the anterior teeth, plus the advantage of using ready-made resin teeth for labial surfaces. These are then hollowed out on the lingual surface to facilitate their permanent attachment to the denture framework with the resin of the same shade.

3. Resin teeth processed to a metal framework in the laboratory. Tooth forms of wax may be carved on the denture framework and tried in the mouth, adjusted for esthetics and occlusion, and then processed in a resin of a suitable shade. There is some question as to whether the shade and durability of such teeth are comparable to those of manufactured plastic teeth, but improvements in materials have led to improved quality and appearance of laboratory-made teeth. Moreover, such teeth may frequently be shaped and characterized to better blend with the adjacent natural teeth.

4. Porcelain or resin facings cemented to the denture framework. These may be tried in the mouth on a baseplate wax base and adjusted for esthetics. Ready-made plastic backings may be used, which become part of the pattern for the partial denture framework, and the teeth are then ultimately cemented to the denture framework. Esthetically these are less satisfactory than other types of anterior teeth, but they have the advantage of greater strength and are easily replaced. A record of the mold and shade of each tooth should be kept, and only the ridge lap of the replacement teeth needs to be ground to fit. When replaceability is the main reason for its use, the stock facing should not be beveled, or difficulty will be encountered in replacing it. Replacement also may be accomplished by waxing and processing a resin facing directly to the metal backing. Stock tube or side-groove teeth are not ordinarily used for anterior teeth on partial dentures because of the horizontal forces that tend to dislodge them.

5. Anterior teeth hollowed out to receive resin veneers, the same as for veneer crowns and veneer pontics on fixed partial dentures. This is

most applicable when the denture framework is to be cast in gold. Then labial surfaces may be waxed and the final carving for esthetics done in the mouth. A modification of this method is the waxing of the veneer coping on a previously cast gold base. These are then cast separately and attached to the framework by soldering. Esthetically the result is comparable to that obtained with resin veneer crowns. This method is particularly applicable when there is a desire to make the replaced teeth match adjacent veneered abutment crowns.

WAXING AND INVESTING THE PARTIAL DENTURE BEFORE PROCESSING RESIN BASES

Waxing the partial denture base. Waxing the partial denture base before investing differs little from waxing a complete denture; the only difference is the waxing to and around exposed parts of the metal framework. Here, undercut finishing lines should be provided whenever possible. Then the waxing is merely butted to the finishing line with a little excess to allow for finishing. Otherwise, small voids in the wax may become filled with investing plaster, or fine edges of the investment may break off during boilout and packing. In either case, small pieces of investment may become embedded in the resin at the finishing lines. This is avoided by slightly overwaxing and then finishing the resin back to the metal finishing line with finishing burs. Abrasive wheels and disks should not be used for this purpose, as they will cut into the metal and may burn the resin. Pumice and a rag wheel should be used sparingly for polishing because it will cut the resin more rapidly than the metal and leave the finishing line elevated above the adjacent resin.

When waxing to polished metal parts not possessing a finishing line, it must be remembered that no attachment will exist and that over a period of time there inevitably will be some seepage, separation, and discoloration of the resin in this area. This may be avoided to some extent by roughening the metal whenever possible to effect some mechanical attachment. The wax should be left thick enough so that the resin will have some bulk at its junction with the polished metal. Thin films of resin over metal should be avoided and, in finishing, these should

be cut back to an area of bulk with finishing burs. Otherwise any thin film of resin will eventually separate and become discolored and unclean as a result of marginal seepage.

Gingival form should be waxed in accordance with modern concepts of cosmetics and should be made as self-cleansing as possible. Dental students should become familiar with normal gingival architecture as found on diagnostic casts of natural dentitions, beginning with the casts of each other's mouths usually made in basic technique exercises. In this manner they may have a better concept of gingival contours to be reproduced on prosthetic restorations.

In general, students and technicians alike seem to lack a clear concept of natural gingival architecture and are prone to leave too much tooth embedded in wax. Artificial teeth ordinarily should be uncovered fully to expose all the anatomic crown and even beyond when gingival recession is to be simulated. Relatively few prosthodontic patients are in an age bracket in which some gingival recession and exposed cementum would not normally be present, and this should be simulated on prosthodontic restorations in proportion to the patient's age. With partial dentures, gingival contours around the remaining natural teeth should be used as a guide to the gingival contours to be reproduced on the prosthesis. However, interproximal spaces are almost always filled, particularly between posterior artificial teeth.

Frush has listed the following rules for varying the height of the gingival tissue at the cervical portion of the teeth:

(a) Slightly below the high lip line at the central incisors.
(b) Lower than the central incisor gum line [gingival margin] at the lateral incisors.
(c) Higher than the central or lateral incisor gum line [gingival margin] at the canine.
(d) Slightly lower than the canine at the premolar and variable for both premolars and molars.*

The correctly formed interdental papilla should be formed so that it will be self-cleansing. It should be carved so that it is in harmony with the interpretation of age and will be the deciding

---

*From Frush, J.P.; Dentogenic restorations and dynesthetics, Los Angeles, 1957, Swissdent Foundation.

factor in the visible outline form of the tooth. As Frush has pointed out, even a drop of wax properly placed can change the appearance of a square tooth to one of tapering or ovoid appearance. A properly formed interdental papilla further enhances the natural appearance by increasing the color in this area.

The rules for forming the interdental papilla were given by Frush as follows:

(a) The papilla must extend to the point of tooth contact for cleanliness.
(b) The papillae must be of various lengths.
(c) The interdental papilla must be convex in all directions.
(d) The papillae must be shaped according to the age of the patient.
(e) The papilla must end near the labial face of the tooth and never slope inward to terminate toward the lingual portion of the interproximal surface.*

The denture should be waxed and carved as for a cast restoration, which it actually is, regardless of the material to be used or the method of processing. The fact that a split-mold technique is used for processing does not alter the fact that the form of the denture base is to be reproduced by a casting procedure. Therefore the denture pattern should be waxed with care in the same form as that desired for the finished restoration rather than attempting to shape facial

*From Frush, J.P.; Dentogenic restorations and dynesthetics, Los Angeles, 1957, Swissdent Foundation.

contours on the prosthesis during the polishing phase (Fig. 17-46). Polishing should consist primarily of trimming away the flash, stippling polished surfaces when desired, and polishing lightly with brush wheels and pumice, followed by final polishing with a soft brush wheel and a nonabrasive shining agent such as "whiting." Gross trimming and polishing with pumice should not be necessary if the denture has been properly waxed before investing.

Since the polished surfaces of any denture play an important part in both retention and the control of the food bolus, buccal and lingual contours generally should be made concave. In most cases, border thickness of the denture should be left as recorded in the impression. The only exceptions are the distolingual aspect of the lower denture base to avoid interference with the tongue, and the distobuccal aspect of the upper denture base to avoid interference with the coronoid process of the mandible. These are the only areas that cannot ordinarily be waxed to final contour before investing and may need to be thinned **by the dentist** at the time of final polishing.

Investing the partial denture. In investing a partial denture for processing a resin base, it must be remembered that the denture cast must be recovered from the flask intact for remounting. The practice of cutting the teeth off the cast to expose the connectors and retainers, which are then embedded in the upper half of the flask, is permissible only when an existing denture

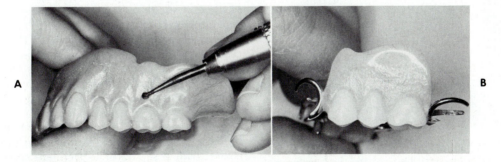

Fig. 17-46. A, Interdental papillae are convex and extend to contact points of adjacent teeth on complete maxillary denture to simulate naturalness. Root indices were carved in wax before denture was processed. Stippling was accomplished with eccentric No. 6 round bur. **B,** Buccal flange of removable partial denture base is similarly treated as in **A.** Finishing of acrylic resin bases is simplified by careful waxing, carving, and investing before processing.

base is being relined and no provision has been made for remounting. (In such case, it seems that this practice has no advantage over investing the denture being so relined upside-down in the lower half of the flask.) Since some increase in vertical dimension has, in the past, been inevitable in any split-mold processing technique, this method results in the denture framework's being raised from the supporting teeth by the amount of increase. Whereas occlusal adjustment in the mouth may temporarily reestablish a harmonious occlusal relation with the opposing teeth, the denture framework must then settle into supporting contact with the abutment teeth at the expense of the underlying ridge.

Changes in vertical dimension may be held to a minimum by using denture resins that can be placed in the mold in a fluid rather than a doughy state or those that may be injected in a fluid state into a closed mold. Dimensional changes occurring during relining may also be held to a minimum by using autopolymerizing resins for this purpose, thus avoiding the thermal expansion of a mold subjected to elevated temperatures.

When two opposing partial dentures are being made concurrently, one is sometimes processed

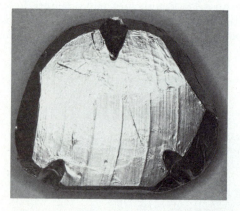

Fig. 17-47. Base of cast has been covered with 0.001 inch tinfoil before investing cast and denture for processing. Base of cast will be free of investing stone when recovered from processing flask and may be conveniently returned to original stone mounting on articulator for occlusal corrections or to preserve original face-bow mounting of maxillary cast.

and placed first and then the final occlusion established on the second denture to a fully restored arch. In such a case, when there are no natural teeth in opposition, it is not necessary that the first denture be remounted after processing. In all other cases, remounting to correct for errors in occlusion is absolutely necessary. Flasking must be accomplished so that the cast may be recovered from the flask undamaged.

Since the partial denture impression (fluid wax) may not be boxed before pouring the cast, metal mounting plates cannot be used as with complete denture impressions. Adding a mounting plate later with additional stone is not dependable, because if the cast separates between the two layers of stone, the mounting record is lost. The base of the stone cast must therefore be keyed by beveling and notching on at least three sides.

Minute voids in the base of the cast will have been reproduced in the stone mounting, and although the obvious larger blebs may be trimmed away, smaller blebs will remain. If the voids in the cast become filled with investing material, the effect is two particles trying to occupy the same space. This may be prevented by covering the base with tinfoil before investing (Fig. 17-47). By coating the base and sides of the cast with petroleum jelly, tinfoil may be easily adapted by burnishing it on with a towel. Not only does this keep the base of the cast isolated from investing material, but the cast also may be more easily recovered from the surrounding investment.

After tinfoiling has been done, the remainder of the cast should be coated with some reliable separator, such as mineral oil, petroleum jelly, sodium silicate, or tinfoil substitute. The entire cast, except for the wax and teeth, may then be invested in the lower half of the flask (Fig. 17-48). As with a complete denture, only the supplied teeth and wax are left exposed to be invested in the upper half. Also, as with a complete denture, the investment in the lower half must be smooth and free of undercuts and must be coated with a separator to facilitate separation of the two halves of the flask.

An alternate and preferred procedure is to invest the cast only to the top of the tinfoiled base, smoothing the investment and applying a reliable separator. Then a second layer of investment is placed around the anatomic portion of the cast, covering the natural teeth and the exposed parts of the denture framework. This is likewise smoothed and made free of undercuts and coated with a separator before pouring the top half of the flask. Recovery of the cast is thus made easier by having a shell of investment over the anatomic portion of the cast, which may be removed separately.

When the denture base is to be characterized by applying tinted resins to the mold, care should be taken not to embed the wax border in the lower half of the flask. Bennett has pointed out the need for investing only to the border of the wax, leaving the entire surface to be tinted reproduced in the upper half of the flask. With this precaution, tinting may be carried all the way to the border, and later removal of the flask will not mar the tinted surface. If tinting is not

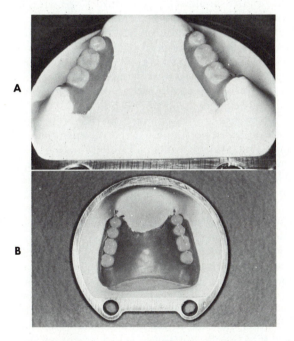

Fig. 17-48. A, Class I mandibular denture invested in lower half of flask. Master cast on which denture will be processed is completely covered with investing stone, exposing only artificial teeth and waxed denture bases. There are *no* undercuts in invested lower half of flask, thus assuring separation of flask halves after investment procedure is completed. **B,** Maxillary Class I denture invested in lower half of investing flask.

to be done or is to be done only at the cervical margins of the teeth and the interdental papillae, the wax border should be embedded in the lower half where it may be faithfully reproduced and preserved during polishing.

The use of resin materials that require trial packing is complicated by the presence of the retentive framework of the partial denture. With their use, trial packing must be done with two sheets of cellophane between two layers of the resin dough; otherwise the flask could not be opened without pulling the resin away from either the teeth in one half of the flask or the metal framework in the other. Resin dough is placed in each half of the flask, the sheets of cellophane placed between them, and the flask closed for trial packing. The flask is then opened, the cellophane removed, and the excess flash trimmed away. Final closure is then effected without the intervening sheets of cellophane.

Resin materials that require no trial packing have been developed. These are mixed as usual but are either poured into the mold or placed into the mold in a soft state. They offer little or no resistance to closure of the flask, yet the finished product is comparable to resin materials packed in a doughy state. They must be used in some excess, with the excess escaping between the halves of the flask. Although they are soft enough to allow the escape of gross excess, the use of a land space is advisable to avoid a thin film on the land area. Any film existing on the land area after deflasking may be interpreted as an opening of the flask by that amount, hence the need for some provision for an intervening space to accommodate the excess and to facilitate its escape as the flask is closed.

To provide such a land space, the land area on the lower half of the flask may be painted with melted baseplate wax before the top half is poured. After wax elimination a space then remains to accommodate any excess resin remaining after the flask is completely closed. It is necessary that no plaster or wax be allowed to remain on the rim of the flask and that the flask make metal-to-metal contact before the second half is poured. Only in this way is it possible to see that the flask is completely closed before it is placed in the curing unit.

The pouring of the top half of the flask follows the same procedure as with a complete denture.

Whereas it is not absolutely necessary that the entire top half be poured in stone, it is necessary that a stone cap of some type be used to prevent tooth movement in an occlusal direction. This is because of the inability of plaster to withstand closing pressures. All plaster remaining on the occlusal surfaces of the teeth should be removed and a separator added before the stone cap is poured to facilitate its removal during deflasking. If the use of stone investment is preferred, a shell of improved stone or die stone may be painted or applied with the fingers onto the wax and teeth and allowed to harden before the remainder of the flask is filled with plaster. If a full stone investment is preferred, some provision should be made for easy separation during deflasking. Not only should a separator stone cap be used, but metal separators or knife cuts radiating out to the walls of the flask should also be placed on the partially set stone. Deflasking is then easily accomplished by removing the stone cap and inserting a knife blade between the sections of stone.

Boilout should be deferred until the investing material has set for several hours or, preferably, overnight. Boilout must effectively eliminate all wax residue; therefore an adequate source of clean hot water must be available. Immersion of a flask containing the invested denture in boiling water for 5 minutes will adequately soften the wax supporting the artificial teeth so that flask halves may be separated and the remaining wax flushed out. After wax elimination with boiling water, the invested denture should be flushed with a solution of grease-dissolving detergent and again with clean boiling water.

Immediately after boilout the warm mold should be painted with a thin film of tinfoil substitute, being careful not to allow it to collect around the cervical portions of the teeth. A second coat should be applied after the first coat has reasonably dried, and packing of the mold should proceed immediately after this film has dried to the touch.

When the master cast for a distal extension partial denture has been repoured from a secondary impression, the supporting "foot" on the retention frame may not necessarily be in contact with the cast. Closing pressure within the flask may distort the unsupported extension of the metal framework, with subsequent rebound on deflasking. The finished denture base will then lack contact with the supporting tissues, resulting in denture rotation about the fulcrum line similar to that occurring after tissue resorption. **To provide support for the distal extension of the metal framework during flask closure, an autopolymerizing resin should be sprinkled or painted around the distal end of the framework and allowed to harden before proceeding with packing the denture resin** (Fig. 4-50).

PROCESSING THE DENTURE

Processing follows the same procedure as that for a complete denture. Denture base characterization may be added just before packing. This is most desirable when denture base material will be visible. Posterior resin bases alone ordinarily do not require characterization, but the dentist should select a denture base material that closely resembles the color of the surrounding tissues. The ideal resin base material for partial dentures is therefore one that (1) may be used without trial packing, (2) possesses a shade that is compatible with surrounding tissues, (3) is dimensionally stable and accurate, and (4) is dense and lends itself to polishing.

There has never been any question concerning the merits of tinfoiling the denture before investing, which results in a tinfoil-lined matrix and eliminates the need for a separating film. The fact remains, however, that the use of a tinfoil substitute has become almost universal.

At best, any tinfoil substitute creates an undesirable film at the gingival margins of the teeth, resulting in microscopic separation between the teeth and the surrounding resin. This may be shown by sectioning a finished denture and by observing the marginal discoloration around the cervical portions of the teeth after several months in the mouth. To some extent, injection molding obviates this objection to the use of a tinfoil substitute—which is one of the principal advantages of injection molding over compression molding.

Since the use of compression molding is widespread and is likely to continue, methods that eliminate the use of a tinfoil substitute are needed. The layered silicone rubber method results in more complete adaptation of the resin around the cervical portions of porcelain teeth and more complete bonding to resin teeth. In addition, denture base tints may be applied directly to the mold without first applying a separating film.

A room-temperature–curing silicone rubber, which has sufficient body and toughness for the purpose, is applied to the wax surface of the denture and over the teeth. To prevent movement of the teeth during processing, the occlusal surfaces should be exposed before the upper half of the flask is poured. The manufacturer's instructions must be followed as to mixing and time elapsed before the outer stone investment is added to ensure curing and bonding to the overlying investment. Boilout is then completed in the usual way.

A further advantage of the layered silicone rubber method is the ease with which deflasking is accomplished. If the wax carving of the denture has been completed with care before flasking, denture tints remain unaltered by unnecessary trimming and polishing of the processed denture.

All resin base materials available up to the present time exhibit some dimensional change, both during processing and in the mouth. The fit of the denture is therefore dependent, to a large extent, on the accuracy, or lack of accuracy, of the denture base material, since impression and cast materials in use today are themselves reasonably accurate. In an attempt to minimize dimensional changes in the denture base, materials and techniques are constantly being improved. Some of these use injection molding to provide a continuous source of material to the mold as curing shrinkage occurs. One technique uses hydraulic pressure within the top half of the flask to limit the shrinkage toward the cast only. It is claimed, by the originator of this technique, that processing by any other means results in both a distorted mold and a distorted cast, because of collapse of the stone or plaster around the myriad of small air voids inevitably present.

Denture base materials that may be poured into the mold or placed into the mold in a soft state are being used. This technique eliminates trial packing and excessive pressures, which leads to open flasks and altered vertical dimension, as is sometimes experienced with compression molding of resin base materials. Activated, or autopolymerizing, resins are frequently used to avoid mold expansions at higher temperatures. Materials other than acrylic resins are used with various techniques, some of these being styrene, vinyl, and, experimentally, epoxy resins. The main objective behind the development of newer techniques and materials is greater dimensional accuracy and stability, combined with strength and better appearance.

The study of the history of denture base materials is a most interesting one that has been covered elsewhere in dental literature. The future of denture base materials promises to be just as fascinating a study, but such a discussion cannot be included within the scope of this book. With newer materials the future of methyl methacrylate as a denture base material is uncertain despite its acceptance as the best material available for this purpose since its introduction in 1937. Although it has made possible the simulation of natural tissue color and contours combined with ease of manipulation, the fact remains that it leaves much to be desired as far as accuracy and dimensional stability are concerned. Whether other and newer materials will eventually supplant methyl methacrylate as a denture base material remains to be seen. The fact is that the denture base of the future (1) must be capable of accurately reproducing natural tissue tones faithfully through the use of characterizing stains and customizing procedures and (2) must not require elaborate processing procedures and equipment, which would make the cost prohibitive for general usage.

REMOUNTING AND OCCLUSAL CORRECTION TO AN OCCLUSAL TEMPLATE

Even with improved denture base materials and processing techniques, some movement of artificial teeth will still occur because of the dimensional instability of the wax in which the artificial teeth were arranged. Until sources of error can be eliminated, remounting will continue to be necessary. How well the occlusion may be perfected by remounting will depend on the manner in which jaw relations were transferred to an instrument and how closely the instrument is capable of reproducing functional occlusion. But even though the articulator is capable of reproducing only a static centric relation, that relation at least should be reestablished before placement of the denture.

Whereas it is admitted that there are limitations to the perfection of eccentric occlusion in the mouth, some believe that it can be done with more accuracy than on an instrument that is incapable of reproducing eccentric positions. Correction for errors in centric occlusion, however, should not be included in this philosophy, for such is based on a premise that centric occlusion may be established satisfactorily by intraoral adjustment, followed then by a perfecting of eccentric occlusion. Because of denture instability and the inaccessibility of the occlusion for analysis, this is presuming more than anyone can justify. Even occlusal adjustment of natural dentition, in which each tooth has its own support, can best be done when preceded by an analysis of articulated diagnostic casts.

One cardinal premise must be accepted if prosthetic dentistry is to be anything more than a haphazard procedure. This is **that it is possible to transfer centric jaw relation to an instrument with accuracy and to maintain this relation throughout the fabrication of the prosthesis.** If this is true, then centric occlusion—coinciding either with centric jaw relation or with centric occlusion of the remaining natural teeth, or both—must have been established before initial placement of the prosthesis. This means that occlusal correction by remounting after final processing is an absolute necessity to the success of the restoration.

Remounting after processing is accomplished by returning the cast to a keyed relationship with the articulator mounting. Whereas the use of metal mounting plates attached to both surfaces may be desirable, it is not practical to do so with a partial denture cast. Stone to stone, properly keyed and free of debris, provides a sufficiently accurate surface for remounting.

Precautions to be taken in remounting. The following precautions should be taken to assure the accuracy of remounting to make final occlusal adjustment before the polishing and initial placement of the denture. These apply to all

types of occlusal relationship records but are directed particularly to remounting to an occlusal template, when stone vertical stops are used.

1. Make sure that the base of the cast has been reduced before keying and mounting are done, so that it will not have to be altered later to get it into the flask.

2. Bevel the margins of the base of the cast so that it will seat in a definite boxlike manner in the articulator mounting.

3. Notch the posterior and the anterior aspects of the base to assure further its return to its original position. Notches at the margins are preferable to depressions within the base, as the former permit a visual check of the accuracy of the remounting.

4. Lubricate lightly the base and sides of the cast before it is mounted to facilitate its easy removal from the mounting stone.

5. Tinfoil the base and sides of the cast before flasking it so that traces of investment will not be present to interfere with remounting.

6. When remounting the cast, secure it to the articulator with sticky wax or modeling plastic, followed by stone over both the mounting and the sides of the cast.

7. Before adjusting the occlusion, make certain that no traces of investment remain on the vertical stops.

8. Take care not to abrade the opposing occlusal surface during occlusal adjustment. The use of marking tape or inked ribbon is preferable to articulating paper. The artificial tooth is less likely to cut through and mar the opposing surface, and ink or dye will not build up a false opposing surface, as will the wax from articulating paper.

9. Occlusal readjustment to an occlusal template is complete when the stone vertical stops are again in contact. With other types of articulator mountings, readjustment is complete when the vertical pin is again in contact and any valid horizontal excursions are freed of interference.

Occlusal readjustment, as was the original articulation, is at the expense of the original tooth anatomy. Occlusal surfaces should be reshaped by adding grooves and spillways and by reducing the area of the occlusal table, thus improving the masticating efficiency of the artificial tooth.

Although this may be done immediately after occlusal readjustment and before initial placement of the denture, it may be deferred until final adjustment has been completed. In any event, it is a necessary step in the completion of any removable prosthesis.

Porcelain teeth may be reshaped with abrasive or diamond mounted points. Plastic teeth lend themselves better to reshaping with small burs to restore functional anatomy. Either type should be repolished judiciously to avoid reduction of cuspal contacts. Although cusps may be narrowed, spillways added, and the total area of contact reduced to improve masticating efficiency, critical areas of contact, both vertical and horizontal, must always be preserved.

The term **remounting** is also applied to the mounting of a completed prosthetic restoration back onto an instrument using some kind of interocclusal records. Discrepancies in occlusion resulting from processing of tooth-borne dentures may be corrected by reattaching the indexed processing cast and denture to the same instrument on which the occlusion was formulated. **However, because of some instability inherent in distal extension removable partial dentures, such dentures should be recovered from processing investment, finished, and polished for performing occlusal corrections by the use of new intraoral records.** A remounting cast must be made by the dentist before occlusal corrections can be accomplished. This is simply done by first placing the denture in the mouth and making an irreversible hydrocolloid (alginate) impression of the denture and remaining teeth in the arch (Fig. 17-49). When the impression is removed, the denture usually will remain in the impression or can be accurately replaced. Undercuts in the denture bases are blocked out, the retentive elements of the framework are covered with a thin layer of molten wax, and a remounting cast is poured in the impression. The remounting casts are than oriented to the articulator by the same type of interocclusal records that were used to orient the casts to formulate the occlusion. These procedures will be covered in Chapter 19 as an integral part of the initial placement appointment.

Occlusal harmony must exist before the patient is given possession of the dentures. De-

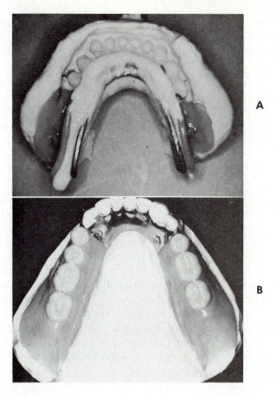

Fig. 17-49. **A,** Stock, perforated tray is used to make irreversible hydrocolloid (alginate) impression of denture and dental arch. Blockout of undercuts in denture base and of tips of direct retainers is necessary so that denture can be readily removed and replaced on resultant remounting cast, as illustrated in **B. B,** Remounting cast poured in stone. Denture can be readily removed and replaced on cast for occlusal correction procedures using articulator.

laying the correction of occlusal discrepancies until the dentures have had a chance to settle is not justifiable.

POLISHING THE DENTURE

The areas to be considered in the polishing of a partial denture are (1) the borders of the denture bases, (2) the facial surfaces, and (3) the teeth and adjacent areas.

The borders on full metal bases will have been established previously. On partial metal bases and full resin bases the accuracy with which the border may be finished will depend on the accuracy of the impression record and how well this was preserved on the stone cast. Edentulous areas recorded from impressions in stock trays generally lack the accuracy at the borders that is found on casts made from impressions in individualized trays and by secondary impression methods. Border accuracy is determined also by whether or not the impression recorded a functional or a static relationship of the bordering tissue attachments.

Denture borders. The principal objectives to be considered in making an impression of edentulous areas of a partially edentulous arch are (1) maximum support for the partial denture base and (2) extension of the borders to obtain maximum coverage compatible with moving tissues. Although this second objective may be obtained with an adequate individualized impression tray, **it is best accomplished with a secondary impression method.** Not only should the **extent** of the border be recorded accurately but also its **width.** Both extent and width as recorded should be preserved on the stone cast. With the exception of certain areas that are arbitrarily thinned in polishing (mentioned previously in this chapter), finishing and polishing the denture borders should consist only of removing any flash and artifactual blebs. Otherwise borders should be left as recorded in the impression.

When the impression is made in a stock tray, both the extent and the width of the border will have been influenced by the tray itself. Some areas will be left short of the total area available for denture support, while others will be extended beyond functional limits by the overextension of the tray. In such areas the technician must attempt to accurately interpret the anatomy of the mouth and arbitrarily trim the denture borders just short of obvious overextension. **This presumes an intimate knowledge of the anatomy of the mouth of the patient for whom the restoration is being made, which the technician does not possess.** Any overextension remaining after arbitrarily trimming the border must be corrected in the mouth. It is preferable that the dentist finish the borders of dentures, having painstakingly developed them during impression procedures.

Facial surfaces. The facial surfaces of the denture base are those polished surfaces lying between the borders and the supplied teeth. Methods have been proposed for making sectional impression records of buccal contours, thereby permitting the denture base to be made to conform to facial musculature. These have never received wide acceptance and may be considered impractical in removable partial prosthodontics.

Facial surfaces may be established in wax or may be carved into the denture base after processing. Generally it is desirable that it be done in wax as part of the wax pattern, because it is easier to do so and because contours can best be established at a time when additions can be made if desired. Buccal surfaces should be made concave to aid in the retention of the denture by border molding, to preserve the border roll and thereby prevent food impaction, and to facilitate return of the food bolus back onto the masticating table. Lingual surfaces should be made concave to provide tongue room and to aid in the retention of the denture. If such contours are established previously in wax, finishing is not only more easily accomplished but border and gingival areas are also less likely to be inadvertently altered. Polishing of concave surfaces is always more difficult than polishing flat and convex surfaces, and this can largely be avoided by taking care to contour and polish the wax pattern before investing.

Finishing gingival and interproximal areas. The contouring of gingival and interproximal areas in the cured resin is difficult and generally unsatisfactory. The practice of doing so dates back to the days when vulcanite rubber was trimmed and shaped with Pearson-type chisels, and a trimming block was a necessary piece of equipment in any dental laboratory. Finishing was done with vulcanite burs and with brush wheels and pumice, creating the vertical interproximal grooves that for many years were typical of the "denture look." Not only is this contrary to modern concepts of denture esthetics but also gingival and interpoximal carving of the denture resin around plastic teeth may not be done without some damage to the teeth themselves.

Modern cosmetic considerations demand that gingival carving be done around each tooth individually, with variations in the height of the gingival curve and in the length of the interdental papillae. Interproximally the papillae should be convex rather than concave. The gingival attachment should be free of grooves and ditches that would accumulate debris and stain and should be as free-cleansing as possible. All this precludes gross shaping and trimming of gingival areas **after** processing. Gingival carving should be done in wax, and investing should be done with care to avoid blebs and artifacts. Finishing should consist only of trimming around the teeth and the interdental papillae with small round burs to create a more natural simulation of living tissue, plus light stippling with an off-center round bur for the same reason. Polishing should consist only of light buffing with brush wheels and pumice and finally with a soft brush wheel and a nonabrasive polishing agent such as tin oxide.

Pumicing of gingival areas can only serve to polish the high spots, and although it may be done lightly, its use should be limited to light buffing of areas already made as smooth as possible by other means. Not only does heavy pumicing of the denture resin create a typical "denture look" but it also alters the surface of any plastic teeth present. If pumicing must be done, protect plastic teeth with adhesive tape during the process.

Any polishing operation on a partial denture done on a lathe is made hazardous by the presence of direct retainers, which can easily become caught in the polishing wheel. Although the least damage that might occur is the distortion of a clasp arm, there is a greater possibility that the denture may be thrown forceably into the lathe pan, with serious damage to the framework or other parts of the denture. The technician must be ever conscious of this possibility and must always cover any projecting clasp with the finger while it is near the polishing wheel. In addition, it is wise to keep a pumice pan well filled with wet pumice to cushion the shock should an accident occur. Any other lathe pan used in polishing should be lined with a towel or with a resilient material such as automobile undercoating material for the same reason.

SELF-ASSESSMENT AIDS

1. The dentist not only must be familiar with laboratory procedures but also must be proficient in executing them. True or false?
2. Although certain laboratory procedures may be delegated to a dental laboratory technician, the dentist must be able to perform those procedures in order to "troubleshoot" and guide and direct the technician. True or false?
3. An intimate knowledge of dental materials employed in the fabrication of removable partial dentures is a must for the dentist. True or false?
4. Duplicate casts are required in many instances in treating partially edentulous patients. Can you name at least three of these instances?
5. What armamentarium and materials are required to duplicate a cast?
6. What is the difference between a reversible and an irreversible hydrocolloid? Which one is most commonly used in duplicating a cast?
7. Is it critical that the duplicating material chosen be compatible with the material from which the duplicate cast will be made?
8. Can you describe a duplicating flask?
9. How is reversible hydrocolloid prepared for duplicating purposes? What temperature of the hydrocolloid is sufficient to duplicate a cast?
10. If a blocked-out master cast is being duplicated, what precautions must be exercised to avoid distortion of the blockout material?
11. Can you give a step-by-step procedure for duplicating a stone cast with reversible hydrocolloid?
12. What is the danger of soaking a stone cast in tap water? A cast must be wet before duplicating it with hydrocolloid. How is this wetting accomplished?
13. Describe the procedure for recovering an investment cast from a duplicating mold and defend your answer.
14. For what reasons should an investment cast not be trimmed on a cast trimmer?
15. An investment cast on which the pattern for the framework will be developed should be oven dried after it is removed from the duplicating material. At what temperature and for how long?
16. An investment cast should be lightly sprayed with a plastic model spray immediately after drying. Can you give three valid reasons for spraying the cast?
17. You should already know the specifications for all components of a removable partial denture framework. Can you describe a logical order of creating the wax or plastic pattern for a mandibular removable partial denture framework to which a wrought-wire retainer arm will be attached?
18. What is meant by an anatomic replica pattern and where is it used?
19. How would you go about making an anatomic replica pattern? What are its advantages over a freehand pattern?
20. Describe the process of spruing a wax pattern for a removable partial denture framework?

21. There are three general rules that should be followed in spruing any wax or plastic pattern for casting. Do you remember what they are?
22. After the pattern has been sprued, it must be covered with an investment (refractory) material to make a mold for casting. The outer investment must be the same material from which the cast was made. What are the purposes of the outer investment?
23. The casting shrinkage of gold alloys from the molten to the cold state is from _____ % to _____ %. The casting shrinkage of chromium-cobalt alloys is about _____ %.
24. A casting ring, with a suitable liner, is used to confine the outer layer of investment around the pattern. The ring is not removed during burnout or casting procedures for gold alloys. What is the purpose of the liner in the ring?
25. After the investment material for a chromium-cobalt alloy casting has set, the ring is removed before burnout. Why?
26. What are the differences in composition of a refractory material for casting gold alloys and one for casting the high-heat type of chromium-cobalt alloys?
27. Give a step-by-step procedure for investing a sprued pattern that will be cast in gold. In chromium-cobalt alloy.
28. The casting mold is prepared to receive the molten alloy by a process known as burnout. Burnout serves three purposes. Can you state the three purposes?
29. Describe a burnout procedure for casting a removable partial denture framework in Type IV gold alloy.
30. Contracture of the mold for plaster-bound refractory investments occurs beyond _____° F.
31. Most refractory investments contain calcium sulfate that begins to break down at _____° F, resulting in a weak and brittle casting.
32. What different methods are used to melt gold alloys for casting? Chromium-cobalt alloys for casting?
33. After the casting is completed, how long should the mold be allowed to bench cool before the mold and casting are plunged in water?
34. What is the purpose of "pickling" a casting? Can you describe a pickling procedure?
35. If the wax pattern for a casting was neatly and properly developed and investing and casting procedures were correctly accomplished, finishing the casting should not be a time-consuming procedure. How would you finish a gold alloy removable partial denture framework. A chromium-cobalt alloy framework?
36. Describe a hardening heat treatment for a Type IV gold alloy framework.
37. Record bases, trial denture bases, and individual impression trays are conveniently made of autopolymerizing acrylic resin. What is an autopolymerizing acrylic resin and how does it differ from a heat-cured acrylic resin?
38. Record bases or trial denture bases should be fabricated by a "sprinkling" technique using autopolymerizing acrylic resin, whereas individual or customized impression trays may be fabricated with "adapted" autopolymerizing acrylic resin. For what reason or reasons are the processes different?
39. Review the procedures for making individualized acrylic resin impression trays as given in Chapter 14.
40. If you use a secondary or altered cast impression tray for a mandibular distal extension denture, you will attach an individualized tray to the framework. Can you give a step-by-step procedure for making such a tray?
41. Record bases and occlusion rims are necessary to record maxillomandibular relations for Class I and II arches and in Class III arches with long edentulous spans. Can you describe a step-by-step procedure for making record bases by the "sprinkling" method to mount diagnostic casts?
42. A record base is attached to the framework for a distal extension mandibular denture and is fabricated after the secondary impression has been made and the master cast has been recovered. Could you make such a record base?
43. What purpose does an occlusion rim serve?
44. If an occlusion rim represents the missing teeth and supporting structures in a partially edentulous arch, should the occlusion rims be wider than the occlusal surfaces of the teeth they are replacing? Should occlusion rims not occupy the same position (buccolingually) the missing teeth occupied? There are several advantages to correctly proportioned occlusion rims as opposed to badly proportioned occlusion rims. Do you know what these advantages are?
45. Artificial posterior teeth were arranged on mandibular and maxillary trial bases (record) of acrylic resin attached to the respective frameworks. The arrangement was acceptable and approved. What procedures must now take place before the final arrangement of teeth and development of the external forms of the bases for processing?
46. Except around metal portions of the framework, should there be any difference in developing gingival contours, root indices, interdental papillae, lingual contours of individual teeth, and so on for

removable partial denture bases and complete denture bases?

47. A partial denture must be so invested for processing acrylic resin bases that the processed denture and its cast can be recovered from the flask intact and unmarred. This procedure will facilitate and simplify correction of occlusal discrepancies resulting from processing. True or false?

48. Before investing the master cast and waxed denture in the lower half of the flask, what should be done to the base of the cast to facilitate recovery of the cast and remounting procedures?

49. After the processing flask containing the invested denture has been separated and residual wax flushed out, and a tinfoil substitute correctly applied, there is one observation that must be made and dealt with in regard to the minor connector for attaching the resin base and its relation to the residual ridge. What is this observation and how is it dealt with before acrylic resin is packed in the mold?

50. Discrepancies in occlusion as a result of processing may be corrected by returning the processed denture and cast (intact) to the instrument on which the occlusion was developed—provided the dentures are tooth borne or the occlusion was developed using an occlusal template. Can you describe this type of process for correcting occlusal discrepancies?

51. Correction of occlusal discrepancies for distal extension dentures should be accomplished by an entirely different procedure than the above procedure. This procedure is described in Chapter 19.

52. Finishing and polishing the removable partial denture may be accomplished in the same manner as for a complete denture. However, polishing the removable partial denture on a lathe is made more hazardous and requires more attention because of the presence of _____.

CHAPTER

18 WORK AUTHORIZATIONS FOR REMOVABLE PARTIAL DENTURES

Work authorization
   Content
   Function
   Characteristics
Definitive instructions by work authorizations
Legal aspects of work authorizations
Delineation of responsibilities by work
     authorizations

A work authorization is a written direction for laboratory procedures to be performed in the fabrication of dental restorations. The responsibility of a dentist to the public and to the dental profession in safeguarding the quality of prosthodontic services is discharged, in part, through meaningful work authorizations. Properly executed, they provide a means for increased professional satisfaction in a removable partial denture service.

A work authorization by a dentist is similar to granting "power of attorney"; it grants authority for others to act in the dentist's behalf. It bears the same relationship to a dental laboratory technician as the sextant does to a navigator—it plots the desired course.

Work authorizations are effective channels of communication when properly executed. They enhance the quality of the completed restorations by eliminating stereotyped production, and in its place provide for individually, scientifically considered prostheses.

WORK AUTHORIZATION
Content

The information contained in a work authorization should include (1) name and address of the dental laboratory, (2) name and address of

the dentist originating the work authorization, (3) date of work authorization, (4) identification of the patient. (5) desired completion date of the request, (6) specific instructions, (7) signature of the dentist, and (8) registered license number of the dentist. All these requirements can be accommodated in a simply designed form (Fig. 18-1).

Function

The following four important functions are performed by a work authorization: (1) It furnishes definite instructions for the laboratory procedures to be accomplished and establishes the acceptable minimum of quality for the services rendered. (2) It provides a means of protecting the public from the illegal practice of dentistry. (3) It is a protective document for both the dentist and dental laboratory technician if they become participants in a lawsuit to resolve matters between them. (4) It completely delineates the responsibilities of the dentist and the dental laboratory technician.

Characteristics

A work authorization must be legible, clear, concise, and readily understood. It is unreasonable to assume that laboratory technicians are

DENTISTRY 16

WORK AUTHORIZATION – REMOVABLE PARTIAL DENTURES
University of Florida College of Dentistry

To: _____ Date: _____

From: _____

Patient Identification: _____

General Request: _____

Date and Time Required: _____

Alloy for Framework: (specific by trade name) _____

Denture Base:　( ) Acrylic Resin　　( ) Metal　　( ) Combination

　Specific by Trade Name: _____

Tooth Selection:

　Anterior:　Make _____　Mold _____　Shade _____

　Posterior:　Make _____　Mold _____　Shade _____

Specific Instructions: _____

_____

_____

_____

_____

_____

_____

_____

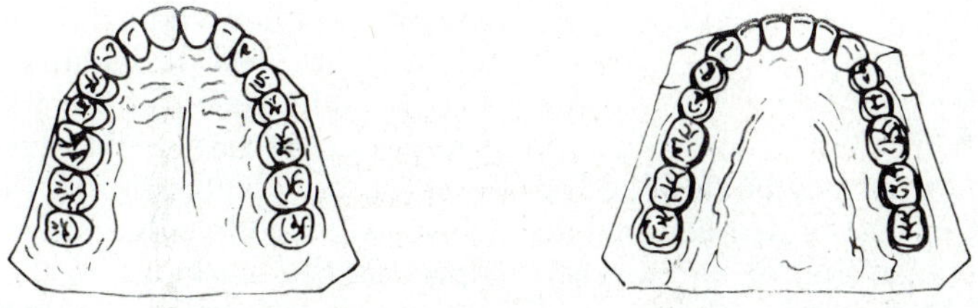

_____

COLOR CODE ON CAST: Design – Green; Survey Lines – Black; Finishing Lines – Red
PLEASE WAX TO FOLLOWING SPECIFICATIONS – TYPE ''D'' GOLD: COBALT-CHROME IN PARENTHESIS

1. Lingual Bar – 6 GA. ½ Pear (1 GA. Sheet
2. Anterior, Posterior, and Single Palatal Bars – Two 26(28) GA. Sheet
3. Linguoplate Aprons
   Cast Bases
   Full Palatal Castings } 24 GA. Sheet
4. Guiding Plane Minor Connector – 22 GA. Sheet
5. Indirect Retainer – 10 GA. ½ RD. Strip

6. Wrought Wire Components – 18 GA. RD. Type II Wire
7. Finishing Lines – 12 GA. ½ RD. Strip Inverted
8. Direct Retainers – Molars, Large Plastic Patterns; Premolars and Canines, Medium Plastic Patterns
9. Master Cast Relief for Retention Mesh – One 20 GA. Sheet
10. Base Retention Mesh – 12 GA. ½ RD. Strip
11. Borders for Cast Base – 14 GA. RD. Strip

Student Dentist's Sig. _____ Instr. Sig. & No. _____

Fig. 18-1. Work authorization form used in undergraduate clinic designed specifically for removable partial dentures to furnish detailed information to laboratory technician. It is available in tablet form so that carbon copy of work authorization can be conveniently made. Original copy is white and goes to laboratory technician. Carbon copy is yellow and is retained in files of dentist.

decoding experts. Sufficient information must be included in a work authorization to enable the technician to study and execute the request. Many dentists are overly presumptive in assuming that a request can be acceptably fulfilled without proper directions.

It is sound practice to provide the dental laboratory technician with adequate written instructions for each required laboratory service in the construction of a restoration. Therefore a new work authorization should accompany the material returned to the laboratory for continuing progress in completing the restoration. In a modern dental practice it is highly improbable that a "one trip" laboratory service is adequate to provide a truly professional removable restoration.

No single work authorization form is adequate to furnish detailed instructions for accomplishing the laboratory phases in the construction of removable partial dentures, crowns and fixed partial dentures, and complete dentures or for accomplishing orthodontic laboratory procedures. Inherent differences in the many types of restorations themselves and differences in the laboratory phases necessary for their construction establish a requirement for individual work authorization forms.

DEFINITIVE INSTRUCTIONS BY WORK AUTHORIZATIONS

Work authorization forms may be designed so that only a minimum of writing is necessary to relay thorough instructions (Fig. 18-2). The form can contain printed listings of materials and specifications that require either a **check mark** or a **fill-in** for authorizing their use.

A reminder space to designate the choice of metal for the framework is included. Frameworks for removable partial dentures are usually cast in either Type "D" gold or a chromium-cobalt alloy. The nature of the material of the denture base may be indicated by a checkmark. It is difficult to elicit this information from the markings on master casts.

Space is reserved on the work authorization form to furnish the technician with information on the dentist's selection of teeth. The responsibility for tooth selection must remain with the dentist. Success of the removable partial den-

ture partly depends on the consideration given to the size, number, and placement of the artificial teeth as well as the material from which they are made.

A display of courtesy deserved by, and a demonstration of respect for, the laboratory technician are indicated. The general request is prefaced by **please** and the specific instructions are ended with **thank you.** Do any other three words promote better relations?

A good work authorization form not only assures clarity, but it also simplifies correct execution. Figures can be provided on which diagrams may be drawn to enhance written descriptions when necessary. These diagrams may show the occlusal and lingual surfaces of the posterior teeth and the lingual surfaces of the anterior teeth. The palatal region of the maxillary arch and the lingual slopes of the mandibular alveolar ridge also can be included. These features allow a clear, diagrammatic representation of the location of major connectors, which will complement the outline of the framework on the master cast.

A color-code index can be used to explain the markings on the master cast when it is submitted to the laboratory for the fabrication of a framework. A green pencil is used to outline the framework; red designates the desired location of finishing lines on the framework; and black lines denote the height of contour on teeth and soft tissues created during the survey of the cast. The color code eliminates confusion in interpreting the markings on the master cast.

Specifications for waxing the framework components for gold or chromium-cobalt alloy castings must be furnished for the technician and are an integral part of the work authorization form. Specifications that are adequate for most removable partial denture frameworks may be listed. This feature alone saves time and effort in preparing the work authorization and **is also a handy reference for the laboratory technician.** The listing of average specifications does not preclude altering a specification when the situation requires other characteristics in a given component.

The specific instructions in a work authorization must be so constructed that they will be a constant source of direction and supervision

DENTISTRY 16

WORK AUTHORIZATION – REMOVABLE PARTIAL DENTURES
University of Florida College of Dentistry

To: *Central Laboratory UFCD*   Date: *6-11-76*

From: *John Resin   Stu. # 92*

Patient Identification: *# 406*

General Request: *Please fabricate a maxillary removable partial denture framework*

Date and Time Required: *6-18-76   10 a.m.*

Alloy for Framework: (specific by trade name) *Jelenko #7 gold*

Denture Base: ( ) Acrylic Resin   ( ) Metal   ( ) Combination

Specific by Trade Name: _____

Tooth Selection:

Anterior: Make _____   Mold _____   Shade _____

Posterior: Make _____   Mold _____   Shade _____

Specific Instructions: *Orient master cast to surveyor by tripod marks. Block out all undercuts parallel to path of placement (except retentive terminals). Provide indices to transfer design to refractory cast. Wax pattern to below specs. Cast and finish. ANATOMIC REPLICA PATTERN. Please return finished framework and blocked out master cast. Thank you.*

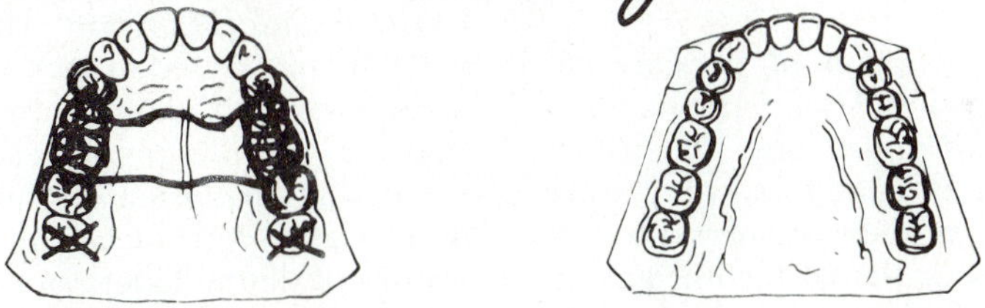

COLOR CODE ON CAST: Design – Green; Survey Lines – Black; Finishing Lines – Red
PLEASE WAX TO FOLLOWING SPECIFICATIONS – TYPE "D" GOLD: COBALT-CHROME IN PARENTHESIS

1. Lingual Bar – 6 GA. ½ Pear : 24 GA. Sheet
2. Anterior, Posterior, and Single Palatal Bars – Two 26(28) GA. Sheet
3. Linguoplate Aprons
   Cast Bases   } 24 GA. Sheet
   Full Palatal Castings }
4. Guiding Plane Minor Connector – 22 GA. Sheet
5. Indirect Retainer – 10 GA. ½ RD. Strip

6. Wrought Wire Components – 18 GA. RD. Type II Wire
7. Finishing Lines – 12 GA. ½ RD. Strip Inverted
8. Direct Retainers – Molars, Large Plastic Patterns; Premolars and Canines, Medium Plastic Patterns
9. Master Cast Relief for Retention Mesh – One 20 GA. Sheet
10. Base Retention Mesh – 12 GA. ½ RD. Strip
11. Borders for Cast Base – 14 GA. RD. Strip

Student Dentist's Sig. *John Resin #92*   Instr. Sig. & No. *A.E. Maser 116*

Fig. 18-2. This work authorization accompanies master cast on which **dentist** has designed and drawn outline for removable partial denture framework. It is simple and non-time-consuming to execute, yet furnishes detailed information so that request can be properly fulfilled.

for the laboratory phases of a removable partial denture service. Instructions should leave no doubt of the dentist's requirements in a request for laboratory services. It is foolish to use undercut dimensions of 0.25 to 0.50 mm when surveying a master cast unless directions for incorporating these dimensions in the finished framework are included.

Work authorization blanks should be available in tablet form so that a carbon duplicate can be conveniently made, supplying a copy for both the dentist and the dental laboratory technician. The original may be of a different color than is the carbon copy for ready identification.

LEGAL ASPECTS OF WORK AUTHORIZATIONS

No national statutory restrictions exist on dental laboratory operations. Regulation of dental laboratories and dental laboratory technicians is invested in the states. Fortunately all states exercise this control.

Interpretations of acts constituting the practice of dentistry are moderately uniform. However, statutory restrictions on dental laboratory operations vary widely from state to state in stringency and requirements for legal operations.

Prosecution and conviction of persons engaged in the illegal practice of dentistry is a time-consuming and difficult proceeding. This situation could be alleviated if duly executed work authorizations were required to be presented by all dental laboratories or dental technicians on demand of a duly authorized agency.

Many states require that work authorizations be made in duplicate and that both the dentist and dental laboratory technician retain a copy for a period of 2 years or more from the date of work authorization. Thus documents are available to substantiate or refute claims and counterclaims concerning the illegal practice of dentistry or to aid in the settlement of misunderstandings between a dentist and a dental laboratory technician.

DELINEATION OF RESPONSIBILITIES BY WORK AUTHORIZATIONS

The dentist is responsible for all phases of a removable partial denture service in the strict sense of the word, although the dental laboratory technician may be requested to perform certain mechanical phases of the service. **However, the laboratory technician is responsible only to the dentist and never to the patient.** A dentist who relegates the design of a removable partial denture to a less qualified individual immediately eliminates the opportunity for a preventive removable partial denture service.

A dentist who imposes on auxiliary personnel responsibilities that legally and morally belong with the dentist does a great injustice to the patients, the technicians, and the dental profession. There is little doubt that the illegal practice of dentistry and the presently existing impasse between dentist and some dental laboratory technicians are partly a result of many individual dentists imposing unrealistic responsibility on their laboratory technicians. Furthermore, this unwelcome relationship may have been caused by the submission of poor impressions, casts, records, and instructions to the laboratory technician with the demand of impossible quality in the returned restoration under threat of economic boycott.

Most dental laboratory technicians are ethical and earnestly desire to contribute their talents to the dental profession. The dental profession is vitally interested in increasing the number of serious-minded dental auxiliary personnel to share in providing oral health. However, until the dental profession elevates itself in the eyes of laboratory technicians and also elevates the stature of dental laboratory technology, greater availability of responsible auxiliary personnel is more fancied than real.

The dental laboratory technician is a member of a team whose objectives are the prevention of oral disease and the maintenance of oral health as adjuncts to the physical and mental well-being of the public. A good dental laboratory technician is a valuable asset to the dentist and contributes much to the team effort in providing oral health for patients. To paraphrase statements by G. P. Smith, the degree and quality of the team effort are the responsibility of the dentist and depend on the knowledge, experience, technical skill, administrative ability, integrity, and ability of the dentist to communicate effectively.

Much of the laboratory phase of a removable partial denture service may be delegated by a dentist. Work authorizations help to fulfill the moral obligation to supervise and direct those technical phases that can be accomplished by dental laboratory technicians.

There are substantial indications that many members of the dental profession either are not cognizant of the rewards of writing good work authorizations or are not proficient in their execution. It is not a secret that some dentists submit no instructions when availing themselves of commercial dental laboratory services.

If the practice of prosthodontics is to remain in the control of dentists, each member of the dental profession must avoid delegating responsibility to those who are less qualified to accept the responsibility.

Movements to legalize illegal dentistry (denturism) are seemingly becoming more prevalent and are being instituted by ill-advised and uninformed persons. Perhaps this current trend could have been avoided had dentists expended as much effort to communicate with technicians in the past as they are now to prevent illegal dentistry.

SELF-ASSESSMENT AIDS

1. What is a work authorization?
2. What are the national (U.S.) statutory regulations regarding work authorizations?
3. Work authorizations go by different names in various parts of the country, such as work order or work order form. What is it called in your state?
4. Do you know of any state dental practice acts that do not include a requirement for work authorizations from dentists to dental laboratory technicians?
5. Are work authorizations legal documents?
6. Properly executed work authorizations are effective channels of communication between a dentist and a dental laboratory technician. What accrues to a dentist who always furnishes the dental laboratory or dental laboratory technician a clear work authorization?
7. The contents of a properly executed work authorization will include eight categories of transmitted data. Do you know what information these eight areas include?
8. A dental work authorization performs four distinct functions. What are they?
9. If you were a dental laboratory technician, what characteristics would you like to see in a work authorization from the dentist?
10. A dentist has a responsibility to the patient and to the dental laboratory technician. A dental laboratory technician has a responsibility to the dentist, never to a patient. True or false?
11. If you, the dentist, present clear instructions and other information to a good dental laboratory technician, should you not expect to receive quality performed laboratory services? What would you expect if your instructions were vague?
12. Whose responsibility is it to select artificial teeth, denture base materials, and metal alloys for frameworks—the dentist's or the technician's?
13. Would you believe that the definitive instructions contained on a work authorization form have been reduced to "make partial" by some dentists? Believe it!
14. Do you feel that a dentist must be responsible for the physical characteristics of framework components? If so, how do you relate your requirements or specifications to the dental laboratory technician?
15. A work authorization, properly executed, will delineate responsibilities. Can you expand this statement in your own words?
16. Do you consider a dental laboratory technician a dental health team member?
17. Should you and your dental laboratory technician have some differences over work returned from the laboratory, would you "second thought" your work authorization for the returned work?
18. Why do states require that a copy of the work authorization be retained by the dentist and dental laboratory technician for certain lengths of time?
19. Do you feel that the words "please" and "thank you" have a place in writing authorizations?
20. Take a good look at the work authorization forms illustrated in this chapter. Do you have suggestions for their improvement?

19 INITIAL PLACEMENT, ADJUSTMENT, AND SERVICING OF THE REMOVABLE PARTIAL DENTURE

Occlusal interference from denture framework
Adjustments to bearing surfaces of denture
    bases
Adjustment of occlusion in harmony with
    natural and artificial dentition
Instructions to the patient
Follow-up services

Initial placement of the completed partial denture, the fifth of six essential phases of partial denture service mentioned in Chapter 2, should never be sandwiched between other scheduled appointments. In too many instances, the restoration is quickly placed and the patient dismissed with instructions to return when soreness or discomfort develops. Perhaps this is where the word **patient** originated, because of the patience required in accommodating to a new denture. Patients should not be given possession of removable restorations until denture bases have been initially adjusted as required, occlusal discrepancies have been eliminated, and patient education procedures have been continued.

Although it is true that some accommodation is a necessary part of adjusting to new dentures, many other factors are also pertinent. Among these are how well the patient has been informed as to the mechanical and biologic problems involved in the fabrication and wearing of a removable prosthetic restoration and how much confidence the patient has acquired in the excellence of the finished product through personal observation of the various steps in its construction. Knowing in advance that every step

has been carefully planned and executed with skill, and having acquired confidence both in the dentist and in the excellence of the restoration, the patient is better able to accept the adjustment period as a necessary, but transient, step in learning to wear the prosthesis. Much of this confidence can be dissipated if the dentist places the prosthesis with an air of finality as though to imply that "my part in the fabrication of this restoration is now completed. The rest is up to you, including payment of the fee on your way out of the office."

The term **adjustment** has two connotations, each of which must be considered separately. First are the adjustments to the bearing surfaces of the denture and the occlusion made by the dentist at the time of initial placement and thereafter. Second is the adjustment or accommodation by the patient, psychologically and biologically, to the presence of a foreign body, which is to serve as a prosthetic restoration of some missing part or parts of the body, in this particular instance, an oral prosthesis.

After processing resin bases the occluding teeth must be altered to perfect the occlusal relationship between opposing artificial dentition or between artificial dentition and an opposing cast or template. Denture bases then must be finished to eliminate excess and to perfect the contours of polished surfaces for the best functional and esthetic result. All these are machining operations made necessary by the inadequacies of casting procedures, for actually both the metal and resin parts of a prosthetic restoration are produced by casting methods. Unfortunately such machining operations in the laboratory rarely eliminate the need for final adjustment in the mouth, which is also, in effect, a machining process to perfect the fit of the restoration to the oral tissues.

Included in this final step in a long sequence of machining procedures necessary to produce a biologically acceptable prosthetic restoration are the adjustment of the occlusion to accommodate the occlusal rests and other metal parts of the denture, the adjustment of the bearing surfaces of the denture bases in harmony with the supporting soft tissues, and the final adjustment of occlusion on the artificial dentition to harmonize with natural occlusion in all mandibular positions.

OCCLUSAL INTERFERENCE FROM DENTURE FRAMEWORK

Any occlusal interference from occlusal rests and other parts of the denture framework should have been eliminated before or during the establishment of occlusal relations. Assuming that the denture framework will have been tried in the mouth before a final jaw relation is established, any such interference should have been detected and eliminated. **Much of this need not exist at all if mouth preparations and the design of the denture framework are carried out with a specific treatment plan in mind.** In any event, occlusal interference from the framework itself should not ordinarily require further adjustment at the time the finished denture is initially placed. **For the dentist to have sent an impression or casts of the patient's mouth to the laboratory and to receive a finished partial denture prosthesis without having once tried the cast framework in the mouth is not only a dereliction of his responsibility to the patient but is also, in effect, handing the practice of prosthetic dentistry over to the dental laboratory technician.** However, when such is done, it is obvious

that occlusal interference from the casting itself must be detected and eliminated before proceeding with other adjustments to the denture.

ADJUSTMENTS TO BEARING SURFACES OF DENTURE BASES

The machining of bearing surfaces to perfect the fit of the denture to the supporting tissues should be accomplished by the use of some indicator paste (Fig. 19-1). The paste must be one that will be readily displaced by positive tissue contact and will not adhere to the tissues of the mouth. Several pressure indicator pastes are commercially available. However, an acceptable paste can be made by combining equal parts of a vegetable shortening (Crisco) and zinc oxide. The components must be thoroughly spatulated to a homogenous mixture. A quantity sufficient to fill several small ointment jars may be mixed at one time.

Rather than dismiss the patient with instructions to return when soreness develops and then overrelieve the denture over a traumatized area to restore patient comfort, the use of pressure indicator paste should be routine with any tissue-bearing prosthetic restoration. The paste should be applied in a thin layer over the bearing surfaces and then both occlusal and digital pressure should be applied to the denture. The patient cannot be expected to apply a heavy enough force to the new denture to register all of the pressure areas present. Therefore the dentist should apply both vertical and horizontal forces with the fingers in excess of that which might be expected of the patient. The denture is then removed and inspected. Any areas heavy enough to displace a thin film of indicator paste should be relieved and the procedure repeated with a new film of indicator until excessive pressure areas have been eliminated. However, an area of the denture base showing through the film of indicator paste may be erroneously interpreted as a pressure spot, when actually the paste had adhered to the tissues in that area. Therefore only those areas showing through an intact film of indicator paste should be interpreted as pressure areas and relieved accordingly.

Pressure areas most frequently encountered are as follows: **in the mandibular arch**—(1) the

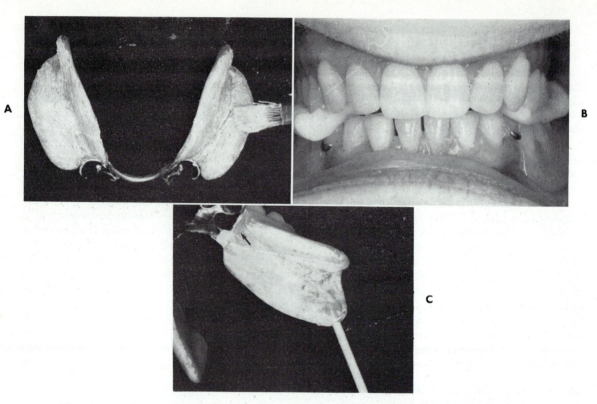

Fig. 19-1. A, Tissue side of finished bases should be carefully inspected, and surface blebs or sharp projections should be eliminated when found. Entire tissue surfaces of bases should be coated with **thin** coat of pressure indicator paste using stiff-bristle brush (glue brush) after the bases have been dried; Brush marks should be evident and should run anteroposteriorly. Thick application of indicator paste will probably give false information regardless of the accuracy of denture base. **B,** Denture should be dipped in cold water before placement in patient's mouth to prevent paste from sticking to oral tissues. After careful seating of denture, patient should close firmly on cotton rolls for few seconds. **C,** Denture is removed and paste is interpreted for pressure spots. Note that brush marks have been eliminated, which indicates that base is contacting tissues of basal seats throughout. Black arrow points to potential pressure spot, since paste has been eliminated from the area. Swab stick points to area where paste was eliminated in placing and removing the denture. This particular area is difficult to evaluate and should not be relieved unless soreness appears. However, area adjacent to abutment should be sparingly relieved. Several placements of denture are usually necessary to evaluate accuracy of bases.

lingual slope of the mandibular ridge in the premolar area, (2) the mylohyoid ridge, (3) the border extension into the retromylohyoid space, and (4) the distobuccal border in the vicinity of the ascending ramus and the external oblique ridge; and **in the maxillary arch**—(1) the inside of the buccal flange of the denture over the tuberosities, (2) the border of the denture lying at the malar prominence, and (3) at the pterygomaxillary notch where the denture may impinge on the pterygomandibular raphe or the pterygoid hamulus itself. In addition, in either arch there may be bony spicules or spicules in the denture base itself that will require specific relief.

The amount of relief by machining that will

be necessary will depend on the accuracy of the impression registration, the master cast, and the denture base. Despite the accuracy of modern impression and cast materials, many denture base materials leave much to be desired in this regard, and the element of technical errors is also always present. It is therefore essential that discrepancies in the denture base be detected and corrected before the tissues of the mouth are subjected to the stress of supporting a prosthetic restoration. This is one of our major responsibilities to the patient, that trauma be always held to a minimum. **Therefore the appointment time for the initial placement of the denture must be adequate to permit such adjustment.**

ADJUSTMENT OF OCCLUSION IN HARMONY WITH NATURAL AND ARTIFICIAL DENTITION

The final step in the adjustment of the partial denture at the time of initial placement is the adjustment of the occlusion to harmonize with the natural occlusion in all mandibular excursions. When opposing partial dentures are placed concurrently, the adjustment of the occlusion will parallel, to some extent, the adjustment of occlusion on complete dentures. This is particularly true when the few remaining natural teeth are out of occlusion. But where **one or more** natural teeth may occlude in any mandibular position, those teeth will influence mandibular movement to some extent. It is necessary therefore that the artificial dentition on the partial denture be made to harmonize with whatever natural occlusion remains.

Occlusal adjustment of tooth-borne removable partial dentures may be performed accurately by any of several intraoral methods. **It has been our experience, however, that occlusal adjustment of distal extension removable partial dentures is accomplished more conveniently and accurately by using an articulator than by any intraoral method.** Since distal extension denture bases will exhibit some movement under a closing force, intraoral indications of occlusal discrepancies, whether by inked ribbon or disclosing waxes, are difficult to interpret. Distal extension dentures, positioned on remounting casts, can conveniently be re-

lated to the articulator with new, nonpressure interocclusal records, and the occlusion can be adjusted accurately at the appointment for initial placement of the dentures (Fig. 19-2).

The methods by which occlusal relations may be established and recorded have been discussed in Chapter 16. In this chapter the advantages of establishing a functional occlusal relationship with an intact opposing arch have been discussed and also the limitations that exist to perfecting harmonious occlusion on the finished prosthesis by intraoral adjustment alone. Even when the occlusion on two opposing partial dentures is being adjusted entirely in the mouth, it is best that one arch be considered an intact arch and the other one adjusted to it. This is accomplished by first eliminating any occlusal interference to mandibular movement imposed by one denture and adjusting any opposing natural dentition to accommodate the prosthetically supplied teeth. Then the opposing partial denture is placed, and occlusal adjustments are made to harmonize with both the natural dentition and the opposing denture, which is now considered part of an intact dental arch. Which denture is adjusted first and which one is made to occlude with it is somewhat arbitrary, with the following exceptions: If one partial denture is entirely tooth supported and the other has a tissue-supported base, the tooth-supported denture is adjusted to final occlusion with any opposing natural teeth and then that arch is treated as an intact arch and the opposing denture adjusted to occlude with it. If both partial dentures are entirely tooth borne, the one occluding with the most natural teeth is adjusted first and the second denture then adjusted to occlude with an intact arch. Tooth-borne segments of a composite (tooth- and tissue-supported) partial denture are likewise adjusted first to harmonize with any opposing natural dentition. The final adjustment of occlusion on opposing tissue-supported bases is usually done on the mandibular denture, since this is the moving member, and the occlusion is made to harmonize with the maxillary denture, which is treated as part of an intact arch.

Intraoral occlusal adjustment is accomplished by using some kind of indicator and suitable mounted points and burs. Diamond or other

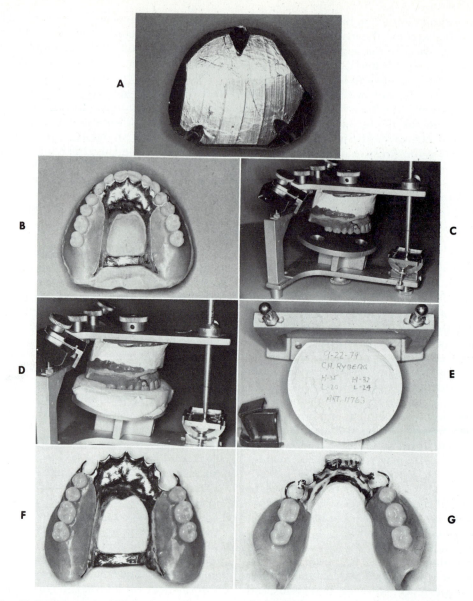

Fig. 19-2. Sequence of laboratory and clinical procedures for correction of occlusal discrepancies as a result of processing restorations. **A,** Maxillary master cast has been removed from indexed mounting on articulator, and base of cast has been covered with tinfoil before investing procedure. **B,** Processed maxillary restoration and master cast is recovered intact from investing medium. **C,** Restoration and indexed cast is attached to original mounting with sticky wax. Remounting jig is attached to lower member of articulator. **D,** Patty of quick-setting stone is placed on remount jig just thick enough to record occlusal and incisal surfaces when articulator is closed. Original face-bow record is thus preserved. **E,** Face-bow record is trimmed and identified with patient's name, articulator number, horizontal and lateral condylar adjustments, and date. **F** and **G,** Maxillary and mandibular restorations are recovered, finished, and polished.

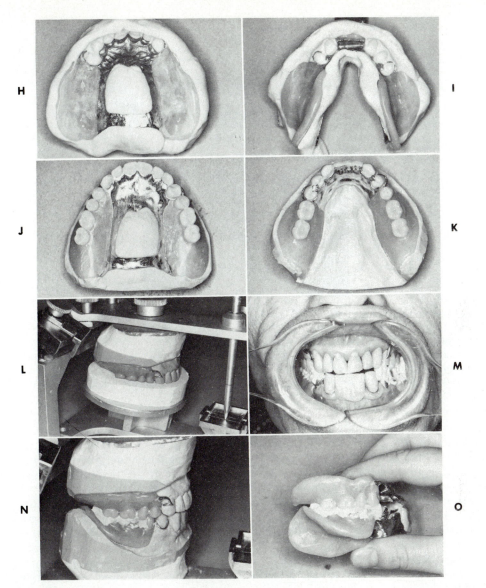

Fig. 19-2, cont'd. H and **I,** After restorations are tried in and adjusted to basal seats, impression is made of placed restorations using perforated stock tray and irreversible hydrocolloid. **J** and **K,** Casts are poured in impressions after undercuts in denture bases are blocked out with wet facial tissue. Dentures are readily removed and replaced on mounting casts. **L,** Maxillary denture and remounting cast is placed in face-bow record on mounting jig, and maxillary cast is attached to upper arm of articulator with stone. **M,** Centric relation is recorded as near vertical dimension of occlusion as possible, avoiding contact of opposing teeth. Recording medium is fast-setting impression plaster. **N,** Mandibular restoration and remounting cast are attached to lower member of articulator with stone using just made centric relation record. **O,** Another intraoral recording of centric relation is made.   *Continued.*

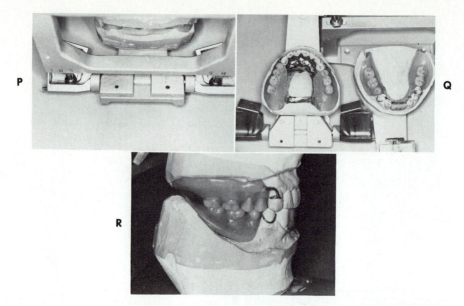

Fig. 19-2, cont'd. P, Restorations and attached record are returned to articulator. If condylar elements are snug against condylar housings, it can be safely assumed that centric relation has been recorded and that casts have been accurately mounted to this maxillomandibular relationship. **Q,** Occlusion may now be harmonized as laboratory procedure on articulator. Original condylar settings may be used since original face-bow transfer record was duplicated. **R,** Patient is not given possession of restorations until occlusion has been refined and occlusal harmony is obtained.

abrasive points must be used to reduce enamel and metal contacts. These also may be used to reduce plastic tooth surfaces, but burs may be used for plastic with greater effectiveness. Articulation paper may be used as an indicator if one recognizes that heavy interocclusal contacts may become perforated, leaving only a light mark, while secondary contacts, being lighter and frequently sliding, may make a heavier mark. Although articulation ribbon does not become perforated, it is not easy to use in the mouth, and the differentiation between primary and secondary contacts is difficult to ascertain.

In general, occlusal adjustment of multiple contacts between natural and artificial dentition when tooth-borne partial dentures are involved follows the same principles as those for natural dentition alone. This is because the partial dentures are retained by devices attached to the abutment teeth, whereas with complete dentures no mechanical retainers are present. The use of more than one color of articulation paper

or ribbon to record and differentiate between centric and eccentric contacts is just as helpful in adjusting partial denture occlusion as natural occlusion, and for the initial adjustment this method may be used.

For final adjustment, however, since one denture will be adjusted to occlude with an intact arch, the use of an occlusal wax may be necessary to establish points of excessive contact and interference. This cannot be done by articulation paper alone. An occlusal wax, such as Kerr occlusal indicator, which is adhesive on one side, or strips of 28-gauge Kerr green casting wax or other similar soft wax, may be used. It should always be used bilaterally, with two strips folded together at the midline. Thus the patient is not as likely to deviate to one side as when wax is introduced unilaterally (Fig. 19-3).

For centric contacts the patient is guided to tap into the wax and then the wax is removed and inspected under transillumination for perforations. All perforated areas are either pre-

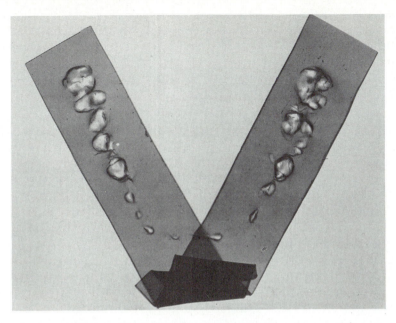

Fig. 19-3. Two strips of 28-gauge soft green (casting) wax are placed in mouth between opposing dentition. These are first folded over anteriorly to unite two halves, and patient is guided to tap in centric occlusion two or three times. Viewed out of mouth, against source of light, uniform contacts free of perforations may be considered to be simultaneous contacts. Perforations in wax represent occlusal prematurities that should be relieved. Accuracy of this method or any other intraoral method depends not only on dentist's interpretation of marks (perforations) but also on stability of denture bases.

mature contacts or excessive contacts and must be adjusted. One of two methods may be used to locate specific areas to be relieved. Articulation ribbon may be used to mark the occlusion, and then those marks representing areas of excessive contact are identified by referring to the wax record and are relieved accordingly. A second method is to introduce the wax strips a second time, this time adapting them to the buccal and lingual surfaces for retention. After having the patient tap into the wax, perforated areas are marked with waterproof pencil. The wax is then stripped off and the penciled areas are relieved.

Whichever method is used, it must be repeated until occlusal balance in centric occlusion has been established and more uniform contacts without perforations are evident from a final interocclusal wax record. After adjustment in centric occlusion has been completed, any remaining areas of interference are then reduced, thus

assuring that there is no interference during the chewing stroke. Adjustments to relieve interference during the chewing stroke should be confined to buccal surfaces of mandibular teeth and lingual surfaces of maxillary teeth. This serves to narrow the cusps so that they will go all the way into the opposing sulci without wedging as they travel into centric contact. Skinner proposed giving a small bite of soft banana to chew rather than to expect the patient to chew without food actually being present. The small bolus of banana promotes normal functional activity of the chewing mechanism, yet by its soft consistency does not itself cause indentations in the soft wax. Any interfering contacts encountered during the chewing stroke are thus detected as perforations in the wax, which are marked with pencil and relieved accordingly.

Adjustments to occlusion should be repeated at a reasonable interval after the dentures have reached a point of equilibrium and the musculature has become adjusted to the changes brought about by restoration of occlusal contacts. This second occlusal adjustment usually may be considered sufficient until such time as tissue-supported denture bases no longer support the occlusion and corrective measures, either reoccluding the teeth or relining the denture, must be employed. **However, a periodic recheck of occlusion at intervals of 6 months is advisable to avoid traumatic interference resulting from changes in denture support or tooth migration.**

After the adjustment of occlusion the anatomy of the artificial teeth should be restored to maximum efficiency by restoring grooves and spillways (food escapeways) and by narrowing the teeth buccolingually to increase the sharpness of the cusps and reduce the width of the food table. Mandibular buccal and maxillary lingual surfaces in particular should be narrowed to assure that these areas will not interfere with closure into the opposing sulci. Since artificial teeth used on partial dentures opposing natural or restored dentition should always be considered **material** out of which a harmonious occlusal surface is created, final adjustment of the occlusion always should be followed by the meticulous restoration of the most functional occlusal anatomy possible. Although this may be done after a subsequent occlusal adjustment at a later date, the possibility that the patient may fail to return on schedule is always present, and in the meantime, broad and inefficient occlusal surfaces may cause an overloading of the supporting structures, which would be traumatogenic. Therefore the restoration of an efficient occlusal anatomy is an essential part of the denture adjustment at the time of placement. Again, this requires that sufficient time be allotted for the initial placement of the partial denture to permit all necessary occlusal corrections to be accomplished.

INSTRUCTIONS TO THE PATIENT

Finally, before the patient is dismissed, the difficulties that may be encountered and the care that must be given the prosthesis and the abutment teeth must be reviewed with the patient.

The patient should be advised that some discomfort or minor annoyance may be experienced initially. Whereas this is to some extent caused by the presence of bulk, which the tongue in particular must become accustomed to, any foreign object, however comfortable, must be accepted biologically and psychologically before it can become an integral part of the oral mechanism.

The patient must be advised of the possibility of soreness developing despite every attempt on the part of the dentist to prevent its occurrence. Since patients vary widely in their ability to tolerate discomfort, it is perhaps best to advise every patient as though soreness is inevitable, with every assurance that any needed adjustments will be made. On the other hand, the dentist should be aware of the fact that some patients are unable to accommodate the presence of a removable prosthesis. Fortunately these are few in any practice. However, the dentist must avoid any positive statements that might be interpreted or construed by the patient to be positive assurance tantamount to a guarantee that the patient will be able to use the prosthesis with comfort and acceptance. Too much depends on the patient's ability to accept a foreign object and to tolerate reasonable pressures to make such assurance possible.

Discussing phonetics with the patient in regard to the new dentures may indicate that this is a unique problem to be overcome because of the influence of the prosthesis on speech. With few exceptions, which usually result from excessive and avoidable bulk in the denture design or improper placement of teeth and the contour of denture bases, the average patient will experience little difficulty in wearing the partial denture. Most of the hindrances to normal speech will disappear in a few days.

Similarly, perhaps little or nothing should be said to the patient about the possibility of gagging or the tongue's reaction to a foreign object. Most patients will experience little or no difficulty in this regard, and the tongue will normally accept smooth, nonbulky contours without objection. Contours that are too thick, too bulky, or improperly placed should be avoided in the construction of the denture, but if present, these should be detected and eliminated at the time of placement of the denture. The dentist should palpate the prosthesis in the mouth and reduce excessive bulk accordingly before the patient has an opportunity to object to it. The area most frequently needing thinning is the distolingual flange of the mandibular denture. Here the denture flange should almost always be thinned during the finishing and polishing of the denture base. Sublingually the denture flange should be reproduced as recorded in the impression, but distal to the second molar the flange should be trimmed somewhat thinner. Then, on placing the denture, the dentist should palpate this area to ascertain that a minimum of bulk exists that might be encountered by the side and base of the tongue. If this needs further reduction, it should be done and the denture repolished before dismissing the patient.

The patient should be advised of the need for keeping the dentures and the abutment teeth meticulously clean. If cariogenic processes are to be prevented, the accumulation of debris should be avoided as much as possible, particularly around abutment teeth and beneath minor connectors. Furthermore, inflammation of gingival tissues is prevented by removing accumulated debris and by substituting toothbrush massage for the normal stimulation of tongue and food contact with areas that will be covered by the denture framework.

The mouth and partial denture should be cleaned after eating and before retiring. Brushing before breakfast also may be effective in reducing the bacterial count, which may help to lessen acid formation in the caries-susceptible individual after eating. A partial denture may be effectively cleaned by using a small, stiff-bristle brush. Debris may be effectively removed through the use of dentifrices, since they contain the essential elements for cleaning. Household cleaners should not be used because they are too abrasive for use on resin surfaces. The patient, and the elderly or the handicapped patient in particular, should be advised to clean the denture over a basin partially filled with water so that the fall will be broken if the denture is dropped accidentally during cleaning.

In addition to brushing with a dentifrice, additional cleaning may be accomplished by using a proprietary denture cleaning solution. The patient should be advised to soak the dentures in the solution for 15 minutes once daily, followed by a thorough brushing with a dentifrice. Al-

though hypochlorite solutions are effective denture cleansers, they have a tendency to tarnish chromium-cobalt frameworks and should be avoided.

In some mouths the precipitation of salivary calculus on the partial denture necessitates taking extra measures for its removal. Thorough daily brushing of the denture will avoid deposits of calculus for many patients. However, any buildup of calculus noted by the patient between scheduled recall appointments should be removed in the dental office. This can be quickly and readily accomplished by using an ultrasonic cleaner.

Since many patients will dine away from home, the informed patient should provide some means of carrying out midday oral hygiene. Simply rinsing the partial denture and the mouth with water after eating is beneficial if brushing is not possible.

Opinion is divided on the question of whether or not a partial denture should be worn during sleep. Conditions should determine the advice given the patient, **although generally the tissues should be allowed to rest by removing the denture at night.** The denture should be placed in a container and covered with water to prevent its dehydration, with subsequent dimensional change. About the only situation that possibly justifies wearing partial dentures at night is when stresses generated by bruxism would be more destructive, since they then would be concentrated on fewer teeth. Broader distribution of the stress load, plus the splinting effect of the partial denture, may make wearing the denture at night advisable. However, an individual latex rubber mouth protector should be worn at night until the cause of the bruxism is eliminated.

Frequently the question arises of whether an opposing complete denture should be worn when a partial denture in the other arch is out of the mouth. The answer is that if the partial denture is to be removed at night, the opposing complete denture should not be left in the mouth. **There is no more certain way of destroying the alveolar ridge, which supports a maxillary complete denture, than to have it occlude with a few remaining anterior mandibular teeth.**

The partial denture patient should not be dismissed as completed without at least one subsequent appointment for evaluation of the response of oral structures to the restorations and minor adjustment if needed. This should be made at an interval of 24 hours after initial placement of the denture. It need not be a lengthy appointment but should be made as a definite rather than a drop-in appointment. Not only does this give the patient assurance that any necessary adjustments will be made and provide the dentist with an opportunity to check on the patient's acceptance of the prosthesis, but it also avoids giving the patient any idea that the dentist's schedule may be interrupted at will and serves to give notice that an appointment is necessary for future adjustments.

FOLLOW-UP SERVICES

The sixth and final phase of removable partial denture service (periodic recall) and its rationale must be understood by the patient. Patients will probably experience only limited success with the treatment and restorations so meticulously accomplished by the dentist unless they return for periodic oral evaluations.

After all necessary adjustments to the partial denture have been made and the patient has been advised as to the proper care of the denture, he must also be advised as to the future care of the mouth to ensure health and longevity of the remaining structures. How often the mouth and denture should be examined by the dentist depends on the oral and physical condition of the patient. Patients who are caries susceptible or who have tendencies toward periodontal disease or alveolar atrophy should be examined more frequently. Every 6 months should be the rule if conditions are normal.

The need for increasing retention on clasp arms to make the denture more secure will depend on the type of clasp that has been used. **Increasing retention should be accomplished by contouring the clasp arm to engage a deeper part of the retentive undercut rather than by forcing the clasp in toward the tooth.** The latter creates only frictional retention, which violates the principle of clasp retention. Being an active force, such retention contributes to tooth or res-

toration movement or both in a horizontal direction, disappearing only when either the tooth has been moved or the clasp arm returns to a **passive** relationship with the abutment tooth. Unfortunately this is almost the only adjustment that can be made to a half-round cast clasp arm. On the other hand, the round wrought-wire clasp arm may be adjusted cervically and brought into a deeper part of the retentive undercut. Thus the passivity of the clasp arm in its terminal position is maintained, but retention is increased by its being forced to flex more to withdraw from the deeper undercut. The patient should be advised that the abutment tooth and the clasp will serve longer if the retention is held to a minimum, which is only that amount necessary to resist reasonable dislodging forces.

Development of denture rocking or looseness in the future may be the result of a change in the form of the supporting ridges rather than lack of retention. This should be detected as early as possible after it occurs and corrected by relining or rebasing. The loss of tissue support is usually so gradual that the patient may be unable to detect the need for relining. This usually must be determined by the dentist at subsequent examinations as evidenced by rotation of the distal extension denture about the fulcrum line. If the partial denture is opposed by natural dentition, the loss of base support causes a loss of occlusal contact, which may be detected by having the patient close on wax strips placed bilaterally. If, however, a complete denture or distal extension partial denture opposes the partial denture, the interocclusal wax test is not dependable, since occlusal contact may have been maintained by posterior closure, changes in the temporomandibular joint, or migration of the opposing denture. In such case, evidence of loss of ridge support is determined solely by the indirect retainer leaving its seat as the distal extension denture rotates about the fulcrum line.

No assurance can be given to the patient that uncrowned abutment teeth will not decay at some future time. Even with full cast crowns there can be no positive assurance that the tooth will not ever decay gingival to the crown, as a result of gingival recession and caries attack of exposed cementum. The patient can be assured, however, that prophylactic measures in the form of meticulous oral hygiene, coupled with routine care by the dentist, will be rewarded by greater health and longevity of the remaining teeth.

The patient should be advised that maximum service may be expected from the partial denture if the following rules are observed:

1. Avoid careless handling of the denture, which may lead to distortion or breakage. Damage to the partial denture occurs while it is out of the mouth, as a result of dropping it during cleaning or an accident occurring when the denture is not being worn. Fractured teeth and denture bases can be repaired, as can broken clasp arms, but a distorted framework can rarely, if ever, be satisfactorily readapted or repaired.

2. Teeth should be protected from caries by proper oral hygiene, proper diet, and frequent dental care. The teeth will be no less susceptible to caries when a partial denture is being worn but may be more so because of the retention of debris. At the same time, the remaining teeth have become all the more important as a result of oral rehabilitation, and abutment teeth have become even more valuable because of their importance to the success of the partial denture. Therefore the need for a rigid regimen of **oral hygiene, diet control,** and **periodic clinical observation and treatment** is essential to the future health of the entire mouth. **Also the patient must be more conscientious about returning periodically for examination and necessary treatment at intervals stated by the dentist.**

3. Periodontal damage to the abutment teeth can be avoided by maintaining tissue support of any distal extension bases. As a result of periodic examination this can be detected and corrected by relining or whatever procedure is indicated.

4. Partial denture treatment must be accepted as something that cannot be considered permanent but must receive regular and continuous care by both the patient and the dentist. The obligations for maintaining caries control and for returning at stated intervals for treatment must be clearly understood, as well as the fact that regular charges will be made by the dentist for whatever treatment is rendered.

SELF-ASSESSMENT AIDS

1. The term **adjustment** has two connotations in relation to removable partial dentures. Do you know these two connotations?
2. At what stage of treatment should any occlusal interference by a framework have been corrected?
3. What is meant by adjustments to the bearing surfaces of denture bases?
4. How do you detect areas of the denture base that may contribute to soreness if not relieved?
5. What is a pressure indicator paste? Can you give a detailed procedure for using a pressure indicator paste? How do you interpret prospective pressure spots when using a pressure indicator paste?
6. Can you interpret overextension or underextension of borders of the denture base with the use of a pressure indicator paste?
7. Can the pterygomandibular raphe be impinged by the borders of either maxillary or mandibular distal extension bases?
8. Some occlusal discrepancies are bound to occur in dentures as a result of the processing of acrylic resin. True or false?
9. The dentist must correct any and all occlusal discrepancies as completely as possible before the patient is given possession of the restorations. True or false?
10. You are initially placing a tooth-borne removable partial denture. How do you correct occlusal discrepancies and assure yourself that occlusal harmony exists?
11. What is the danger in trying to correct occlusal discrepancies of distal extension dentures by an intraoral technique?
12. What is a remount cast? How is it made?
13. Can you give a detailed procedure for correction of occlusal discrepancies by remounting distal extension removable partial dentures on an articulator?
14. What are the several advantages in using an articulator to correct occlusal discrepancies?
15. After correction of occlusal discrepancies, should the occlusal anatomy of prosthetically supplied teeth be restored by ensuring that adequate grooves and spillways are present? How do you determine where and where not to recontour?
16. By what procedures do you restore the "glaze" on occlusal surfaces of vacuum-fired porcelain artificial teeth attached to an acrylic resin denture base?
17. An informed patient will adjust to new restorations better than an uninformed patient. At what

phase of treatment should patient education begin?

18. What instructions do you review with the patient before ending the initial placement appointment?

19. Why should an appointment be made for 24 hours after the initial placement of restorations?

20. Does your responsibility in the treatment of a patient end after the 24-hour evaluation appointment?

21. How do you feel about providing the patient with printed suggestions relative to the care and use of restorations before the initial placement appointment?

22. What length of time should you schedule for the initial placement of distal extension removable partial dentures?

23. How would you safely adjust the following types of clasp arms to make them more retentive and to make them remain passive? A cast circumferential clasp; a combination clasp.

20 RELINING AND REBASING THE REMOVABLE PARTIAL DENTURE

Relining tooth-borne denture bases
Relining distal extension denture bases
Methods of reestablishing occlusion on a
  relined partial denture

Differentiation between relining and rebasing has been discussed previously in Chapter 1. Briefly, **relining** is the resurfacing of a denture base with new material to make it fit the underlying tissues more accurately, whereas **rebasing** is the replacement of a denture base with new material without changing the occlusal relations of the teeth. Relining removable restorations is a frequent occurrence in many dental practices; however, rebasing is seldom performed, comparatively speaking.

In either case a new impression registration is necessary, using the existing denture base as an impression tray for either a closed-mouth* or an open-mouth impression procedure. One of several types of impression materials may be used. The impression may be made with a metallic oxide impression paste, with one of the rubber-base or silicone impression materials, with an activated resin used as an impression material, or with a mouth-temperature wax.

In making the decision between a closed-mouth and an open-mouth impression method for relining, one must first consider the reasons for doing so and the objectives to be obtained. Again, it is necessary to differentiate between

the two basic types of partial dentures, one being the all–tooth-borne restoration and the other being the tooth- and tissue-supported restoration.

Before relining or rebasing is undertaken, the oral tissues should be returned to a state of health. For more information refer to the Chapter 15 discussion about conditioning abused and irritated tissues.

RELINING TOOTH-BORNE DENTURE BASES

When total abutment support is available, but for one reason or another a removable partial denture has been the restoration of choice, support for that restoration is derived entirely from the abutment teeth at each end of each edentulous span. This support may be effective through the use of occlusal rests, boxlike internal rests, internal attachments, or supporting ledges on abutment restorations. Except for intrusion of abutment teeth under functional stress, settling of the restoration toward the tissues of the residual ridge is prevented by the supporting abutments. Tissue changes occurring beneath tooth-borne denture bases do not affect the support of the denture, and therefore relining or rebasing is usually done for other reasons including the following: (1) unhygienic conditions and the trapping of debris between the denture and the residual ridge, (2) an unsightly condition

---

*"An impression made while the mouth is closed and with the patient's muscular activity molding the borders." From Zwemer, T.J., editor: Boucher's clinical dental terminology, ed. 3, St. Louis, 1982, The C.V. Mosby Co.

resulting from the space that has developed, or (3) patient discomfort associated with lack of tissue contact arising from open spaces between the denture base and the tissues. Anteriorly, some loss of support beneath a denture base may lead to some denture movement, despite occlusal support and direct retainers located posteriorly. Rebasing might be the treatment of choice if the artificial teeth are to be replaced or rearranged or if the denture base needs to be replaced for esthetic reasons or because it has become defective.

For either relining or rebasing to be accomplished, the original denture base must have been made of a resin material that can be relined or replaced. Frequently tooth-borne partial denture bases are made of metal as part of the cast framework. These cannot be satisfactorily relined, although they may sometimes be altered by drastic grinding to provide mechanical retention for the attachment of an entirely new resin base. Ordinarily a metal base, with its several advantages, is not used in a tooth-borne area in which early tissue changes are anticipated. A metal base should not be used after recent extractions or other surgery, nor for a long span when relining to provide secondary tissue support may become necessary. (A distal extension metal base is ordinarily used only when a partial denture is being made over tissues that have become conditioned to supporting a previous denture base.)

Since the tooth-borne denture base cannot be depressed beyond its terminal position with the occlusal rests seated and the teeth in occlusion and since it cannot rotate about a fulcrum, a closed-mouth impression method is used. Virtually any impression material may be used, provided sufficient space is allowed beneath the denture base to permit the excess material to flow to the borders, at which it is either turned by the bordering tissues or, as in the palate, is allowed to escape through holes without unduly displacing the underlying tissues. The qualities of each type of impression material must be kept in mind when one is selecting the material to be used for this purpose. Ordinarily an impression material is used that will record the anatomic form of the oral tissues.

A word should be said in favor of relining a tooth-borne resin base with autopolymerizing acrylic resin as an intraoral procedure. When one or more relatively short spans are to be relined, the making of an impression for that purpose requires that the denture be flasked and processed. The possibility that the vertical dimension of occlusion may be increased and that the denture may be distorted during laboratory procedures must be weighed against the disadvantages of using a direct reline material. Fortunately these materials are constantly being improved with greater predictability and color stability. The possibility that the original denture base will become crazed or distorted by the action of the activated monomer is minimal when the base is made of modern cross-linked resin. However, for this reason, earlier resin bases should not be subjected to relining with direct reline resins.

When relining in the mouth with a resin reline material is done with a definite technique, the results can be quite satisfactory, with complete bonding to the existing denture base, with good color stability, and with permanence and accuracy. The procedure for applying a direct reline of an existing resin base is as follows:

1. Relieve generously the tissue side of the denture base and just over the borders. This not only provides space for an adequate thickness of new material but also eliminates the possibility of tissue impingement because of confinement of the material.

2. Apply masking or adhesive tape over the polished surfaces from the relieved border to the occlusal surfaces of the teeth.

3. Mix the powder and liquid in a glass jar according to the proportions recommended by the manufacturer.

4. While the material is reaching the desired consistency, have the patient rinse the mouth with cold water. At the same time, wipe the fresh surfaces of the dried denture base with a cotton pellet saturated with some of the monomer. This facilitates bonding and makes sure that the surface is free of any contamination.

5. When the material has first begun to take on some body, but while it is still quite fluid, apply it to the tissue side of the denture base

and over the borders. Immediately place the denture in the mouth in its terminal position and have the patient close into occlusion. Then, with the patient's mouth open, manipulate the cheeks to turn the excess at the border and establish harmony with bordering attachments. If a mandibular denture is being relined, have the patient move the tongue into each cheek and then against the anterior teeth to establish a functional lingual border. It is necessary that the direct retainers be effective to prevent displacement of the denture while molding of the borders is accomplished. Otherwise the denture must be held in its terminal position with finger pressure on the occlusal surfaces.

6. Immediately remove the denture from the mouth and with fine curved iris scissors trim away gross excess material and any material that has flowed onto proximal tooth surfaces and other components of the denture framework. While this is being done, have the patient again rinse the mouth with cold water. Then replace the denture in its terminal position, bringing the teeth into occlusion. Then repeat the border movements with the patient's mouth open. By this time or soon thereafter the material will have become firm enough to maintain its form out of the mouth.

7. Remove the denture, rinse it quickly in water, and dry the relined surface with compressed air. Apply a generous coat of glycerine or Tect-ol with a brush or cotton pellet to prevent frosting of the surface because of evaporation of monomer. The material is then allowed to bench cure, thus eliminating patient discomfort and tissue damage from exothermic heat or prolonged contact with raw monomer. Although it is preferable that 20 to 30 minutes elapse before trimming and polishing, it may be done as soon as the material hardens. The masking tape must be removed before trimming is done but should be replaced over the teeth and polished surfaces below the junction of the new and old materials to protect those surfaces during final polishing.

Properly done, a direct reline is entirely acceptable for most **tooth-borne** partial denture bases made of a resin material, **except when some tissue support may be obtained for long spans between abutment teeth.** In the latter case a reline impression in wax may be accomplished, the denture may then be flasked, and a processed reline may be added for optimal tissue contact and support.

RELINING DISTAL EXTENSION DENTURE BASES

A distal extension partial denture, deriving its major support from the tissues of the residual ridge, requires relining much more frequently than does a tooth-supported denture. Because of this, distal extension bases are usually made of a resin material that can be relined to compensate for loss of support because of tissue changes. Whereas tooth-supported areas are relined for other reasons, the sole reason for relining a distal extension base is to reestablish tissue support for that base.

The need for relining a distal extension base is determined by evaluating the stability and occlusion at reasonable intervals after initial placement of the denture. Before initial placement of the denture the patient must be advised (1) that periodic examination and also relining, when it becomes necessary, are imperative, (2) that the success of the partial denture and the health of the remaining tissues and abutment teeth depend on periodic examination and servicing of both the denture and the abutment teeth, and (3) that a charge will be made for these visits in proportion to the treatment required.

There are two indications of the need for relining a distal extension partial denture base. **First,** a loss of occlusal contact between opposing dentures or between the denture and opposing natural dentition may be evident (Fig. 8-15). This is determined by having the patient close on two strips of 28-gauge soft green or blue (casting) wax. If occlusal contact between artificial dentition is weak or lacking while the remaining natural teeth in opposition are making firm contact, the distal extension denture needs to have occlusion reestablished on the present base either by altering the occlusion, or by reestablishing the original position of the denture framework and base, or sometimes both. In most instances, reestablishing the original relationship of the denture is necessary, and the occlusion will automatically be reestablished.

Second, a loss of tissue support causing rotation and settling of the distal extension base or bases is obvious when alternate finger pressure is applied on either side of the fulcrum line (Fig. 8-16). Although checking for occlusal contact alone may be misleading, such rotation is positive proof that relining is necessary. If occlusal inadequacy is detected without any evidence of denture rotation toward the residual ridge, all that need be done is to reestablish occlusal contact by rearranging the teeth or by adding to the occlusal surfaces with resin or cast gold onlays. On the other hand, if occlusal contact is adequate but denture rotation can be demonstrated, it is usually a result of migration or extrusion of opposing teeth or a shift in position of an opposing maxillary denture, thus maintaining occlusal contact at the expense of the stability and tissue support of that denture. This is frequently the situation when a partial denture is opposed by a maxillary complete denture. It is not unusual for a patient to complain of looseness of the maxillary complete denture and request relining of that denture when actually it is the partial denture that needs relining. Relining and thus repositioning the partial denture results in repositioning of the maxillary complete denture with a return of stability and retention in that denture. **Therefore evidence of rotation of a distal extension partial denture about the fulcrum line must be the deciding factor as to whether relining needs to be done.**

Rotation tissueward about the fulcrum line always results in a lifting of the indirect retainer(s). The framework of any distal extension partial denture must be in its original terminal position with indirect retainers fully seated during and at the end of any relining procedure. Any possibility of rotation about the fulcrum line because of occlusal influence must be prevented, and therefore the framework must be held in its original terminal position during the time the impression is being made. This all but eliminates the practicability of using a closed-mouth impression procedure effectively when relining unilateral or bilateral distal extension bases.

Therefore the only sure method of making a reline impression for a distal extension partial denture is with an open-mouth procedure done in exactly the same manner as the original secondary impression (Fig. 15-13). The denture to be relined is first relieved generously on the tissue side and then is treated the same as the original impression base for a functional impression. The step-by-step procedure is the same, with the dentist's three fingers placed on the two principal occlusal rests and at a third point between, preferably at an indirect retainer farthest from the axis of rotation. The framework is thus returned to its original terminal position, with all tooth-supported components fully seated. The tissues beneath the distal extension base are then registered in a relationship to the original position of the denture that will assure (1) the denture framework being returned to its intended relationship with the supporting teeth, (2) the reestablishment of optimum tissue support for the distal extension base, and (3) the restoration of the original occlusal relationship with the opposing teeth.

Although it is true that the teeth are not allowed to come into occlusion during an open-mouth impression procedure, the original position of the denture is positively determined by its relationship with the supporting abutment teeth. Since this is the relationship on which the original occlusion was established, returning the denture to that position should bring about a return to the original occlusal relationship if two conditions are satisfied. First of these is that the laboratory procedures during relining must be done accurately without any increase in vertical dimension. This is essential with any reline procedure, but particularly with a partial denture because any change in vertical dimension will prevent occlusal rests from seating and will result in overloading and trauma to the underlying tissues. The second condition is that the opposing teeth have not extruded or migrated or that the position of an opposing denture has not become irreversibly altered. In the latter situation some adjustment of the occlusion will be necessary, but this should be deferred until the opposing teeth or denture and the structures associated with the temporomandibular joint have had a chance to return to their original position before denture settling occurred. One of the greatest satisfactions of a job well done is to be found in the execution of an open-mouth reline procedure as described previously, which results in the restoration not only of the original denture relationship and tissue support but the original occlusal relationship as well.

METHODS OF REESTABLISHING OCCLUSION ON A RELINED PARTIAL DENTURE

Occlusion on a relined partial denture may be reestablished by several methods depending on whether the relining results in an increase in the vertical dimension of occlusion or a lack of opposing occlusal contacts. In either instance, it is usually necessary to make a remounting cast for the relined partial denture so that the denture can be correctly related to an opposing cast on an articulator as described in Chapter 19 (Fig. 19-2).

In rare instances, after the relining of a distal extension partial denture by the method previously described, the occlusion is found to be negative rather than positive or the same as it was before relining. This may be a result of wear of occlusal surfaces over a period of time, the original occlusion being high with resulting depression of opposing teeth, or other reasons. In such a case, occlusion on the denture must be restored to reestablish an even distribution of occlusal loading over both natural and artificial dentition. Otherwise, the natural dentition must carry the burden of mastication unaided, and the denture becomes only a space-filling or cosmetic device.

If the artificial teeth to be corrected are acrylic resin, the occlusion can be reestablished either by adding autopolymerizing acrylic resin to occlusal surfaces or by fabricating gold occlusal surfaces, which can be attached to the original replaced teeth. The original teeth also may be removed from the denture base and replaced by new teeth arranged to harmonize with the opposing occlusal surfaces. Baseplate wax may be used to support the teeth as they are being arranged. The wax should be carved to restore the lingual anatomy of the teeth and the portion of the denture base that was eliminated when the original teeth were removed. A stone matrix is made covering the occlusal and lingual surfaces of the teeth and denture flange. Then wax may be removed from the denture base and teeth. Those areas on the stone matrix, intimate to the new acrylic resin to be added, should be painted with a tinfoil substitute. The new teeth are placed in the stone matrix, and the matrix is accurately attached to the denture base with sticky wax. Autopolymerizing acrylic resin is then used to attach the teeth and is conveniently sprinkled on by a buccal approach. The buccal surface of the denture base adjacent to the teeth should be overfilled slightly so that the correct shape may be restored to this portion of the base during finishing and polishing procedures. Occlusal discrepancies as a result of this procedure should be corrected on the articulator by new jaw relation records if the denture involved has a distal extension base.

A second method is to remove the original teeth and replace them with a hard inlay wax occlusion rim on which a functional registration of occlusal pathways is then established (Chapter 16). Either the original teeth or new teeth may then be arranged to occlude with the template thus obtained and subsequently attached to the denture base with processed or autopolymerizing resin. If the latter is used, the need for flasking may be eliminated by securing the teeth to a stone matrix while the resin attachment is applied with a brush technique. Regardless of the method used for reattaching the teeth, the occlusion thus established should require little adjustment in the mouth and should be typical of the occlusal harmony that is possible by this method.

SELF-ASSESSMENT AIDS

1. What is the difference between relining and rebasing an acrylic resin denture base?
2. On occasion, tissue changes beneath tooth-borne denture bases require correction of the bases to reestablish intimate contact of the base and residual ridge. Can you think of three indications which would lead you to believe that intimate contact must be restored?
3. In any relining procedure, sufficient space between the denture base and residual ridge must

be provided to accommodate new material. True or false?

4. Tooth-borne removable partial denture bases may often be relined with a color-matching, autopolymerizing acrylic resin as a chairside procedure. Can you describe such a procedure, including preparation of the bases as well as the precautions that must be observed for patient comfort?

5. When relining a tooth-borne base, should the anatomic or functional form of the ridge be used?

6. Suppose you discover that rests are not correctly seated in their prepared seats when you are accomplishing a chairside reline procedure. What must you do?

7. Suppose you must reline a Class III, modification 1, type of removable restoration and the edentulous areas of the residual ridge are from canine to third molar on each side and you desire some support of the bases by the residual ridges. What procedure should you then undertake to acceptably reline the restoration? Include your impression procedure, impression material, processing, and correction of any occlusal discrepancies encountered.

8. There are two indications of the need for relining a distal extension removable partial denture. Can you state these two indications?

9. There is little difference in relining a distal extension denture base and making a secondary impression with a tray attached to the framework. Can you describe the procedures, both clinical and laboratory, that must be performed in relining a distal extension base?

10. After completion of the reline procedure and finishing of the restoration, occlusal discrepanancies invariably occur. They must be corrected before the patient is given possession of the restoration. How do you go about correcting occlusal discrepancies for a relined distal extension denture?

11. Should the same adjustment procedures of the denture base to residual ridge be undertaken for a relined base as was performed for initial placement of a new denture?

12. Does adjustment of the denture base to the basal seat precede or follow correction of occlusal discrepancies?

13. Suppose that after relining a distal extension denture base you find that occlusal contacts of opposing posterior artificial teeth are minimal or nonexistent. What then?

14. Before relining or rebasing is undertaken, the oral tissues should be returned to a state of health. True or false? Rationalize your answer please.

21 REPAIRS AND ADDITIONS TO REMOVABLE PARTIAL DENTURES

Broken clasp arms
Fractured occlusal rests
Distortion or breakage of other components—
   major and minor connectors
Loss of an additional tooth or teeth not involved
   in the support or retention of the restoration

Loss of an abutment tooth necessitating its
   replacement and making a new direct
   retainer
Other types of repairs
Repairing by soldering

The need for repairing or adding to a partial denture will occasionally arise. However, the frequency of this occurring should be held to a minimum by careful diagnosis, intelligent treatment planning, adequate mouth preparations, and carrying out an effective partial denture design with all component parts properly constructed. Any need for repairs or additions will then be the result of unforeseen complications arising in abutment or other teeth in the arch or to breakage or distortion of the denture through accident or careless handling by the patient rather than to faulty design or construction.

It is important that the patient be instructed in the proper placement and removal of the restoration so that undue strain is not placed on clasp arms or other parts of the denture nor on the abutment teeth contacted. The patient also should be advised that care must be given the restoraton when it is out of the mouth and that any distortion may be irreparable. It should be made clear that there can be no guarantee against breakage or distortion from causes other than obvious structural defects.

BROKEN CLASP ARMS

There are several reasons for breakage of clasp arms (Fig. 21-1, *A* and *B*):

1. Breakage may result from repeated flexure into and out of too severe an undercut. If the periodontal support is greater than the fatigue limit of the clasp arm, failure of the metal occurs first; otherwise the abutment tooth is loosened and eventually lost because of the persistent strain placed on it. This type of breakage can be avoided by locating clasp arms only where an acceptable minimum of retention exists, as determined by an accurate survey of the master cast.

2. Breakage may occur as a result of structural failure of the clasp arm itself. A cast clasp arm that is not properly formed or is subjected to careless finishing and polishing will eventually break at its weakest point. This can be avoided by providing a uniform taper to flexible retentive clasp arms and uniform bulk to all rigid nonretentive clasp arms.

Wrought-wire clasp arms may eventually fail because of repeated flexure at the point at which a nick or constriction occurred as a result of careless use of contouring pliers. They also may break at the point of origin from the casting as a result of excessive manipulation during initial adaptation to the tooth or subsequent readaptation. The latter can best be avoided by cautioning the patient against repeatedly lifting the clasp arm away from the tooth by application of the fingernail during removal of the denture. A wrought-wire clasp arm can normally be adjusted several times over a period of years without

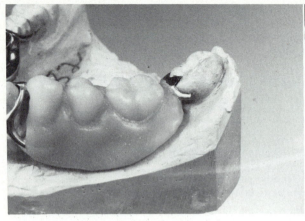

A

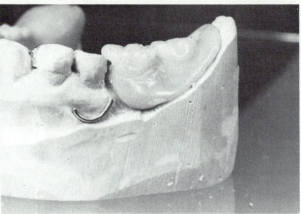

B

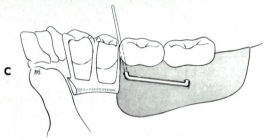

C

Fig. 21-1. **A,** Broken direct retainer on molar abutment. Reason for breakage should be determined. Denture must be evaluated for prospective serviceability if retainer arm is repaired. In many instances, patient will best be served by replacing denture with new restoration. **B,** Fractured wrought-wire retainer arm. **C,** Lingual view of technique for replacing broken retentive clasp arm with 18-gauge wrought wire. Wrought wire is embedded securely with autopolymerizing acrylic resin in groove cut in resin base.

failure. It is only when the number of adjustments are excessive that breakage is likely to occur.

Wrought-wire clasp arms also may break at the point of origin because of recrystallization of the metal. This can be prevented by proper selection of wrought wire, by avoiding burnout temperatures exceeding 1300° F, and by avoiding excessive casting temperatures when a cast-to method is used. When wrought wire is attached to the framework by soldering, the soldering technique must avoid recrystallization of the wire. For this reason, it is best that soldering be done electrically to prevent overheating the wrought wire. A low-fusing (1420° to 1500° F) triple-thick color-matching gold solder should be used rather than a solder possessing a higher fusing temperature.

3. Breakage may occur because of careless handling by the patient. Any clasp arm will become distorted or will break if subjected to excessive abuse by the patient. The most common cause of failure of a **cast clasp arm** is distortion caused by accidentally dropping the denture

into the lavatory basin or onto other hard surfaces.

A broken retentive clasp arm, regardless of its type, may be replaced with a wrought-wire retentive arm embedded in a resin base or attached to a metal base by electric soldering. Frequently this avoids the necessity of constructing an entirely new clasp arm (Fig. 21-1, *C*).

FRACTURED OCCLUSAL RESTS

Breakage of an occlusal rest almost always occurs where it crosses the marginal ridge. Improperly prepared occlusal rest seats are usually the cause of such weakness: an occlusal rest crossing a marginal ridge that was not lowered sufficiently during mouth preparations is either made too thin or is thinned by adjustment in the mouth to avoid occlusal interference. Failure of an occlusal rest rarely results from a structural defect in the metal and rarely if ever is caused by accidental distortion. **Therefore the blame for such failure must frequently be assumed by the dentist for not having provided sufficient space for the rest during mouth preparations.**

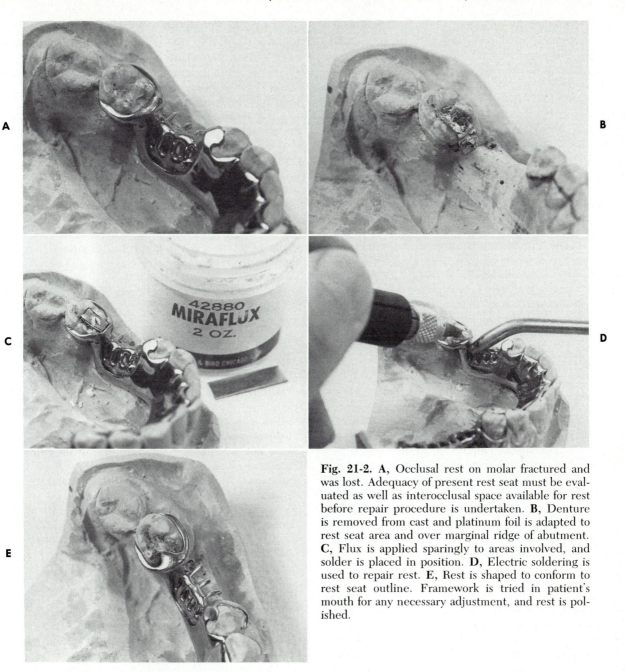

Fig. 21-2. A, Occlusal rest on molar fractured and was lost. Adequacy of present rest seat must be evaluated as well as interocclusal space available for rest before repair procedure is undertaken. **B,** Denture is removed from cast and platinum foil is adapted to rest seat area and over marginal ridge of abutment. **C,** Flux is applied sparingly to areas involved, and solder is placed in position. **D,** Electric soldering is used to repair rest. **E,** Rest is shaped to conform to rest seat outline. Framework is tried in patient's mouth for any necessary adjustment, and rest is polished.

Broken occlusal rests may be repaired by soldering as illustrated in Fig. 21-2. In preparation for the repair it may be necessary to alter the rest seat of the broken rest or relieve occlusal interferences. With the partial denture in its terminal position, an impression is made in irreversible hydrocolloid and then removed, with the partial denture remaining in the impression. Dental stone is poured into the impression and allowed to set. The partial denture is then removed from the cast, and platinum foil is adapted to the rest seat, the marginal ridge, and overlaps the guiding plane. The partial denture is returned to the cast, and with a fluoride flux, gold solder is electrically fused to the platinum foil and minor connector in sufficient bulk to form an occlusal rest.

An alternative solder to use is an industrial brazing alloy, which is higher fusing, but responds excellently to electrical soldering and does not tarnish. An example of such a solder is Electric Solder.*

DISTORTION OR BREAKAGE OF OTHER COMPONENTS—MAJOR AND MINOR CONNECTORS

Assuming that these components were made with adequate bulk originally, distortion usually occurs from abuse by the patient (Fig. 21-3). All such components should be designed and fabricated with sufficient bulk to assure their rigidity and permanence of form under normal circumstances.

Major and minor connectors occasionally become weakened by adjustment to avoid or eliminate tissue impingement. Such adjustment at the time of initial placement is a result of either inadequate survey of the master cast or faulty design or fabrication of the casting. This is inexcusable and reflects on the dentist; such a restoration should be remade rather than further weakening the restoration by attempting to compensate for its inadequacies by relieving the metal. Similarly, tissue impingement arising from inadequately relieved components results from faulty planning, and the casting should be remade with enough relief to avoid impingement. Failure of any component that was weak-

*J.F. Jelenko Co., Armonk, N.Y.

ened by adjustment at the time of initial placement is the responsibility of the dentist. However, adjustment made necessary by settling of the restoration because abutment teeth have become intruded under functional loading may be unavoidable. Subsequent failure resulting from the weakening effect of such adjustment may necessitate making a new restoration as a consequence of tissue changes. Frequently, repeated adjustment to a major or minor connector results in a loss of rigidity to the point that the connector can no longer function effectively. In such cases either a new restoration must be made or that part replaced by casting a new section and then reassembling the denture by soldering. This occasionally requires disassembly of denture bases and artificial teeth. The cost and probable success must then be weighed against the cost of a new restoration. Frequently the latter course is advisable.

LOSS OF AN ADDITIONAL TOOTH OR TEETH NOT INVOLVED IN THE SUPPORT OR RETENTION OF THE RESTORATION

Additions to a partial denture are usually simply made when the bases are made of resin. The addition of teeth to metal bases is more complex and necessitates either casting a new component, and attaching it by soldering, or creating retentive elements for the attachment of a resin extension. In most instances, when a distal extension denture base is extended, the need for subsequent relining of the entire base should be considered. **After the extension of the denture base, a relining procedure of both the new and old base then should be carried out to provide optimal tissue support for the restoration.**

LOSS OF AN ABUTMENT TOOTH NECESSITATING ITS REPLACEMENT AND MAKING A NEW DIRECT RETAINER

A lost abutment tooth will usually be the next adjacent tooth, which may or may not have to undergo restorative treatment (Fig. 21-4). In the latter case, any new restoration should be done to conform to the original path of placement, with proximal guiding plane, occlusal rest seat, and suitable retentive areas. Otherwise, modi-

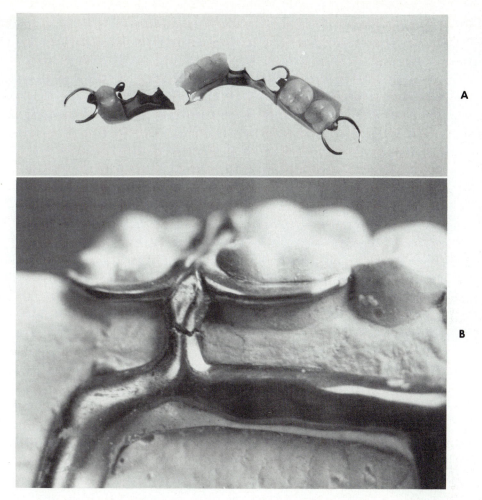

Fig. 21-3. A, Mandibular major connector completely fractured. Thinness of metal at fracture site contributed to eventual strain hardening. Major connectors must be carefully planned and laboratory procedures properly executed to avoid such occurrences. **B,** Fractured minor connector of embrasure clasp for maxillary partial denture. Repair of this component requires that platinum foil be adapted under fracture site on cast and that electric soldering be used.

fications to the existing tooth should be done the same as during any other mouth preparations, with proximal recontouring, preparation of an adequate occlusal rest seat, and any reduction in tooth contours necessary to accommodate retentive and stabilizing components. A new clasp assembly then may be cast for this tooth and the denture reassembled with the new replacement tooth added.

OTHER TYPES OF REPAIRS

Other types of repairs may include the replacement of a broken or lost prosthetically supplied tooth, the repair of a broken resin base, or the reattachment of a loosened resin base to the metal framework (Fig. 21-5). Breakage is sometimes the result of poor design, faulty fabrication, or the use of the wrong material for a given situation. Other times it results from an

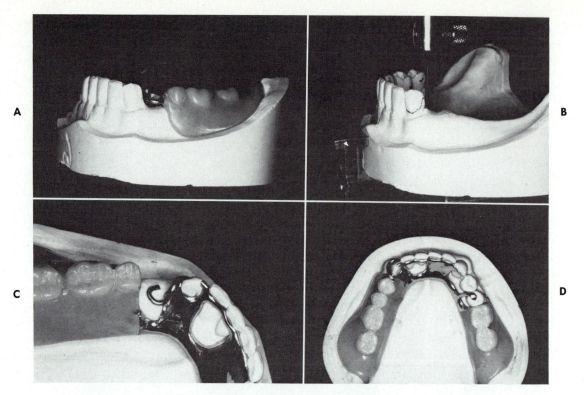

Fig. 21-4. **A,** First premolar abutment had to be extracted. This Class I restoration could be returned to service by using canine as abutment and replacing lost first premolar. **B,** Cast was surveyed to determine modifications required for added retainer compatible with original design of restoration. **C,** Necessary recontouring of canine abutment was accomplished. New retainer assembly was cast and soldered to major connector. Wrought-wire retentive arm was employed as part of retainer assembly. **D,** Left first premolar was replaced, and patient was given possession of restoration after occlusal adjustment was accomplished.

accident that will not necessarily repeat itself. If the latter occurs, repair or replacement usually suffices. On the other hand, if fracture has occurred because of structural defects or if it occurs a second time after the denture has been repaired once before, then some change in the design, either by modification of the original denture or with a new denture, may be necessary.

REPAIRING BY SOLDERING

It has been said that 80% of all soldering in dentistry can be done electrically. Electric soldering units are available for this purpose, and most dental laboratories are so equipped (Fig. 21-6). Electric soldering permits soldering close

to a resin base without removing that base, because of the rapid localization of heat at the electrode. The resin base needs only to be protected with a wet casting ring liner during soldering.

Color-matching gold solder may be used for soldering both gold and chromium-cobalt alloys. A solder for gold alloys that melts between 1420° and 1500° F is entirely adequate to solder gold alloys to chromium-cobalt alloys, thereby lessening the chance of recrystallizing gold wrought wire by excessive and prolonged heat. For electric soldering, triple-thick solder should be used so that the additional bulk of the solder will retard melting momentarily while the carbon electrode conducts heat to the area being soldered. For soldering chromium-cobalt alloys a color-

A 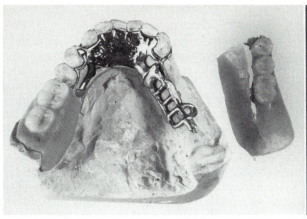 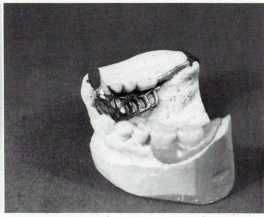 B

Fig. 21-5. A, Fractured denture base became completely detached from framework. Remaining portion of denture was placed in patient's mouth, impression was made in irreversible hydrocolloid, and cast was poured. **B,** Buccal portion of denture base contained artificial teeth and could be accurately related to minor connector. Index was made in stone. Right basal seat area of cast was painted with separating medium, and cast, denture, and index were assembled. New base was made of autopolymerizing acrylic resin by sprinkling method. Denture was relined after broken retainer on left second premolar was repaired.

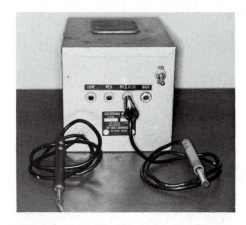

Fig. 21-6. Electric soldering machine with adjustment for low, medium, medium high, or high heat. Carbon electrode that furnishes heat for soldering is on right. Electrode on left completes electric circuit when touched to framework being soldered. Carbon electrode should be placed first on framework and removed last when soldering.

matching white 19K gold solder, which melts at about 1676° F, is used. An application of flux is essential to the success of any soldering operation to prevent oxidation of the parts being joined as well as the solder itself. A borax-type flux is used when soldering gold alloys. Fluoride-type flux must be used when soldering chromium-cobalt alloys. When a gold alloy is to be soldered to a chromium-cobalt alloy, a fluoride-type flux should be chosen.

The following is a procedure for electric soldering:

1. Roughen both sections to be joined.

2. Adapt platinum foil to the master cast to serve as a backing on which the solder will flow. Lift the edges of the foil to form a trough to confine the flow of the solder.

3. Seat the pieces to be soldered onto the master cast and secure them temporarily with sticky wax. Over each piece add enough soldering investment to secure them after the sticky wax is eliminated, but leave as much metal exposed as possible.

4. After flushing off the sticky wax with hot water, secure the cast to the soldering stand. Cut sufficient solder and place conveniently nearby.

5. Flux both sections. Put sufficient triple-thick solder on or in the joint to complete the soldering in one operation, always starting with enough solder to complete the job.

6. Wet the carbon tip with water to aid conduction of the current and then touch the carbon tip to the solder. Place the other electrode on any portion of the framework to complete the electric circuit and heat the carbon electrode. Do not push the solder with the carbon tip, but let the heat alone make the solder flow. Do not remove the carbon tip from the solder while the soldering operation is in progress, as this will cause surface pitting because of arcing. After the solder has flowed, remove the electrodes, **removing the carbon tip electrode last,** and proceed to remove the work from the cast for finishing.

Torch soldering requires an entirely different approach. It is used when the solder joint is long or unusually bulky and when a larger quantity of solder has to be used. Torch soldering cannot be undertaken to repair a removable restoration having acrylic resin denture bases or artificial teeth supported by acrylic resin. The procedure for torch soldering is as follows:

1. Roughen both sections to be joined.
2. Adapt platinum foil to the master cast so that it extends under both sections.
3. Seat the sections on the master cast in the correct relationship and secure them temporarily with sticky wax. Flow sticky wax also into the joint to be soldered.
4. Attach a dental bur or nail over the two sections with a liberal amount of sticky wax. Attach a second and even a third nail or bur across other areas to lend additional support. Never use pieces of wood for this purpose because the wood will swell if it gets wet, thus distorting the relationship of the two sections.
5. Remove the assembled casting from the master cast carefully. Adapt a stock of utility wax directly under each section, on either side of the platinum foil. After boilout is done, investment will remain in the center to support the platinum foil.
6. Invest the casting in sufficient soldering investment to secure it, leaving as much of the area to be soldered exposed as possible. When the investment has set, boil out the sticky and utility waxes. Then place the investment in a drying oven at a temperature not exceeding 200° F until the contained moisture has been eliminated. Do not preheat the investment with a

torch, or oxides will be formed that will interfere with the flow of the solder.

7. Use the reducing part of the flame, which is that feathery part just outside the blue inner cone. Flux the joint thoroughly and dry out the flux with the outer part of the flame until it has a powdery appearance. Heat the casting until it is dull red and then, holding a strip of solder in the soldering tweezers, dip it into the flux and feed it into the joint while the casting is being held at a dull red heat with the torch. Once the soldering operation has begun, do not remove the flame, as any cooling will cause oxides to be formed. The heat from the casting should be sufficient to melt the solder; therefore do not put the flame directly on the solder or it will become overheated, resulting in pitting.

8. After the soldering has been completed, allow the investment to cool slowly before quenching and proceeding with finishing. Remember that any soldering operation that heats the entire casting is in effect a softening heat-treating operation, and heat-hardening of a repaired gold alloy casting is desirable to restore its optimal physical properties.

SELF-ASSESSMENTS AIDS

1. The need for repairing a component of a removable partial denture may arise occasionally. How may the frequency of breakage of components be minized?
2. For what three reasons may breakage of a direct retainer arm occur?
3. An occlusal or incisal rest may fracture in use and invariably occurs at marginal ridge or incisal areas. What is the predominant reason for lack of strength at the junction of the rest and minor connector?
4. Have you ever tried to adjust a distorted major connector? What problems, if any, did you encounter?
5. Other than by accident, for what reasons could a major connector become distorted?
6. An abutment with a guarded prognosis is sometimes used to avoid an extension-type denture. Loss of such abutments requires extension of denture bases and inclusion of an artificial tooth replacing the abutment. Suppose the denture was not designed anticipating eventual loss of the posterior abutment. Would this influence your decision to repair or remake the denture?
7. Extension of a base in replacing an abutment

tooth usually requires relining of the entire base. True or false?

8. When a terminal abutment for a distal extension removable partial denture is lost, can the existing denture be modified with a new clasp assembly on another abutment?

9. Porcelain artificial teeth that have been excessively ground or that were not arranged in occlusal harmony sometimes fracture in use and have to be replaced. Can you perform this procedure? Is an impression necessary? If the replaced tooth is on an extension base, how do you adjust the occlusion?

10. What is a distinct advantage of electric soldering over torch soldering for the repair of a metallic element of a removable partial denture?

11. Suppose a rest broke at its junction with the minor connector. How could you create a new rest by soldering? Would you perform a clinical procedure on the old rest seat preparation first?

12. You are soldering chromium-cobalt alloy. What solder should you use? Any special type of flux required?

13. What solder and flux would you use to repair a Type IV gold alloy framework?

14. When using an electric soldering unit, why must the carbon electrode be removed from the work last?

15. What is the purpose of using a flux when performing soldering operations?

16. Should torch soldering be attempted on a restoration with acrylic resin bases?

17. After you have repaired a framework by either electric or torch soldering, should a heat-hardening treatment be performed? Why or why not?

22 TEMPORARY REMOVABLE PARTIAL DENTURES

Appearance
Space maintenance
Reestablishing occlusal relationships
Conditioning teeth and residual ridges
Interim restoration during treatment
Conditioning the patient for wearing a prosthesis

Removable partial dentures designed to be used for short intervals often must be fabricated as a part of a total prosthodontic treatment. These are the various types of prosthetic restorations for the partially edentulous mouth that are, and must be, considered temporary restorations. Such restorations serve many useful purposes. It is important, however, that patients be made aware that such restorations are temporary and may jeopardize the integrity of adjacent teeth and health of supporting tissues if worn for extended periods without supportive care.

Temporary restorations may be indicated as a part of total treatment for

1. The sake of appearance
2. Maintenance of a space
3. Reestablishing occlusal relationships
4. Conditioning teeth and residual ridges
5. An interim restoration during treatment
6. Conditioning the patient for wearing a prosthesis.

APPEARANCE

For the sake of appearance a temporary denture may replace only one or more missing anterior teeth, or it may replace several teeth, both anterior and posterior. Such a restoration is usually made of acrylic resin, either by a sprinkling method or by waxing, flasking, and processing with either autopolymerizing or thermal-curing resin (Fig. 22-1). It may be retained by wraparound wrought-wire clasps, Crozat-type clasps, interproximal spurs, or wire loops. In rare instances, separate cast circumferential type clasps may be used by attaching them to the resin base with a retaining lug.

SPACE MAINTENANCE

When a space results from recent extractions or traumatic loss of teeth, it is usually prudent to maintain the space while tissues heal. In younger patients the space should be maintained until the adjacent teeth have reached sufficient maturity to be used as abutments for fixed restorations (Fig. 22-2). In adult patients the maintenance of the space can prevent undesirable migration and extrusion of adjacent or opposing teeth until definitive treatment can be accomplished (Fig. 22-3).

REESTABLISHING OCCLUSAL RELATIONSHIPS

Temporary partial dentures are used for the following reasons: (1) to establish a new occlusal relationship or vertical dimension and (2) to condition teeth and ridge tissues to support better the partial denture to follow.

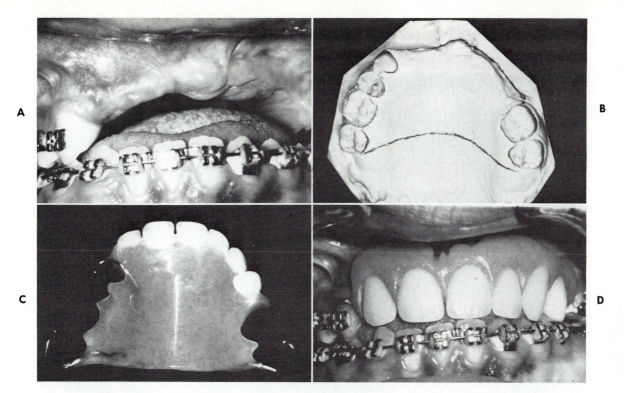

Fig. 22-1. A, Fifteen-year-old female involved in automobile accident resulting in loss of several maxillary teeth. She was undergoing orthodontic treatment at time of accident. **B,** Design of temporary partial denture on cast. **C,** Temporary restoraton fabricated by sprinkling on autopolymerizing acrylic resin. Wrought-wire retainers are located on maxillary right canine and second molars. **D,** Temporary removable partial denture in position.

Temporary partial dentures may be used as occlusal splints in much the same manner as cast or resin occlusal splints are used on natural teeth (Figs. 22-4 and 22-5). When total tooth support is available, there is little difference between a fixed and a removable occlusal splint, except that a removable splint is too likely to be left out of the mouth unless the patient is actually made more comfortable by its presence. This is usually true when temporomandibular joint pathology is alleviated by wearing an occlusal splint. In other situations it may be advisable to cement the removable restoration to the teeth until such time as the patient has become accustomed to, and dependent on, the jaw relationship provided by the splint.

Both fixed and removable tooth-supported occlusal splints have much in common. Either of them may be eliminated sectionally as restorative treatment is being done, thus maintaining the established jaw relation until all restorative treatment has been completed. The dentist decides whether these are to be fixed or removable and whether they are made of a cast (silver or gold) alloy or of a resin material.

When one or more distal extension bases exist on an occlusal splint, a different situation exists. The establishment of a new occlusal or vertical relation depends too much on the quality of support the splint receives to ignore the need for the best possible support for any existing distal extension base. Both broad coverage and functional basing of tissue-supported bases are desirable, as well as some type of occlusal rest on the nearest abutments. Any tissue-supported occlusal splint should be at least be relined in the

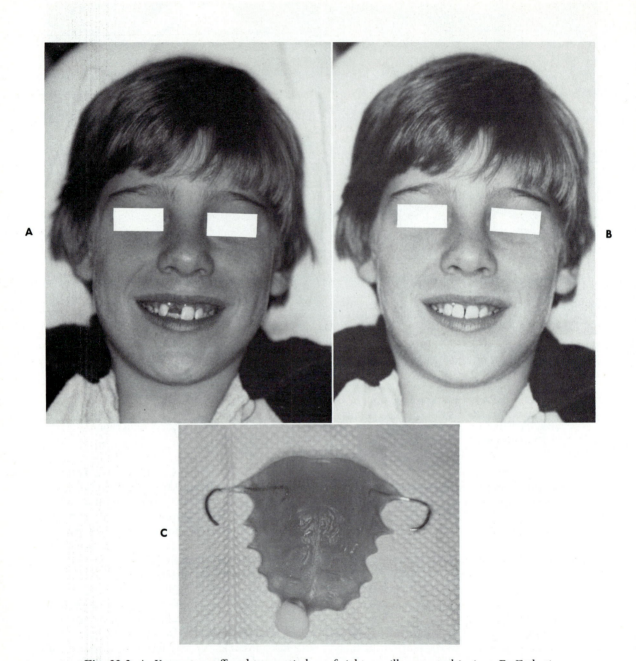

Fig. 22-2. A, Youngster suffered traumatic loss of right maxillary central incisor. **B,** Esthetic result obtained with temporary denture. **C,** Temporary restoration for replacement of central incisor. Note wrought-wire retainers for first molars. (Courtesy Department of Pedodontics, University of Alabama School of Dentistry, Birmingham, Ala.)

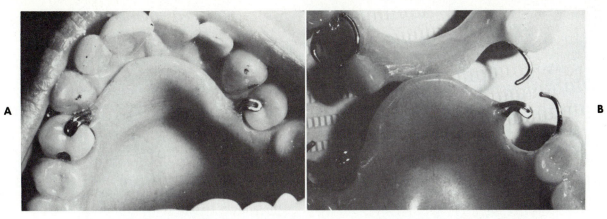

Fig. 22-3. A, Temporary maxillary partial denture for adult. Note use of wrought-wire occlusal rests on first premolars to suppport anterior portion of restoration. **B,** Opposing temporary prostheses for patient in **A.** Not only will residual ridge areas be conditioned for more definitive prosthesis, but anticipated abutments will also be conditions. Restorations will prevent migration and eruption of remaining natural teeth until definitive treatment is begun.

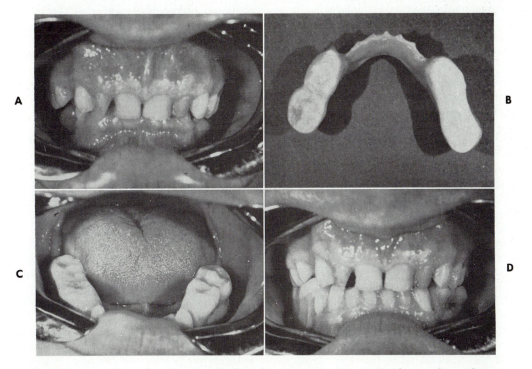

Fig. 22-4. Four views showing use of removable occlusal splint. **A,** Evidence of overclosure to be corrected by occlusal reconstruction. **B,** Removable occlusal splint for lower arch, using tooth-colored acrylic resin for occlusal surfaces. **C,** Removable splint in mouth. Occlusal anatomy is result of occlusal registration done in wax on resin base, which is then invested, and to which tooth-colored resin is added to reproduce functional occlusal surfaces that were recorded in wax. **D,** Resulting occlusion with removable splint. This may be adjusted until satisfactory, and then it signifies vertical dimension to be maintained by oral rehabilitation.

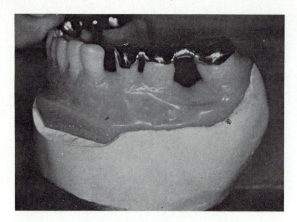

Fig. 22-5. Cast gold occlusal splints. Following occlusal adjustment, splints are cemented to teeth. Since these are made to fit unprepared natural teeth, they cannot extend beyond height of contour of each tooth. Surveying is therefore necessary before their construction. Splints may be eliminated tooth by tooth as subsequent restorations are being done, thus maintaining established vertical relationship.

mouth with a autopolymerizing reline resin to afford optimal coverage and support for the distal extension base.

CONDITIONING TEETH AND RESIDUAL RIDGES

O.C. Applegate, in an article on the choice of partial or complete denture treatment, has emphasized the advantages of conditioning edentulous areas to provide stable support for distal extension partial dentures. This is accomplished by having the patient wear a temporary partial denture for a period of time before construction of the final base (Fig. 22-6, *A*). In the absence of opposing occlusion, stimulation of the underlying tissues by applying intermittent finger pressure to the denture base is advised. Whether the stimulation is from occlusal or finger pressure, there seems to be little doubt that the tissues of the residual ridge become more capable of supporting a distal extension partial denture when they have been conditioned by the wearing of a previous restoration.

Abutment teeth also benefit from the wearing of a temporary restoration when such a resto-

ration applies an occlusal load to those teeth, either through occlusal coverage or through occlusal rests (Fig. 22-6, *B*). Frequently a tooth that is to be used as an abutment for a partial denture has been out of occlusion for some time. Immediately on applying an occlusal load to that tooth sufficient to support any type of removable prosthesis, some intrusion of the tooth will occur. If such intrusion is allowed to occur after initial placement of the final prosthesis, the occlusal relationship of the prosthesis and its relation to the adjacent gingival tissues will be altered. Perhaps this is one reason for gingival impingement, which occurs after the denture has been worn for some time, even though seemingly adequate relief had been provided initially. When a temporary partial denture is worn, such abutment teeth have an opportunity to become stabilized under the loading of the temporary restoration, and intrusion will have occurred before the making of the impression for the master cast. There is sufficient reason to believe that both abutment teeth and supporting ridge tissues are better capable of providing continuing support for the partial denture when they have been previously conditioned by the wearing of a temporary restoration.

INTERIM RESTORATION DURING TREATMENT

In some instances an existing partial denture can be used with modifications as an interim partial denture. Such modifications may include relining and adding teeth and clasps to an existing denture. In other instances an existing partial denture may be converted to a transitional complete denture for immediate placement while tissues heal and an opposing arch is prepared to receive a partial denture. Sometimes a temporary partial denture must be made to replace missing anterior teeth in a partially edentulous arch, which are ultimately to be replaced with fixed restorations. On occasion the anterior portion of the restoration is cut away when the fixed restorations are placed, leaving the remainder of the denture to be worn while posterior abutment teeth are being prepared.

Still another type of temporary denture is one on which missing posterior teeth are replaced

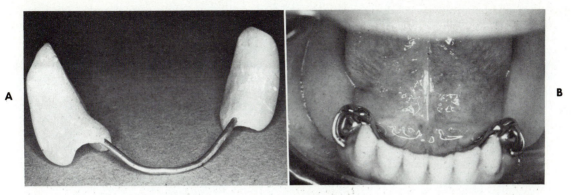

Fig. 22-6. A, Typical exercise prosthesis, designed by O.C. Applegate to condition residual ridges before making final impressions. **B,** Exercise restoration to condition both residual ridges and abutment teeth.

temporarily with a resin occlusion rim rather than with occluding teeth. In dental school clinics it is sometimes impossible to complete treatment in a school year, and the continuing student may desire to resume treatment after the summer recess. In such instances, occlusion may be maintained, and the tissues may be conditioned by having the patient wear a temporary restoration with posterior occlusion rims that have been adjusted to occlusal harmony.

CONDITIONING THE PATIENT FOR WEARING A PROSTHESIS

A temporary restoration may be made to aid the patient in making a transition to complete dentures when the total loss of teeth is inevitable. Such a partial denture also may be considered a valid part of the treatment, since the patient is at the same time being conditioned to wear a removable prosthesis. It should be considered strictly a temporary measure that provides the patient with a restoration for the remaining life of the natural teeth when further restorative treatment of those teeth is impractical or economically or technically impossible.

This type of a partial denture may be worn for prolonged periods, in the meantime undergoing revision, modification to include additional teeth lost, or relining when such becomes necessary or advisable. The dentist should agree to provide such a partial denture only under the following conditions: (1) that a definite fee for the treatment is appropriate and that the fee will depend on the servicing necessary and (2) that when further wearing of the transitional denture is unwise and jeopardizes the health of the remaining tissues, the transition to complete dentures will proceed.

It is imperative that a distinction be made between temporary restorations and a true partial denture service and that the patient be advised of the purposes and limitations of such restorations.

SELF-ASSESSMENT AIDS

1. Removable partial dentures designed to be used for short intervals are temporary restorations and serve definite purposes. They must not be represented to the patient as other than temporary. True or false?
2. Temporary removable partial dentures may jeopardize the integrity of adjacent teeth and health of supporting tissues if worn for extended periods without supportive care. True or false? Rationalize your answer.
3. Temporary removable partial dentures serve many useful purposes. Two of these are (1) to maintain appearance and (2) to reestablish occlusal relationships. Name the other four purposes.
4. In adult patients the placement of a temporary partial denture to maintain a space can prevent undesirable migration and extrusion of adjacent or opposing teeth until definitive treatment can be accomplished. True or false?

5. The use of a temporary partial denture as an occlusal splint to reestablish the occlusal relationship for a Class I partial denture requires broad coverage and functional basing of the tissue-supported bases. What is the best method of achieving functional basing?

6. One of the functions that a temporary denture provides is to condition teeth and residual ridges. Why is it important to condition teeth and residual ridges?

7. The construction of temporary partial dentures requires that prosthodontic principles not be violated and that procedures be meticulously executed. True or false?

23 MAXILLOFACIAL APPLICATIONS OF REMOVABLE PARTIAL PROSTHODONTICS

WILLIAM R. LANEY, B.S., D.M.D., M.S.*

The prosthetic replacement of tissue defects, which were either traumatically or developmentally acquired, often depends on removable prostheses that are retained by clasps on the teeth. Certain considerations will be discussed that do not supplant but rather supplement those general principles of design that apply to the usual removable pratial denture. Such components as the obturator that closes the defect resulting from a hemisection of the maxilla and the pharyngeal portion of a cleft palate prosthesis impose further burdens on the usual designs. Resultant dislodging forces must be considered and provided for in the design that will be used for any particular patient.

Several types of prostheses depend on a partial denture framework for their retention. An attempt to describe only a representative few is made, since the variations are myriad and do not lend themselves to easy classification.

*Consultant in Prosthodontics and Chairman, Department of Dentistry, Mayo Clinic and Mayo Foundation; Professor of Dentistry, Mayo Graduate School of Medicine, Rochester, Minnesota.

PROSTHESES FOR ACQUIRED DEFECTS

Acquired defects of the jaws are those occurring postnatally and are usually related to a traumatic incident or surgical treatment for the elimination of disease processes. Treatment approaches for the replacement of lost oral structures are predicated on such factors as disease prognosis, size and location of the defect, presence or absence of teeth, residual bony support, maxillomandibular jaw relationships, esthetic requirements, and adjunctive therapeutic modalities such as irradiation. Treatment planning for the prosthodontic restoration of acquired oral defects should begin before surgical intervention and is coordinated with the surgeon. Presurgical planning involves a review of radiographs, photographs, diagnostic casts, and the contemplated surgical reconstructive procedures.

Maxillary defects

In instances where maxillary surgical treatment will not be extensive, it is usually desirable to use a revised existing prosthesis or prefabricated splint for immediate insertion. Regardless of configuration, the prosthetic device temporarily closes the defect and provides support for border tissues during the immediate postsurgical healing phase. The temporary obturator will likely require revision during the subsequent 2- to 3-month period so as to maintain appropriate adaptation at the border.

When teeth are present in the mouth, fabrication of the more definitive prosthesis is divided into three phases:

1. Complete restoration of all remaining teeth in the affected arch and treatment of the periodontal tissues
2. Design and casting of the metal framework
3. Fabrication of the tissue replacement section of the prosthesis

The first phase should include full crown coverage for at least the abutment teeth. These restorations should provide protection from carious processes and, when properly surveyed, should provide optimal location of the retentive and stabilizing components. The loss of any teeth places a burden on the remaining teeth and the loss of all teeth is catastrophic. The dentist should resort to any measures that will preserve the integrity of the remaining teeth, including the splinting together of all or groups of teeth.

Defect configuration can range from small localized palatal perforations to large cavities involving the palate, maxillary sinuses, and nose (Fig. 23-1). The minor defect may be obturated by an extension from a more conventional removable partial denture. A more typical defect results from hemisection of the maxilla, and the prosthesis designed for its obturation must separate the oral from the antral-nasal cavities. It should be planned to take advantage of the physical opportunities for retention provided by the configuration of the defect itself as well as the teeth (Fig. 23-2). The structures usually involved in defects that can be considered for augmentation of prosthesis retention and stability include

1. The rim of the soft palate
2. The anterior wall of the temporal bone in the infratemporal fossa
3. The skin-mucosal band of scar tissue on the internal surface of the cheek
4. The anterior nasal spine
5. The floor of the nose above the hard palate along the midline

Although the detailed design of the metal framework will vary for each patient, two general principles must be considered. First, the stabilizing aspects of the design must be emphasized. For example, every molar and premolar tooth remaining after hemimaxillectomy should have a stabilizing arm to distribute

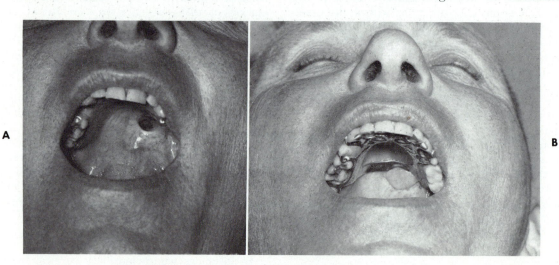

Fig. 23-1. A, Localized palatal defect. **B,** Palatal defect obturated with extension of conventional removable partial denture. (From Laney, W.R., and Gibilisco, J.A., editors; Diagnosis and treatment is prosthodontics, Philadelphia, 1983, Lea & Febiger.)

torque forces adequately. Second, retentive clasp arms should be designed so that they resist the displacement forces of the finished prosthesis (Fig. 23-3). It must be remembered that weight alone is often an important displacing force for these restorations. The design of the

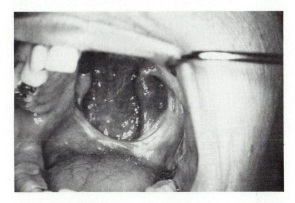

Fig. 23-2. Maxillary defect resulting from hemimaxillectomy: surgical area to be prosthetically restored involves oral, antral, and nasal cavities. (From Laney, W.R., and Gibilisco, J.A., editors; Diagnosis and treatment in prosthodontics, Philadelphia, 1983, Lea & Febiger.)

cast framework as the primary vehicle for supporting the prosthesis and for distribution of stress may need to be altered to take advantage of inclination and distribution of the teeth. Fig. 23-4 illustrates the use of a buccal bar connector in combination with circumferential clasps and lingual guiding planes to provide positive retention and better functional control of the prosthesis.

The tissue replacement section of the prosthesis is important because it serves the primary function of this type of restoration. When the framework has been checked in the mouth for accurate fit, an acrylic resin tray is adapted to the retentive grid in the defect area. This impression tray is underextended 1 to 2 mm in all directions, and the border is recorded with a low-fusing modeling plastic. During this procedure, care is taken to extend the base into all soft tissue and bony areas that can provide support or retention for the finished prosthesis and are compatible with the path of placement. Following border molding, all modeling plastic areas that contact tissue are reduced 0.5 mm,

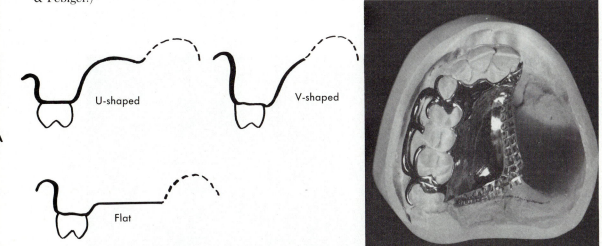

Fig. 23-3. A, Palate and defect configuration affect displacement forces of obturator prosthesis. U-shaped palate coupled with tooth as extension of alveolar ridge provides good stabilization and resistance to obturator rotation. Other palate or ridge shapes do not contribute as effectively to stabilization. **B,** Prosthesis design maximizing use of deep buccal tooth undercuts for retention, occlusal rests for support, and lingual surface contact for reciprocation. (From Laney, W.R., and Gibilisco, J.A., editors; Diagnosis and treatment in prosthodontics, Philadelphia, 1983, Lea & Febiger.)

and the final impression is made with rubber-base or mouth-temperature wax impression material. Where tray manipulation is difficult, undercuts are not extensive, or facial tissue support requires additional bulk, wax may be the material of choice because it can be readily altered.

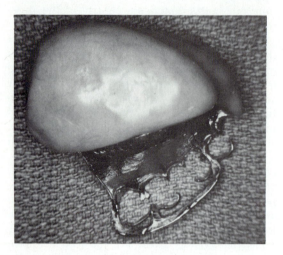

Fig. 23-4. Prosthesis using both obturator and cast framework components to provide optimal retention and stability.

The original cast is now altered by removing all of the tissue-born section, retaining only the teeth and adjacent gingival ridge–palatal portions involved in the casting (Fig. 23-5). After scoring the residual cast section, the framework and impression are seated accurately on the cast, and a new tissue section is poured into the final impression. Thus a corrected cast is available for processing.

Mandibular defects

Defects caused by surgical intervention to eradicate or control disease frequently involve jaw resection. Discontinuity of the mandible following loss of a segment will result in impaired muscular control of the residual segment or segments. Disruption of mandibular continuity permits deviation of the remaining jaw segment medially and posteriorly toward the defect and rotation on occlusal contact. As the anterior surgical margin approaches the midline and beyond, stability of the residual fragment diminishes.

Unilateral loss of the mandible, to include teeth, their periodontium, alveolar ridge with soft tissue covering, muscle attachments, and temporomandibular joint function, significantly

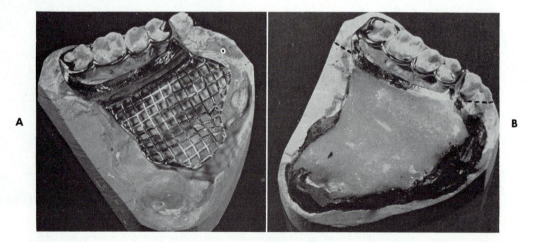

Fig. 23-5. Prosthetic treatment of maxillary hemisection. **A,** All posterior teeth remaining after hemisection of maxilla should have reciprocal arms to distribute widely the downward dislodging force of unsupported side. **B,** When corrected impression is obtained, all original cast except teeth and adjacent gingival tissues is cut away, and new cast is poured into corrected impression. Dotted line separates new section from original section of cast.

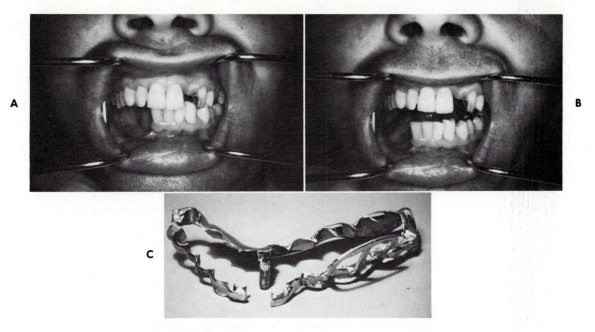

Fig. 23-6. A, Right mandibular resection resulting in discontinuity defect. **B,** Note midline deviation of residual mandibular segment to defect side on opening. **C,** Type of cast framework for lateral guide flange used to control mandibular deviation. (**C** from Laney, W.R., and Gibilisco, J.A., editors; Diagnosis and treatment in prosthodontics, Philadelphia, 1983, Lea & Febiger.)

reduces the proprioceptive influence on positional control. Strength and precision of function are significantly reduced.

Mandibular resection frequently involves the sacrifice of portions of adjacent structures that influence position and function. These include the floor of the mouth, tongue, pharyngeal and palatal musculature, and buccal mucosa. All may be involved in closure of the surgical wound, and their compromise may adversely affect mastication, deglutition, speech, and facial appearance.

Without surgical reconstruction to restore continuity, control of the residual mandibular segment to improve its alignment and occlusal functional potential is a prosthodontic procedure. The method selected for stabilization depends on the following: (1) the extent and location of resected bone, (2) the extent of soft tissue excision, and (3) the presence of teeth. One approach involves the use of a removable vertical guide flange attached to remaining man-

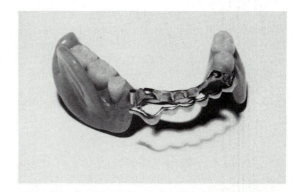

Fig. 23-7. Definitive type of removable partial prosthesis incorporating lateral guide flange and hinged labial bar.

dibular teeth with a removable cast framework (Fig. 23-6). This guidance device is advantageous in the immediate postoperative period, since it permits mandibular opening and closing but controls medioposterior deviation by engaging the maxillary dentition. Its effectiveness depends on design criteria, which include rigidity, multiple rests for stress distribution, maximum retention, and reciprocation. It should be emphasized that removable guidance devices are generally used as temporary control or training entities. If after a 6- to 12-month therapy period the patient is unable to position the residual segment in an acceptable occluding position, consideration may need to be given before further use of such designs in a more definitive partial prostheses (Fig. 23-7).

Undesirable sequelae

The following are factors that directly affect the treatment of patients with maxillary or mandibular oral defects.

Irradiation. Many patients having a defect resulting from cancer therapy have received radiation therapy combined with surgical procedures. This therapy greatly diminishes the normal blood supply and makes the tissues particularly susceptible to infections and traumatic injury. Because the original blood supply to the maxilla is greater than that to the mandible, the effects of radiation are more common on the mandible. Patient responses to a therapeutic dose of 6000 rad (supervoltage externally delivered) vary considerably, so that an individual assessment of the patient should guide the placement of a prosthesis. The degree and duration of the acute reaction to the therapy along with the appearance of the tissues as it relates to blood supply dictate the prosthetic treatment. The surgery usually diminishes the sensory nerve supply to the area so that these patients may develop a mucosal ulcer without the usual symptom of pain. Therefore all patients who have been irradiated should be closely followed for possible trauma caused by the prosthesis.

The major and minor salivary glands are frequently involved in head and neck irradiation treatment fields. Early glandular response includes interstitial edema and duct obstruction. As gland function is compromised, the patient experiences a reduction in saliva production. Early loss of the serous component results in thickened saliva after the fourth or fifth day, and the mouth becomes progressively drier until xerostomia is a persistent symptom after the dose

has exceeded 2000 rads. Although temporarily compromised, salivary function will usually return if the dose is not larger. As therapy progresses with a curative dose, interstitial fibrosis and degeneration of small blood vessels occur. In total these changes further compromise mucosal integrity and render the tissues more susceptible to trauma.

It follows naturally that there is a correlation between the tissue resistance and the amount of trauma required to produce a breakdown in the tissues. The amount of time the prosthesis is worn and the way it is used (speech, deglutition, mastication) will influence the total amount of trauma produced. Each patient should therefore gradually increase the time and activities performed with the prosthesis until it is determined how much trauma can be safely tolerated.

Prosthesis factors. As mentioned previously, weight is a considerable displacing factor, and when prostheses demand thickness and bulk they should be constructed in such a way that they are hollow. This is an easy process today with the autopolymerizing resins. These resins enable one to process hollow restorations that may be capped and sealed with additional autopolymerizing resin.

When arranging teeth for a restoration replacing a hemisection of the maxilla, it should be remembered that the remaining tissue bearing the force of occlusion is of poor quality. Therefore the occlusion should be arranged to contact just lightly on the affected side. In some instances it may be preferable to eliminate occlusal contact entirely, to avoid any pressure. The patient should be instructed to avoid chewing on the affected side. In this difficult situation, it is better to eat only on one side without soreness than to eat on both and develop constantly irritated tissue areas.

Surgery. When constructing prostheses after radical surgery of the face and neck, one must be prepared to alter them to accommodate for changes in tissue topography. These changes result from altered physiology in connection with lymph drainage in general. Sometimes these patients will have a marked difference in the tissue-fluid content of their facial tissues from morning to night. This may prove difficult for the prosthodontist because if the prosthesis fits in the morning, it will be loose in the afternoon, and if it fits in the afternoon, it may cause sore spots in the morning. In general, the former situation is preferred. Accordingly it may be better to make all impressions in the morning.

Furthermore the process of scar contraction may continue for several weeks or months, which will demand periodic revision of the prosthesis. Restoration of facial contour should never be attempted when considerable pressure against scar tissue is required to do so. This again may cause ulceration, displacement of the restoration, movement of the teeth, or all three.

Psychological considerations. It must be realized that these particular patients have been through a difficult period. The thoughts of losing large parts of the face are matters of concern to even the most callous. The realization that the resultant defects in speech or appearance may be permanent does not encourage the patient. Therefore the individual should be informed that the prostheses are available, and a clear assessment of their role should be offered.

The dentist should neither dispel hope with talk of failure nor build false hope with talk of great success. Rather, the dentist should consider personal chances of creating a successful prosthesis. Then the patient should be encouraged to cooperate in the construction of the restoration and be encouraged to wear it. Negative approaches are poor. If one dwells unduly on the chance of failure, a bad mistake is made. Instead, the dentist should tell the truthful story of the many people who wear these restorations successfully.

Sharry has noted that there is a great deal of difference between the following statements:
1. There are many people who wear these restorations happily and successfully.
2. There are many people who cannot wear these restorations.

The former is encouraging, the latter deadening. Use of a positive bright approach, being careful not to build up false hopes, is best. Painting a bleak picture can seriously affect the patient's attitude toward the prosthesis.

Years of fabricating maxillofacial prostheses have suggested that it is perhaps the most rewarding branch of prosthetic dentistry. Affected patients are not petty, arrogant people; they are appreciative, cooperative, and a pleasure to know. The patient can often tell the dentist much about how the restoration should serve and can offer constructive suggestions concerning its design. The dentist should always listen to, and weigh carefully, these suggestions. Experience suggests that near failures have been converted to successful restorations by following the patient's directions in certain aspects of fabrication.

PROSTHESES FOR CONGENITAL DEFECTS

Congenital defects of the orofacial complex are those defects that exist at, and usually before, birth. Perhaps the most common of these are the cleft lip and palate. The cleft palate obturator is one of the most common prostheses associated with congenital oral defects and is probably the one about which most has been written in the past.

Classification

Cleft palates lend themselves to morphologic classifications. The simplest and perhaps the most easily remembered is that of Veau, who proposed four classes (Fig. 23-8):

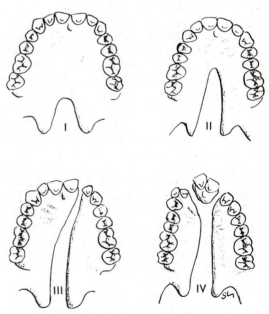

Fig. 23-8. Veau's classification of cleft palates.

Class I, which involves only the soft palate

Class II, which involves the soft and hard palates but not the alveolus

Class III, which involves the soft and hard palates, continuing through the alveolus on one side of the premaxillary area

Class IV, which involves the soft and hard palates, the cleft continuing through the alveolus on both sides, leaving a free premaxilla

The latter two classes are usually, though not always, associated with a cleft lip. The cleft lip is usually surgically closed by the sixth to twelfth week of life. To permit undisturbed growth, surgical closure of the cleft palate is usually delayed until the child is about 18 months old.

Etiology

The etiology of cleft palate is not clear but seems at the present time to have some basis in heredity, although many other factors have been mentioned, such as infectious disease of the mother, nutritional inadequacies, and various other changes in the intrauterine environment.

Personality evaluation

The personality range of individuals with a cleft palate is not much different from that of the general population. Perhaps more of them fall into the quiet, unresponsive, withdrawn category and a few exhibit a brashness or bravado (which generally disappears on continued association with them). However, a large share are well-adjusted, pleasant people. Sometimes one wonders how so many can be happy when the attitude of the parents and the public is often such that a considerable degree of overprotection or rejection is the fate of these individuals when they are children.

It should be noted here that so many factors influence diagnosis and treatment of these patients that a "team approach" (dentist, surgeon, pediatrician, speech pathologist and therapist, psychologist, audiologist, medical social worker, vocational counselor, and so on) to management of these patients is essential.

Anatomy

During examination of clefts that have not been treated surgically, the dentist should observe the nasal and pharyngeal cavities and their component structures and, using a blunt instrument or finger, ascertain the tissue consistency of various areas. It should be noted here that the gag reflex of the person with a cleft palate is markedly diminished and does not usually hinder palpatory examination.

Knowledge of the anatomic structure of these cavities serves not merely to satisfy intellectual curiosity but, more importantly, to place the dentist on familiar ground when and if it becomes necessary to remove impression materials that may inadvertently be forced through the cleft or perforation while obtaining an impression of the dental arches.

The normal soft palate either closes the nasal cavity from the pharynx or the oral cavity from the pharynx, or it just relaxes as the occasion demands (Fig. 23-9). If this "valve" is not whole, it cannot effectively perform these closing functions but rather allows food to enter the nasopharynx during deglutition and allows air to enter the nasal cavity during the production of those speech sounds wherein the air should be directed into the oral cavity. Further, it makes the production of such sounds as /puh/ and /kuk/ practically impossible.

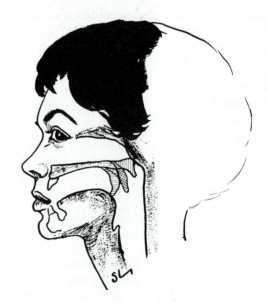

Fig. 23-9. Three positions of soft palate during normal activity.

A group of muscles is attached to the soft palate and is responsible for the closure of the nasal cavity. This total action (closing off the nasal cavity) is called **palatopharyngeal closure.** To accomplish this, the following, more or less simultaneous, muscular contractions take place.

The levator veli palatini muscle originates on the petrous portion of the temporal bone and the cartilage of the eustachian tube. It runs downward and forward to insert into the palatine aponeurosis and contracts, pulling the soft palate upward and backward (Fig. 23-10). This is a paired muscle, and on entering the soft palate it merges with its fellow of the opposite side, forming a sling. At the same time, the tensor veli palatini, which arises from the scaphoid fossa, the sphenoid spine, and eustachian cartilage, travels downward and forward to the lateral aspect of the hamulus (which is used as a pulley). It then swings medially to enter the soft palate, contracts, and effects tension on the soft palate. Now the soft palate has been pulled backward and upward.

However, the pull is not sufficient to close the gap between the distal limits of the soft palate and pharynx, so the pharynx accommodates by moving forward and medially. This is accomplished by the joint action of three muscles. The pterygopharyngeal portion of the superior constrictor, which originates usually on the medial pterygoid plate, travels backward fanwise to terminate in a median raphe in the posterior pharynx. It contracts and pulls the posterior pharyngeal wall forward to meet the soft palate (Fig. 23-11). Meanwhile, since this action may not be quite enough in certain instances, the palatopharyngeus muscle comes into play. This muscle can be seen in the throat as the posterior pillars of the tonsils and has two parts, the thyropalatal and pharyngopalatal portions. The pharyngopalatal portion of the muscle arises in the palatal aponeurosis and travels backward and downward to insert in a fanwise fashion into the posterior pharynx anterior to, but interlaced with, the superior constrictor fibers. This portion contracts strongly, is more or less circular, and produces a ridge or "bunching up" of the posterior pharyngeal musculature called Passavant's cushion in an attempt to approximate the soft palate and pharynx (Fig. 23-12). This is usually visible in the patient with a cleft palate. It is located at levels varying from as high as the region of the vertebral atlas to as low as the level of the distally projected mandibular occlusal plane. Now the soft palate is touching the posterior pharyngeal wall, but there is a leak when the lateral aspect of the soft palate does not meet the lateral aspect of the pharynx. This will be closed by the salpingopharyngeus muscle. This muscle rises from the cartilage of the eustachian tube and travels downward and laterally to fan out and insert into the lateral pharyngeal wall. When it contracts it pulls the lateral wall medially, thus closing the last gap in palatopharyngeal closure. All of these muscle contractions take place almost simultaneously. The palatopharyngeal mechanism has now closed the nasal cavity from the oral cavity and pharynx. This movement is used in deglutition to prevent food from entering the nose and in speech when pronouncing the so-called plosive sounds—/puh/, /buh/, /tuh/, /duh/, /kuh/, and /guh/. These sounds are produced by closing off the nose and building up pressure in the mouth and suddenly releasing it. Thus the name **plosive.**

The second position, the closure of the oral cavity, is a result of the contraction of the thyropalatal portion of the palatopharyngeus muscle. This portion arises from the posterolateral rim of the thyroid cartilage and courses upward through the posterior pillar to insert into the

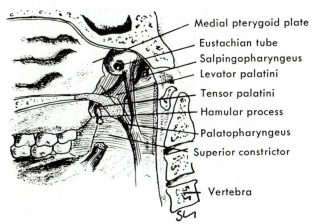

Medial pterygoid plate

Eustachian tube

Salpingopharyngeus

Levator palatini

Tensor palatini

Hamular process

Palatopharyngeus

Superior constrictor

Vertebra

Fig. 23-10. Dissection of velopharyngeal area as seen from side.

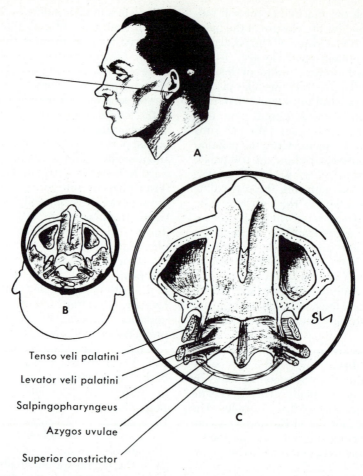

Tenso veli palatini

Levator veli palatini

Salpingopharyngeus

Azygos uvulae

Superior constrictor

Fig. 23-11. Musculature of soft palate as seen from above. **A,** Area of section. **B,** Portion of section used. **C,** Detail of section.

palatine aponeurosis, where it merges with its fellow of the opposite side, forming an inverted U. When it contracts it pulls the soft palate down toward the tongue. Meanwhile, the tensor is flattening the dome of the soft palate to bring down the portion of the structure that may not come down with the action of the thyropalatal muscle. Concurrently the tongue is forced upward and backward. To finally eliminate the possibility of a leak, the palatoglossus muscle, which is attached superiorly to the palate and inferiorly to the tongue, forming more or less a sphincteric structure in this motion, contracts and com-

pletes the approximation. Therefore it can now be seen that palatopharyngeal closure **is not** a simple sphincteric action of the superior constrictor and palatopharyngeus muscles (which run in a nearly horizontal direction), but is instead the resultant contraction of these and others, such as the levator, the tensor, and the salpingopharyngeus muscles, running in a vertical direction. The second position is used in sucking and in the pronunciation of sounds such as /ng/ in the word *sing*.

The third position finds the palate relaxed as in normal breathing.

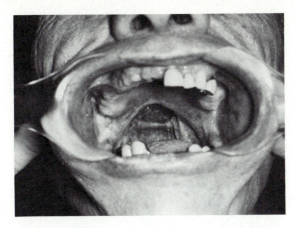

Fig. 23-12. Well-developed Passavant's pad on posterior pharyngeal wall. (From Laney, W.R., editor: Maxillofacial prosthetics, Littleton, Mass., 1979, Publishing Sciences Group.)

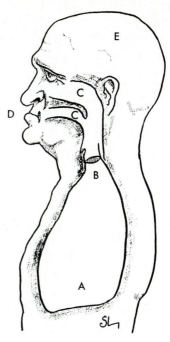

Fig. 23-13. Mechanisms of speech. *A,* Respiratory organ (lungs). *B,* Phonating organ (vocal cords). *C,* Resonating chambers (oral and nasal cavities). *D,* Articulating organs (lips, tongue, and teeth). *E,* Integrating center (brain).

Pathology

The patient with a cleft palate, because of an inability to close off the nose, is frequently the victim of nasal infections and middle ear infections, sometimes resulting in deafness. Being unable to pronounce correctly the plosive sounds, the patient tries to overcompensate with the tongue. Thus the attempt is made to obturate the cleft with the tongue and articulate at the same time. These habits are an obstacle to the speech therapist who must attempt to train the patient to forget them and learn a new set of movements.

Physiology of speech

Speech is a function of respiration, phonation, resonation, articulation, and integration. Respiration is concerned with the exchange of air by the lungs; phonation is accomplished by the abduction and adduction of the vocal cords, which change the pitch of the voice; resonation is realized in the nasal, oral, and pharyngeal cavities, which are the prime resonation chambers. The teeth, tongue, lips, and palate serve as articulatory mechanisms, and all of these components of speech would be nothing without the integrating facilities of the human brain (Fig. 23-13).

The soft palate performs any one of the following basic functions in speech. It closes off the nasal cavity, as in producing /k/ and hard /g/; it closes off the oral cavity for production of the sounds /m/, /n/, and /ng/ (as in *ring*), or it may close neither cavity completely, allowing varying portions of the airstream to enter the appropriate resonating chambers.

Although the soft palate is but one part of the palatopharyngeal mechanism (the other part being the pharyngeal muscles), it is of such importance that when cleft, the palate is incompetent.

Surgical treatment

Two general types of physical treatment can restore partially or completely the function of the soft palate. The first concerns surgical procedures to close the soft palate (and the hard

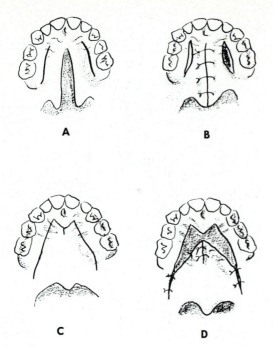

Fig. 23-14. Surgical procedures in cleft palate therapy. **A,** Relaxing incisions in palatal mucosa. **B,** Mucosa elevated and displaced medially where freshened edges of cleft are sutured together. **C,** Incision for push-back operation. **D,** Push-back completed and sutured.

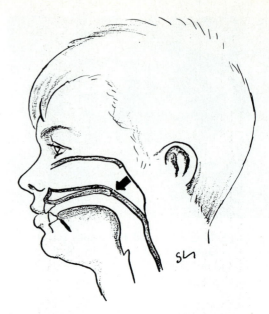

Fig. 23-15. Pharyngeal flap operation viewed from side. Flap is based below.

palate when involved). The other uses an artificial restoration or obturator, which serves not to close the soft palate but rather to fill the space between the palatal remnants. Both the surgical and prosthetic approaches are usually of little avail without speech therapy, given previously, concurrently, or subsequently. It must be noted that given the choice of a highly skilled surgeon's efforts or those of an equally skilled prosthodontist, the surgeon is preferred, for being highly skilled, the surgeon should know the chances for success in a surgical procedure and will recommend a prosthodontist if it is in the best interest of the patient. The surgical approach is generally concerned with the closure and, in many instances, the lengthening of the palate (Fig. 23-14).

When palatoplasty does not provide adequate palatal length, the surgeon may perform a pharyngeal flap operation, wherein a longitudinal

flap is dissected from the posterior pharyngeal wall (its attachment being located either below or above) and is brought forward and sutured to the denuded posterior edge of the soft palate (Fig. 23-15). This then forms a continuous tissue bridge between the soft palate and the pharynx, which functions well as part of the palatopharyngeal mechanism. The flap, as dissected, tends to curl medially, leaving lateral space for air transmission through the nasal cavity. Since much of the pharyngeal closing movement is in a medial direction, one can see that this action can aid in velopharyngeal closure because the lateral walls converge medially toward the flap. There are more definitive surgical approaches to the cleft palate, but they are generally concerned with either of these two aims.

Prosthetic treatment

The prosthetic approach uses a metal framework that is similar to a partial denture framework in which is included a posterior latticework extension into the area of the cleft (Fig. 23-16). This extension supports an acrylic resin bulb, which is the obturator.

The **preservation** of the patient's teeth is of

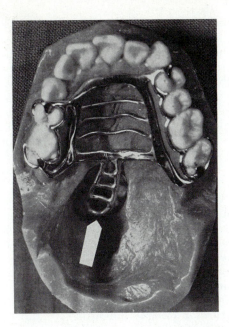

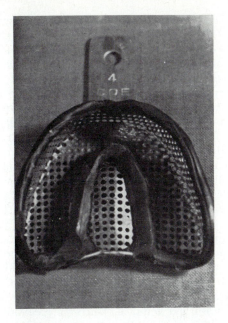

Fig. 23-16. Ladderlike extension of framework into area of cleft (arrow).

Fig. 23-17. Use of utility wax to confine impression material to tissues.

prime importance, because although obturators have been made for edentulous patients, they can never be as efficient as those that use the teeth for stabilization. Therefore all necessary restorative dentistry must be accomplished immediately. In a large percentage of patients the dentist is faced with the problem of restoring occlusal harmony, and therefore the patient may first require orthodontic treatment. However, an obturator often can be combined with the orthodontic appliance. When a patient has good occlusion, no active caries, and no periodontal disease or other oral lesions, fabrication of a more permanent prosthetic restoration may be undertaken. It is imperative that these patients be recalled for examination every 6 months and that signs of disease be treated immediately. Obturators suspected of contributing to disease must be redesigned.

Impressions with irreversible hydrocolloid impression material. An examination will reveal the nature of the unrepaired cleft or, if repaired, those perforations that sometimes result from tissue breakdown. One should look particularly in the anterior mucobuccal fold for minute oro-nasal perforations after the repair of Class III and IV clefts.

A resilient impression material must be used because of the many tissue undercuts. The irreversible (alginate) hydrocolloid impression materials serve this purpose adequately.

The problems incident to impressions are divided into two groups, the unrepaired cleft presenting one situation and the repaired cleft another. The unrepaired cleft palate, Classes II, III, and IV, will be considered first. (The method of obtaining impressions of the teeth is not modified by Class I clefts.) When one is using a hydrocolloid impression material, the posterior portion of the tray should be modified with boxing or utility wax to prevent material from flowing down the patient's throat. In addition, the use of this wax adjacent to the cleft or perforation will record more accurately the mucosal detail by confining the impression material to those areas (Fig. 23-17).

The material should be prevented from entering the nasal cavity in such a large quantity that it may fracture from the main body of material. Such an accident requires a tedious process of fragmentation and removal. To prevent this, the tray should be underloaded in the area of the cleft. The tooth-bearing section of the tray is completely filled with the alginate, but the area corresponding to the cleft is loaded to a height of only 2 to 3 mm. Thus when the tray is seated, the material is not likely to be forced upward into the cleft in sufficient quantity to lock. Cleft palates previously repaired present slightly different problems. The palatal repair itself may look adequate, and yet an oronasal perforation may exist in the labial mucobuccal fold, as previously mentioned. Since impression material would be forced into smaller perforations under more pressure, it is best to pack them with cotton or petroleum jelly and gauze.

Amounts of impression material small enough to be dislodged by blowing the nose should not be of concern. Larger amounts, however, require a considerable degree of skill in their fragmentation and removal, since they cannot be pushed into the mouth as in unrepaired defects and must be manipulated within the nasal cavity.

Those perforations that may exist on the palate itself should be approached in a similar manner. If the area is large enough to pack off with lubricated gauze, this is the method of choice. If the diameter is 12 mm or more, then perhaps it is better to handle it like an open cleft, using utility wax to dam and underload the tray in that area.

Framework. The design of the framework is of primary importance, as it must be balanced to eliminate harmful torque effects on the teeth as much as possible. The essential requirements for the casting consist of the following: (1) The metal to be used should be as thin as possible

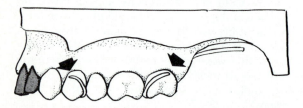

Fig. 23-18. When anterior replacements are necessary (shaded teeth), clasp on anterior abutments should engage mesial undercut. Clasp on distal abutments should engage distal undercut.

commensurate with strength so that metal bulk does not present an added obstacle to speech. (2) The tip of the clasp should engage a distal undercut on the posterior abutments to support the obturator. On abutments further anterior the clasp should engage mesial undercuts when anterior replacements are necessary (Fig. 23-18). If proper undercuts are not present or if the teeth must be restored with complete crowns because of caries or for other reasons such as fixed splinting, adequate embrasure crossing space must be planned in the restorations. It is wise to use continuous lingual stabilization or guiding planes, even on teeth not used for retentive clasps, to distribute widely the torquing forces often developed by these restorations.

The pharyngeal portion is usually attached to the framework by a distal loop or grid from the casting. The superoinferior position of the loop will vary according to the type of prosthesis.

Obturator design. Following are the three main types of obturators: the hinge or movable type, the fixed type, and the meatus type (Fig. 23-19). The hinged type is connected to the main framework by means of a hinge. Its bulk is located above the cleft edges and supposedly serves an anatomic purpose in that it moves up and back, supported by the soft palatal edges, as does the normal soft palate to effect velopharyngeal closure. Theoretically this is workable, but in practice it is not quite true because many cleft palates have limited motion. The fixed type is stationary and is directed toward the area of maximum constriction of the palatopharyngeal musculature in the oronasopharynx. This usually occurs at the level of the plane of the hard palate. The fixed type is the obturator in most general use today and, if made well, is relatively efficient. The meatus obturator will be discussed later because of the difference in construction.

Pharyngeal impressions. The methods of obtaining impressions for the hinge type or the fixed type are essentially the same and are secondary impression procedures using the framework as a tray. They involve the following steps: A mound of modeling plastic approximating the pharyngeal defect in shape and size is placed on the distal extension and warmed. This bulk is directed posteriorly above the palatal plane and after tempering is placed into the patient's

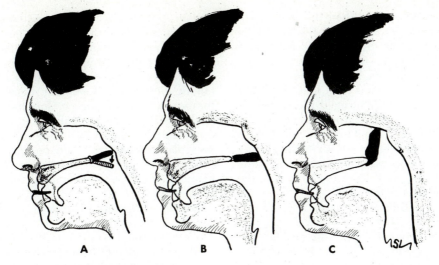

Fig. 23-19. Location of pharyngeal portion of several obturators. **A,** Hinge type. **B,** Fixed type. **C,** Meatus type.

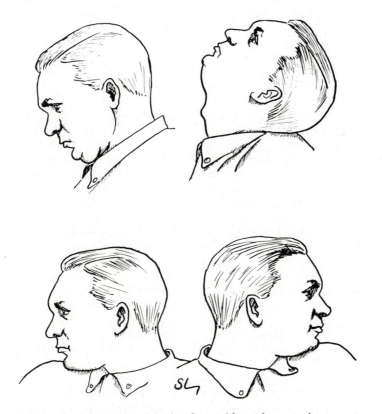

Fig. 23-20. Positions of head for border-molding pharyngeal impressions.

mouth while still warm. When the framework is seated properly on the teeth, the patient is instructed to swallow, tilt the head back, and then place the chin on the chest; from there, the head is turned from left shoulder to right shoulder (Fig. 23-20). This total routine should be accomplished quickly to mold the modeling plastic while it is still warm. The resultant impression is then removed from the mouth and compared with the defect. Gross inadequacies are noted, and if necessary more material is added. The modeling plastic impression is then removed and all excess trimmed.

It should have sufficient height and width to provide a positive soft tissue contact during palatopharyngeal function. These dimensions are confirmed by the patient's speech and by clinical judgments of hypernasality or hyponasality. Vowel sounds such as /a/ or /ee/ and /s/ or other sibilants aid in assessing palatopharyngeal competence. Refinements in the modeling plastic obturator are made in response to patient performance.

When acceptable extension has been achieved, the functionally molded impression surface is reduced 1 to 2 mm uniformly and covered with mouth-temperature wax (Iowa formula*) that has been melted and tempered in a water bath. The tempered impression is placed in the mouth and prosthesis is seated. Immediately the patient is instructed to repeat the head movements previously described, and to repeat the speech sounds on command. The patient then remains relaxed for 15 to 20 minutes, periodically repeating this routine as requested by the dentist. Care must be taken to avoid overtrimming the impression during this stage. At the conclusion of the period allowed for wax flow, the impression is examined and additions or corrections are made until it is acceptable for speech and comfort. The composite palatal and pharyngeal sections are then invested, and the obturator is processed in clear acrylic resin.

Experience in making impressions for a fixed type of restoration (and occasionally the hinge type) has demonstrated that attempts to obtain accurate detail in impression by means of the **wash** materials may be abandoned. There is a

certain amount of leakage that will occur around any obturator, and this leakage does not materially affect the efficiency of the restoration. When the patient swallows, there is a vigorous excursion of the pharyngeal musculature; when talking there is less movement. Because the restoration must be made comfortable enough to enable the patient to swallow, an air leak will occur during ordinary speech. Furthermore, the musculature changes its shape, and the detail obtained from a wash impression will not be maintained on tissue topography for any length of time.

Meatus obturator. The pharyngeal impression for a meatus obturator is considered as a separate section here. It is rarely used; the classic design is difficult to achieve in most patients but, when achieved, has dramatic results. The meatus obturator is formulated on the presumption that complete occlusion of the oropharynx from the nasopharynx is not necessary for good cleft-palatal speech. It is believed, rather, that the partial occlusion of the nasal cavity will result in a marked diminution and, in many instances, complete elimination of the nasal sound that is so apparent and objectionable in the patient with a cleft palate. If the restoration fulfills this objective, the logopedist, who when using other appliances has to train certain muscles to reduce the hypernasality and others to conquer the articulative defects, need direct efforts only toward correcting the latter. Muscle training incident to reducing nasality is unnecessary.

Whereas the usual fixed type of obturator is directed in a line more or less parallel to, and continuous with the palate, this type is inclined perpendicularly to the palate (Fig. 23-21).

The construction is not complicated. The casting is finished with the usual loop projecting into the cleft and is checked in the mouth for accuracy. With this framework as a vehicle, softened modeling plastic is molded around the distal loop with its greatest bulk directly above the loop. When the modeling plastic is hard, it is removed. More softened material is added, and the denture framework is repositioned in the mouth. Then the patient attempts to blow air through the nose. If air escapes, small amounts of modeling plastic are added in likely areas until no air escapes through the nose and the patient

---

*Kerr Mfg. Co., Romulus, Mich.

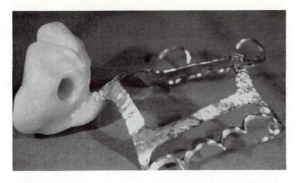

Fig. 23-21. Side view of meatus obturator showing its relation to framework.

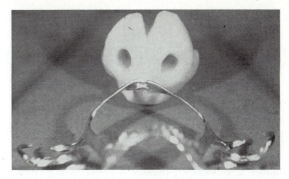

Fig. 23-22. Frontal view of meatus obturator showing vents.

talks as though afflicted with a bad cold (the so-called rhinolalia clausa). The impression is removed from the mouth, and at this time any projection of material into the eustachian tubes should be cut from the impression to allow free interchange of air.

The completed impression is invested, boiled out, and processed in clear acrylic resin. After being polished, it is placed in the patient's mouth to check for gross errors in processing. When it is satisfactory, a vent about 3 mm in diameter is cut in an anterior-posterior direction, approximately in the center and free of turbinates and vomer. If the latter is very large, it may be necessary to make two smaller vents (Fig. 23-22).

This opening serves as a means of breathing through the nose. The restoration is put back into the mouth, and the patient is instructed to speak. If the voice sounds "closed," the aperture is enlarged until a balance between the closed and open "nose" is reached. Immediately on placing the prosthesis and balancing the size of the hole, the resultant nasality should improve. Only the articulative defects remain, and these are not as unpleasant because of the normal nasal quality. There is usually no gagging tendency and no irritation of the mucous membrane.

Occlusion. The typical cleft-palate facial appearance is related to midface underdevelopment exaggerated by the relative mandibular prognathism. Current treatment planning rationale avoids early palatal surgery to encourage optimum maxillary bony growth and develop-

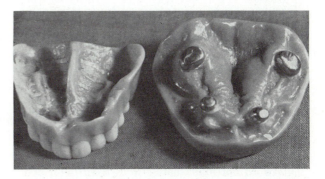

Fig. 23-23. Model of repaired cleft palate with its restoration. Four remaining maxillary teeth, which do not occlude with mandibular teeth, are crowned and act as retentive mechanism for overdenture. Occlusion is established entirely on denture.

ment. In some situations early maxillary orthopedic treatment has been effective in aligning residual jaw segments even before tooth eruption. When combined with later cleft bone-grafting procedures to stabilize more desirable positional relationships, which have been obtained, these measures can moderate developing malocclusion.

Despite such efforts, restoration of the vertical dimension of occlusion and provision of adequate support for the lip frequently pose treatment problems. When occlusal vertical and facial dimension cannot be restored with the dentition alone following orthodontic treatment, fabrication of an overdenture supported by teeth restored with metal copings usually is the treatment of choice (Fig. 23-23).

SELECTED READING RESOURCES

Rarely, if ever, is a textbook found to be all inclusive in subject matter related to a dental clinical discipline or subdiscipline. Therefore this section, listing other textbooks and articles from dental periodical literature, may assist in broadening a student's perspectives in principles and concepts in removable partial prosthodontics.

Some of the articles have historic significance and are considered classics. Contemporary selections are included, and many of the articles are current to the submission of the manuscript for this seventh edition. A background and progress of removable partial prosthodontics over the years may be extracted from this section by the serious student of dentistry.

We do not infer that sources have been exhausted in compiling the lists of either textbooks or articles. We have attempted to correctly classify listed articles for ready reference, however, the length of the *Miscellaneous* section attests to the difficulties encountered.

TEXTBOOKS

Applegate, O.C.: Essentials of removable partial denture prosthesis, Philadelphia, 1965, W.B. Saunders Co.

Baker, J.L., and Goodkind, R.J.: Theory and practice of precision attachment removable partial dentures, St. Louis, 1981, The C.V. Mosby Co.

Beumer, J., Curtis, T.A., and Firtell, D.N.: Maxillofacial prosthetics, St. Louis, 1979, The C.V. Mosby Co.

Boucher, L.J.: A comprehensive review of dentistry, Philadelphia, 1979, W.B. Saunders Co.

Boucher, L.J., and Renner, R.P.: Treatment of partially edentulous patients, St. Louis, 1982, The C.V. Mosby Co.

Brewer, A.A., and Morrow, R.M.: Overdentures, ed. 2, St. Louis, 1980, The C.V. Mosby Co.

Craig, R.G.: Restorative dental materials, ed. 6, St. Louis, 1980, The C.V. Mosby Co.

Dawson, P.E.: Evaluation, diagnosis, and treatment of occlusal problems, St, Louis, 1974, The C.V. Mosby Co.

Dolder, E.J., and Durrer, G.T.: The bar-joint denture, Chicago, 1978, Quintessence Publishing Company, Inc.

Dubrul, E.L.: Sicher's oral anatomy, ed. 7, St. Louis, 1980, The C.V. Mosby Co.

Dykema, R.W., Cunningham, D.M., and Johnston, J.F.: Modern practice in removable partial prosthodontics, Philadelphia, 1969, W.B. Saunders Co.

Ellinger, C.W., Rayson, J.H., Terry, J.M., and Unger, J.W.: Synopsis of complete dentures, Lexington, Ky., 1983, C & J Publishing Co.

Farrell, J.: Partial denture designing, London, 1970, Henry Kimpton Medical Publisher and Bookseller.

Gaerny A.: Removable closure of the interdental space (C.I.S.), Berlin and Chicago, 1972, Quintessence Publishing Company, Inc.

Goldman, H.M., and Cohen, D.W.: Periodontal therapy, ed. 6, St. Louis, 1979, The C.V. Mosby Co.

Heartwell, C.M., Jr., and Rahn, A.O.: Syllabus of complete dentures, ed. 3, Philadelphia, 1980, Lea & Febiger.

Hickey, J.C., and Zarb, G.A.: Boucher's prosthodontic treatment for edentulous patients, ed. 8, St. Louis, 1980, The C.V. Mosby Co.

Johnson, D.L., and Stratton, R.J.: Fundamentals of removable prosthodontics, Chicago, 1980, Quintessence Publishing Company, Inc.

Johnston, J.F., Phillips, R.W., and Dykema, R.W.: Modern practice in crown and bridge prosthodontics, Philadelphia, 1971, W.B. Saunders Co.

Krol, A.J.: Removable partial denture design outline syllabus, ed. 3, San Francisco, 1981, Bookstore, University of the Pacific School of Dentistry.

Laney, W.R., Desjardins, R.P., Chalian, V.A., and Gillis, R.E., Jr.: Maxillofacial prosthetics, Littleton, Mass, 1979, PSG Publishing Co.

Laney, W.R., and Gibilisco, J.A.: Diagnosis and treatment in prosthodontics, Philadelphia, 1983, Lea and Febiger.

Miller, E.L.: Removable partial prosthodontics, Baltimore, 1972, The Williams & Wilkins Co.

Osborne, J., and Lammie, G.A.: Partial dentures, ed. 4, Oxford, 1974, Blackwell Scientific Publications.

Phillips, R.W.: Skinner's science of dental materials, ed. 7, Philadelphia, 1973, W.B. Saunders Co.

Preiskel, H.W.: Precision attachments in dentistry, ed. 3, St. Louis, 1980, The C.V. Mosby Co.

Ramfjord, S.P., and Ash, M.M., Jr.: Occlusion, ed. 2, Philadelphia, 1971, W.B. Saunders Co.

Rudd, K.D., Eissman, H.F., and Morrow, R.M.: Dental laboratory procedures, vol. III, Removable partial dentures, St. Louis, 1981, The C.V. Mosby Co.

Sharry, J.J., editor: Complete denture prosthodontics, ed. 3, New York, 1974, McGraw-Hill Book Co.

Singer, F., and Schön, F.: Partial dentures, Chicago, 1973, Quintessence Publishing Company, Inc.

Stewart, K.L., Kueliker, W.A., and Rudd, K.D.: Clinical removable partial prosthodontics, St. Louis, 1982, The C.V. Mosby Co.

Tylman, S.D., and Malone, W.P.F.: Tylman's theory and practice of fixed prosthodontics, ed. 7, St. Louis, 1978, The C.V. Mosby Co.

Yalisove, I.L., and Dietz, J.B., Jr.: Telescopic prosthetic therapy, Philadelphia, 1979, George F. Stickley Co.

Zarb, G.A., Bergman, B., Clayton, J.A., and MacKay, H.F.: Prosthodontic treatment for partially edentulous patients, St. Louis, 1978, The C.V. Mosby Co.

Zwemer, T.J., editor: Boucher's clinical dental terminology, ed. 3, St. Louis, 1982, The C.V. Mosby Co.

ABUTMENT RETAINERS: EXTERNAL AND INTERNAL ATTACHMENTS

Adisman, I.K.: The internal clip attachment in fixed-removable partial denture prosthesis, N.Y. J. Dent. **32**:125-129, 1962.

Ainamo, J.: Precision removable partial dentures with pontic abutments, J. Prosthet. Dent. **23**:289-295, 1970.

Augsburger, R.H.: The Gilmore attachment, J. Prosthet. Dent. **16**:1090-1102, 1966.

Becker, C.M., Campbell, M.C., and Williams, D.L.: The Thompson dowel-rest system modified for chrome-cobalt removable partial denture frameworks, J. Prosthet. Dent. **39**:384-391, 1978.

Berg, T., Jr.: I-bar: myth and countermyth, Dent. Clin. North Am. **23**:1, 65-75, 1979.

Blatterfein, L.: Study of partial denture clasping, J. Am. Dent. Assoc. **43**:169-185, 1951.

Blatterfein, L.: Design and positional arrangement of clasps for partial dentures, N.Y. J. Dent. **22**:305-306, 1952.

Breisach, L.: Esthetic attachments for removable partial dentures, J. Prosthet. Dent. **17**:261-265, 1967.

Brodbelt, R.H.W.: A simple paralleling template for precision attachments, J. Prosthet. Dent. **27**:285-288, 1972.

Brudvik, J.S., and Wormley, J.H.: Construction techniques for wrought wire retentive clasp arms are related to clasp flexibility, J. Prosthet. Dent. **30**:769-774, 1973.

Caldarone, C.V.: Attachments for partial dentures without clasps, J. Prosthet. Dent. **7**:206-208, 1957.

Clayton, J.A.: A stable base precision attachment removable partial denture (PARPD): theories and principles, Dent. Clin. North Am. **24**:3-29, 1980.

Cooper, H.: Practice management related to precision attachment prostheses, Dent. Clin. North Am. **24**:45-61, 1980.

DeVan, M.M.: Fortn. Rev. Chic. Dent. Soc. **27**:7-12 (portrait), 1954.

DeVan, M.M.: Preserving natural teeth through the use of clasps, J. Prosthet. Dent. **5**:208-214, 1955.

Dietz, W.H.: Modified abutments for removable and fixed prosthodontics, J. Prosthet. Dent. **11**:1112-1116, 1961.

Dolder, E.J.: The bar joint mandibular denture, J. Prosthet. Dent. **11**:689-707, 1961.

Eliason, C.M.: RPA clasp design for distal-extension removable partial dentures, J. Prosthet. Dent. **49**:25-27, 1983.

Farrell, J.: Wrought wire retainers—a method of increasing their flexibility, Br. Dent. J. **131**:327, 1971.

Frank, R.P., Brudvik, J.S., and Nicholls, J.I.: A comparison of the flexibility of wrought wire and cast circumferential clasps, J. Prosthet. Dent. **49**:471-476, 1983.

Garver, D.G.: A new clasping system for unilateral distal-extension removable partial dentures, J. Prosthet. Dent. **39**:268-273, 1978.

Gillings, B.R.D.: Co-Sm closed-field magnets as retentive aids in sectional dentures and removable sectional bridges, J. Dent. Res. (I.A.D.R. abstract 222a) **59**:entire issue, 1980.

Gilson, T.D.: A fixable-removable prosthetic attachment, J. Prosthet. Dent. **9**:247-255, 1959.

Gindea, A.E.: A retentive device for removable dentures, J. Prosthet. Dent. **27**:501-508, 1972.

Grasso, J.E.: A new removable partial denture clasp assembly, J. Prosthet. Dent. **43**:618-21, 1980.

Green, J.H.: The hinge-lock abutment attachment, J. Am. Dent. Assoc. **47**:175-180, 1953.

Handlers, M., Lenchner, N.H., and Weissman, B.: A retaining device for partial dentures, J. Prosthet. Dent. **7**:483-488, 1957.

Hekneby, M.: The spring-slide joint for lower free end removable partial dentures, J. Prosthet. Dent. **11**:256-263, 1961.

Highton, R., Caputo, A.A., and Matyas, J.: Retention and stress characteristics for a magnetically-retained partial denture, J. Dent. Res. (I.A.D.R. abstract 279) **62**:entire issue, 1982.

Isaacson, G.O.: Telescope crown retainers for removable partial dentures, J. Prosthet. Dent. **22**:436-448, 1969.

James, A.G.: Self-locking posterior attachment for removable tooth-supported partial dentures, J. Prosthet. Dent. **5**:200-205, 1955.

Johnson, J.F.: The application and construction of the pin-ledge retainer, J. Prosthet. Dent. **3**:559-567, 1953.

Knodle, J.M.: Experimental overlay and pin partial denture, J. Prosthet. Dent. **17**:472-478, 1967.

Knowles, L.E.: A dowel attachment removable partial denture, J. Prosthet. Dent. **13**:679-687, 1963.

Koper, A.: Retainer for removable partial dentures—the Thompson dowel, J. Prosthet. Dent. **30**:759-768, 1973.

Kotowicz, W.E.: Clinical procedures in precision attachment removable partial denture construction, Dent. Clin. North Am. **24**:143-164, 1980.

Kotowicz, W.E., Fisher, R.L., Reed, R.A., and Jaslow, C.: The combination clasp and the distal extension removable partial denture, Dent. Clin. North Am. **17**:651-660, 1973.

Krol, A.J.: Clasp design for extension base removable partial dentures, J. Prosthet. Dent. **29**:408-415, 1973.

Krol, A.J.: RPI clasp retainer and its modifications, Dent. Clin. North Am. **17**:631-649, 1973.

Langer, A.: Combinations of diverse retainers in removable partial dentures, J. Prosthet. Dent. **40**:378-384, 1978.

Lubovich, R.P., and Peterson, T.: The fabrication of a ceramic-metal crown to fit an existing removable partial denture clasp, J. Prosthet. Dent. **37**:610-614, 1977.

Mann, A.W.: The lower distal extension partial denture using the Hart-Dunn attachment, J. Prosthet. Dent. **8**:282-288, 1958.

McLeod, N.S.: A theoretical analysis of the mechanics of the Thompson dowel semiprecision intracoronal retainer, J. Prosthet. Dent. **37**:19-27, 1977.

McLeod, N.S.: Improved design for the Thompson dowel rest semiprecision intracoronal retainer, J. Prosthet. Dent. **40**:513-516, 1978.

Mensor, M.C., Jr.: Attachment fixation for overdentures, I. J. Prosthet. Dent. **37**:366-373, 1977.

Mensor, M.C., Jr.: Attachment fixation of the overdenture. II. J. Prosthet. Dent. **39**:16-20, 1978.

Morrison, M.L.: Internal precision attachment retainers for partial dentures, J. Am. Dent. Assoc. **64**:209-215, 1962.

Morrow, R.M.: Tooth-supported complete dentures: an approach to preventive prosthodontics, J. Prosthet. Dent. **21**:513-522, 1969.

Myers, G.E., Wepfer, G.G., and Peyton, F.A.: The thiokol rubber base impression materials, J. Prosthet. Dent. **8**:330-339, 1958.

Oddo, V.J., Jr.: The movable-arm clasp for complete passivity in partial denture construction, J. Am. Dent. Assoc. **74**:1009-1015, 1967.

Plotnik, I.J.: Internal attachment for fixed removable partial dentures, J. Prosthet. Dent. **8**:85-93, 1958.

Pound, E.: Cross-arch splinting vs. premature extractions, J. Prosthet. Dent. **16**:1058-1068, 1966.

Preiskel, H.: Precision attachments for free-end saddle prostheses, Br. Dent. J. **127**:462, 468, 1969.

Preiskel, H.: Screw retained telescopic prosthesis, Br. Dent. J. **130**:107-112, 1971.

Prince, I.B.: Conservation of the supportive mechanism, J. Prosthet. Dent. **15**:327-338, 1965.

Singer, F.: Improvements in precision—attached removable partial dentures, J. Prosthet. Dent. **17**:69-72, 1967.

Smith, R.A., and Rymarz, F.P.: Cast clasp transitional removable partial dentures, J. Prosthet. Dent. **22**:381-385, 1969.

Stankewitz, C.G., Gardner, F.M., and Butler, G.V.: Adjustment of cast clasps for direct retention, J. Prosthet. Dent. **45**:344, 1981.

Stansbury, B.E.: A retentive attachment for overdentures, J. Prosthet. Dent. **35**:228-230, 1976.

Stewart, B.L., and Edwards, R.O.: Retention and wear of precision-type attachments, J. Prosthet. Dent. **49**:28-34, 1983.

Strohaver, R.A., and Trovillion, H.M.: Removable partial overdentures, J. Prosthet. Dent. **35**:624-629, 1976.

Tautin, F.S.: Abutment stabilization using a nonresilient gingival bar connector, J. Am. Dent. Assoc. **99**:988-989, 1979.

Vasic, S., et al.: An aesthetic clasp for acrylic partial dentures, J. Can. Dent. Assoc. **37**:38-39, 1971.

Vig. R.G.: Splinting bars and maxillary indirect retainers for removable partial dentures, J. Prosthet. Dent. **13**:125-129, 1963.

Walter, J.D.: Anchor attachments used as locking devices in two-part removable prostheses,[1] J. Prosthet. Dent. **33**:628-632, 1975.

Waltz, M.E.: Ceka extracoronal attachments, J. Prosthet. Dent. **29**:167-171, 1973.

Wands, D.: The semi-precision dowel rest retainer for removable partial dentures. In Clark, J.W., editor: Clinical dentistry, vol. 5, New York, 1976, Harper & Row, Publishers, Inc.

White, J.T.: Visualization of stress and strain related to removable partial denture abutments, J. Prosthet. Dent. **40**:143-151, 1978.

Williams, A.G.: Technique for provisional splint with attachment, J. Prosthet. Dent. **21**:555-559, 1969.

Willis, L.M., and Swoope, C.C.: Precision attachment partial dentures. In Clark, J.W., editor: Clinical dentistry, vol. 5, New York, 1976, Harper & Row, Publishers, Inc.

Zakler, J.M.: Intracoronal precision attachments, Dent. Clin. North Am. **24**:131-141, 1980.

Zinner, I.D.: Semiprecision rest system for distal extension removable partial denture design, J. Prosthet. Dent. **42**:131-134, 1979.

ANATOMY

Barker, B.C.W.: Dissection of regions of interest to the dentist from a medical approach, Aust. Dent. J. **16**:163-171, 1971.

Bennett, N.G.: A contribution to the study of the movements of the mandible, J. Prosthet. Dent. **8**:41-54, 1958.

Boucher, C.O.: Anatomy of the mouth in relation to complete dentures, J. Wis. State Dent. Soc. **19**:161-166, 1943.

Boucher, C.O.: Complete denture impressions based upon the anatomy of the mouth, J. Am. Dent. Assoc. **31**:1174-1181, 1944.

Brodie, A.G.: Anatomy and physiology of head and neck musculature, Am. J. Orthod. **36**:831-844, 1950.

Casey, D.M.: Palatopharyngeal anatomy and physiology, J. Prosthet. Dent. **49**:371-378, 1983.

Craddock, F.W.: Retromolar region of the mandible, J. Am. Dent. Assoc. **47**:453-455, 1953.

Haines, R.W., and Barnett, S.G.: The structure of the mouth in the mandibular molar region, J. Prosthet. Dent. **9**:962-974, 1959.

Last, R.J.: The muscles of the mandible, Dent. Dig. **61**:165-169, 1955.

Martone, A.L., et al.: Anatomy of the mouth and related structures. I. J. Prosthet. Dent. **11**:1009-1018, 1961; II. **12**:4-27, 1962; III. **12**:206-219, 1962; IV. **12**:409-419, 1962; V. **12**:629-636, 1962; VI. **12**:817-834, 1962; VII. **13**:4-33, 1963; VIII. **13**:204-228, 1963.

Merkeley, H.J.: The labial and buccal accessory muscles of mastication, J. Prosthet. Dent. **4**:327-334, 1954.

Merkeley, H.J.: Mandibular rearmament. I. Anatomic considerations, J. Prosthet. Dent. **9**:559-566, 1959.

Pendleton, E.C.: Anatomy of the face and mouth from the standpoint of the denture prosthetist, J. Am. Dent. Assoc. **33**:219-234, 1946.

Pendleton, E.C.: Changes in the denture supporting tissues, J. Am. Dent. Assoc. **42**:1-15, 1951.

Pietrokovski, J.: The bony residual ridge in man, J. Prosthet. Dent. **34**:456-462, 1975.

Pietrokovski, J., Sorin, S., and Zvia, H.: The residual ridge in partially edentulous patients, J. Prosthet. Dent. **36**:150-158, 1976.

Preti, G., Bruscagin, C., and Fava, C.: Anatomic and statistical study to determine the inclination of the condylar long axis, J. Prosthet. Dent. **49**:572-575, 1983.

Roche, A.F.: Functional anatomy of the muscles of mastication, J. Prosthet. Dent. **13**:548-570, 1963.

Silverman, S.I.: Denture prosthesis and the functional anatomy of the maxillofacial structures, J. Prosthet. Dent. **6**:305-331, 1956.

BIOMECHANICS

Applegate, O.C.: Use of the paralleling surveyor in modern partial denture construction, J. Am. Dent. Assoc. **27**:1397-1407, 1940.

Avant, W.E.: Factors that influence retention of removable partial dentures, J. Prosthet. Dent. **25**:265-270, 1971.

Avant, W.E.: Fulcrum and retention lines in planning removable partial dentures, J. Prosthet. Dent. **25**:162-166, 1971.

Aydinlik, E., and Akay, H.U.: Effect of a resilient layer in a removable partial denture base on stress distribution to the mandible, J. Prosthet. Dent. **44**:17-20, 1980.

Brudevold, F.: Basic study of the chewing forces of a denture wearer, J. Am. Dent. Assoc. **43**:45-51, 1951.

Brudvik, J.S., and Morris, H.F.: Stress-relaxation testing. Part III: Influence of wire alloys, gauges, and lengths on clasp behavior, J. Prosthet. Dent. **46**:374-379, 1981.

Cecconi, B.T.: Effect of rest design on transmission of forces to abutment teeth, J. Prosthet. Dent. **32**:141-151, 1974.

Cecconi, B.T., Asgar, K., and Dootz, E.: The effect of partial denture clasp design on abutment tooth movement, J. Prosthet. Dent. **25**:44-56, 1971.

Cecconi, B.T., Asgar, K., and Dootz, E.: Removable partial denture abutment tooth movement as affected by inclination of residual ridges and types of loading, J. Prosthet. Dent. **25**:375-381, 1971.

Cecconi, B.T., Asgar, K., and Dootz, E.: Clasp assembly modifications and their effect on abutment tooth movement, J. Prosthet. Dent. **27**:160-167, 1972.

Clayton, J.A., and Jaslow, C.: A measurement of clasp forces on teeth, J. Prosthet. Dent. **25**:21-43, 1971.

Craig, R.G., and Farah, J.W.: Stresses from loading distal extension removable partial dentures, J. Prosthet. Dent. **39**:274-277, 1978.

DeVan, M.M.: The nature of the partial denture foundation: suggestions for its preservation, J. Prosthet. Dent. **2**:210-218, 1952.

Fisher, R.L.: Factors that influence the base stability of mandibular distal-extension removable partial dentures: a longitudinal study, J. Prosthet. Dent. **50**:167-171, 1983.

Frank, R.P., and Nicholls, J.I.: A study of the flexibility of wrought wire clasps, J. Prosthet. Dent. **45**:259-267, 1981.

Frechette, A.R.: The influence of partial denture design on distribution of force to abutment teeth, J. Prosthet. Dent. **6**:195-212, 1956.

Fujita, T., and Caputo, A.A.: Photo-elastic stress analysis of occlusal force distribution with peridontally involved teeth, J. Dent. Res. (I.A.D.R. abstract 122) **59**:entire issue, 1980.

Goodkind, R.J.: The effects of removable partial dentures on abutment tooth mobility, J. Prosthet. Dent. **30**:139-146, 1973.

Goodman, J.J., and Goodman, H.W.: Balance of force in precision free-end restorations, J. Prosthet. Dent. **13**:302-308, 1963.

Hall, W.A.: Variations in registering interarch transfers in removable partial denture construction, J. Prosthet. Dent. **30**:548-553, 1973.

Harrop, J., and Javid, N.: Reciprocal arms of direct retainers in removable partial dentures, J. Canad. Dent. Assoc. **4**:208-211, 1976.

Henderson, D., and Seward, T.E.: Design and force distribution with removable partial dentures; a progress report, J. Prosthet. Dent. **17**:350-364, 1967.

Highton, R., and Caputo, A.A.: Force transmission by labial and lingual I-bar partial dentures, J. Dent. Res. (I.A.D.R. abstract) **59**:entire issue, 1980.

Hindels, G.W.: Stress analysis in distal extension partial dentures, J. Prosthet. Dent. **7**:197-205, 1957.

Johnson, D.L., Stratton, R.J., and Duncanson, M.G.J.: The effect of single plane curvature on half-round cast clasps, J. Dent. Res. **62**:833-836, 1983.

Kaires, A.K.: Partial denture design and its relation to force distribution and masticatory performance, J. Prosthet. Dent. **6**:672-683, 1956.

Khalil, M.F., et al.: Three dimensional photo-elastic analysis of cantilever bridge and precision attachment removable partial denture, J. Dent. Res. (I.A.D.R. abstract 1009) **59**:entire issue, 1980.

Knowles, L.E.: The biomechanics of removable partial dentures and its relationship to fixed prosthesis, J. Prosthet. Dent. **8**:426-430, 1958.

Kratochvil, F.J.: Influence of occlusal rest position and clasp design on movement of abutment teeth, J. Prosthet. Dent. **13**:114-124, 1963.

Kratochvil, F.J., Thompson, W.D., and Caputo, A.A.: Photoelastic analysis of stress patterns on teeth and bone with attachment retainers for removable partial dentures, J. Prosthet. Dent. **46**:21-28, 1981.

Lofbers, P.G., Ericson, G., and Eliasson, S.: A clinical and radiographic evaluation of removable partial dentures retained by attachments to alveolar bars, J. Prosthet. Dent. **47**:126-132, 1982.

Lowe, R.O., et al.: Swallowing and resting forces related to lingual flange thickness in removable partial dentures, J. Prosthet. Dent. **23**:279-288, 1970.

MacGregor, A.R., Miller, T.P.G., and Farah, J.W.: Stress analysis of partial dentures, J. Dent. **6**:125-132, 1978.

Maroso, D.J., Schmidt, J.R., and Blustein, R.: A preliminary study of wear of porcelain when subjected to functional movements of retentive clasp arms, J. Prosthet. Dent. **45**:14-17, 1981.

McCartney, J.W.: Motion vector analysis of an abutment for a distal-extension removable partial denture, J. Prosthet. Dent. **43**:15-21, 1980.

McDowell, G.C.: Force transmission by indirect retainers during unilateral loading, J. Prosthet. Dent. **39**:616-621, 1978.

McDowell, G.C., and Fisher, R.L.: Force transmission by indirect retainers when a unilateral dislodging force is applied, J. Prosthet. Dent. **47**:360-365, 1982.

McLeod, N.S.: An analysis of the rotational axes of semi-precision and precision distal-extension removable partial dentures, J. Prosthet. Dent. **48**:130-134, 1982.

Morris, H.F., Asgar, K., and Tillitson, E.: Stress-relaxation testing. Part I: A new approach to the testing of removable partial denture alloys, wrought wires, and clasp behavior, J. Prosthet. Dent. **46**:133-141, 1981.

Morris, H.F., et al.: Stress-relaxation testing. Part IV: Clasp pattern dimensions and their influence on clasp behavior, J. Prosthet. Dent. **50**:319-326, 1983.

Nery, E.B., et al.: Functional loading of bioceramic augmented alveolar ridge—a pilot study, J. Prosthet. Dent. **43**:338-343, 1980.

Plotnick, I.J., Beresin, V.E., and Simkins, A.B.: The effects of variations in the opposing dentition on changes in the partially edentulous mandible. I. J. Prosthet. Dent. **33**:278-286, 1975; II. **33**:403-406, 1975; III. **33**:529-534, 1975.

Shohet, H.: Relative magnitudes of stress on abutment teeth with different retainers, J. Prosthet. Dent. **21**:267-282, 1969.

Smith, B.H.: Changes in occlusal face height with removable partial dentures, J. Prosthet. Dent. **34**:278-285, 1975.

Smith, B.J., and Turner, C.H.: The use of crowns to modify abutment teeth of removable partial dentures, J. Dent. **7**:52-56, 1979.

Smyd, E.S.: Bio-mechanics of prosthetic dentistry, J. Prosthet. Dent. **4**:368-383, 1954.

Smyd, E.S.: The role of tongue, torsion, and bending in prosthodontic failures, J. Prosthet. Dent. **11**:95-111, 1961.

Stern, W.J.: Guiding planes in clasp reciprocation and retention, J. Prosthet. Dent. **34**:408-414, 1975.

Swoope, C.C., and Frank, R.P.: Stress control and design. In Clark, J.W., editor: Clinical dentistry, vol. 5, New York, 1976, Harper & Row, Publishers, Inc.

Taylor, D.T., Pflushoeft, F.A., and McGivney, G.P.: Effect of two clasping assemblies on arch integrity as modified by base adaptation, J. Prosthet. Dent. **47**:120-125, 1982.

Wills, D.J., and Manderson, R.D.: Biomechanical aspects of the support of partial dentures, J. Dent. **5**:310-318, 1977.

Yurkstas, A., Fridley, H.H., and Manly, R.S.: A functional evaluation of fixed and removable bridgework, J. Prosthet. Dent. **1**:570-577, 1951.

Zoeller, G.N.: Block form stability in removable partial dentures, J. Prosthet. Dent. **22**:633-637, 1969.

Zoeller, G.N., and Kelly, W.J., Jr.: Block form stability in removable partial prosthodontics, J. Prosthet. Dent. **25**:515-519, 1971.

CLASSIFICATION

Applegate, O.C.: The rationale of partial denture choice, J. Prosthet. Dent. **10**:891-907, 1960.

Avant, W.E.: A universal classification for removable partial denture situations, J. Prosthet. Dent. **16**:533-539, 1966.

Bailyn, M.: Tissue support in partial denture construction, Dent. Cosmos **70**:988-997, 1928.

Beckett, L.S.: The influence of saddle classification on the design of partial removable restoration, J. Prosthet. Dent. **3**:506-516, 1953.

Costa, E.: A simplified system for identifying partially edentulous arches, J. Prosthet. Dent. **32**:639-645, 1974.

Cummer, W.E.: Partial denture service. In Anthony, L.P., editor: American textbook of prosthetic dentistry, Philadelphia, 1942, Lea & Febiger.

Friedman, J.: The ABC classification of partial denture segments, J. Prosthet. Dent. **3**:517-524, 1953.

Godfrey, R.J.: Classification of removable partial dentures, J. Am. Coll. Dent. **18**:5-13, 1951.

Mensor, M.C., Jr.: Classification and selection of attachments, J. Prosthet. Dent. **29**:494-497, 1973.

Miller, E.L.: Systems for classifying partially dentulous arches, J. Prosthet. Dent. **24**:25-40, 1970.

Skinner, C.N.: A classification of removable partial dentures based upon the principles of anatomy and physiology, J. Prosthet. Dent. **9**:240-246, 1959.

CLEFT PALATE

Aram, A., and Subtelny, J.D.: Velopharyngeal function and cleft palate prostheses, J. Prosthet. Dent. **9**:149-158, 1959.

Baden, E.: Fundamental principles of orofacial prosthetic therapy in congenital cleft palate, J. Prosthet. Dent. **4**:420-433, 1954.

Bixler, D.: Heritability of clefts of the lips and palate, J. Prosthet. Dent. **33**:100-108, 1975.

Buckner, H.: Construction of a denture with hollow obturator, lid and soft acrylic lining, J. Prosthet. Dent. **31**:95-99, 1974.

Calvan, J.: The error of Gustan Passavant, Plast. Reconstr. Surg. **13**:275-289, 1954.

Cooper, H.K.: Integration of service in the treatment of cleft lip and cleft palate, J. Am. Dent. Assoc. **47**:27-32, 1953.

Dalston, R.M.: Prosthodontic management of the cleft-palate patient: a speech pathologist's view, J. Prosthet. Dent. **37**:327-329, 1978.

Ettinger, R.L.: Use of teeth with a poor prognosis in cleft palate prosthodontics, J. Am. Dent. Assoc. **94**:910-914, 1977.

Fox, A.: Prosthetic correction of a severe acquired cleft palate, J. Prosthet. Dent. **8**:542-546, 1958.

Gibbons, P., and Bloomer, H.: A supportive-type prosthetic speech aid, J. Prosthet. Dent. **8**:362-369, 1958.

Graber, T.M.: Oral and nasal structures in cleft palate speech, J. Am. Dent. Assoc. **53**:693-706, 1956.

Harkins, C.S.: Modern concepts in the prosthetic rehabilitation of cleft palate patients, J. Oral Surg. **10**:298-312, 1952.

Harkins, C.S., and Ivy, R.H.: Surgery and prosthesis in the rehabilitation of cleft palate patients, J. South. Calif. Dent. Assoc. **19**:16-24, 1951.

Immekus, J.E., and Aramy, M.A.: A fixed-removable partial denture for cleft palate patients, J. Prosthet. Dent. **34**:286-291, 1975.

Landa, J.S.: The prosthodontist views the rehabilitation of the cleft palate patient, J. Prosthet. Dent. **6**:421-427, 1956.

Lavelle, W.E., and Zach, G.E.: The tissue bar and Ceka anchor as aids in cleft palate rehabilitation, J. Prosthet. Dent. **30**:321-325, 1973.

Lloyd, R.S., Pruzansky, S., and Subtelny, J.D.: Prosthetic rehabilitation of a cleft palate patient subsequent to multiple surgical and prosthetic failures, J. Prosthet. Dent. **7**:216-230, 1957.

Merkeley, H.J.: Cleft palate prosthesis, J. Prosthet. Dent. **9**:506-513, 1959.

Nidiffer, T.J., and Shipmon, T.H.: The hollow-bulb obturator for acquired palatal openings, J. Prosthet. Dent. **7**:126-134, 1957.

Olinger, N.A.: Cleft palate prosthesis rehabilitation, J. Prosthet. Dent. **2**:117-135, 1952.

Rosen, M.S.: Prosthetics for the cleft palate patient, J. Am. Dent. Assoc. **60:**715-721, 1960.

Rothenberg, L.I.A.: Overlay dentures for the cleft-palate patient, J. Prosthet. Dent. **37:**190-195, 1977.

Schneiderman, C.R., and Maun, M.B.: Air flow and intelligibility of speech of normal speakers and speakers with a prosthodontically repaired cleft palate, J. Prosthet. Dent. **39:**193-199, 1978.

Sharry, J.J.: The meatus obturator in cleft palate prosthesis, Oral Surg. **7:**852-855, 1954.

Sharry, J.J.: Meatus obturator in particular and pharyngeal impressions in general, J. Prosthet. Dent. **8:**893-896, 1958.

Tautin, F.S., and Schaaf, N.A.: Superiorly based obturator, J. Prosthet. Dent. **33:**96-99, 1975.

COMPLETE MOUTH AND OCCLUSAL REHABILITATION

Brewer, A.A., and Fenton, A.H.: The overdenture, Dent. Clin. North Am. **17:**723-746, 1973.

Bronstein, B.R.: Rationale and technique of biomechanical occlusal rehabilitation, J. Prosthet. Dent. **4:**352-367, 1954.

Cohn, L.A.: Occluso-rehabilitation, Principles of diagnosis and treatment planning, Dent. Clin. North Am., pp. 259-281, March, 1962.

Dubin, N.A.: Advances in functional occlusal rehabilitation, J. Prosthet. Dent. **6:**252-258, 1956.

Kazis, H.: Functional aspects of complete mouth rehabilitation, J. Prosthet. Dent. **4:**833-841, 1954.

Kornfeld, M.: The problem of function in restorative dentistry, J. Prosthet. Dent. **5:**670-676, 1955.

Landa, J.S.: An analysis of current practices in mouth rehabilitation, J. Prosthet. Dent. **5:**527-537, 1955.

Mann, A.W., and Pankey, L.D.: Oral rehabilitation utilizing the Pankey-Mann instrument and a functional bite technique, Dent. Clin. North Am., pp. 215-230, March, 1959.

Mann, A.W., and Pankey, L.D.: Oral rehabilitation. I. Use of the P-M instrument in treatment planning and restoring the lower posterior teeth, J. Prosthet. Dent. **10:**135-150, 1960.

Mann, A.W., and Pankey, L.D.: Oral rehabilitation. II. Reconstruction of the upper teeth using a functionally generated path technique, J. Prosthet. Dent. **10:**151-162, 1960.

McCartney, J.W.: Occlusal reconstruction and rebase procedure for distal extension removable partial dentures, J. Prosthet. Dent. **43:**695-698, 1980.

Rubinstein, M.N.: Approach to mouth reconstruction, Dent. Dig. **61:**24-28, 1955.

Schuyler, C.H.: An evaluation of incisal guidance and its influence on restorative dentistry, J. Prosthet. Dent. **9:**374-378, 1959.

Schweitzer, J.M.: Open bite from the prosthetic point of view, Dent. Clin. North Am., pp. 269-283, March, 1957.

CROWNS AND FIXED PARTIAL DENTURES

Alexander, P.C.: Analysis of the cuspid protective occlusion, J. Prosthet. Dent. **13:**309-317, 1963.

Beeson, P.E.: The use of acrylic resins as an aid in the development of patterns for two types of crowns, J. Prosthet. Dent. **13:**493-498, 1963.

Caplan, J.: Maintenance of full coverage fixed-abutment bridges, J. Prosthet. Dent. **5:**852-854, 1955.

Coelho, D.H.: The ultimate goal in fixed bridge procedures, J. Prosthet. Dent. **4:**667-672, 1954.

Coelho, D.H.: Criteria for the use of fixed prosthesis, Dent. Clin. North Am., pp. 299-311, March, 1957.

Cooper, T.M., et al.: Effect of venting on cast gold full crowns, J. Prosthet. Dent. **26:**621-626, 1971.

Cowgen, G.T.: Retention, resistance and esthetics of the anterior three-quarter crown, J. Am. Dent. Assoc. **62:**167-171, 1961.

Culpepper, W.D., and Moulton, P.S.: Considerations in fixed prosthodontics, Dent. Clin. North Am. **23:**21-35, 1979.

Ewing, J.E.: Re-evaluation of the cantilever principle, J. Prosthet. Dent. **7:**78-92, 1957.

Freese, A.S.: Impressions for temporary acrylic resin jacket crowns, J. Prosthet. Dent. **7:**99-101, 1957.

Goldberg, A., and Jones, R.D.: Constructing cast crowns to fit existing removable partial denture clasps, J. Prosthet. Dent. **36:**382-386, 1976.

Guyer, S.E.: Nonrigid subocclusal connector for fixed partial dentures, J. Prosthet. Dent. **26:**433-436, 1971.

Hagerman, D.A., and Arnim, S.S.: The relation of new knowledge of the gingiva to crown and bridge procedures, J. Prosthet. Dent. **5:**538-542, 1955; Dent. Abstr. **1:**44, 1956.

Henderson, D., et al.: The cantilever type of posterior fixed partial dentures: a laboratory study, J. Prosthet. Dent. **24:**47-67, 1970.

Hill, G.M.: Construction of a crown to fit a removable partial denture clasp, J. Prosthet. Dent. **38:**226-228, 1977.

Johnson, E.A., Jr.: Combination of fixed and removable partial dentures, J. Prosthet. Dent. **14:**1099-1106, 1964.

Johnston, J.F., Dykeman, R.W., Mumford, G., and Phillips, R.W.: Construction and assembly of porcelain veneer gold crowns and pontics, J. Prosthet. Dent. **12:**1125-1137, 1962.

Kahn, A.E.: Reversible hydrocolloids in the construction of the unit-built porcelain bridge, J. Prosthet. Dent. **6:**72-79, 1956.

Kunisch, W.H., and Dodd, J.: A conversion alternative to ceramics in a crown-and-sleeve coping prosthesis, J. Prosthet. Dent. **49:**581-582, 1983.

Leff, A.: New concepts in the preparation of teeth for full coverage, J. Prosthet. Dent. **5:**392-400, 1955.

Leff, A.: Reproduction of tooth anatomy and positional relationship in full cast or veneer crowns, J. Prosthet. Dent. **6:**550-557, 1956.

Malson, T.S.: Anatomic cast crown reproduction, J. Prosthet. Dent. **9:**106-112, 1959.

Mueninghoff, K.A., and Johnson, M.H.: Fixed-removable partial dentures, J. Prosthet. Dent. **48:**547-550, 1982.

Nuttal, E.B.: Clinical and technical aspects of crown and bridge prosthesis, Bull. Phila. Cty. Dent. Soc. **14:**128-133, 1950.

Patur, B.: The role of occlusion and the periodontium in restorative procedures, J. Prosthet. Dent. **21:**371-379, 1969.

Phillips, R.W., and Biggs, D.H.: Distortion of wax patterns as influenced by storage time, storage temperature, and temperature of wax manipulation, J. Am. Dent. Assoc. **41**:28-37, 1950.

Phillips, R.W., and Price, R.R.: Some factors which influence the surface of stone dies poured in alginate impressions, J. Prosthet. Dent. **5**:72-79, 1955.

Phillips, R.W., and Swartz, M.L.: A study of adaptation of veneers to cast gold crowns, J. Prosthet. Dent. **7**:817-822, 1957.

Pound, E.: The problem of the lower anterior bridge, J. Prosthet. Dent. **5**:543-545, 1955.

Preston, J.D.: Preventing ceramic failures when integrating fixed and removable prostheses, Dent. Clin. North Am. **23**:37-52, 1979.

Pruden, K.C.: A hydrocolloid technique for pin-ledge bridge abutments, J. Prosthet. Dent. **6**:65-71, 1956.

Pruden, W.H.: Full coverage, partial coverage, and the role of pins, J. Prosthet. Dent. **26**:302-306, 1971.

Rhoads, J.E.: The fixed-removable partial denture, J. Prosthet. Dent. **48**:122-129, 1982.

Rubin, M.K.: Full coverage: the provisional and final restorations made easier, J. Prosthet. Dent. **8**:664-672, 1958.

Sheets, C.E.: Dowel and core foundations, J. Prosthet. Dent. **23**:58-65, 1970.

Shooshan, E.D.: The reverse pin-porcelain facing, J. Prosthet. Dent. **9**:284-301, 1959.

Smith, G.P.: The marginal fit of the full cast shoulderless crown, J. Prosthet. Dent. **7**:231-243, 1957.

Smith, G.P.: Objectives of a fixed partial denture, J. Prosthet. Dent. **11**:463-473, 1961.

Staffanou, R.S., and Thayer, K.E.: Reverse pin-porcelain veneer and pontic technique, J. Prosthet. Dent. **12**:1138, 1145, 1962.

Sulek, W.D., and Plekovich, E.J.: A scanning electron microscopic comparison of porcelain polishing techniques, J. Dent. Res. (I.A.D.R. abstract 1104) **59**:entire issue, 1980.

Talkov, L.: The copper band splint, J. Prosthet. Dent. **6**:245-251, 1956.

Thurgood, B.W., Thayer, K.E., and Lee, R.E.: Complete crowns constructed for an existing partial denture, J. Prosthet. Dent. **29**:507-512, 1973.

Treppo, K.W., and Smith, F.W.: A technique for restoring abutments for removable partial dentures, J. Prosthet. Dent. **40**:398-401, 1978.

Troxell, R.R.: The polishing of gold castings, J. Prosthet. Dent. **9**:668-675, 1959.

Wagman, S.S.: Tissue management for full cast veneer crowns, J. Prosthet. Dent. **15**:106-117, 1965.

Wagner, A.W., Burkhart, J.W., and Fayle, H.E., Jr.: Contouring abutment teeth with cast gold inlays for removable partial dentures, J. Prosthet. Dent. **201**:330-334, 1968.

Wallace, F.H.: Resin transfer copings, J. Prosthet. Dent. **8**:289-292, 1958.

Welsh, S.L.: Complete crown construction for a clasp-bearing abutment, J. Prosthet. Dent. **34**:320-323, 1975.

Wheeler, R.C.: Complete crown form and the periodontium, J. Prosthet. Dent. **11**:722-734, 1961.

Yalisove, I.L.: Crown and sleeve-coping retainers for removable partial prostheses, J. Prosthet. Dent. **16**:1069-1085, 1966.

DENTAL LABORATORY PROCEDURES

Asgar, K., and Peyton, F.A.: Casting dental alloys to embedded wires, J. Prosthet. Dent. **15**:312-321, 1965.

Becker, C.M., Smith, E.E., and Nicholls, J.I.: The comparison of denture-base processing techniques. I. Material characteristics, J. Prosthet. Dent. **37**:330-338, 1977.

Benfield, J.W., and Lyons, G.V.: Precision dies from elastic impressions, J. Prosthet. Dent. **12**:737-752, 1962.

Blanchard, C.H.: Filling undercuts on refractory casts with investment, J. Prosthet. Dent. **3**:417-418, 1953.

Bolouri, A., Hilger, T.C., and Gowrylok, M.D.: Modified flasking technique for removable partial dentures, J. Prosthet. Dent. **34**:221-223, 1975.

Brudvik, J.S., and Nicholls, J.I.: Soldering of removable partial dentures, J. Prosthet. Dent. **49**:762-765, 1983.

Casey, D.M., Crowther, D.S., and Lauciello, F.R.: Strengthening abutment or isolated teeth on removable partial denture master casts, J. Prosthet. Dent. **46**:105-106, 1981.

Collett, H.A.: Casting chrome-cobalt alloys in small laboratories, J. Prosthet. Dent. **21**:2-266, 1969.

Dirksen, L.C., and Campagna, S.J.: Mat surface and rugae reproduction for upper partial denture castings, J. Prosthet. Dent. **4**:67-72, 1954.

Dootz, E.R., Craig, R.G., and Peyton, F.A.: Influence of investments and duplicating procedures on the accuracy of partial denture castings J. Prosthet. Dent. **15**:679-690, 1965.

Dootz, E.R., Craig, R.G., and Peyton, F.A.: Aqueous acrylamide gel duplicating material, J. Prosthet. Dent. **17**:570-577, 1967.

Dootz, E.R., Craig, R.G., and Peyton, F.A.: Simplification of the chrome-cobalt partial denture casting procedure, J. Prosthet. Dent. **17**:464-471, 1967.

Elbert, C.A., and Ryge, G.: The effect of heat treatment on hardness of a chrome-cobalt alloy, J. Prosthet. Dent. **15**:873-879, 1965.

Elliott, R.W.: The effects of heat on gold partial denture castings, J. Prosthet. Dent. **13**:688-698, 1963.

Enright, C.M.: Dentist-dental laboratory harmony, J. Prosthet. Dent. **11**:393-394, 1961.

Fiebiger, G.E., Parr, G.R., and Goldman, B.M.: Remount casts for removable partial dentures, J. Prosthet. Dent. **48**:106-107, 1982.

Fowler, J.A., Jr., Kuebker, W.A., and Escobedo, J.J.: Laboratory procedures for the maintenance of a removable partial overdenture, J. Prosthet. Dent. **50**:121-126, 1983.

Garfield, R.E.: Replacing an abutment crown for an existing removable partial denture, J. Prosthet. Dent. **45**:103-107, 1981.

Garver, D.G.: Updated laboratory procedure for the subpontic clasping system, J. Prosthet. Dent. **48**:734-735, 1982.

Gay, W.D.: Laboratory procedures for fitting removable partial denture frameworks. J. Prosthet. Dent. **40**:227-229, 1978.

Gilson, T.D., Asgar, K., and Peyton, F.A.: The quality of union formed in casting gold to embedded attachment metals, J. Prosthet. Dent. **15**:464-473, 1965.

Grunewald, A.H., Paffenbarger, G.C., and Dickson, G.:

The effect of molding processes on some properties of denture resins, J. Am. Dent. Assoc. 44:269-284, 1952.

Grunewald, A.H., Paffenbarger, G.C., and Dickson, G.: Dentist, dental laboratory, and the patient, J. Prosthet. Dent. **8**:55-60, 1958.

Gruenwald, A.H., Paffenbarger, G.C., and Dickson, G.: The role of the dental technician in a prosthetic service, Dent. Clin. North Am., pp. 359-370, July, 1960.

Haller, B., Stankewitz, C.G., and Gardner, F.M.: Technique for mounting altered cast using initial anatomic plaster records, J. Prosthet. Dent. **45**:681, 1981.

Hanson, J.G., et al.: Effect on dimensional accuracy when reattaching fractured lone standing teeth of a cast, J. Prosthet. Dent. **47**:488-492, 1982.

Johnson, H.B.: Technique for packing and staining complete or partial denture bases, J. Prosthet. Dent. **6**:154-159, 1956.

Jones, D.W.: Thermal analysis and stability of refractory investments, J. Prosthet. Dent. **18**:234-241, 1967.

Jordan, R.D., Turner, K.A., and Taylor, T.D.: Multiple crowns fabricated for an existing removable partial denture, J. Prosthet. Dent. **48**:102-105, 1982.

Kazanoglu, A., and Smith, E.H.: Replacement technique for a broken occlusal rest, J. Prosthet. Dent. **48**:621-623, 1982.

Lanier, B.R., et al.: Making chromium-cobalt removable partial dnetures: a modified technique, J. Prosthet. Dent. **25**:197-205, 1971.

Lauciello, F.R.: Technique for remounting removable partial dentures opposing maxillary complete dentures, J. Prosthet. Dent. **45**:336-340, 1981.

Mahler, D.B., and Ady, A.B.: The influence of various factors on the effective setting expansion of casting investments, J. Prosthet. Dent. **13**:365-373, 1963.

McCartney, J.W.: The acrylic resin base maxillary removable partial denture: technical considerations, J. Prosthet. Dent. **43**:467-468, 1980.

Morris, H.F., Asgar, K., Rowe, A.P., and Nasjleti, C.E.: The influence of heat treatments on several types of base-metal removable partial denture alloys, J. Prosthet. Dent. **41**:388-395, 1979.

Perry, C.K.: Transfer base for removable partial dentures, J. Prosthet. Dent. **31**:582-584, 1974.

Peyton, F.A., and Anthony, D.H.: Evaluation of dentures processed by different techniques, J. Prosthet. Dent. **13**:269-281, 1963.

Quinlivan, J.T.: Fabrication of a simple ball-socket attachment, J. Prosthet. Dent. **32**:222-225, 1974.

Radue, J.T., and Unser, J.W.: Constructing stable record bases for removable partial dentures. J. Prosthet. Dent. **46**:463, 1981.

Raskin, E.R.: An indirect technique for fabricating a crown under an existing clasp, J. Prosthet. Dent. **50**:580-581, 1983.

Reitz, P.V., and Weiner, M.G.: Fabrication of interim acrylic resin removable partial dentures with clasps, J. Prosthet. Dent. **40**:686-688, 1978.

Ryge, G., Kozak, S.F., and Fairhurst, C.W.: Porosities in dental gold castings, J. Am. Dent. Assoc. **54**:746-754, 1957.

Sarnat, A.E., and Klugman, R.S.: A method to record the path of insertion of a removable partial denture, J. Prosthet. Dent. **46**:222-223, 1981.

Scandrett, F.R., Hanson, J.G., and Unsicker, R.L.: Layered silicone rubber technique for flasking removable partial dentures, J. Prosthet. Dent. **40**:349-350, 1978.

Schmidt, A.H.: Repairing chrome-cobalt castings, J. Prosthet. Dent. **5**:385-387, 1955.

Schneider, R.L.: Custom metal occlusal surfaces for acrylic resin denture teeth, J. Prosthet. Dent. **46**:98-101, 1981.

Schneider, R.L.: Adapting ceramometal restorations to existing removable partial dentures, J. Prosthet. Dent. **49**:279-281, 1983.

Schwalm, C.A., and LaSpina, F.Y.: Fabricating swinglock removable partial denture frameworks, J. Prosthet. Dent. **45**:216-220, 1981.

Shay, J.S., and Mattingly, S.L.: Technique for the immediate repair of removable partial denture facings, J. Prosthet. Dent. **47**:104-106, 1982.

Simmons, E.B., Wagner, A.G., and Traweek, F.C.: Processing acrylic resin bases for removable partial dentures on a hydrocolloid cast, J. Prosthet. Dent. **39**:692-696, 1978.

Smith, G.P.: The responsibility of the dentist toward laboratory procedures in fixed and removable partial denture prosthesis, J. Prosthet. Dent. **13**:295-301, 1963.

Smith, R.A.: Clasp repair for removable partial dentures, J. Prosthet. Dent. **29**:231-234, 1973.

Stankewitz, C.G.: Acrylic resin blockout for interim removable partial dentures, J. Prosthet. Dent. **40**:470-471, 1978.

Swoope, C.C., and Frank, R.P.: Fabrication procedures. In Clark, J.W., editor: Clinical dentistry, vol. 5, New York, 1976, Harper & Row, Publishers, Inc.

Sykora, O.: A new tripoding technique, J. Prosthet. Dent. **44**:463-464, 1980.

Teppo, K.W., and Smith, F.W.: A method of immediate clasp repair, J. Prosthet. Dent. **30**:77-80, 1975.

Tuccillo, J.J., and Nielsen, J.P.: Compatibility of alginate impression materials and dental stones, J. Prosthet. Dent. **25**:556-566, 1971.

Ulmer, F.C., and Ward, J.E.: Simplified technique for production of a distal-extension removable partial denture remounting cast, J. Prosthet. Dent. **41**:473-474, 1979.

Williams, H.N., Falkler, W.A., Jr., and Hasler, J.F., Acinetobacter contamination of laboratory dental pumice, J. Dent. Res. **62**:1073-1075, 1983.

DENTURE ESTHETICS: TOOTH SELECTION AND ARRANGEMENT

Askinas, S.W.: Facings in removable partial dentures, J. Prosthet. Dent. **33**:633-636, 1975.

Culpepper, W.D.: A comparative study of shade-matching procedures, J. Prosthet. Dent. **24**:166-173, 1971.

DeVan, M.M.: The appearance phase of denture construction, Dent. Clin. North Am., pp. 255-268, March, 1957.

Fields, H., Jr., Birtles, J.T., and Shay, J.: Combination prosthesis for optimum esthetic appearance, J. Am. Dent. Assoc. **101**:276-279, 1980.

French, F.A.: The selection and arrangement of the anterior

teeth in prosthetic dentures, J. Prosthet. Dent. **1**:587-593, 1951.

Frush, J.P., and Fisher, R.D.: Introduction to dentogenic restorations, J. Prosthet. Dent. **5**:586-595, 1955.

Frush, J.P., and Fisher, R.D.: How dentogenic restorations interpret the sex factor, J. Prosthet. Dent. **6**:160-172, 1956.

Frush, J.P., and Fisher, R.D.: How dentogenics interprets the personality factor, J. Prosthet. Dent. **6**:441-449, 1956.

Hughes, G.A.: Facial types and tooth arrangement, J. Prosthet. Dent. **1**:82-95, 1951.

Krajicek, D.D.: Natural appearance for the individual denture patient, J. Prosthet. Dent. **10**:205-214, 1960.

Levin, E.I.: Dental esthetics and the golden proportion, J. Prosthet. Dent. **40**:244-252, 1978.

Lombardi, R.E.: Factors mediating against excellence in dental esthetics, J. Prosthet. Dent. **38**:243-248, 1977.

Myerson, R.L.: The use of porcelain and plastic teeth in opposing complete dentures, J. Prosthet. Dent. **7**:625-633, 1957.

Payne, A.G.L.: Factors influencing the position of artificial upper anterior teeth, J. Prosthet. Dent. **26**:26-32, 1971.

Pound, E.: Lost—fine arts in the fallacy of the ridges, J. Prosthet. Dent. **4**:6-16, 1954.

Pound, E.: Recapturing esthetic tooth position in the edentulous patient, J. Am. Dent. Assoc. **55**:181-191, 1957.

Pound, E.: Applying harmony in selecting and arranging teeth, Dent. Clin. North Am., pp. 241-258, March, 1962.

Roraff, A.R.: Instant photographs for developing esthetics, J. Prosthet. Dent. **26**:21-25, 1971.

Smith, B.J.: Esthetic factors in removable partial prosthodontics, Dent. Clin. North Am. **23**:53-63, 1979.

Tillman, E.J.: Molding and staining acrylic resin anterior teeth, J. Prosthet. Dent. **5**:497-507, 1955; Dent. Abstr. **1**:111, 1956.

Van Victor, A.: Positive duplication of anterior teeth for immediate dentures, J. Prosthet. Dent. **3**:165-177, 1953.

Van Victor, A.: The mold guide cast—its significance in denture esthetics, J. Prosthet. Dent. **13**:406-415, 1963.

Vig, R.G.: The denture look, J. Prosthet. Dent. **11**:9-15, 1961.

Wallace, D.H.: The use of gold occlusal surfaces in complete and partial dentures, J. Prosthet. Dent. **14**:326-333, 1964.

Wolfson, E.: Staining and characterization of acrylic teeth, Dent. Abstr. **1**:41, 1956.

Young, H.A.: Denture esthetics, J. Prosthet. Dent. **6**:748-755, 1956.

Zarb, G.A., and MacKay, H.F.: Cosmetics and removable partial dentures—the class IV partially edentulous patient, J. Prosthet. Dent. **46**:360-368, 1981.

DIAGNOSIS AND TREATMENT PLANNING

Applegate, O.C.: Evaluating oral structures for removable partial dentures, J. Prosthet. Dent. **11**:882-885, 1961.

Bartels, J.C.: Diagnosis and treatment planning, J. Prosthet. Dent. **7**:657-662, 1957.

Bennett, C.G.: Transitional restorations for function and esthetics, J. Prosthet. Dent. **15**:867-872, 1965.

Blatterfein, L.: The planning and contouring of acrylic resin veneer crowns for partial denture clasping, J. Prosthet. Dent. **6**:386-404, 1956.

Blatterfein, L., and Kaufman, E.G.: Prevention of problems with removable partial dentures. Council on Dental Materials, Instruments, and Equipment, J. Am. Dent. Assoc. **100**:919-921, 1980.

Bolender, C.L., Swenson, R.D., and Yamane, G.: Evaluation of treatment of inflammatory papillary hyperplasia of the palate, J. Prosthet. Dent. **15**:1013-1022, 1965.

Casey, D.M., and Lauciello, F.R.: A review of the submerged-root concept, J. Prosthet. Dent. **43**:128-132, 1980.

Contino, R.M., and Stallard, H.: Instruments essential for obtaining data needed in making a functional diagnosis of the human mouth, J. Prosthet. Dent. **7**:66-77, 1957.

Dreizen, S.: Nutritional changes in the oral cavity, J. Prosthet. Dent. **16**:1144-1150, 1966.

Dummer, P.M.H., and Gidden, J.: The upper anterior sectional denture, J. Prosthet. Dent. **41**:146-152, 1979.

Dunn, B.W.: Treatment planning for removable partial dentures, J. Prosthet. Dent. **11**:247-255, 1961.

Foster, T.D.: The use of the face-bow in making permanent study casts, J. Prosthet. Dent. **9**:717-721, 1959.

Frechette, A.R.: Partial denture planning with special reference to stress distribution, J. Prosthet. Dent. **1**:700-707 (disc., 208-209), 1951.

Friedman, S.: Effective use of diagnostic data, J. Prosthet. Dent. **9**:729-737, 1959.

Garver, D.G., and Fenster, R.K.: Vital root retention in humans: a final report, J. Prosthet. Dent. **43**:368-373, 1980.

Garver, D.G., et al.: Vital root retention in humans: a preliminary report, J. Prosthet. Dent. **40**:23-28, 1978.

Guyer, S.E.: Selectively retained vital roots for partial support of overdentures: a patient report, J. Prosthet. Dent. **33**:258-263, 1975.

Harvey, W.L.: A transitional prosthetic appliance, J. Prosthet. Dent. **14**:60-70, 1964.

Heintz, W.D.: Treatment planning and design: prevention of errors of ommission and commission, Dent. Clin. North Am. **23**:3-12, 1979.

Henderson, D., Hickey, J.C., and Wehner, P.J.: Prevention and preservation—the challenge of removable partial denture service, Dent. Clin. North Am., pp. 459-473, July, 1965.

House, M.M.: The relationship of oral examination to dental diagnosis, J. Prosthet. Dent. **8**:208-219, 1958.

Kabcenell, J.L.: Planning for individualized prosthetic treatment, J. Prosthet. Dent. **34**:405-407, 1975.

Killebrew, R.F.: Crown construction and splinting of mobile partial denture abutments, J. Am. Dent. Assoc. **70**:334-338, 1965.

Krikos, A.A.: Preparing guide planes for removable partial dentures, J. Prosthet. Dent. **34**:152-155, 1975.

Lambson, G.O.: Papillary hyperplasia of the palate, J. Prosthet. Dent. **16**:636-645, 1966.

Lopes, I., and Norlau, L.A.: Specific mechanics for abutment uprighting, Aust. Dent. J. **25**:273-278, 1980.

McCracken, W.L.: Differential diagnosis: fixed or removable partial dentures, J. Am. Dent. Assoc. **63**:767-775, 1961.

McGill, W.J.: Acquiring space for partial dentures, J. Prosthet. Dent. **17**:163-165, 1967.

Miller, E.L.: Planning partial denture construction, Dent. Clin. North Am. **17**:571-584, 1973.

Miller, E.L.: Critical factors in selecting removable prosthesis, J. Prosthet. Dent. 34:486-490, 1975.

Mopsik, E.R., Buck, R.P., Connors, J.O., and Watts, L.N.: Surgical intervention to reestablish adequate intermaxillary space before fixed or removable prosthodontics, J. Am. Dent. Assoc. 95:957-960, 1977.

Moulton, G.H.: The importance of centric occlusion in diagnosis and treatment planning, J. Prosthet. Dent. 10:921-926, 1960.

Nassif, J., and Blumenfeld, W.L.: Joint consultation services by the periodontist and prosthodontist, J. Prosthet. Dent. 29:55-60, 1973.

Nassif, J., Blumenfeld, W.L., and Tarsitano, J.T.: Dialogue—a treatment modality, J. Prosthet. Dent. 33:696-700, 1975.

Payne, S.H.: Diagnostic factors which influence the choice of posterior occlusion, Dent. Clin. North Am., pp. 203-213, March, 1957.

Rudd, K.D., and Dunn, B.W.: Accurate removable partial dentures, J. Prosthet. Dent. 18:559-570, 1967.

Saunders, T.R., Gillis, R.E., and Desjardins, R.P.: The maxillary complete denture opposing the mandibular bilateral distal-extension partial denture: treatment considerations, J. Prosthet. Dent. 41:124-128, 1979.

Sauser, C.W.: Pretreatment evaluation of partially edentulous arches, J. Prosthet. Dent. 11:886-893, 1961.

Seiden, A.: Occlusal rests and rest seats, J. Prosthet. Dent. 8:431-440, 1958.

Swoope, C.C., and Frank, R.P.: Removable partial dentures indications and planning. In Clark, J.E., editor: Clinical dentistry, vol. 5, New York, 1976, Harper & Row, Publishers, Inc.

Turner, C.E., and Shaffer, F.W.: Planning the treatment of the complex prosthodontic case, J. Am. Dent. Assoc. 97:992-993, 1978.

Uccellani, E.L.: Evaluating the mucous membranes of the edentulous mouth, J. Prosthet. Dent. 15:295-303, 1965.

Wagner, A.G.: Instructions for the use and care of removable partial dentures, J. Prosthet. Dent. 26:481-490, 1971.

Waldron, C.A.: Oral leukoplakia, carcinoma, and the prosthodontist, J. Prosthet. Dent. 15:367-376, 1965.

Walker, W.A., and Kramer, D.C.: Claspless chrome-cobalt transitional removable partial dentures, J. Am. Dent. Assoc. 96:814-818, 1978.

Waller, M.I.: The root seat and the removable partial denture: a clinical investigation, J. Prosthet. Dent. 34:1623, 1975.

Welker, W.A., and Kramer, D.C.: Claspless chrome-cobalt transitional removable partial dentures, J. Am. Dent. Assoc. 96:814-818, 1978.

Young, H.A.: Diagnostic survey of edentulous patients, J. Prosthet. Dent. 5:5-14, 1955.

IMPRESSION MATERIALS AND METHODS; THE PARTIAL DENTURE BASE

Akerly, W.B.: A combination impression and occlusal registration technique for extension-base removable partial dentures, J. Prosthet. Dent. 39:226-229, 1978.

Appleby, D.C., Cohen, S.R., Racowsky, L.P., and Mingledorff, E.B.: The combined reversible hydrocolloid/irreversible hydrocolloid impression system: clinical application, J. Prosthet. Dent. 46:48-58, 1981.

Applegate, O.C.: The partial denture base, J. Prosthet. Dent. 5:636-648, 1955.

Applegate, O.C.: An evaluation of the support for the removable partial denture, J. Prosthet. Dent. 10:112-123, 1960.

Bailey, L.R.: Acrylic resin tray for rubber base impression materials, J. Prosthet. Dent. 5:658-662, 1955.

Bailey, L.R.: Rubber base impression techniques, Dent. Clin. North Am., pp. 156-166, March, 1957.

Bauman, R., and DeBoer, J.: A modification of the altered cast technique, J. Prosthet. Dent. 47:212-213, 1982.

Beaumont, A.J.: Sectional impression for maxillary Class I removable partial dentures and maxillary immediate dentures, J. Prosthet. Dent. 49:438-441, 1983.

Blatterfein, L., Klein, I.E., and Miglino, J.C.: A loading impression technique for semiprecision and precision removable partial dentures, J. Prosthet. Dent. 43:9-14, 1980.

Chase, W.W.: Adaptation of rubber-base impression materials to removable denture prosthetics, J. Prosthet. Dent. 10:1043-1050, 1960.

Chong, M.P., et al.: The tear test as a means of evaluating the resistance to rupture of alginate impression materials, Aust. Dent. J. 16:145-151, 1971.

Clark, R.J., and Phillips, R.W.: Flow studies of certain dental impression materials, J. Prosthet. Dent. 7:259-266, 1957.

DeFreitas, J.F.: Potential toxicants in alginate powders, Aust. Dent. J. 25:224-228, 1980.

Dootz, E.R.: Fabricating non-precious metal bases, Dent. Clin. North Am. 24:113-122, 1980.

Ellio, B., and Lamb, D.J.: The setting characteristics of alginate impression materials, Br. Dent. J. 151:343-346, 1981.

Frank, R.P.: Analysis of pressures produced during maxillary edentulous impression procedures, J. Prosthet. Dent. 22:400-403, 1969.

Fusayama, T., and Nakazato, M.: The design of stock trays and the retention of irreversible hydrocolloid impressions, J. Prosthet. Dent. 21:136-142, 1969.

Gilmore, W.H., Schnell, R.J., and Phillips, R.W.: Factors influencing the accuracy of silicone impression materials, J. Prosthet. Dent. 9:304-314, 1959.

Harris, W.T., Jr.: Water temperature and accuracy of alginate impressions, J. Prosthet. Dent. 21:613-617, 1969.

Harrison, J.D.: Prevention of failures in making impressions and dies, Dent. Clin. North Am. 23:13-20, 1979.

Heartwell, C.M., et al.: Comparison of impressions made in perforated and nonperforated rimlocks trays, J. Prosthet. Dent. 27:494-500, 1972.

Herfort, T.W., et al.: Viscosity of elastomeric impression materials, J. Prosthet. Dent. 38:396-404, 1977.

Holmes, J.B.: Influence of impression procedures and occlusal loading on partial denture movement, J. Prosthet. Dent. 15:474-481, 1965.

Hudson, W.C.: Clinical uses of rubber impression materials and electroforming of casts and dies in pure silver, J. Prosthet. Dent. 8:107-114, 1958.

Huggett, R., Jagger, R.G., and Bates, J.F.: Strength of the acrylic denture base tooth bond, Br. Dent. J. 153:187-190, 1982.

Johnston, J.F., Cunningham, D.M., and Bogan, R.G.: The

dentist, the patient, and ridge preservation, J. Prosthet. Dent. **10**:288-295, 1960.

Jarvis, R.G., and Earnshaw, R.: The effect of alginate impressions on the surface of cast gypsum. II. The role of sodium sulphate in incompatibility, Aust. Dent. J. **26**:12-17, 1981.

Koran, A., III: Impression materials for recording the denture bearing mucosa, Dent. Clin. North Am. **24**:97-111, 1980.

Kramer, H.M.: Impression technique for removable partial dentures, J. Prosthet. Dent. **11**:84-92, 1961.

Leach, C.D., and Donovan, T.E.: Impression technique for maxillary removable partial dentures, J. Prosthet. Dent. **50**:283-286, 1983.

Lee, R.E.: Mucostatics, Dent. Clin. North Am. **24**:81-96, 1980.

Leupold, R.J.: A comparative study of impression procedures for distal extension removable partial dentures, J. Prosthet. Dent. **16**:708-720, 1966.

Leupold, R.J., and Kratochvil, F.J.: An altered-cast procedure to improve support for removable partial dentures, J. Prosthet. Dent. **15**:672-678, 1965.

McCrorie, J.W.: Corrective impression waxes. A simple formula, Br. Dent. J. **152**:95-96, 1982.

Mitchell, J.V., and Damele, J.J.: Influence of tray design upon elastic impression materials, J. Prosthet. Dent. **23**:51-57, 1970.

Morrow, R.M., et al.: Compatibility of alginate impression materials and dental stones, J. Prosthet. Dent. **25**:556-566, 1971.

Myers, G.E.: Electroformed die technique for rubber base impressions, J. Prosthet. Dent. **8**:531-535, 1958.

O'Brien, W.J.: Base retention, Dent. Clin. North Am. **24**:123-130, 1980.

Pfeiffer, K.A.: Clinical problems in the use of alginate hydrocolloid, Dent. Abstr. **2**:82, 1957.

Phillips, R.W.: Factors influencing the accuracy of reversible hydrocolloid impressions, J. Am. Dent. Assoc. **43**:1-17, 1951.

Phillips, R.W.: Factors affecting the surface of stone dies poured in hydrocolloid impressions, J. Prosthet. Dent. **2**:390-400, 1952.

Phillips, R.W.: Elastic impression materials—a second progress report of a recent conference, J. South. Calif. Dent. Assoc. **26**:150-153, 1958.

Phillips, R.W.: Physical properties and manipulation of rubber impression materials, J. Am. Dent. Assoc. **59**:454-458, 1959.

Prieskel, H.W.: Impression techniques for attachment-retained distal extension removable partial dentures, J. Prosthet. Dent. **25**:620-628, 1971.

Rapuano, J.A.: Single tray dual-impression technique for distal extension partial dentures, J. Prosthet. Dent. **24**:41-46, 1970.

Rehberg, H.J.: The impression tray—an important factor in impression precision, Int. Dent. J. **27**:146-153, 1977.

Rosenstiel, E.: Rubber base elastic impression materials, Dent. Abstr. **1**:55, 1956.

Rudd, K.D., Morrow, R.M., and Bange, A.A.: Accurate casts, J. Prosthet. Dent. **21**:545-554, 1969.

Rudd, K.D., Morrow, R.M., and Strunk, R.R.: Accurate alginate impressions, J. Prosthet. Dent. **22**:294-300, 1969.

Rudd, et al.: Comparison of effects of tap water and slurry water on gypsum casts, J. Prosthet. Dent. **24**:563-570, 1970.

Silver, M.: Impressions and silver-plated dies from a rubber impression material, J. Prosthet. Dent. **6**:543-549, 1956.

Smith, P.K.: The effect on the accuracy of polysulphide impression material after treating preparations with various agents, Aust. Dent. J. **16**:337-339, 1971.

Smith, R.A.: Secondary palatal impressions for major connector adaptation, J. Prosthet. Dent. **24**:108-110, 1976.

Stafford, G.D., and MacCulloch, W.T.: Radiopaque denture base materials, Br. Dent. J. **131**:22-24, 1971.

Steffel, V.L.: Relining removable partial dentures for fit and function, J. Prosthet. Dent. **4**:496-509, 1954; J. Tenn. Dent. Assoc. **36**:35-43, 1956.

Storer, R., and McCabe, J.F.: An investigation of methods available for sterilizing impressions, Br. Dent. J. **151**:217-219, 1981.

Vahidi, F.: Vertical displacement of distal-extension ridges by different impression techniques, J. Prosthet. Dent. **40**:374-377, 1978.

Wilson, J.H.: Partial dentures—relining the saddle supported by the mucosa and alveolar bone, J. Prosthet. Dent. **3**:807-813, 1953.

Young, J.M.: Surface characteristics of dental stone: impression orientation, J. Prosthet. Dent. **33**:336-341, 1975.

MAXILLOFACIAL PROSTHESIS

Ackerman, A.J.: Maxillofacial prosthesis, Oral Surg. **6**:176-200, 1953.

Ackerman, A.J.: The prosthetic management of oral and facial defects following cancer surgery, J. Prosthet. Dent. **5**:413-432, 1955.

Brown, K.E.: Fabrication of a hollow-bulb obturator, J. Prosthet. Dent. **21**:97-103, 1969.

Brown, K.E.: Reconstruction considerations for severe dental attrition, J. Prosthet. Dent. **44**:384-388, 1980.

Cantor, R., et al.: Methods for evaluating prosthetic facial materials, J. Prosthet. Dent. **21**:324-332, 1969.

Curtis, T.A., and Cantor, R.: The forgotten patient in maxillofacial prosthesis, J. Prosthet. Dent. **31**:662-680, 1974.

Desjardins, R.P.: Prosthodontic management of the cleft palate patient, J. Prosthet. Dent. **33**:655-665, 1975.

Firtell, D.N., and Curtis, T.A.: Removable partial denture design for the mandibular resection patient, J. Prosthet. Dent. **48**:437-443, 1982.

Firtell, D.N., and Grisius, R.J.: Retention of obturator—removable partial dentures: a comparison of buccal and lingual retention, J. Prosthet. Dent. **43**:211-217, 1980.

Gay, W.D., and King, G.E.: Applying basic prosthodontic principles in the dentulous maxillectomy patient, J. Prosthet. Dent. **43**:433-435, 1980.

Goll, G.: Design for maximal retention of obturator prosthesis for hemimaxillectomy patients (letter), J. Prosthet. Dent. **48**:108-109, 1982.

Immekus, J.E., and Aramy, M.: Adverse effects of resilient denture liners in overlay dentures, J. Prosthet. Dent. **32**:178-181, 1974.

Kelley, E.K.: Partial denture design applicable to the maxillofacial patient, J. Prosthet. Dent. **15**:168-173, 1965.

King, G.E., and Martin, J.W.: Cast circumferential and wire clasps for obturator retention, J. Prosthet. Dent. **49**:799-802, 1983.

Metz, H.H.: Mandibular staple implant for an atrophic mandibular ridge: solving retention difficulties of a denture, J. Prosthet. Dent. **32**:572-578, 1974.

Monteith, G.G.: The partially edentulous patient with special problems, Dent. Clin. North Am. **23**:107-115, 1979.

Moore, D.J.: Cervical esophagus prosthesis, J. Prosthet. Dent. **30**:442-445, 1973.

Nethery, W.J., and Delclos, L.: Prosthetic stent for gold-grain implant to the floor of the mouth, J. Prosthet. Dent. **23**:81-87, 1970.

Shifman, A., and Lepley, J.B.: Prosthodontic management of postsurgical soft tissue deformities associated with marginal mandibulectomy. Part I: Loss of the vestibule, J. Prosthet. Dent. **48**:178-183, 1982.

Smith, E.H., Jr.: Prosthetic treatment of maxillofacial injuries, J. Prosthet. Dent. **5**:112-128, 1955.

Strain, J.C.: A mechanical device for duplicating a mirror image of a cast or moulage in three dimensions, J. Prosthet. Dent. **5**:129-132, 1955.

Toremalm, N.G.: A disposable obturator for maxillary defects, J. Prosthet. Dent. **29**:94-96, 1973.

Weintraub, G.S., and Yalisove, I.L.: Prosthodontic therapy for cleidocranial dysostosis: report of cast, J. Am. Dent. Assoc. **96**:301-305, 1978.

Wright, S.M., Pullen-Warner, E.A., and LeTissier, D.R.: Design for maximal retention of obturator prosthesis for hemimaxillectomy patients, J. Prosthet. Dent. **47**:88-91, 1982.

Young, J.M.: The prosthodontist's role in total treatment of patients, J. Prosthet. Dent. **27**:399-412, 1972.

MISCELLANEOUS

Abere, D.J.: Post-placement care of complete and removable partial dentures, Dent. Clin. North Am. **23**:143-151, 1979.

Academy of Denture Prosthetics: Principles, concepts and practices in prosthodontics, J. Prosthet. Dent. **37**:204-221, 1977.

Adisman, I.K.: What a prosthodontist should know, J. Prosthet. Dent. **21**:409-416, 1969.

American Association of Dental Schools: Curricular guidelines for removable prosthodontics, J. Dent. Educ. **44**:343-346, 1980.

Applegate, O.C.: Conditions which may influence the choice of partial or complete denture service, J. Prosthet. Dent. **7**:182-196, 1957.

Applegate, O.C.: The removable partial denture in the general practice of tomorrow, J. Prosthet. Dent. **8**:609-622, 1958.

Applegate, O.C.: Factors to be considered in choosing an alloy, Dent. Clin. North Am., pp. 583-590, Nov., 1960.

Asgar, K., et al.: A new alloy for partial dentures, J. Prosthet. Dent. **23**:36-43, 1970.

Atwood, D.A.: Practice of prosthodontics: past, present, and future, J. Prosthet. Dent. **21**:393-401, 1970.

Augsburger, R.H.: Evaluating removable partial dentures by mathematical equations, J. Prosthet. Dent. **22**:528-543, 1969.

Backenstose, W.M., and Wells, J.G.: Side effects of immersion-type cleansers on the metal components of dentures, J. Prosthet. Dent. **37**:615-621, 1977.

Baker, C.R.: Difficulties in evaluating removable partial dentures, J. Prosthet. Dent. **17**:60-62, 1967.

Baker, C.R.: Occlusal reactive prosthodontics, J. Prosthet. Dent. **17**:566-569, 1967.

Barrett, D.A., and Pilling, L.O.: The restoration of carious clasp-bearing teeth, J. Prosthet. Dent. **15**:309-311, 1965.

Barsby, M.J., and Schwarz, W.D.: A survey of the teaching of partial denture construction in dental schools in the United Kingdom, J. Dent. **7**:1-8, 1979.

Bates, J.F.: Studies related to fracture of partial dentures, Br. Dent. J. **120**:79-83, 1966.

Bauman, R.: Survey of dentists' attitudes regarding instructions for home care for patients who wear dentures, J. Am. Dent. Assoc. **100**:206-208, 1980.

Beck, H.O.: A clinical evaluation of the arcon concept of articulation, J. Prosthet. Dent. **9**:409-421, 1959.

Beck, H.O.: Alloys for removable partial dentures, Dent. Clin. North Am., pp. 591-596, Nov., 1960.

Beck, H.O., and Morrison, W.E.: Investigation of an arcon articulator, J. Prosthet. Dent. **6**:359-372, 1956.

Becker, C.M., and Bolender, C.L.: Designing swinglock partial dentures, J. Prosthet. Dent. **46**:126-132, 1981.

Becker, C.M., and Swoope, C.C.: Swinglock partial dentures. In Clark, J.W., editor: Clinical dentistry, vol. 5, New York, 1976, Harper & Row, Publishers, Inc.

Bergman, B., Hugoson, A., and Olsson, C.O.: Caries, periodontal and prosthetic findings in patients with removable partial dentures: a ten-year longitudinal study, J. Prosthet. Dent. **48**:506-514, 1982.

Blanco-Dalmau, L.: The nickel problem, J. Prosthet. Dent. **48**:99-101, 1982.

Blatterfein, L.: Role of the removable partial denture in the restoration of lost vertical dimension, N.Y. Univ. J. Dent. **10**:274-276, 1952.

Blatterfein, L., et al.: Minimum acceptable procedures for satisfactory removable partial denture service, J. Prosthet. Dent. **27**:84-87, 1972.

Bolender, C.L., and Becker, C.M.: Swinglock removable partial dentures: where and when, J. Prosthet. Dent. **45**:4-10, 1981.

Boucher, C.O.: Writing as a means for learning, J. Prosthet. Dent. **27**:229-234, 1972.

Boucher, L.J., et al.: Guidelines for advanced prosthodontic education, J. Prosthet. Dent. **23**:104-110, 1970.

Breitbart, A.R.: Converting a tooth-supported denture to a distal extension removable partial denture, J. Prosthet. Dent. **18**:233, 1967.

Brockhurst, P.J.: Comparison of the performance of materials for spring members in dental appliances, using the theory of simple bending, Aust. Dent. J. **15**:119-125, 1970.

Cavalaris, C.J.: Pathologic considerations associated with partial dentures, Dent. Clin. North Am. **17**:585-600, 1973.

Cecconi, B.C.: Removable partial denture research and its clinical significance, J. Prosthet. Dent. **39**:203-210, 1978.

Charbeneau, G.T., et al.: Report of the Committee on Scientific Investigation of the American Academy of Restorative Dentistry, J. Prosthet. Dent. **36**:441-467, 1976.

Cheraskin, E., and Ringsdorf, W.M., Jr.: The ecology of the prosthodontic problem, J. Am. Dent. Assoc. **92**:133-139, 1976.

Cotmore, J.M., Mingledorf, E.B., Pomerantz, J.M., and Grasso, J.E.: Removable partial denture survey: clinical practice today, J. Prosthet. Dent. **49**:321-327, 1983.

Coy, R.E., and Arnold, P.D.: Survey and design of diagnostic casts for removable partial dentures, J. Prosthet. Dent. **32**:103-106, 1974.

Cunningham, D.M.: Comparison of base metal alloys and Type IV gold alloys for removable partial denture frameworks, Dent. Clin. North Am. **17**:719-722, 1973.

Cutright, D.E.: Morphogenesis of inflammatory papillary hyperplasia, J. Prosthet. Dent. **33**:380-385, 1975.

Dale, J.W.: A full and partial denture survey, Aust. Dent. J. **15**:225-227, 1970.

Derry, A., and Bertram, U.: A clinical survey of removable partial dentures after 2 years usage, Acta Odontol. Scand. **28**:581-598, 1970.

DeVan, M.M.: The additive partial denture: its principles and design (partial dentures), North West Dent. **35**:303-307, 312, 1956; Dent. Abstr. **2**:468, 1957.

Dukes, B.S., and Fields, H., Jr.: Comparison of disclosing media used for adjustment of removable partial denture frameworks, J. Prosthet. Dent. **45**:380-382, 1981.

Elliott, R.W.: The effects of heat on gold partial denture castings, J. Prosthet. Dent. **13**:688-698, 1963.

Ettinger, R.L.: The acrylic removable partial denture, J. Am. Dent. Assoc. **95**:945-949, 1977.

Ewing, J.E.: Temporary cementation in fixed partial prosthesis, J. Prosthet. Dent. **5**:388-391, 1955.

Ewing, J.E.: The construction of accurate full crown restorations for an existing clasp by using a direct metal pattern technique, J. Prosthet. Dent. **15**:889-899, 1965.

Farah, J.W., MacGregor, A.R., and Miller, T.P.G.: Stress analysis of disjunct removable partial dentures, J. Prosthet. Dent. **42**:271-275, 1979.

Federation of Prosthodontic Organizations: Guidelines for evaluation of completed prosthodontic treatment for removable partial dentures, J. Prosthet. Dent. **27**:326-328, 1972.

Fenton, A.H., and Jeffrey, J.D.: Allergy to a partial denture casting: case report, J. Canad. Dent. Assoc. **10**:446-468, 1978.

Fenton, A.H., Zarb, G.A., and MacKay, H.F.: Overdenture oversights, Dent. Clin. North Am. **23**:117-130, 1979.

Fields, H., and Campfield, R.W.: Removable partial prosthesis partially supported by an endosseous blade implant, J. Prosthet. Dent. **31**:273-278, 1974.

Fish, S.F.: Partial dentures, Br. Dent. J. **128**:243-246, 289-293, 339-344, 398-402, 446-453, 495-502, 547-551, 590-592, 1970.

Fish, S.F., et al.: A study of prosthetic dentistry, Br. Dent. J. **127**:59-70, 1969.

Fisher, R.: Relation of removable partial denture base stability to sex, age, and other factors, J. Dent. Res. (A.A.D.R. abstract 613) **49**:entire issue, 1980.

Frank, R.P.: Fabrication of temporary and treatment partial dentures, J. Prosthet. Dent. **30**:215-221, 1973.

Frank, R.P.: Evaluating refractory cast wax-ups for removable partial dentures, J. Prosthet. Dent. **35**:388-392, 1976.

Gilmore, H.W., et al.: Report of the Committee on Scientific Investigation of the American Academy of Restorative Dentistry, J. Prosthet. Dent. **40**:192-206, 1978.

Girardot, R.L.: The physiologic aspects of partial denture restorations, J. Prosthet. Dent. **3**:689-698, 1953.

Glossary of prosthodontic terms, J. Prosthet. Dent. **38**:70-109, 1977.

Hamilton, A.I., et al.: Report of the Committee on Scientific Investigation of the American Academy of Restorative Dentistry, J. Prosthet. Dent. **34**:86-110, 1975.

Hardcourt, H.J., et al.: The properties of nickel-chromium casting alloys containing boron and silicon, Br. Dent. J. **129**:419-423, 1970.

Harrison, W.M., and Stansbury, B.E.: The effect of joint surface contours on the transverse strength of repaired acrylic resin, J. Prosthet. Dent. **23**:464-472, 1970.

Heintz, W.D.: Principles, planning, and practice for prevention, Dent. Clin. North Am. **17**:705-718, 1973.

Herlands, R.E.: Removable partial denture terminology, J. Prosthet. Dent. **8**:964-972, 1958.

Hickey, J.C.: Responsibility of the dentist in removable partial dentures, J. Ky. Dent. Assoc. **17**:70-87, 1965.

Hickey, J.C.: Charge to workshop on advanced prosthodontic training, J. Prosthet. Dent. **21**:388-392, 1969.

Hobdell, M.H., et al.: The prevalence of full and partial dentures in British populations, Br. Dent. J. **128**:437-442, 1970.

Jankelson, B.H.: Adjustment of dentures at time of insertion and alterations to compensate for tissue changes, J. Am. Dent. Assoc. **64**:521-531, 1962.

Jones, R.R.: The lower partial denture, J. Prosthet. Dent. **2**:219-229, 1952.

Kaaber, S.: Twelve year changes in mandibular bone level in free end saddle denture wearers, J. Dent. Res. (A.A.D.R. abstract 1367) **60**:entire issue, 1981.

Kaires, A.K.: A study of partial denture design and masticatory pressures in a mandibular bilateral distal extension case, J. Prosthet. Dent. **8**:340-350, 1958.

Kelly, E.: Fatigue failure in denture base polymers, J. Prosthet. Dent. **21**:257-266, 1969.

Kelly, E.: Changes caused by a mandibular removable partial denture opposing a maxillary complete denture, J. Prosthet. Dent. **27**:140-150, 1972.

Kelly, E.K.: The physiologic approach to partial denture design, J. Prosthet. Dent. **3**:699-710, 1953.

Kessler, B.: An analysis of the tongue factor and its functioning areas in dental prosthesis, J. Prosthet. Dent. **5**:629-635, 1955.

Klein, I.E., et al.: Minimum clinical procedures for satisfactory complete denture, removable partial denture, and fixed partial denture services, J. Prosthet. Dent. **22**:4-10, 1969.

Kratochvil, F.J.: Maintaining supporting structures with a removable partial prosthesis, J. Prosthet. Dent. **25**:167-174, 1971.

Kratochvil, F.J., and Caputo, A.A.: Photoelastic analysis of pressure on teeth and bone supporting removable partial dentures, J. Prosthet. Dent. **32**:52-61, 1974.

Kratochvil, F.J., Davidson, P.N., and Guijt, J.: Five-year survey of treatment with removable partial dentures. Part I, J. Prosthet. Dent. **48:**237-244, 1982.

Landa, J.S.: The troublesome transition from a partial lower to a complete lower denture, J. Prosthet. Dent. **4:**42-51, 1954.

Lanser, A.: Tooth-supported telescope restorations, J. Prosthet. Dent. **45:**515-520, 1981.

Levin, B.: Removable prosthodontics in the United Kingdom and Scandinavia, J. Prosthet. Dent. **33:**224-232, 1975.

Lewis, A.J.: Failure of removable partial denture castings during service, J. Prosthet. Dent. **39:**147-149, 1978.

Lewis, A.J.: Radiographic evaluation of porosities in removable partial denture castings, J. Prosthet. Dent. **39:**278-281, 1978.

Lopuck, S.E., Reitz, P.V., and Altadonna, J.: Hinge for a unilateral maxillary arch prosthesis, J. Prosthet. Dent. **45:**446-448, 1981.

Lorton, L.: A method of stabilizing removable partial denture castings during clinical laboratory procedures, J. Prosthet. Dent. **39:**344-345, 1978.

Love, W.B.: Prosthodontics—past, present, and future, J. Prosthet. Dent. **36:**261-264, 1976.

MacEntee, M.I.: Integration of fixed and removable prosthodontics in an undergraduate curriculum, J. Dent. Educ. **45:**204-206, 1981.

MacEntee, M.I., Hawbolt, E.B., and Zahel, J.I.: The tensile and shear strength of a base metal weld joint used in dentistry, J. Dent. Res. **60:**154-158, 1981.

Maetani, T., et al.: Effect of T.F.E. coating on plaque accumulation on dental castings, J. Dent. Res. (A.A.D.R. abstract 1359) **60:**entire issue, 1981.

Maison, W.G.: Instructions to denture patients, J. Prosthet. Dent. **9:**825-831, 1959.

Makrauer, F.L., and Davis, J.S.: Gastroscopic removal of a partial denture, J. Am. Dent. Assoc. **94:**904-906, 1977.

Margolese, S., Swoope, C.C., and Pettapiece, G.: Attitudes of dentists in British Columbia toward removable prosthodontics, J. Prosthet. Dent. **43:**22-25, 1980.

Martone, A.L.: The effects of oral prostheses on the production of speech sounds, Ohio State Univ. Dent. Abstr. **2:**508, 1957.

Martone, A.L.: The fallacy of saving time at the chair, J. Prosthet. Dent. **7:**416-419, 1957.

Martone, A.L.: The challenge of the partially edentulous mouth, J. Prosthet. Dent. **8:**942-954, 1958.

Massler, M.: Geriatric nutrition: the role of taste and smell in appetite, J. Prosthet. Dent. **32:**247-250, 1980.

McCracken, W.L.: Auxiliary uses of cold-curing acrylic resins in prosthetic dentistry, J. Am. Dent. Assoc. **47:**298-304, 1953.

McCracken, W.L.: A comparison of tooth-borne and tooth-tissue–borne removable partial dentures, J. Prosthet. Dent. **3:**375-381, 1953.

McCracken, W.L.: A philosophy of partial denture treatment, J. Prosthet. Dent. **13:**889-900, 1963.

Means, C.R., and Flenniken, I.E.: Gagging—a problem in prosthetic dentistry, J. Prosthet. Dent. **23:**614-620, 1970.

Mehringer, E.J.: The saliva as it is related to the wearing of dentures, J. Prosthet. Dent. **4:**312-318, 1954.

Michell, D.L., and Wilke, N.D.: Articulators through the years. I. Up to 1940, J. Prosthet. Dent. **39:**330-338, 1978. II. From 1940, **39:**451-458, 1978.

Miller, E.L.: Critical factors in selecting removable prostheses, J. Prosthet. Dent. **34:**486-490, 1975.

Miller E.L.: Clinical management of denture-induced inflammations, J. Prosthet. Dent. **38:**362-365, 1977.

Mohamed, S.E., Schmidt, J.R., and Harrison, J.D.: Articulators in dental education and practice, J. Prosthet. Dent. **36:**319-325, 1976.

Morris, H.F., and Asgar, K.: Physical properties and microstructure of four new commercial partial denture alloys, J. Prosthet. Dent. **33:**36-46, 1975.

Morse, P.K., and Boucher, L.J.: What a prosthodontist does, J. Prosthet. Dent. **21:**402-408, 1969.

Neufeld, J.O.: Changes in the trabecular pattern of the mandible following the loss of teeth, J. Prosthet. Dent. **8:**685-697, 1958.

Öatlund, S.G.: Saliva and denture retention, J. Prosthet. Dent. **10:**658-663, 1960.

Osborne, J., and Lammie, G.A.: The bilateral free-end saddle lower denture, J. Prosthet. Dent. **4:**640-652, 1954.

Overton, R.G., and Bramblett, R.M.: Prosthodontic services: a study of need and availability in the United States, J. Prosthet. Dent. **27:**329-339, 1972.

Pascoe, D.F., and Wimmer, J.: A radiographic technique for the detection of internal defects in dental castings, J. Prosthet. Dent. **39:**150-157, 1978.

Phillips, R.W., and Leonard, L.J.: A study of enamel abrasion as related to partial denture clasps, J. Prosthet. Dent. **6:**657-671, 1956.

Plainfield, S.: Communication distortion. The language of patients and practitioners of dentistry, J. Prosthet. Dent. **22:**11-19, 1969.

Prieskel, H.W.: The distal extension prosthesis reappraised, J. Dent. **5:**217-230, 1977.

Ramsey, W.O.: The relation of emotional factors to prosthodontic service, J. Prosthet. Dent. **23:**4-10, 1970.

Raybin, N.H.: The polished surface of complete dentures, J. Prosthet. Dent. **13:**236-239, 1963.

Reynolds, J.M.: Crown construction for abutments of existing removable partial dentures, J. Am. Dent. Assoc. **69:**423-426, 1964.

Rissen, L., et al.: Effect of fixed and removable partial dentures on the alveolar bone of abutment teeth, J. Dent. Res. (A.A.D.R. abstract 1368) **60:**entire issue, 1981.

Rothman, R.: Phonetic considerations in denture prosthesis, J. Prosthet. Dent. **11:**214-223, 1961.

Rudd, K.D., and Dunn, B.W.: Accurate removable partial dentures, J. Prosthet. Dent. **18:**559-570, 1967.

Rushford, C.B.: A technique for precision removable partial denture construction. J. Prosthet. Dent. **31:**377-383, 1974.

Ruyter, I.E., and Svendsen, S.A.: Flexural properties of denture base polymers, J. Prosthet. Dent. **43:**95-104, 1980.

Savage, R.D., and MacGregor, A.R.: Behavior therapy in prosthodontics, J. Prosthet. Dent. **24:**126-132, 1970.

Schabel, R.W.: Dentist-patient communication—a major factor in treatment prognosis, J. Prosthet. Dent. **21:**3-5, 1969.

Schabel, R.W.: The psychology of aging, J. Prosthet. Dent. **27:**569-573, 1972.

Schole, M.L.: Management of the gagging patient, J. Prosthet. Dent. **9**:578-583, 1959.

Schoper, A.F.: Removable appliances for the preservation of the teeth, J. Prosthet. Dent. **4**:634-639, 1954.

Schopper, A.F.: Loss of vertical dimension: causes and effects: diagnosis and various recommended treatments, J. Prosthet. Dent. **9**:428-431, 1959.

Schulte, J.K., and Smith, D.E.: Clinical evaluation of swing-lock removable partial dentures, J. Prosthet. Dent. **44**:595-603, 1980.

Schuyler, C.H.: Stress distribution as the prime requisite to the success of a partial denture, J. Am. Dent. Assoc. **20**:2148-2154, 1963.

Schuyler, A.F.: Planning the removable partial denture to restore function and maintain oral health, N.Y. Dent. J. **13**:4-10, 1947.

Schwarz, W.D., and Barsby, M.J.: Design of partial dentures in dental practice, J. Dent. **6**:166-170, 1978.

Sears, V.H.: Comprehensive denture service, J. Am. Dent. Assoc. **64**:531-552, 1962.

Skinner, E.W., and Gordon, C.C.: Some experiments on the surface hardness of dental stones, J. Prosthet. Dent. **6**:94-100, 1956.

Skinner, E.W., and Jones, P.M.: Dimensional stability of self-curing denture base acrylic resin, J. Am. Dent. Assoc. **51**:426-431, 1955.

Smith, B.H.: Changes in occlusal face height with removable partial prostheses, J. Prosthet. Dent. **34**:278-285, 1975.

Smith, F.W., and Applegate, O.C.: Roentgenographic study of bone changes during exercise stimulation of edentulous areas, J. Prosthet. Dent. **11**:1086-1097, 1961.

Stendahl, C.G., and Grob, D.J.: Detection of binding areas on removable partial denture frameworks, Dent. Clin. North Am. **23**:101-106, 1979.

Sweeney, W.T., Myerson, R.L., Rose, E.E., and Semmelman, J.O.: Proposed specification for plastic teeth, J. Prosthet. Dent. **7**:420-424, 1957.

Swoope, C.C., and Frank, R.P.: Insertion and post-insertion care. In Clark, J.W., editor: Clinical dentistry, vol. 5, New York, 1976, Harper & Row, Publishers, Inc.

Sykora, O.: Extracoronal removable partial denture service in Canada, J. Prosthet. Dent. **39**:37-41, 1978.

Tallgren, A.: Alveolar bone loss in denture wearers as related to facial morphology, Acta Odontol. Scand. **28**:251-270, 1970.

Teppo, K.W., and Smith, F.W.: A method of immediate clasp repair, J. Prosthet. Dent. **34**:77-80, 1975.

Tomlin, H.R., and Osborne, J.: Cobalt-chromium partial dentures; a clinical survey, Br. Dent. J. **110**:307-310, 1961.

Trainor, J.E., and Elliott, R.W., Jr.: Removable partial dentures designed by dentists before and after graduate level instruction: a comparative study, J. Prosthet. Dent. **27**:509-514, 1972.

Wagner, A.G.: Maintenance of the partially edentulous mouth and care of the denture, Dent. Clin. North Am. **17**:755-768, 1973.

Wagner, A.G., and Forgue, E.G.: A study of four methods of recording the path of insertion of removable partial dentures, J. Prosthet. Dent. **35**:267-272, 1976.

Wallace, D.H.: The use of gold occlusal surfaces in complete and partial dentures, J. Prosthet. Dent. **14**:326-333, 1964.

Walter, J.D.: Partial denture technique. I. Introduction, Br. Dent. J. **147**:241-243, 1979. II. The purpose of the denture: choice of material, **147**:302-304, 1979. III. Supporting the denture, **148**:13-16, 1980. IV. Guide planes, **148**:70-72, 1980.

Weaver, R.E., and Goebel, W.M.: Reactions to acrylic resin dental prostheses, J. Prosthet. Dent. **43**:138-142, 1980.

Williams, E.O., and Hartman, G.E.: Instructional aid for teaching removable partial denture design, J. Prosthet. Dent. **48**:222, 1982.

Wilson, J.H.: Some clinical and technical aspects of partial dentures, Dent. J. Aust. **26**:176-183, 1954.

Wise, H.B., and Kaiser, D.A.: A radiographic technique for examination of internal defects in metal frameworks, J. Prosthet. Dent. **42**:594-595, 1979.

Young H.A.: Factors contributory to success in prosthodontic practice, J. Prosthet. Dent. **5**:354-360, 1955.

Young, L., Jr.: Try-in of the removable partial denture framework, J. Prosthet. Dent. **46**:579-580, 1981.

Zach, G.A.: Advantages of mesial rests for removable partial dentures, J. Prosthet. Dent. **33**:32-35, 1975.

Zerosi, C.: A new type of removable splint: its indications and function, Dent. Abstr. **1**:451-452, 1956.

MOUTH PREPARATIONS

Alexander, J.M., and Van Sickels, J.E.: Posterior maxillary osteotomies: an aid for a difficult prosthodontic problem, J. Prosthet. Dent. **41**:614-617, 1979.

Atwood, D.A.: Reduction of residual ridges in the partially edentulous patient, Dent. Clin. North Am. **17**:745-754, 1973.

Axinn, S.: Preparation of retentive areas for clasps in enamel, J. Prosthet. Dent. **34**:405-407, 1975.

Belinfante, L.S., and Abney, J.M., Jr.: A teamwork approach to correct a severe prosthodontic problem, J. Am. Dent. Assoc. **91**:357-359, 1975.

Boitel, R.H.: The parallelometer, a precision instrument for the prosthetic laboratory, J. Prosthet. Dent. **12**:732-736, 1962.

Gaston, G.W.: Rest area preparations for removable partial dentures, J. Prosthet. Dent. **10**:124-134, 1960.

Glann, G.W., and Appleby, R.C.: Mouth preparations for removable partial dentures, J. Prosthet. Dent. **10**:698-706, 1960.

Johnston, J.F.: Preparation of mouths for fixed and removable partial dentures, J. Prosthet. Dent. **11**:456-462, 1961.

Kahn, A.E.: Partial versus full coverage, J. Prosthet. Dent. **10**:167-178, 1960.

Laney, W.R., and Desjardins, R.P.: Comparison of base metal alloys and Type IV gold alloys for removable partial denture framework, Dent. Clin. North Am. **17**:611-630, 1973.

Lorey, R.E.: Abutment considerations, Dent. Clin. North Am. **24**:63-79, 1980.

Marquardt, G.L.: Dolder bar joint mandibular overdenture: a technique for nonparallel abutment teeth, J. Prosthet. Dent. **36**:101-111, 1976.

McArthur, D.R., and Turvey, T.A.: Maxillary segmental osteotomies for mandibular removable partial denture patients, J. Prosthet. Dent. **41**:381-387, 1979.

McCarthy, J.A., and Moser, J.B.: Mechanical properties of

tissue conditioners. Part I: theoretical considerations, behavioral characteristics and tensile properties, J. Prosthet. Dent. **40**:89-97, 1978.

McCarthy, J.A., and Moser, J.B.: Mechanical properties of tissue conditioners, part II: creep characteristics, J. Prosthet. Dent. **40**:334-342, 1978.

McCracken, W.L.: Mouth preparations for partial dentures, J. Prosthet. Dent. **6**:39-52, 1956.

Mills, M.: Mouth preparation for removable partial denture, J. Am. Dent. Assoc. **60**:154-159, 1960.

Mopsik, E.R., Buck, R.P., Connors, J.O., and Watts, L.N.: Surgical intervention to reestablish adequate intermaxillary space before fixed or removable prosthodontics, J. Am. Dent. Assoc. **95**:957-960, 1977.

Phillips, R.W.: Report of the Committee on Scientific Investigation of the Academy of Restorative Dentistry, J. Prosthet. Dent. **13**:515-535, 1963.

Schorr, L., and Clayman, L.H.: Reshaping abutment teeth for reception of partial denture clasps, J. Prosthet. Dent. **4**:625-633, 1954.

Sollé, W.: The parallelo-facere: a parallel drilling machine for use in the oral cavity, J. Am. Dent. Assoc. **63**:344-352, 1961.

Stamps, J.T., and Tanquist, R.A.: Restoration of removable partial denture rest seats using dental amalgam, J. Prosthet. Dent. **41**:224-227, 1979.

Stern, W.J.: Guiding planes in clasp reciprocation and retention, J. Prosthet. Dent. **34**:408-414, 1975.

Swoope, C.C., and Frank, R.P.: Mouth preparation. In Clark, J.W., editor: Clinical dentistry, vol. 5, New York, 1976, Harper & Row, Publishers, Inc.

Tucker, K.M., and Heget, H.S.: The incidence of inflammatory papillary hyperplasia, J. Am. Dent. Assoc. **93**:610-613, 1976.

Wong, R., Nicholls, J.I., and Smith, D.E.: Evaluation of prefabricated lingual rest seats for removable partial dentures, J. Prosthet. Dent. **48**:521-526, 1982.

OCCLUSION; JAW RELATION RECORDS; TRANSFER METHODS

Applegate, O.C.: Loss of posterior occlusion, J. Prosthet. Dent. **4**:197-199, 1954.

Baraban, D.J.: Establishing centric relation and vertical dimension in occlusal rehabilitation, J. Prosthet. Dent. **12**:1157-1165, 1962.

Bauman, R.: Minimizing postinsertion problems: a procedure for removable partial denture placement, J. Prosthet. Dent. **42**:381-385, 1979.

Beck, H.O.: A clinical evaluation of the arcon concept of articulation, J. Prosthet. Dent. **9**:409-421, 1959.

Beck, H.O.: Selection of an articulator and jaw registration, J. Prosthet. Dent. **10**:878-886, 1960.

Beck, H.O.: Choosing the articulator, J. Am. Dent. Assoc. **64**:468-475, 1962.

Beckett, L.S.: Accurate occlusal relations in partial denture construction, J. Prosthet. Dent. **4**:487-495, 1954.

Berke, J.D., and Moleres, I.: A removable appliance for the correction of maxillomandibular disproportion, J. Prosthet. Dent. **17**:172-177, 1967.

Berman, M.H.: Accurate interocclusal records, J. Prosthet. Dent. **10**:620-630, 1960.

Beyron, H.L.: Occlusal relationship, Int. Dent. J. **2**:467-496, 1952.

Beyron, H.L.: Characteristics of functionally optimal occlusion and principles of occlusal rehabilitation, J. Am. Dent. Assoc. **48**:648-656, 1954.

Beyron, H.L.: Occlusal changes in adult dentition, J. Am. Dent. Assoc. **48**:674-686, 1954.

Block, L.S.: Preparing and conditioning the patient for intermaxillary relations, J. Prosthet. Dent. **2**:599-603, 1952.

Block, L.S.: Tensions and intermaxillary relations, J. Prosthet. Dent. **4**:204-207, 1954.

Boos, R.H.: Occlusion from rest position, J. Prosthet. Dent. **2**:575-588, 1952.

Boos, R.H.: Basic anatomic factors of jaw position, J. Prosthet. Dent. **4**:200-203, 1954.

Boos, R.H.: Maxillomandibular relations, occlusion, and the temporomandibular joint, Dent. Clin. North Am., pp. 19-35, March, 1962.

Borgh, O., and Posselt, U.: Hinge axis registration: experiments on the articulator, J. Prosthet. Dent. **8**:35-40, 1958.

Boucher, C.O.: Occlusion in prosthodontics, J. Prosthet. Dent. **3**:633-656, 1953.

Braly, B.V.: Occlusal analysis and treatment planning for restorative dentistry, J. Prosthet. Dent. **27**:168-171, 1972.

Cerveris, A.R.: Vibracentric equilibration of centric occlusion, J. Am. Dent. Assoc. **63**:476-483, 1961.

Christensen, P.B.: Accurate casts and positional relation records, J. Prosthet. Dent. **8**:475-482, 1958.

Clayton, J.A., et al.: Pantographic tracings of mandibular movements and occlusion, J. Prosthet. Dent. **25**:389-396, 1971.

Cohn, L.A.: Factors of dental occlusion pertinent to the restorative and prosthetic problem, J. Prosthet. Dent. **9**:256-277, 1959.

Collett, H.A.: Balancing the occlusion of partial dentures, J. Am. Dent. Assoc. **42**:162-168, 1951.

Colman, A.J.: Occlusal requirements for removable partial dentures, J. Prosthet. Dent. **17**:155-162, 1967.

D'Amico, A.: Functional occlusion of the natural teeth of man, J. Prosthet. Dent. **11**:899-915, 1961.

Draper, D.H.: Forward trends in occlusion, J. Prosthet. Dent. **13**:724-731, 1963.

Emmert, J.H.: A method for registering occlusion in semi-edentulous mouths, J. Prosthet. Dent. **8**:94-99, 1958.

Fedi, P.F.: Cardinal differences in occlusion of natural teeth and that of artificial teeth, J. Am. Dent. Assoc. **62**:482-485, 1962.

Fountain, H.W.: Seating the condyles for centric relation records, J. Prosthet. Dent. **11**:1050-1058, 1961.

Gilson, T.D.: Theory of centric correction in natural teeth, J. Prosthet. Dent. **8**:468-474, 1958.

Goodfriend, D.J.: New facebow for dentist-laboratory cooperation, J. Am. Dent. Assoc. **68**:866-872, 1964.

Granger, E.R.: The articulator and the patient, Dent. Clin. North Am., pp. 527-539, Nov., 1960.

Hausman, M.: Interceptive and pivotal occlusal contacts, J. Am. Dent. Assoc. **66**:165-171, 1963.

Henderson, D.: Occlusion in removable partial prosthodontics, J. Prosthet. Dent. **27**:151-159, 1971.

Hindels, G.W.: Occlusion in removable partial denture prosthesis, Dent. Clin. North Am., pp. 137-146, March, 1962.

Hughes, G.A., and Regli, C.P.: What is centric relation? J. Prosthet. Dent. **11**:16-22, 1961.

Jaffe, V.N.: The functionally generated path in full denture construction, J. Prosthet. Dent. **4**:214-221, 1954.

Jankelson, B.: Considerations of occlusion on fixed partial dentures, Dent. Clin. North Am., pp. 187-203, March, 1959.

Jeffreys, F.E., and Platner, R.L.: Occlusion in removable partial dentures, J. Prosthet. Dent. **10**:912-920, 1960.

Kapur, K.K.: The comparison of different methods of recording centric relation, 1956, Tufts Univ. Dent. Abstr. **2**:508, 1957.

Lauritzen, A.G., and Bodner, G.H.: Variations in location of arbitrary and true hinge axis points, J. Prosthet. Dent. **11**:224-229, 1961.

Lindblom, G.: Balanced occlusion with partial reconstructions, Int. Dent. J. **1**:84-98, 1951.

Lindblom, G.: The value of bite analysis, J. Am. Dent. Assoc. **48**:657-664, 1954.

Long, J.H., Jr.: Location of the terminal hinge axis by intraoral means, J. Prosthet. Dent. **23**:11-24, 1970.

Lucia, V.O.: Centric relation—theory and practice, J. Prosthet. Dent. **10**:849-956, 1960.

Lucia, V.O.: The gnathological concept of articulation, Dent. Clin. North Am., pp. 183-197, March, 1962.

Lundquist, D.O., and Fiebiger, G.E.: Registration for relating to the mandibular cast to the maxillary cast based on Kennedy's classification system, J. Prosthet. Dent. **35**:371-375, 1976.

Mann, A.W., and Pankey, L.D.: The P.M. philosophy of occlusal rehabilitation, Dent. Clin. North Am., pp. 621-636, Nov., 1963.

McCollum, B.B.: The mandibular hinge axis and a method of locating it, J. Prosthet. Dent. **10**:428-435, 1960.

McCracken, W.L.: Functional occlusion in removable partial denture construction, J. Prosthet. Dent. **8**:955-963, 1958.

McCracken, W.L.: Impression materials in prosthetic dentistry, Dent. Clin. North Am., pp. 671-684, Nov., 1958.

McCracken, W.L.: Occlusion in partial denture prosthesis, Dent. Clin. North Am., pp. 109-119, March, 1962.

Mehta, J.D., and Joglekar, A.P.: Vertical jaw relations as a factor in partial dentures, J. Prosthet. Dent. **21**:618-625, 1969.

Meyer, F.S.: The generated path technique in reconstruction dentistry. I and II. J. Prosthet. Dent. **9**:354-366, 432-440, 1959.

Millstein, P.L., et al.: Determination of the accuracy of wax interocclusal registrations, J. Prosthet. Dent. **25**:189-196, 1971.

Moore, A.W.: Ideal versus adequate dental occlusion, J. Am. Dent. Assoc. **55**:51-56, 1957.

Moulton, G.H.: The importance of centric occlusion in diagnosis and treatment planning, J. Prosthet. Dent. **10**:921-926, 1960.

Nayyar, A., Bill, J.A., Jr., and Twiggs, S.W.: Comparison of interocclusal recording materials for mounting a working cast, J. Dent. Res. (A.A.D.R. abstract 1216) **60**:entire issue, 1981.

Nuttall, E.B.: Establishing posterior functional occlusion for fixed partial dentures, J. Am. Dent. Assoc. **66**:341-348, 1963.

O'Leary, T.J., et al.: Tooth mobility in cuspid-protected and group-function occlusions, J. Prosthet. Dent. **27**:21-25, 1972.

Olsson, A., and Posselt, U.: Relationship of various skull reference lines, J. Prosthet. Dent. **11**:1045-1049, 1961.

Reitz, P.V.: Technique for mounting removable partial dentures on an articulator, J. Prosthet. Dent. **22**:490-494, 1969.

Reynolds, J.M.: Occlusal wear facets, J. Prosthet. Dent. **24**:367-372, 1970.

Ricketts, R.M.: Occlusion—the medium of dentistry, J. Prosthet. Dent. **21**:39-60, 1969.

Robinson, M.J.: Centric position, J. Prosthet. Dent. **1**:384-386, 1951.

Scaife, R.R., Jr., and Holt, J.E.: Natural occurrence of cuspid guidance, J. Prosthet. Dent. **22**:225-229, 1969.

Scandrett, F.R., and Hanson, J.G.: Technique for attaching the master cast to its split mounting index, J. Prosthet. Dent. **40**:467-469, 1978.

Schireson, S.: Grinding teeth for masticatory efficiency and gingival health, J. Prosthet. Dent. **13**:337-345, 1963.

Schuyler, C.H.: Fundamental principles in the correction of occlusal disharmony—natural and artificial (grinding), J. Am. Dent. Assoc. **22**:1193-1202, 1935.

Schuyler, C.H.: Correction of occlusal disharmony of the natural dentition, N.Y. Dent. J. **13**:445-462, 1947.

Schuyler, C.H.: Factors of occlusion applicable to restorative dentistry, J. Prosthet. Dent. **3**:772-782, 1953.

Schuyler, C.H.: An evaluation of incisal guidance and its influence in restorative dentistry, J. Prosthet. Dent. **9**:374-378, 1959.

Schuyler, C.H.: Factors contributing to traumatic occlusion, J. Prosthet. Dent. **11**:708-715, 1961.

Sears, V.H.: Occlusion: the common meeting ground in dentistry, J. Prosthet. Dent. **2**:15-21, 1952.

Sears, V.H.: Occlusal pivots, J. Prosthet. Dent. **6**:332-338, 1956.

Sears, V.H.: Centric and eccentric occlusions, J. Prosthet. Dent. **10**:1029-1036, 1960.

Sears, V.H.: Mandibular equilibration, J. Am. Dent. Assoc. **65**:45-55, 1962.

Shanahan, T.E.J., and Leff, A.: Interocclusal records, J. Prosthet. Dent. **10**:842-848, 1960.

Silverman, M.M.: Determination of vertical dimension by phonetics, J. Prosthet. Dent. **6**:465-471, 1956; Dent. Abstr. **2**:221, 1957.

Skurnik, H.: Accurate interocclusal records, J. Prosthet. Dent. **21**:154-165, 1969.

Stuart, C.E.: Accuracy in measuring functional dimensions and relations in oral prosthesis, J. Prosthet. Dent. **9**:220-236, 1959.

Teteruck, W.R., and Lundeen, H.C.: The accuracy of an ear face-bow, J. Prosthet. Dent. **16**:1039-1046, 1966.

Wagner, A.G.: A technique to record jaw relations for distally edentulous dental arches, J. Prosthet. Dent. **29**:405-407, 1973.

Weinberg, L.A.: The transverse hinge axis: real or imaginary, J. Prosthet. Dent. **9**:775-787, 1959.

Weinberg, L.A.: An evaluation of the face-bow mounting, J. Prosthet. Dent. **11**:32-42, 1961.

Weinberg, L.A.: Arcon principle in the condylar mechanism of adjustable articulators, J. Prosthet. Dent. **13**:263-268, 1963.

Weinberg, L.A.: An evaluation of basic articulators and their concepts. I and II. J. Prosthet. Dent. **13**:622-663, 1963.

Wilson, J.H.: The use of partial dentures in the restoration of occlusal standards, Aust. Dent. J. **1**:93-101, 1956.

PARTIAL DENTURE DESIGN

Antos, E.W., Jr., Tenner, R.P., and Foerth, D.: The swinglock partial denture: an alternative approach to conventional removable partial denture service, J. Prosthet. Dent. **40**:257-262, 1978.

Askinas, S.W.: Facings in removable partial dentures, J. Prosthet. Dent. **33**:633-636, 1975.

Avant, E.W.: Indirect retention in partial denture design, J. Prosthet. Dent. **16**:1103-1110, 1966.

Axinn, S., O'Connor, R.P., Jr., and Kopp, E.N.: Immediate removable partial denture frameworks, J. Am. Dent. Assoc. **95**:583-585, 1977.

Becker, C.W., and Bolender, C.L.: Designing swinglock partial dentures, J. Prosthet. Dent. **46**:126-132, 1981.

Berg, T., Jr.: I-bar: myth and counterymyth, Dent. Clin. North Am. **23**:65-75, 1979.

Berg, T., Jr., and Caputo, A.A.: Anterior rests for maxillary removable partial dentures, J. Prosthet. Dent. **39**:139-146, 1978.

Blatterfein, L.: A systematic method of designing upper partial denture bases, J. Am. Dent. Assoc. **46**:510-525, 1953.

Blatterfein, L.: The use of the semiprecision rest in removable partial dentures, J. Prosthet. Dent. **22**:301-306, 1969.

Bolouri, A.: Removable partial denture design for a few remaining natural teeth, J. Prosthet. Dent. **39**:346-348, 1978.

Campbell, L.D.: Subjective reactions to major connector designs for removable partial dentures, J. Prosthet. Dent. **36**:507-516, 1977.

Casey, D.M., and Lauciello, F.R.: A method for marking the functional depth of the floor of the mouth, J. Prosthet. Dent. **43**:108-111, 1980.

Cecconi, B.T.: Lingual bar design, J. Prosthet. Dent. **29**:635-639, 1973.

Chick, A.O.: Correct location of clasps and rests on dentures without stress-breakers, Br. Dent. J. **95**:303-309, 1953.

Collett, H.A.: Biologic approach to clasp partial dentures, Dent. Dig. **61**:309-313, 1955.

Cowles, K.R.: Partial denture design: a simple teaching aid, J. Prosthet. Dent. **47**:219, 1982.

Demer, W.J.: An analysis of mesial rest-I-bar clasps designs, J. Prosthet. Dent. **36**:243-253, 1976.

Dunny, J.A., and King, G.E.: Minor connector designs for anterior acrylic resin bases: a preliminary study, J. Prosthet. Dent. **34**:496-497, 1975.

Ettinger, R.L.: The acrylic removable partial denture, J. Am. Dent. Assoc. **95**:945-949, 1977.

Firtell, D.N.: Effect of clasp design upon retention of removable partial dentures, J. Prosthet. Dent. **20**:43-52, 1968.

Firtell, D.N., Herzberg, T.W., and Walsh, J.F.: Root retention and removable partial denture design, J. Prosthet. Dent. **42**:131-134, 1979.

Fisher, R.L., and Jaslow, C.: The efficiency of an indirect retainer, J. Prosthet. Dent. **33**:24-30, 1975.

Frank, R.P.: An investigation of the effectiveness of indirect retainers, J. Prosthet. Dent. **38**:494-506, 1977.

Frantz, W.R.: Variations in a removable maxillary partial denture design by dentists, J. Prosthet. Dent. **34**:625-633, 1975.

Frechette, A.R.: Partial denture planning with special reference to stress distribution, J. Ont. Dent. Assoc. **30**:318-329, 1953.

Ghamrawy, E.: Oral ecologic response caused by removable partial dentures, J. Dent. Res. (I.A.D.R. abstract 2898) **62**:entire issue, 1982.

Ghamrawy, E.: Plaque formation and crevicular temperature relation to minor connector position, J. Dent. Res. (I.A.D.R. abstract 387) **61**:entire issue, 1982.

Giradot, R.L.: History and development of partial denture design, J. Am. Dent. Assoc. **28**:1399-1408, 1941.

Henderson, D.: Major connectors for mandibular removable partial dentures, J. Prosthet. Dent. **30**:532-548, 1973.

Henderson, D.: Major connectors—united it stands, Dent. Clin. North Am. **17**:661-668, 1973.

Highton, R., Caputo, A.A., and Rhodes, S.: Force transmission and retentive capabilities utilizing labial and palatal I-bar partial dentures, J. Dent. Res. (A.A.D.R. abstract 1214) **60**:entire issue, 1981.

Holt, J.E.: Guilding planes: when and where, J. Prosthet. Dent. **46**:4-6, 1981.

Jacobson, T.E., and Krol, A.J.: Rotational path removable partial denture design, J. Prosthet. Dent. **48**:370-376, 1982.

Jordan, L.G.: Designing removable partial dentures with external attachments (clasps), J. Prosthet. Dent. **2**:716-722, 1952.

Kelly, E.K.: The physiologic approach to partial denture design, J. Prosthet. Dent. **3**:699-710, 1953.

King, G.E.: Dual-path design for removable partial dentures, J. Prosthet. Dent. **39**:392-395, 1978.

King, G.E., Barco, M.T., and Olson, R.J.: Inconspicuous retention for removable partial dentures, J. Prosthet. Dent. **39**:505-507, 1978.

Knodle, J.M.: Experimental overlay and pin partial denture, J. Prosthet. Dent. **17**:472-478, 1967.

Krikos, A.A.: Artificial undercuts for teeth which have unfavorable shapes for clasping, J. Prosthet. Dent. **22**:301-306, 1969.

Krikos, A.A.: Preparing guide planes for removable partial dentures, J. Prosthet. Dent. **34**:152-155, 1975.

Lanser, A.: Telescope retainers for removable partial dentures, J. Prosthet. Dent. **45**:37-43, 1981.

LaVere, A.M., and Freda, A.L.: A simplified procedure for survey and design of diagnostic casts, J. Prosthet. Dent. **37**:680-683, 1977.

LaVere, A.M., and Krol, A.J.: Selection of a major connector for the extension base removable partial denture, J. Prosthet. Dent. **30**:102-105, 1973.

Lorencki, S.F.: Planning precision attachment restorations, J. Prosthet. Dent. **21**:506-508, 1969.

MacKinnon, K.P.: Indirect retention in partial denture construction, Dent. J. Aust. **27**:221-225, 1955.

Maxfield, J.B., Nicholls, J.E., and Smith, D.E.: The measurement of forces transmitted to abutment teeth of removable partial dentures, J. Prosthet. Dent. **41**:134-142, 1979.

McCartney, J.W.: Lingual plating for reciprocation, J. Prosthet. Dent. **42**:624-625, 1979.

McCracken, W.L.: Contemporary partial denture designs, J. Prosthet. Dent. **8**:71-84, 1958.

McCracken, W.L.: Survey of partial denture designs by commercial dental laboratories, J. Prosthet. Dent. **12**:1089-1110, 1962.

Moore, D.S.: Some fundamentals of partial denture design to conserve the supporting structures, J. Ont. Dent. Assoc. **32**:238-240, 1955.

Nairn, R.I.: The problem of free-end denture bases, J. Prosthet. Dent. **16**:522-532, 1966.

Perry, C.: Philosophy of partial denture design, J. Prosthet. Dent. **6**:775-784, 1956.

Pipko, D.J.: Combinations in fixed-removable prostheses, J. Prosthet. Dent. **26**:481-490, 1971.

Potter, R.B., Appleby, R.C., and Adams, C.D.: Removable partial denture design: a review and a challenge, J. Prosthet. Dent. **17**:63-68, 1967.

Ryan, J.: Technique of design in partial denture construction. J. Dent. Assoc. S. Afr. **9**:123-133, 1954.

Rybeck, S.A., Jr.: Simplicity in a distal extension partial denture, J. Prosthet. Dent. **4**:87-92, 1954.

Schmidt, A.H.: Planning and designing removable partial dentures, J. Prosthet. Dent. **3**:783-806, 1953.

Schuyler, C.H.: The partial denture as a means of stabilizing abutment teeth, J. Am. Dent. Assoc. **28**:1121-1125, 1941.

Scott, D.C.: Suggested designs for metal partial dentures, Dent. Tech. **2**:21, 26, 1954.

Shohet, H.: Relative magnitudes of stress on abutment teeth with different retainers, J. Prosthet. Dent. **21**:267-282, 1969.

Steffel, V.L.: Simplified clasp partial dentures designed for maximum function, J. Am. Dent. Assoc. **32**:1093-1100, 1945.

Steffel, V.L.: Fundamental principles involved in partial denture design, J. Am. Dent. Assoc. **42**:534-544, 1951.

Steffel, V.L.: Fundamental principles involved in partial denture designs—with special reference to equalization of tooth and tissue support, Aust. J. Dent. **54**:328-333, 1950; Dent. J. Aust. **23**:68-77, 1951.

Sykora, O.: Fabrication of a posterior shade guide for removable partial dentures, J. Prosthet. Dent. **50**:287-8, 1983.

Sykora, O., and Calikkocaoglu, S.: Maxillary removable partial denture designs by commercial dental laboratories, J. Prosthet. Dent. **22**:633-640, 1970.

Tautin, F.S.: Abutment stabilization using a nonresilient gingival bar connector, J. Am. Dent. Assoc. **99**:988-998, 1979.

Thompson, W.D., Kratochvil, F.J., and Caputo, A.A.: Evaluation of photoelastic stress patterns produced by various designs of bilateral distal-extension removable partial dentures, J. Prosthet. Dent. **38**:261-273, 1977.

Tsao, D.H.: Designing occlusal rests using mathematical princples, J. Prosthet. Dent. **23**:154-163, 1970.

Vofa, M., and Kotowicz, W.E.: Plaque retention with lingual bar and lingual plate major connectors, J. Dent. Res. (A.A.D.R. abstract 609) **59**:entire issue, 1980.

Wagner, A.G., and Traweek, F.C.: Comparison of major connectors for removable partial dentures, J. Prosthet. Dent. **47**:242-245, 1982.

Waller, N.I.: The root rest and the removable partial denture, J. Prosthet. Dent. **33**:16-23, 1975.

Warren, A.B., and Caputo, A.A.: Load transfer to alveolar bone as influenced by abutment design for tooth-supported dentures, J. Prosthet. Dent. **33**:137-148, 1975.

Weinberg, L.A.: Lateral force in relation to the denture base and clasp design, J. Prosthet. Dent. **6**:785-800, 1956.

Zach, G.A.: Advantages of mesial rests for removable partial dentures, J. Prosthet. Dent. **33**:32-35, 1975.

PERIODONTAL CONSIDERATIONS

Amsterdam, M., and Fox, L.: Provisional splinting—principles and technics, Dent. Clin. North Am., pp. 73-99, March, 1959.

App, G.R.: Periodontal treatment for the removable partial prosthesis patient. Another half century? Dent. Clin. North Am. **17**:601-610, 1973.

Applegate, O.C.: The interdependence of periodontics and removable partial denture prosthesis, J. Prosthet. Dent. **8**:269-281, 1958.

Aydinlik, E., Dayangac, B., and Celik, E.: Effect of splintings on abutment tooth movement, J. Prosthet. Dent. **49**:477-480, 1983.

Bates, J.F., and Addy, M.: Partial dentures and plaque accumulation, J. Dent. **6**:285-293, 1978.

Becker, C.M., and Kaldahl, W.B.: Using removable partial dentures to stabilize teeth with secondary occlusal traumatism, J. Prosthet. Dent. **47**:587-594, 1982.

Brill, N., et al.: Ecologic changes in the oral cavity caused by removable partial dentures, J. Prosthet. Dent. **38**:138-148, 1977.

Clarke, N.G.: Treatment planning for fixed and removable partial dentures; a periodontal view, J. Prosthet. Dent. **36**:44-50, 1976.

Dello Russo, N.M.: Gingival autografts as an adjunct to removable partial dentures, J. Am. Dent. Assoc. **104**:179-181, 1982.

Gilson, C.M.: Periodontal considerations, Dent. Clin. North Am. **24**:31-44, 1980.

Gomes, B.C., Renner, R.P., and Bauer, P.N.: Periodontal considerations in removable partial dentures, J. Am. Dent. Assoc. **101**:496-498, 1980.

Gomes, B.C., et al.: A clinical study of the periodontal status of abutment teeth supporting swinglock removable partial dentures—a pilot study, J. Prosthet. Dent. **46**:7-13, 1981.

Hall, W.B.: Periodontal preparation of the mouth for restoration, Dent. Clin. North. Am. **24**:195-213, 1980.

Ivancie, G.P.: Interrelationship between restorative dentistry and periodontics, J. Prosthet. Dent. **8**:819-830, 1958.

Jordan, L.G.: Treatment of advanced periodontal disease by prosthodontic procedures, J. Prosthet. Dent. **10**:908-911, 1960.

Kimball, H.D.: The role of periodontia in prosthetic dentistry, J. Prosthet. Dent. **1**:286-294, 1951.

Krogh-Poulsen, W.: Partial denture design in relation to occlusal trauma in periodontal breakdown, Int. Dent. J. **4**:847-867, 1954; also Acad. Rev. **3**:18-23, 1955.

McCall, J.O.: The periodontal element in prosthodontics, J. Prosthet. Dent. **16**:585-588, 1966.

McKenzie, J.S.: Mutual problems of the periodontist and prosthodontist, J. Prosthet. Dent. **5**:37-42, 1955.

Morris, M.L.: Artificial crown contours and gingival health, J. Prosthet. Dent. **12**:1146-1155, 1962.

Mulcahy, D.F.: Using removable partial dentures to stabilize teeth with secondary occlusal traumatism (letter), J. Prosthet. Dent. **49**:448-449, 1983.

Nevin, R.B.: Periodontal aspects of partial denture prosthesis, J. Prosthet. Dent. **5**:215-219, 1955.

Orban, B.S.: Biologic principles in correction of occlusal disharmonies, J. Prosthet. Dent. **6**:637-641, 1956.

Overby, G.E.: Esthetic splinting of mobile periodontally involved teeth by vertical pinning. J. Prosthet. Dent. **11**:112-118, 1961.

Perel, M.L.: Periodontal consideration of crown contours, J. Prosthet. Dent. **26**:627-630, 1971.

Picton, D.C.A., and Wills, D.J.: Viscoelastic properties of the periodontal ligament and mucous membrane, J. Prosthet. Dent. **40**:263-272, 1978.

Rissin, L., et al.: Effect of age and removable partial dentures on gingivitis and periodontal disease, J. Prosthet. Dent. **42**:217-223, 1979.

Rudd, K.D., and O'Leary, T.J.: Stabilizing periodontally weakened teeth by using guide plane removable partial dentures: a preliminary report, J. Prosthet. Dent. **16**:721-727, 1966.

Schuyler, C.H.: The partial denture and a means of stabilizing abutment teeth, J. Am. Dent. Assoc. **28**:1121-1125, 1941.

Schwalm, C.A., Smith D.E., and Erickson, J.D.: A clinical study of patients 1 to 2 years after placement of removable partial dentures, J. Prosthet. Dent. **38**:380-391, 1977.

Sternlicht, H.C.: Prosthetic treatment planning for the periodontal patient, Dent. Abstr. **2**:81-82, 1957.

Stipho, H.D.K., Murphy, W.M., and Adams, D.: Effect of oral prostheses on plaque accumulation, Br. Dent. J. **145**:47-50, 1978.

Talkov, L.: Survey for complete periodontal prosthesis, J. Prosthet. Dent. **11**:124-131, 1961.

Tebrock, O.C., et al.: The effect of various clasping systems on the mobility of abutment teeth for distal-extension removable partial dentures, J. Prosthet. Dent. **41**:511-516, 1979.

Thayer, H.H., and Kratochvil, F.J.: Periodontal considerations with removable partial dentures, Dent. Clin. North. Am. **24**:195-213, 1980.

Thomas, B.O.A., and Gallager, J.W.: Practical management of occlusal dysfunctions in periodontal therapy, J. Am. Dent. Assoc. **46**:18-31, 1953.

Trapozzano, V.R., and Winter, G.R.: Periodontal aspects of partial denture design, J. Prosthet. Dent. **2**:101-107, 1952.

Waerhaug, J.: Justification for splinting in periodontal therapy, J. Prosthet. Dent. **22**:201-208, 1969.

Ward, H.L., and Weinberg, L.A.: An evaluation of periodontal splinting, J. Am. Dent. Assoc. **63**:48-54, 1961.

White, J.T.: Abutment stress in overdenture, J. Prosthet. Dent. **40**:13-17, 1978.

PHYSIOLOGY; MANDIBULAR MOVEMENT

Brekke, C.A.: Jaw function. I. Hinge rotation, J. Prosthet. Dent. **9**:600-606, 1959. II. Hinge axis, hinge axes, **9**:936-940, 1959. III. Condylar placement and condylar retrusion. **10**:78-85, 1960.

Brotman, D.N.: Contemporary concepts of articulation, J. Prosthet. Dent. **10**:221-230, 1960.

Emig, G.E.: The physiology of the muscles of mastication, J. Prosthet. Dent. **1**:700-707, 1951.

Fountain, H.W.: The temporomandibular joints—a fulcrum, J. Prosthet. Dent. **25**:78-84, 1971.

Gibbs, C.H., et al.: Functional movements of the mandible, J. Prosthet. Dent. **26**:604-620, 1971.

Jankelson, B.: Physiology of human dental occlusion, J. Am. Dent. Assoc. **50**:664-680, 1955.

Jemt, T., Hedegard, B., and Wickberg, K.: Chewing patterns before and after treatment with complete maxillary and bilateral distal-extension mandibular removable partial dentures, J. Prosthet. Dent. **50**:566-569, 1983.

Kurth, L.E.: Mandibular movement and articulator occlusion, J. Am. Dent. Assoc. **39**:37-46, 1949.

Kurth, L.E.: Centric relation and mandibular movement, J. Am. Dent. Assoc. **50**:309-315, 1955.

McMillen, L.B.: Border movements of the human mandible, J. Prosthet. Dent. **27**:524-532, 1972.

Messerman, T.: A concept of jaw function with a related clinical application, J. Prosthet. Dent. **13**:130-140, 1963.

Naylor, J.G.: Role of the external pterygoid muscles in temporomandibular articulation, J. Prosthet. Dent. **10**:1037-1042, 1960.

Plotnick, I.J., Beresin, V.E., and Simkins, A.B.: The effects of variations in the opposing dentition on changes in the partially edentulous mandible. I. Bone changes observed in serial radiographs, J. Prosthet. Dent. **33**:278-286, 1975.

Plotnick, I.J., Beresin, V.E., and Simkins, A.B.: The effects of variations in the opposing dentition on changes in the partially edentulous mandible. III. Tooth mobility and chewing efficiency with various maxillary dentitions, J. Prosthet. Dent. **33**:529-534, 1975.

Posselt, U.: Studies in the mobility of the human mandible, Acta Odontol. Scand. **10**(supp. 10):19-160, 1952.

Posselt, U.: Movement areas of the mandible, J. Prosthet. Dent. **7**:375-385, 1957.

Posselt, U.: Terminal hinge movement of the mandible, J. Prosthet. Dent. **7**:787-797, 1957.

Saizar, P.: Centric relation and condylar movement, J. Prosthet. Dent. **26**:581-591, 1971.

Schweitzer, J.M.: Masticatory function in man, J. Prosthet. Dent. **11**:625-647, 1961.

Shanahan, T.E.J.: Dental physiology for dentures: the direct application of the masticatory cycle to denture occlusion, J. Prosthet. Dent. **2**:3, 1952.

Shore, N.A.: Educational program for patients with temporomandibular joint dysfunction (ligaments), J. Prosthet. Dent. **23**:691-695, 1970.

Sicher, H.: Positions and movements of the mandible, J. Am. Dent. Assoc. **48**:620-625, 1954.

Skinner, C.N.: Physiology of the occlusal coordination of natural teeth, complete dentures, and partial dentures, J. Prosthet. Dent. **17**:559-565, 1967.

Söstenbö, H.R.: C.E. Luce's recordings of mandibular movement, J. Prosthet. Dent. **11**:1068-1073, 1961.

Ulrich, J.: The human temporomandibular joint: kinematics and actions of the masticatory muscles, J. Prosthet. Dent. **9**:399-406, 1959.

Vaughan, H.C.: The external pterygoid mechanism, J. Prosthet. Dent. **5**:80-92, 1955.

REBASING AND RELINING

Beckett, L.S.: Partial denture. The rebasing of tissue borne saddles; theory and practice, Aust. Dent. J. **16**:340-346, 1971.

Blatterfein, L.: Rebasing procedures for removable partial dentures, J. Prosthet. Dent. **8**:441-467, 1958.

Grady, R.D.: Objective criteria for relining distal-extension removable partial dentures: a preliminary report, J. Prosthet. Dent. **49**:178-181, 1983.

McGivney, G.P.: A reline technique for extension base removable partial dentures. In Lefkowitz, W., editor: Proceedings of the Second International Prosthodontic Congress, St. Louis, 1979, The C.V. Mosby Co.

Steffel, V.L.: Relining removable partial dentures for fit and function, J. Prosthet. Dent. **4**:496-509, 1954.

Wilson, J.H.: Partial dentures—rebasing the saddle supported by the mucosa and alveolar bone, Dent. J. Aust. **24**:185-188, 1952.

Wilson, J.H.: Partial dentures—relining the saddle supported by the mucosa and alveolar bone, J. Prosthet. Dent. **3**:807-813, 1953.

Yasuda, N., et al.: New adhesive resin to metal in removable prosthodontics field, J. Dent. Res. (I.A.D.R. abstract 213) **59**:entire issue, 1980.

STRESSBREAKER DESIGNS

Bartlett, A.A.: Duplication of precision attachment partial dentures, J. Prosthet. Dent. **16**:1111-1115, 1966.

Bickley, R.W.: Combined splint-stress breaker removable partial denture, J. Prosthet. Dent. **21**:509, 512, 1969.

Cecconi, B.T., Kaiser, G., and Rahe, A.: Stress-breakers and the removable partial denture, J. Prosthet. Dent. **34**:145-151, 1975.

Hirschtritt, E.: Removable partial dentures with stress-broken extension bases, J. Prosthet. Dent. **7**:318-324, 1957.

James, A.G.: Stress breakers which automatically return the saddle to rest position following displacement. Mandibular distal extension partial dentures, J. Prosthet. Dent. **4**:73-81, 1954.

Kabcenell, J.L.: Stress breaking for partial dentures, J. Am. Dent. Assoc. **63**:593-602, 1961.

Kane, B.E.: Buoyant stress equalizer, J. Prosthet. Dent. **14**:698-704, 1964.

Kane, B.E.: Improved buoyant stress equalizer, J. Prosthet. Dent. **17**:365-371, 1967.

Levin, B.: Stressbreakers: a practical approach, Dent. Clin. North Am. **23**:77-86, 1979.

Levitch, H.C.: Physiologic stress-equalizer, J. Prosthet. Dent. **3**:232-238, 1953.

Marris, F.N.: The precision dowel rest attachment, J. Prosthet. Dent. **5**:43-48, 1955.

Neill, D.J.: The problem of the lower free-end removable partial denture, J. Prosthet. Dent. **8**:623-634, 1958.

Parker, H.M.: Impact reduction in complete and partial dentures, a pilot study, J. Prosthet. Dent. **16**:227-245, 1966.

Plotnik, I.J.: Stress regulator for complete and partial dentures, J. Prosthet. Dent. **17**:166-171, 1967.

Simpson, D.H.: Considerations for abutments, J. Prosthet. Dent. **5**:375-384, 1955.

Terrell, W.H.: Split bar technic applicable to both precision attachment and clasp cases, J. South. Calif. Dent. Assoc. **9**:10-14, 1942.

SURVEYING

Applegate, O.C.: Use of paralleling surveyor in modern partial denture construction, J. Am. Dent. Assoc. **27**:1317-1407, 1940.

Atkinson, H.F.: Partial denture problems: surveyors and surveying, Aust. J. Dent. **59**:28-31, 1955.

Chestner, S.G.: A methodical approach to the analysis of study cases, J. Prosthet. Dent. **4**:622-624, 1954.

Hanson, J.G.: Surveying, J. Am. Dent. Assoc. **91**:826-828, 1975.

Katulski, E.M., and Appleyard, W.N.: Biological concepts of the use of the mechanical cast surveyor, J. Prosthet. Dent. **9**:629-634, 1959.

Knapp, J.G., Shotwell, J.L., and Kotowicz, W.E.: Technique for recording dental cast–surveyor relations, J. Prosthet. Dent. **41**:352-354, 1979.

Sollé, W.: An improved dental surveyor, J. Am. Dent. Assoc. **60**:727-731, 1960.

Wagner, A.G., and Forque, E.G.: A study of four methods of recording the path of insertion of removable partial dentures, J. Prosthet. Dent. **35**:267-272, 1976.

Yilmaz, G.: Optical surveying of casts for removable partial dentures, J. Prosthet. Dent. **34**:292-296, 1975.

WORK AUTHORIZATIONS

Brown, E.T.: The dentist, the laboratory technician, and the prescription law, J. Prosthet. Dent. **15**:1132-1138, 1965.

Dutton, D.A.: Standard abbreviations (and definitions) for use in dental laboratory work authorizations, J. Prosthet. Dent. **27**:94-95, 1972.

Gehl, D.H.: Investment in the future, J. Prosthet. Dent. **18**:190-201, 1968.

Henderson, D.: Writing work authorizations for removable partial dentures, J. Prosthet. Dent. **16**:696-707, 1966.

Henderson, D., and Frazier, Q.: Communicating with dental laboratory technicians, Dent. Clin. North Am., pp. 603-615, July, 1970.

Leeper, S.H.: Dentist and laboratory: a "love-hate" relationship, Dent. Clin. North Am. **23**:87-99, 1979.

Quinn, I.: Status of the dental laboratory work authorization, J. Am. Dent. Assoc. **79**:1189-1190, 1969.

Travaglini, E.A., and Jannetto, L.B.: A work authorization format for removable partial dentures, J. Am. Dent. Assoc. **96**:429-431, 1978.

INDEX